AF565592

1997
YEAR BOOK OF
DIAGNOSTIC
RADIOLOGY®

Statement of Purpose

The YEAR BOOK Service

The YEAR BOOK series was devised in 1901 by practicing health professionals who observed that the literature of medicine and related disciplines had become so voluminous that no one individual could read and place in perspective every potential advance in a major specialty. In the final decade of the 20th century, this recognition is more acutely true than it was in 1901.

More than merely a series of books, YEAR BOOK volumes are the tangible results of a unique service designed to accomplish the following:

- to *survey* a wide range of journals of proven value
- to *select* from those journals papers representing significant advances and statements of important clinical principles
- to provide *abstracts* of those articles that are readable, convenient summaries of their key points
- to provide *commentary* about those articles to place them in perspective

These publications grow out of a unique process that calls on the talents of outstanding authorities in clinical and fundamental disciplines, trained literature specialists, and professional writers, all supported by the resources of Mosby, the world's preeminent publisher for the health professions.

The Literature Base

Mosby and its Editors survey more than 1,000 journals published worldwide, covering the full range of the health professions. On an annual basis, the publisher examines usage patterns and polls its expert authorities to add new journals to the literature base and to delete journals that are no longer useful as potential YEAR BOOK sources.

The Literature Survey

The publisher's team of literature specialists, all of whom are trained and experienced health professionals, examines every original, peer-reviewed article in each journal issue. More than 250,000 articles per year are scanned systematically, including title, text, illustrations, tables, and references. Each scan is compared, article by article, to the search strategies that the publisher has developed in consultation with the 270 outside experts who form the pool of YEAR BOOK editors. A given article may be reviewed by any number of editors, from one to a dozen or more, regardless of the discipline for which the paper was originally published. In turn, each editor who receives the article reviews it to determine whether or not the article should be included in the YEAR BOOK. This decision is based on the article's inherent quality, its probable usefulness to readers of that YEAR BOOK, and the editor's goal to represent a balanced picture of a given field in each volume of the YEAR BOOK. In addition, the editor indicates when to include figures and tables from the article to help the YEAR BOOK reader better understand the information.

Of the quarter million articles scanned each year, only 5% are selected for detailed analysis within the YEAR BOOK series, thereby assuring readers of the high value of every selection.

The Abstract

The publisher's abstracting staff is headed by a seasoned medical professional and includes individuals with training in the life sciences, medicine, and other areas, plus extensive experience in writing for the health professions and related industries. Each selected article is assigned to a specific writer on this abstracting staff. The abstracter, guided in many cases by notations supplied by the expert editor, writes a structured, condensed summary designed so that the reader can rapidly acquire the essential information contained in the article.

The Commentary

The YEAR BOOK editorial boards, sometimes assisted by guest commentators, write comments that place each article in perspective for the reader. This provides the reader with the equivalent of a personal consultation with a leading international authority—an opportunity to better understand the value of the article and to benefit from the authority's thought processes in assessing the article.

Additional Editorial Features

The editorial boards of each YEAR BOOK organize the abstracts and comments to provide a logical and satisfying sequence of information. To enhance the organization, editors also provide introductions to sections or individual chapters, comments linking a number of abstracts, citations to additional literature, and other features.

The published YEAR BOOK contains enhanced bibliographic citations for each selected article, including extended listings of multiple authors and identification of author affiliations. Each YEAR BOOK contains a Table of Contents specific to that year's volume. From year to year, the Table of Contents for a given YEAR BOOK will vary depending on developments within the field.

Every YEAR BOOK contains a list of the journals from which papers have been selected. This list represents a subset of the more than 1,000 journals surveyed by the publisher and occasionally reflects a particularly pertinent article from a journal that is not surveyed on a routine basis.

Finally, each volume contains a comprehensive subject index and an index to authors of each selected paper.

The 1997 Year Book Series

Year Book of Allergy, Asthma, and Clinical Immunology: Drs. Rosenwasser, Borish, Gelfand, Leung, Nelson, and Szefler

Year Book of Anesthesiology and Pain Management®: Drs. Tinker, Abram, Chestnut, Roizen, Rothenberg, and Wood

Year Book of Cardiology®: Drs. Schlant, Collins, Gersh, Graham, Kaplan, and Waldo

Year Book of Chiropractic®: Dr. Lawrence

Year Book of Critical Care Medicine®: Drs. Parrillo, Balk, Calvin, Franklin, and Shapiro

Year Book of Dentistry®: Drs. Meskin, Berry, Kennedy, Leinfelder, Roser, Summitt, and Zakariasen

Year Book of Dermatologic Surgery®: Drs. Greenway, Papadopoulos, and Whitaker

Year Book of Dermatology®: Drs. Sober and Fitzpatrick

Year Book of Diagnostic Radiology®: Drs. Federle, Clark, Gross, Dalinka, Maynard, Rebner, Smirniotopoulos, and Young

Year Book of Digestive Diseases®: Drs. Greenberger and Moody

Year Book of Drug Therapy®: Drs. Lasagna and Weintraub

Year Book of Emergency Medicine®: Drs. Wagner, Dronen, Davidson, King, Niemann, and Roberts

Year Book of Endocrinology®: Drs. Bagdade, Braverman, Hass, Horton, Kannan, Landsberg, Molitch, Morley, Nathan, Odell, Poehlman, Rogol, and Ryan

Year Book of Family Practice®: Drs. Berg, Bowman, Davidson, Dexter, and Scherger

Year Book of Geriatrics and Gerontology®: Drs. Beck, Burton, Ostwald, Rabins, Reuben, Roth, Shapiro, and Whitehouse

Year Book of Hand Surgery®: Drs. Amadio and Hentz

Year Book of Hematology®: Drs. Spivak, Bell, Ness, Quesenberry, Wiernik, and Blume

Year Book of Infectious Diseases®: Drs. Keusch, Barza, Bennish, Poutsiaka, Skolnik, and Snydman

Year Book of Medicine®: Drs. Klahr, Cline, Petty, Frishman, Greenberger, Malawista, Mandell, and O'Rourke

Year Book of Neonatal and Perinatal Medicine®: Drs. Fanaroff and Klaus

Year Book of Nephrology, Hypertension, and Mineral Metabolism: Drs. Schwab, Bennett, Emmett, Hostetter, Kumar, and Toto

Year Book of Neurology and Neurosurgery®: Drs. Bradley and Wilkins

Year Book of Nuclear Medicine®: Drs. Gottschalk, Blaufox, Neumann, Strauss, and Zubal

Year Book of Obstetrics, Gynecology, and Women's Health: Drs. Mishell, Herbst, and Kirschbaum

Year Book of Occupational and Environmental Medicine®: Drs. Emmett, Frank, Gochfeld, and Hessl

Year Book of Oncology®: Drs. Ozols, Cohen, Glatstein, Loehrer, Tallman, and Wiersma

Year Book of Ophthalmology®: Drs. Wilson, Augsburger, Cohen, Eagle, Flanagan, Grossman, Laibson, Maguire, Nelson, Penne, Rapuano, Sergott, Spaeth, Tipperman, and Ms. Salmon

Year Book of Orthopedics®: Drs. Sledge, Poss, Cofield, Dobyns, Griffin, Springfield, Swiontkowski, Wiesel, and Wilson

Year Book of Otolaryngology—Head and Neck Surgery®: Drs. Paparella and Holt

Year Book of Pain®: Drs. Gebhart, Haddox, Jacox, Janjan, Marcus, Rudy, and Shapiro

Year Book of Pathology and Laboratory Medicine: Drs. Mills, Bruns, Gaffey, and Stoler

Year Book of Pediatrics®: Dr. Stockman

Year Book of Plastic, Reconstructive, and Aesthetic Surgery®: Drs. Miller, Cohen, McKinney, Robson, Ruberg, Smith, and Whitaker

Year Book of Podiatric Medicine and Surgery®: Dr. Kominsky

Year Book of Psychiatry and Applied Mental Health®: Drs. Talbott, Ballenger, Breier, Frances, Meltzer, Schowalter, and Tasman

Year Book of Pulmonary Disease®: Dr. Petty

Year Book of Rheumatology®: Drs. Sergent, LeRoy, Meenan, Panush, and Reichlin

Year Book of Sports Medicine®: Drs. Shephard, Drinkwater, Eichner, Torg, Anderson, and Mr. George

Year Book of Surgery®: Drs. Copeland, Bland, Deitch, Eberlein, Howard, Luce, Seeger, Souba, and Sugarbaker

Year Book of Thoracic and Cardiovascular Surgery®: Drs. Ginsberg, Wechsler, and Williams

Year Book of Urology®: Drs. Andriole and Coplin

Year Book of Vascular Surgery®: Dr. Porter

1997
The Year Book of DIAGNOSTIC RADIOLOGY®

Editor-in-Chief
Michael P. Federle, M.D.
Professor, Department of Radiology, Chief of Abdominal Imaging, University of Pittsburgh Medical Center, Pittsburgh, Pennsylvania

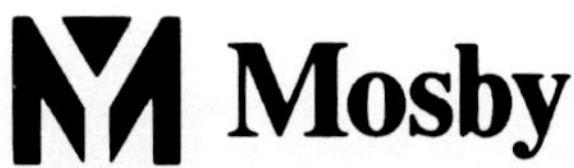

St. Louis Baltimore Boston Carlsbad Chicago Naples New York Philadelphia Portland
London Madrid Mexico City Singapore Sydney Tokyo Toronto Wiesbaden

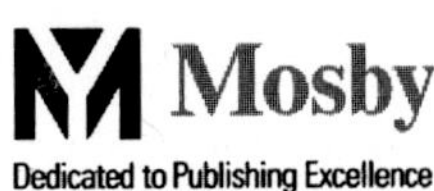

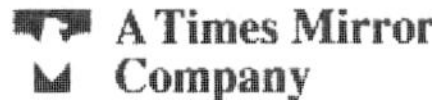

Vice President and Publisher, Continuity Publishing: Kenneth H. Killion
Director, Editorial Development: Gretchen C. Murphy
Developmental Editor: Anna Blazevic
Acquisitions Editor: Li Wen Huang
Director, Continuity—EDP: Maria Nevinger
Project Manager, Editing: Jill C. Waite
Assistant Project Supervisor, Production: Laura M. Higgins
Freelance Staff Supervisor: Barbara M. Kelly
Illustrations and Permissions Coordinator: Steven J. Ramey
Director, Editorial Services: Edith M. Podrazik, B.S.N., R.N.
Information Specialist: Kathleen Moss, R.N.
Information Specialist: Terri Santo, R.N.
Circulation Manager: Lynn D. Stevenson

1997 EDITION

Printed in the United States of America
Composition by Reed Technology and Information Services, Inc.
Printing/binding by Maple-Vail

Mosby–Year Book, Inc.
11830 Westline Industrial Drive
St. Louis, MO 63146

Editorial Office:
Mosby–Year Book, Inc.
161 North Clark Street
Chicago, IL 60601

International Standard Serial Number: 0098–1672
International Standard Book Number: 0–8151–9615–6

Associate Editors

Murray K. Dalinka, M.D.

Professor of Radiology; Chief, Musculoskeletal Radiology, University of Pennsylvania Medical Center, University of Pennsylvania School of Medicine, Hospital of the University of Pennsylvania, Philadelphia, Pennsylvania

Barry H. Gross, M.D.

Professor; Department of Radiology, University of Michigan Hospitals, Ann Arbor, Michigan

C. Douglas Maynard, M.D.

Professor and Chairman, Department of Radiology, Bowman Gray School of Medicine, Wake Forest University, Winston-Salem, North Carolina

Murray Rebner, M.D.

Director, Section of Breast Imaging, Henry Ford Hospital, Detroit, Michigan

Lionel W. Young, M.D.

Professor and Director, Division of Pediatric Radiology, Loma Linda University Children's Hospital, Loma Linda, California

James G. Smirniotopoulos, M.D.

Professor and Chairman, Department of Radiology and Nuclear Medicine, Uniformed Services University of the Health Services, Bethesda, Maryland

Guest Contributor

John H. Rees, M.D.

Junior Scientist in Neuroradiology at the AFIP; Assistant Professor of Radiology at Uniformed Services University of the Health Sciences; Instructor in Neuroradiology, University of Maryland Medical System, Baltimore, Maryland

Table of Contents

Journals Represented

Mosby and its Editors survey more than 1,000 journals for its abstract and commentary publications. From these journals, the Editors select the articles to be abstracted. Journals represented in this YEAR BOOK are listed below.

Abdominal Imaging
Academic Emergency Medicine
Academic Radiology
Acta Neurochirurgica
Acta Radiologica
Administrative Radiology
American Journal of Emergency Medicine
American Journal of Gastroenterology
American Journal of Medicine
American Journal of Neuroradiology
American Journal of Orthopedics
American Journal of Roentgenology
American Journal of Sports Medicine
American Journal of the Medical Sciences
Angiology: The Journal of Vascular Diseases
Annals of Emergency Medicine
Annals of Internal Medicine
Annals of Oncology
Annals of Surgery
Annals of Thoracic Surgery
Archives of Orthopaedic and Trauma Surgery
Breast Journal
British Heart Journal
British Journal of Radiology
British Journal of Surgery
British Journal of Urology
British Medical Journal
Canadian Association of Radiologists Journal
Cancer
Cardiovascular and Interventional Radiology
Chest
Clinical Imaging
Clinical Infectious Diseases
Clinical Nuclear Medicine
Clinical Radiology
Critical Care Medicine
Developmental Medicine and Child Neurology
European Journal of Nuclear Medicine
Foot & Ankle International
Hepatology
Injury
Intensive Care Medicine
Journal of Arthroplasty
Journal of Bone and Joint Surgery (American Volume)
Journal of Bone and Joint Surgery (British Volume)
Journal of Clinical Endocrinology and Metabolism
Journal of Clinical Ultrasound

Journal of Computer Assisted Tomography
Journal of Digital Imaging
Journal of Family Practice
Journal of Hand Surgery (American)
Journal of Neurosurgery
Journal of Nuclear Medicine
Journal of Orthopaedic Research
Journal of Orthopaedic Trauma
Journal of Pediatric Surgery
Journal of Pediatrics
Journal of Rheumatology
Journal of Trauma: Injury, Infection, and Critical Care
Journal of Ultrasound in Medicine
Journal of Urology
Journal of the American Medical Association
Journal of the Neurological Sciences
Kidney International
Magnetic Resonance Imaging
Magnetic Resonance in Medicine
Neurology
Neuroradiology
Neurosurgery
New England Journal of Medicine
Pediatric Nephrology
Pediatric Neurology
Pediatric Radiology
Quarterly Journal of Medicine
Radiology
Skeletal Radiology
Spine
Stroke
The Endocrinologist
Thorax
Ultrasound in Obstetrics and Gynecology
World Journal of Surgery

Standard Abbreviations

The following terms are abbreviated in this edition: acquired immunodeficiency syndrome (AIDS), cardiopulmonary resuscitation (CPR), central nervous system (CNS), cerebrospinal fluid (CSF), computed tomography (CT), deoxyribonucleic acid (DNA), electrocardiography (ECG), health maintenance organization (HMO), human immunodeficiency virus (HIV), intensive care unit (ICU), intramuscular (IM), intravenous (IV), magnetic resonance (MR) imaging (MRI), and ribonucleic acid (RNA).

Note

The Year Book of Diagnostic Radiology® is a literature survey service providing abstracts of articles published in the professional literature. Every effort is made to assure the accuracy of the information presented in these pages. Neither the editors nor the publisher of the Year Book of Diagnostic Radiology® can be responsible for errors in the original materials. The editors' comments are their own opinions. Mention of specific products within this publication does not constitute endorsement.

To facilitate the use of the YEAR BOOK OF DIAGNOSTIC RADIOLOGY® as a reference tool, all illustrations and tables included in this publication are now identified as they appear in the original article. This change is meant to help the reader recognize that any illustration or table appearing in the YEAR BOOK OF DIAGNOSTIC RADIOLOGY® may be only one of many in the original article. For this reason, figure and table numbers will often appear to be out of sequence within the YEAR BOOK OF DIAGNOSTIC RADIOLOGY®.

1 Thorax

Introduction

Last year, I initially thought I was finishing my term on the editorial board of the YEAR BOOK OF DIAGNOSTIC RADIOLOGY with the 1996 YEAR BOOK. Then I thought I would be doing 2 more editions, through 1998. Now I know that this (1997) is my last contribution. My status on the editorial board mirrors the topsy-turvy world of radiology since I began work on the 1992 YEAR BOOK OF DIAGNOSTIC RADIOLOGY. Changes in reimbursement, insurance, and federal policy have filtered into our daily lives as changes in the practice environment; I have personally witnessed major changes in the workload and remuneration of large group practice and academic radiologists, and I assume that private practice radiologists are no less affected. It is probably natural to approach change as a negative, but in my best Deming-speak, I will instead emphasize the opportunities we get to shake our old, stale routines and look for new ways to do things.

Workplace change doesn't faze me as much now because I have children. When I started selecting articles, my oldest daughter was 11; my youngest son is now about to turn 11, and the former 11-year-old is now 16. We share a car; I think I have a turn coming up again in 2 or 3 weeks. In any event, when I started, I still had a preschooler, and now I have someone about to apply to college. Perspective is important. With that in mind, let me emphasize how much I've enjoyed writing these 6 editions' worth of comments. Thanks again to everyone involved, especially to Mike Federle and Murray Rebner.

This year I am demonstrating my ability to accommodate change by starting with 2 new sections. First is "The Pleura." I recommend the first article on how best to detect pneumothorax as an exercise for us all in letting go of preconceptions. The article on peripheral bronchopleural fistula is also worth a special look.

The second section is "Nuclear Medicine." Positron emission tomography (PET) staging of lung cancer is "like a snowball rolling down the side of a snow-covered hill" (what song is that from?), building momentum. Bedside scintigraphy for suspected pulmonary embolism is also a very helpful technique.

One of my favorite articles of the year, on CT's role in sarcoidosis, leads off "Topics in CT." I am in the process of writing a talk that I will entitle, "Chest CT: Utility or Futility," and I know that this article's authors will be sympathetic. The articles on high resolution CT in lupus and in uncommon pneumoconioses are also very interesting.

"Recent Advances in Diagnosis and Therapy" includes a minisymposium on reduction pneumoplasty. Evaluation of lung nodule enhancement using MR also deserves your attention.

The concluding section is, as always, "Pulmonary: General Topics." There are interesting articles on lung cancer staging and on outcome as predicted by imaging, but my favorites (as usual) are the 3 offbeat articles that end the chapter. (The song is "It's Growing," by The Temptations; how neat to conclude with a mention of my favorite singing group!)

Barry H. Gross, M.D.

Breast Cancer and Breast Imaging

INTRODUCTION:

"To everything there is a season." As I write these comments in September 1996, politicians are eagerly or reluctantly anticipating the November election. Fall is in the air and I wonder, as I do every September, where did the summer go? For my co-editor, Dr. Barry Gross, this is his final season with the YEAR BOOK OF DIAGNOSTIC RADIOLOGY. Barry was kind enough to ask me to review the breast imaging and breast cancer articles way back in 1992, and we have continued to collaborate on this project. Barry's superb knowledge of chest radiology, as well as his keen wit and ability to place issues in their proper perspective, have served him and the YEAR BOOK readers well. I will miss his insightful comments and I want to publicly thank him for allowing me to be a member of the YEAR BOOK team.

The articles I have selected for the 1997 edition cover a wide spectrum of topics. More data continue to support screening mammography, especially in women younger than age 50. It is highly likely that both the American Cancer Society and the American College of Radiology will alter their screening guidelines and recommend annual screening mammograms for all women 40 years and older. The United Kingdom multicenter randomized control trial article shows that 2 screening views are better than 1, with little increase in cost per cancer detected. Unfortunately, not all women undergo screening mammography, particularly the elderly. Dr. Blustein's article examines some of the barriers to screening mammography for older women.

Dr. Berg and her colleagues compare MRI and ultrasound in a prospective evaluation of single and double-lumen silicone breast implants. Drs. Weinreb, Stomper, and Orel contribute information on the role of breast MR for cancer staging, differentiation of benign and malignant lesions, and evaluation of silicone implant integrity. Dr. Dowlat and his colleagues' work-in-progress on the value of the axillary sentinel lymph node for breast cancer staging is exciting. The concept of less morbidity with accurate staging of the axilla with this technique appeals to all.

Stereotactic core needle biopsy (SCNB) continues to grow in popularity. Three articles by Drs. Dershaw, Liberman, and Nath discuss the problems of nondiagnostic core biopsies, how recurrent carcinoma of the breast after conservative therapy can be diagnosed with SCNB and how 14-, 16-, and 18-gauge core needles perform with respect to the size and quality of the biopsy samples.

Other articles include an examination of the artificial neural network based on BI-RADS lexicon for probability of breast cancer, and observer variability in lesion description with the BI-RADS lexicon. Finally, an article on the sternalis muscle and case reports that describe some rare birds (breast sparganosis, paraffinomas, and mammographic features of unilateral breast-feeding) complete this year's selections. I hope you enjoy them.

Murray Rebner, M.D.

UKCCCR Multicentre Randomised Controlled Trial of One and Two View Mammography in Breast Cancer Screening

Wald NJ, Murphy P, Major P, et al (St. Bartholomew's Hosp, London)
BMJ 311:1189–1193, 1995 1–1

Background.—An oblique view is necessary in mammographic screening for breast cancer, but the added value of a craniocaudal view is unknown. Retrospective studies have suggested that the addition of a second view could increase the cancer detection rate by 9%. One-view and 2-view mammography were compared for their effectiveness in breast cancer screening in a randomized, controlled trial.

Methods.—The study included 40,163 women aged 50–64 years who were undergoing their first breast screening program. They were randomized into 3 groups: 1 group had 1-view mammography, another group had 2-view mammography, and another had 2-view mammography with 1 view read by 1 reader and both views read by another reader. The 1-view and 2-view approaches were compared for the prevalence of cancers detected, recall rate, and cost and marginal cost per cancer detected.

Results.—The 2-view approach detected 24% more patients with breast cancer than the 1-view approach (95% confidence interval, 16% to 31%). The prevalence of detected cancers was 6.84/1,000 patients with the 2-view approach vs. 5.52/1,000 with the 1-view approach. The recall rate was 6.97% with the 2-view approach vs. 8.16% with the 1-view approach. The 2-view approach was more expensive; however, there was little difference in the average cost per cancer detected. The marginal cost of detecting an extra cancer by the 2-view approach was comparable to the average cost. The estimated reduction in breast cancer mortality was 34% with the 2-view approach compared to 27% with a 1-view approach.

Conclusions.—Two-view mammography—with a craniocaudal view added to the oblique view—detects more breast cancers than the traditional 1-view approach. The 2-view approach increases the cancer detection rate by 24%, reduces the recall rate by 15%, and is financially cost-effective. At least at the initial screening examination—and probably at subsequent examinations as well—the two-view approach is recommended over the 1-view approach.

▶ This study shows the benefit of 2 views compared with 1 view for breast cancer screening. The following are benefits of using a craniocaudal and MLO view instead of the MLO view alone:

- Increased breast cancer detection
- Lower recall rate
- Average cost per cancer detected and marginal cost per extra cancer detected similar for 2 views vs. 1 view

We screen to find breast cancer at its earliest stage of development. This technique detected 24% more cancers (statistically significant at the 95% confidence level). The authors do not provide staging information about the cancers detected. One would expect that the majority of these tumors would be either stage 0 or stage 1. A 15% decrease in the recall rate is also important. One does not want to perform extra imaging studies and, in many cases, the benefit of a second craniocaudal view can turn an indeterminate finding on the MLO view into one that is definitely benign. Finally, in these days of cost containment, the average cost per instance of cancer detected and the marginal cost per extra cancer detected were similar for a 2-view and a 1-view screening study. This study will hopefully convince those who still use only 1 view to add the second craniocaudal view.

M. Rebner, M.D.

Medicare Coverage, Supplemental Insurance, and the Use of Mammography by Older Women

Blustein J (Columbia Univ, New York)

N Engl J Med 332:1138–1143, 1995 1–2

Background.—Medicare began to provide reimbursement for biennial screening mammography in 1991. The use of mammography by women insured by Medicare in 1991 and 1992 was investigated.

Methods.—A nationally representative sample of 4,110 women aged 65 years and older was included in the study. The degree of compliance with accepted guidelines for screening mammography and the extent to which mammography use was associated with having supplemental insurance, which covers the out-of-pocket expenses associated with Medicare benefits, were assessed.

Findings.—In the first 2 years after Medicare established benefits for screening mammography, 36.9% of the sample underwent mammography. Only 14.4% of women without supplemental insurance had the screening, compared with 44.7% with employer-sponsored supplemental insurance, 40.1% with self-purchased supplemental insurance, and 23.9% with Medicaid supplemental insurance. Women with employment-based supplemental insurance were more likely to have mammography than women without supplemental insurance. This was also true for women with self-purchased supplemental insurance and those with Medicaid supplemental insurance.

Conclusions.—In the first 2 years of Medicare coverage, the use of screening mammography was markedly below recommended levels. Women without supplemental insurance were particularly unlikely to have mammography. Effective mass screening of older women is being hindered by copayment requirements.

▶ Dr. Blustein has examined the use of mammography by older women with Medicare and supplemental insurance. The fact that the use of mammography was substantially below recommended levels during the first 2 years of Medicare coverage is disturbing to me. None of the various subgroups reached 50% compliance with screening guidelines. Only 14% of women without supplemental insurance received a screening mammogram!

Simply making a test available does not guarantee a high rate of usage. There are many barriers to screening mammography. Although cost is one, I believe others are more important, such as the referring physician and the patient. Despite all of the existing data, many physicians still doubt the benefits of screening mammography and fear the radiation risk.[1] Also, as the author points out, the patient may have the perception that the referring physician did not recommend the mammogram.

Certainly, costs to the patient need to be minimized. There also needs to be a clear conviction on the part of the referring physician that screening mammography works. Perhaps then, more patients would partake of this potentially lifesaving examination.

M. Rebner, M.D.

Reference

1. Fox SA, Murata PI, Stein JA: The impact of physician compliance on screening mammography in older women. *Arch Intern Med* 51:150–156, 1991.

Single- and Double-Lumen Silicone Breast Implant Integrity: Prospective Evaluation of MR and US Criteria

Berg WA, Caskey CI, Hamper UM, et al (Johns Hopkins Univ, Baltimore, Md; Univ of Wisconsin, Madison)

Radiology 197:45–52, 1995 1–3

Objective.—Patients with silicone breast implants were examined with MR and US for integrity of the implant. Ruptured silicone breast implants should be removed, but implant rupture is often clinically silent and women with these devices need to be monitored.

Methods.—Study participants included 282 women with 534 implants (427 single-lumen silicone, 26 polyurethane-covered silicone, 73 bilumen outer saline and inner silicone, and 8 expander-type outer silicone and inner saline lumen implants). Surface coil MR images and US scans were reviewed for indications of rupture. Magnetic resonance criteria for rupture were a collapsed implant shell, foci of silicone outside the shell, and extracapsular gel. A collapsed shell, low-level echoes within the gel, and "snowstorm" echoes of extracapsular silicone were US indications of implant failure. Additional data obtained included type and age of the implant, previous implant rupture, breast trauma, breast symptoms, and reports of recent mammograms.

Results.—Clinical criteria were not predictive of implant failure, although implants of more than 10 years' duration were more likely to have failed than newer implants. Among single-lumen implants, MR correctly interpreted 49 of 54 intact implants and detected 39 of 40 ruptures, including 14 of 28 with minimal leakage. Of the 23 implants showing foci of silicone outside the shell (Fig 2), only 3 were intact. Ultrasound was less

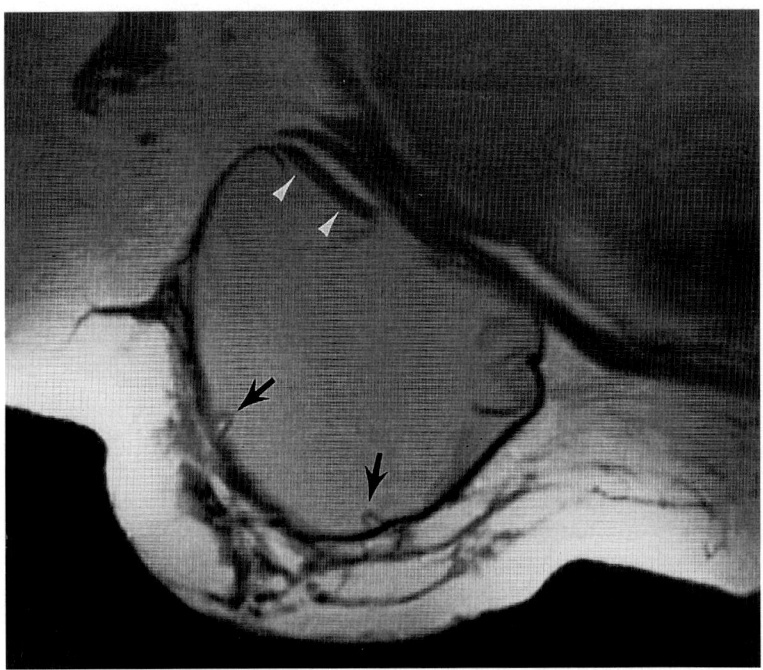

FIGURE 2.—Rupture without shell collapse. An axial fast spin-echo T2-weighted MR image of a 22-year-old left subglandular silicone implant shows multiple areas where a small amount of gel is outside the shell (noose sign, *arrows*). Dacron patches (DuPont, Wilmington, Del) along the back wall of the Cronin-type implant (Dow Corning, Midland, Mich) are also evident (*arrowheads*). (Courtesy of Berg WA, Caskey CI, Hamper UM, et al: Single- and double-lumen silicone breast implant integrity: Prospective evaluation of MR and US criteria. *Radiology* 197:45–52, 1995. Radiological Society of North America.)

accurate, demonstrating 30 of 54 intact implants, 26 of 40 ruptured implants, and only 4 of 28 with minimal leakage. In patients with bilumen implants, MR identified 4 of 5 ruptures in both lumina and depicted 9 of 10 as intact; US showed 1 rupture and identified 2 of 10 as intact. Both mammography and MR demonstrated the integrity of bilumen implants.

Discussion.— The accuracy of MR in evaluating implant integrity in this series of patients was 84%; in contrast, US had an accuracy of only 49%. Ruptures in bilumen implants can be identified with mammography, but MR shows more subtle changes. The bilumen devices are particularly difficult to evaluate with US. Neither MR nor US reliably identified small leaks.

► Like it or not, breast implant imaging is not going to go away. Breast imagers need to be capable of evaluating both single- and double-lumen breast implants. This paper substantiates prior reports, which note that MRI is more accurate than US for implant integrity. Dr. Berg and her colleagues also note that neither MRI nor US was reliable for the detection of minimal silicone leakage with intracapsular rupture. Previous studies showed that mammography was not very helpful in evaluating implant integrity. However, this study suggests that mammography may be of use in screening bilumen implants.

The management of women who may have ruptured breast implants becomes an issue. Should patients undergo screening with US prior to MRI? Should all patients with double-lumen implants undergo mammography and, if negative, then MRI? Should US be performed at all? To this reviewer, cost aside, it seems that if the plastic surgeon has sufficient concern regarding the integrity of the patient's breast implants to warrant explanation, the patient should undergo mammography first and, if negative, breast MRI. At my institution, we have advised our plastic surgeons to go straight from mammography to MRI if there is sufficient clinical concern to suggest a ruptured implant.

M. Rebner, M.D.

Suspect Breast Lesions: Findings at Dynamic Gadolinium-Enhanced MR Imaging Correlated With Mammographic and Pathologic Features

Stomper PC, Herman S, Klippenstein DL, et al (State Univ at New York, Buffalo)

Radiology 197:387–395, 1995 1–4

Introduction.—Gadolinium enhanced MR imaging of the breast is a new technique. It is being studied to determine whether breast carcinomas not seen at mammography can be depicted and if MR imaging can help differentiate malignant from benign breast lesions. Few studies have compared MR imaging with mammographic, clinical, and pathologic findings.

Dynamic contrast enhancement at MR imaging was prospectively correlated with mammographic and pathologic findings of suspect breast lesions.

Methods.—Gadolinium enhanced spoiled gradient-recalled echo MR imaging at 1.5 T was performed on 49 women with 51 breast lesions. The patients also underwent excisional biopsy or cyst aspiration. Associations between pathologic features of invasive carcinomas and enhancement features at MR imaging were explored to determine the prognostic significance of breast carcinoma enhancements.

Results.—There was a high sensitivity of gadolinium enhanced breast MR imaging for invasive carcinomas identified at mammography or physical examination and found to be at least 8 mm in diameter at pathologic examination. Twenty-two of 22, or 100%, of carcinomas evident on dense mammograms enhanced 2.0 or more times the unenhanced intensity. Within 2 minutes after injection of contrast material, each lesion enhanced. However, 1 of 3 (33%) predominantly ductal carcinomas in situ and 20 of 26, or 38%, benign lesions enhanced 2.0 or more times. One of the ductal carcinomas in situ that did not enhance measured 40 mm in diameter and contained a microscopic focus of invasive ductal carcinoma measuring less than 1 mm in diameter. Carcinomas, fibroadenomas, and other benign lesions could not be differentiated with the use of time-intensity curve parameters. No statistically significant correlations were found with nodal status, pathologic size, or hormone receptor status of invasive carcinomas.

Conclusion.—For invasive carcinomas 8 mm or more in diameter, MR imaging enhancement had a sensitivity of 100% and specificity of 65%. No significant difference was seen between enhancement of malignant and benign lesions with time-intensity curves. For a population of women at high risk for breast carcinoma in whom dense parenchyma is seen at mammography, breast MR imaging may be a screening examination. Larger clinical trials should be conducted in the clinical usefulness of breast MR imaging.

▶ The more research that is done on breast MRI, the more apparent it becomes to me that its utility has marked limitations. Thanks to Dr. Stomper and his colleagues at SUNY at Buffalo, data noting the benefits and limitations of breast MRI are presented. At this point in time, I believe breast MRI has practical use for the workup of metastatic adenocarcinoma of unknown primary site when there is a negative mammogram. Also, with a negative mammogram, MRI of the breast is the study of choice to diagnose either intra- or extracapsular rupture of silicone implants. It can also help detect multifocal or multicentric carcinoma when there already is a known primary malignancy of the breast.

However, as far as being able to differentiate benign vs. malignant for a given mammographic lesion, it still has limited specificity. With the advent of stereotactic large core needle biopsy (SCNB) of the breast—a highly accurate procedure—it remains debatable whether breast MRI would be as accurate with respect to specificity for a given mammographic abnormality. To this reviewer, so far the answer is no.

M. Rebner, M.D.

Staging of Suspected Breast Cancer: Effect of MR Imaging and MR-Guided Biopsy

Orel SG, Schnall MD, Powell CM, et al (Univ of Pennsylvania, Philadelphia; Fox Chase Cancer Ctr, Philadelphia)

Radiology 196:115–122, 1995 1–5

Introduction.—Mammography is currently the primary imaging modality used to detect early breast cancer. However, its sensitivity can be as low as 85%. Studies evaluating contrast material-enhanced MRI have reported sensitivity of 100% in detecting breast cancer. However, its cost, lengthy imaging time, and low specificity limit its value as a screening modality. Its value as an adjunctive imaging modality to stage suspected breast cancer and guide treatment planning was evaluated.

Methods.—A total of 176 patients with suspected cancer based on mammographic or clinical findings underwent MRI before excisional biopsy or cyst aspiration. Breast cancer was diagnosed in 64 patients after biopsy or aspiration. Of these 64 patients, 29 (45%) had lesions detected only by mammography, 24 (38%) had lesions detected both clinically and mammographically, 6 (9%) had palpable lesions with no mammographic evidence, and 5 (8%) had lesions detected neither physically nor mammo-

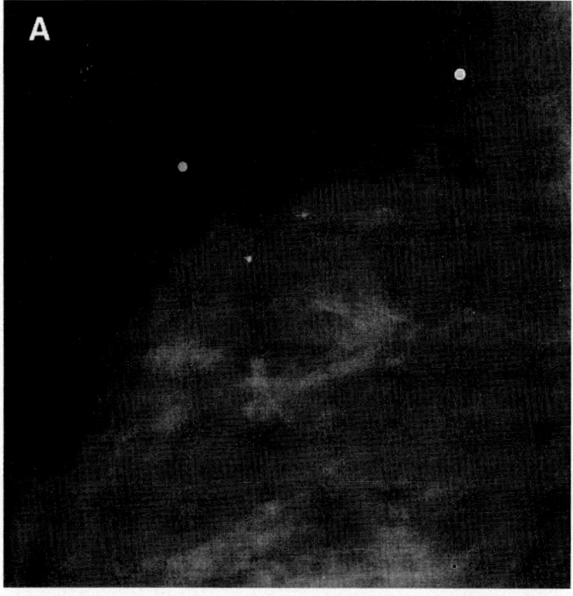

(*Continued*)

FIGURE 2 (cont.)

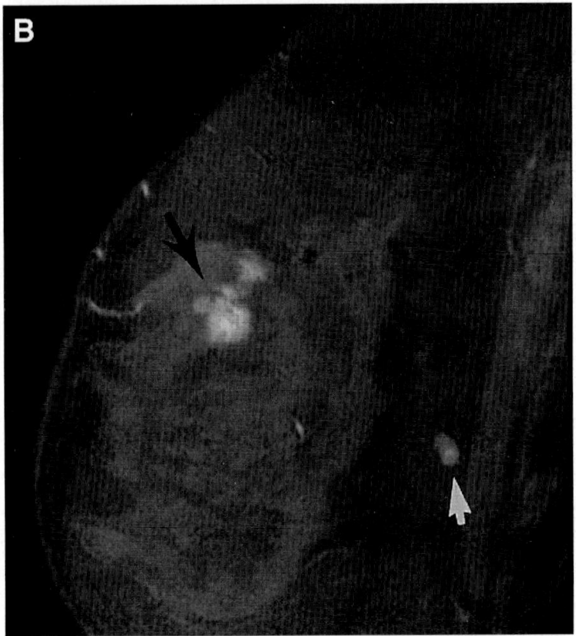

FIGURE 2.—Images obtained in a 53-year-old woman with a palpable mass in the area of prior lumpectomy. A, mediolateral oblique mammogram with skin dots that mark the ends of the scar reveals dense tissue. Additional spot-compression view revealed an ill-defined, 1-cm mass in the lumpectomy bed. B, sagittal contrast-enhanced MR imaging (fast spoiled gradient, 26.2/4.5, 30° flip angle) shows an irregular 1.8-cm area of enhancement (*black arrow*) in the lumpectomy bed and a 5-mm enhancing lesion in the retroglandular fat (*white arrow*). At mastectomy, a 1.5-cm invasive ductal carcinoma was confirmed in the lumpectomy bed and a 4-mm invasive ductal carcinoma in the retroglandular fat. (Courtesy of Orel SG, Schnall MD, Powell CM, et al: Staging of suspected breast cancer: Effect of MR imaging and MR-guided biopsy. *Radiology* 196:115–122, 1995. Radiological Society of North America.)

graphically. Magnetic resonance images were obtained at 1.5 T; they were interpreted prospectively by 2 radiologists before the biopsies were performed. The MRI findings in patients with positive biopsies were reviewed.

Results.—The MR images revealed all 48 invasive cancers and 4 of the 6 purely or predominantly ductal carcinomas in situ (DCIS). Of the 48 invasive cancers, 34 were unifocal and 14 were multifocal or diffuse, 45 had irregular borders, and 3 had well-defined borders. A ductal pattern was seen in 3 of the DCIS lesions. Of the 9 patients with both invasive cancer and DCIS, the MR images identified all of the invasive tumors in all 9, but revealed the DCIS foci in only 5. The MRI and mammographic findings agreed in 33 patients (52%). Of these 33, multifocal cancer was identified with both modalities in 8 patients. There were discrepancies in the mammographic, MRI, and/or pathologic findings in 31 patients (48%), with MRI detecting cancers not identified by mammography in 22 patients (34%). Multifocal or diffuse disease was discovered on MRI in 10 patients with only 1 mammographically identified lesion. Of the 7 patients with multifocal cancer, the additional foci were in the same quadrant as the mammographically detected tumor in 5 patients, but were in different quadrants in 2 patients (Fig 2). Magnetic resonance imaging detected cancer in 11 patients (17%) with normal mammograms. In 1 patient with a mammographically detected comedo-type DCIS, MRI revealed another unsuspected lesion in another quadrant, which was invasive lobular cancer. Biopsy findings correlated more closely with mammographic than with MRI findings in 4 patients (6%). False positive MR images occurred in 5 patients with MRI findings of multifocal cancer. Of the 112 patients with biopsy-proven benign breast lesions, MRI showed suspicious lesions in 10 patients (9%) and multifocal lesions in 3 (3%).

Conclusions.—Magnetic resonance imaging can detect unifocal and multifocal carcinoma that is undetected clinically and mammographically, which can alter treatment planning. It therefore has potential as an adjunctive imaging modality for the staging of suspected breast cancer.

▶ This paper discusses the role of MRI and MR-guided biopsy for the staging of suspected breast cancer. Dr. Orel and her colleagues offer potential benefits of MRI and MR-guided biopsy for patients with known breast cancer.

This study and others have shown that contrast-enhanced MRI can detect additional breast cancers. In addition, in this series, 20% of these cancers represented multifocal or diffuse disease. These data altered therapy in 7 patients (11%). In 2 of 3 patients with axillary lymph node metastases and no mammographically detectable primary carcinoma, MRI found the primary tumor and allowed conservative therapy instead of mastectomy to be performed.

Although these results are promising, certain caveats need to be remembered. First, very few centers in the United States have MR-guided capability. If MRI is the only imaging modality able to detect an abnormality, then radiologists must be able to localize it for the surgeon, and an MR-guided biopsy system is required. Also, MRI only detected 9 of 15 noninvasive breast cancers. Currently, most cases of DCIS that manifest as calcifications are best managed with stereotactic core needle biopsy or excisional biopsy. The authors also note an 81% specificity for multifocal disease. Will surgeons feel comfortable performing a re-excision in an attempt to find more tumor when 19% of the time, the pathology result will be benign?

Other questions from this study that need to be answered include the role of MRI in high risk patients with dense breasts as well as the potential MRI has for staging the axilla in patients with breast carcinoma. Dr. Orel's group has started the research in the right direction!

M. Rebner, M.D.

MR Imaging of the Breast

Weinreb JC, Newstead G (New York Univ)
Radiology 196:593–610, 1996 1–6

Background.—Breast cancer is the second leading cause of cancer-related mortality among women in the United States. Studies have suggested that MRI may play several useful roles in the detection and management of breast disease, although this has been widely debated. In the present report, the authors review the limitations of mammography, as well as the current state of breast MRI and its potential applications in clinical practice.

Discussion.—Although standard mammography is very useful, it also is associated with several disadvantages. Approximately 5% to 15% of palpable breast cancers are not detected on mammography. Additional subclinical cancers may be found only at histopathologic evaluation, meaning that some small but potentially curable lesions go undetected at mammography. Inherent limitations of x-ray mammography, observer limitations, suboptimal mammographic technique, and the size and nature of the lesion and surrounding breast tissue all contribute to unidentified lesions on mammographic studies. In addition, many detected abnormalities on x-ray mammography are indeterminate, necessitating subsequent biopsies for diagnosis and exclusion of cancer. These well-known drawbacks have prompted an increasing interest in breast MRI.

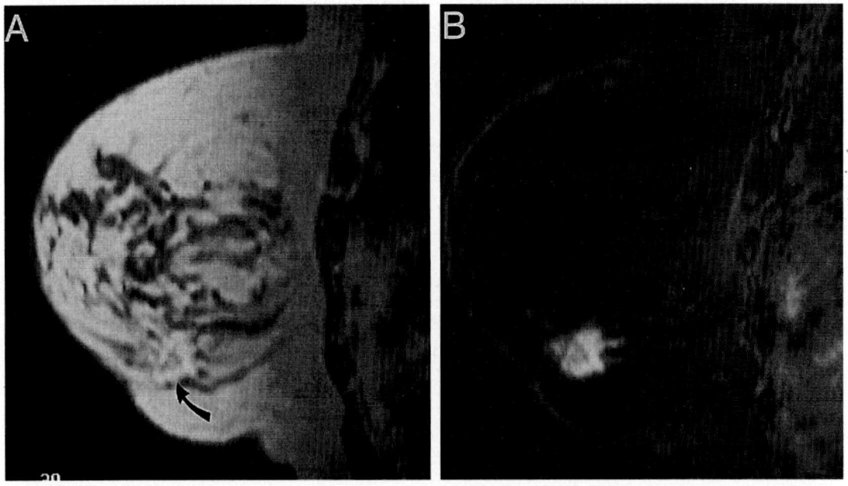

FIGURE 5.—Use of subtraction technique to make enhancing lesions more conspicuous. (**A**), contrast-enhanced sagittal 3D spoiled gradient echo image (12/5, 30° flip angle) shows intensely enhanced mass (*arrow*) with spiculated margins. Mass is minimally hyperintense compared with fat. (**B**), on subtracted image, the spiculated mass is much more obvious. (Courtesy of Weinreb JC, Newstead G: MR imaging of the breast. *Radiology* 196:593–610, 1996. Radiological Society of North America.)

Although earlier studies showed that breast masses could be detected on MRI, poor resolution, the inability to differentiate between benign tissues and malignancies on the basis of signal intensity traits, and lack of sensitivity to cancers suggested that MRI offered few advantages over mammographic studies. The emergence of IV, nonspecific, extracellular, gadolinium-based contrast agents, dedicated breast RF coils, faster and improved imaging capabilities, and approaches that eliminate high-signal-intensity fat have put to rest some of these previous concerns, prompting researchers to reconsider breast MRI (Fig 5). Potential clinical roles include treatment planning, assessment of the posttreatment breast, evaluation of breast implants, characterization of breast masses, MRI-guided biopsy, and cancer screening, although these possible applications are still in the investigational stage.

Conclusions.—Although there have been favorable reports about the use of breast MRI, many mammographers, clinicians, oncologists, and breast surgeons remain skeptical. Despite reservations, however, contrast-enhanced MRI may play an active role in the detection, localization, biopsy, and possibly even treatment of breast cancers in the future.

► Like Drs. Stomper's and Orel's articles (1–4, 1–5), this fine state-of-the-art review of breast MRI describes the current status of this imaging technique. Drs. Weinreb and Newstead point out the limitations of mammography and techniques for performing breast MRI, as well as their advantages and disadvantages.

Clearly, MRI of the breast has a role in detecting intracapsular or extracapsular rupture in women with silicone implants. It also may be beneficial in detecting an occult primary carcinoma of the breast when a patient is seen with positive axillary lymph nodes, and the results of other imaging techniques and the physical examination are negative. It also can detect unsuspected multifocal or multicentric carcinoma in a patient with known breast carcinoma when other imaging modalities depict negative results for the rest of the breast and the contralateral breast. However, as I previously wrote, breast MRI needs further investigation before we substitute it for stereotactic or ultrasound-guided core needle biopsy or excisional biopsy. The authors properly note that the negative predictive value and the false positive rate have to be significantly improved. Perhaps in vivo spectroscopy will help to differentiate benign from malignant lesions. May the magnetic force be with the investigator!

M. Rebner, M.D.

Diagnostic Value of Axillary Sentinel Node in Operative Breast Cancer—Work in Progress

Dowlat K, Fan M, Rayudu G, et al (Rush Univ, Chicago)
Breast J 2:26, 1996 1–7

Introduction.—Greater numbers of breast cancers smaller than 1.0 cm with less than 10% chance of lymph node metastasis have been detected with screening mammography. Alternative methods of staging to axillary adenectomy have been suggested, such as identification and excision of the primary, or sentinel, axillary node rather than full nodal dissection. The metastatic status of the axillary sentinel nodes was correlated to the rest of the lymph nodes in operative breast cancers.

Methods.—Fourteen women, ages 32–73 years, with breast cancer underwent axillary adenectomy. A gamma probe was used to mark the axillary hot spot or the area of radioactivity. The hot nodes were removed with the remainder of the level I and II axillary node dissection and examined for metastasis.

Results.—In 2 women, no hot spots were found. The metastatic status of sentinel nodes ranged from 1 to 5 with a mean of 2. The axillary sentinel nodes represent the metastatic status in operative breast cancer.

Conclusion.—A larger clinical trial should be conducted. If results of a larger trial confirm these results, excision of the primary sentinel axillary node rather than full nodal dissection may be preferred, particularly in T1 breast cancers.

► Staging the axilla with lymph node dissection for invasive breast carcinoma less than 1 cm remains controversial. Does a minimal cancer warrant a full axillary lymph node dissection? If this technique (which has shown promise with other tumors such as melanoma) is accurate, then patients may be spared a full axillary lymph node dissection. The procedure of sentinel node dissection is performed with local anesthesia and has lower cost and morbidity. However, this test's degree of accuracy must be equal to axillary lymph node dissection for it to replace the latter. It remains to be seen whether the false negative and false positive rates will be low enough to warrant the use of this procedure.

M. Rebner, M.D.

Nondiagnostic Stereotaxic Core Breast Biopsy: Results of Rebiopsy

Dershaw DD, Morris EA, Liberman L, et al (Mem Sloan-Kettering Cancer Ctr, New York)
Radiology 198:323–325, 1996 1–8

Introduction.—An accurate, cost-effective method of diagnosing breast disease is the stereotaxic breast biopsy. However, this technique should be correlated with imaging, clinical findings, and histopathologic results. Little has been written on the results of performing a repeat biopsy after

TABLE.—Initial and Repeat Stereotaxic Core Biopsy Findings

Initial Findings	Repeat-Biopsy Sample Histopathologic Findings: Malignant (n = 22)	Repeat-Biopsy Sample Histopathologic Findings: Benign (n = 28)	No Surgical Follow-up (n = 6)
Atypia (n = 30 [54])	15	13	2
Discordant imaging and histopathologic findings (n = 15 [27])	7	4	4
Unusual benign diagnosis (n = 10 [18])	0	10	0
Radial scar (n = 1 [2])	0	1	0

Note: Numbers in brackets are percentages.

(Courtesy of Dershaw DD, Morris EA, Liberman L, et al: Nondiagnostic stereotaxic core breast biopsy: Results of rebiopsy. *Radiology* 198:323–325, 1996. Radiological Society of North America.)

stereotaxic core biopsy. After stereotaxic core biopsy, the indications for and results of second biopsy performed have been determined.

Methods.—During a 29-month period, 314 women, ages 33 to 82 years, underwent stereotaxic core biopsy, and 56, or 18%, were advised to have a second biopsy after stereotaxic core biopsy. In 50 women, repeat biopsy was performed. The stereotaxic core biopsy was conducted with digital imaging and a dedicated, prone stereotaxic table. Specimen radiography was performed when calicifications were present to determine if calcium could be seen in the core biopsy specimens.

Results.—The most common reason for performing a repeat biopsy was diagnosis of ductal atypia in 30 women at stereotaxic core biopsy (Table). Fifteen women had discordant imaging and histopathologic findings, 10 had unusual benign diagnosis, and 1 had a radial scar. Carcinoma was found in 22 of the 56 women, or 39%. Among the 30 women with ductal atypia, 15 had carcinoma, or 50%. Among the 15 women with discordant imaging and histopathologic findings, 7 had carcinoma, or 47%. There was no detection of any other cancer.

Conclusion.—For stereotaxic core biopsy to be optimally effective, rebiopsy is necessary for those lesions with a high incidence of coexistent malignancy or for which results are nonconcordant. A missed diagnosis should be rare when stereotaxic core biopsy is performed in this fashion. Malignancy was found in 39% of the 56 women recommended for a rebiopsy.

▶ Dr. Dershaw and his colleagues have written another important paper for radiologists who perform stereotaxtic core needle biopsy (SCNB) of the breast. In 18% of their 314 patients, a repeat SCNB was recommended. It is noteworthy that the most common cause of rebiopsy was ductal atypia. In one half of these patients, carcinoma was subsequently diagnosed. The next most common cause for rebiopsy was discordance between the mammographic findings and the pathology results. Sampling error likely was the cause for this discordance.

No technique is 100% accurate. It is vital for radiologists who perform SCNB to correlate the mammographic findings and the pathology results. Discordance requires further action—either repeat core biopsy or excisional biopsy. At our institution, the discordant rate for the 170 cases performed to date is 3%. We prefer that our patients with ductal atypia or discordant mammographic and pathologic findings undergo excisional biopsy. This is simply a preference our surgeons and radiologists have agreed upon. Our rebiopsy rate is 12%.

Regardless of what type of second biopsy is done, the patient should not be allowed to "fall through the cracks." Proper communication between surgeon, pathologist, radiologist, and referring physician is required for effective care to be delivered to the patient.

M. Rebner, M.D.

Recurrent Carcinoma After Breast Conservation: Diagnosis With Stereotaxic Core Biopsy

Liberman L, Dershaw DD, Durfee S, et al (Mem Sloan-Kettering Cancer Ctr, New York)

Radiology 197:735–738, 1995 1–9

Background.—Although stereotaxic core biopsy (SCB) has been increasingly used in the tissue diagnosis of indeterminate or suspicious lesions found at mammography, no one has assessed its use in conservatively treated breasts. The efficacy of SCB in distinguishing carcinoma from benign breast lesions after breast-conserving treatment (BCT) was investigated.

Methods.—Seventeen of 316 patients with SCB had nonpalpable lesions in breasts previously treated with BCT. In 14 patients, surgical correlation was obtained. Patients underwent SCBs in prone position using digital stereotaxic equipment.

Findings.—Carcinomas were identified on SCB in 11 of 14 patients. Infiltrating ductal carcinoma (IFDC) was detected in 5 patients, ductal carcinoma in situ (DCIS) in 5, and infiltrating lobular carcinoma (ILC) in 1. In 10 of these patients, surgical histopathologic findings were in accord with core biopsy findings. One patient with 2 foci of IFDC on SCB had 1 found at mastectomy. In 2 patients with atypical ductal hyperplasia on SCB, DCIS was identified at surgery. In another patient, fat necrosis was identified at surgical biopsy as well as SCB (Fig 1).

Conclusions.—Stereotaxic core biopsy appears to be useful for the diagnosis of local tumor recurrence after breast-conserving treatment. When recurrent carcinoma is diagnosed on SCB, patients may proceed directly to definitive surgical treatment, usually mastectomy. Further research is needed to confirm the efficacy of SCB for the diagnosis of benign masses in conservatively treated breasts.

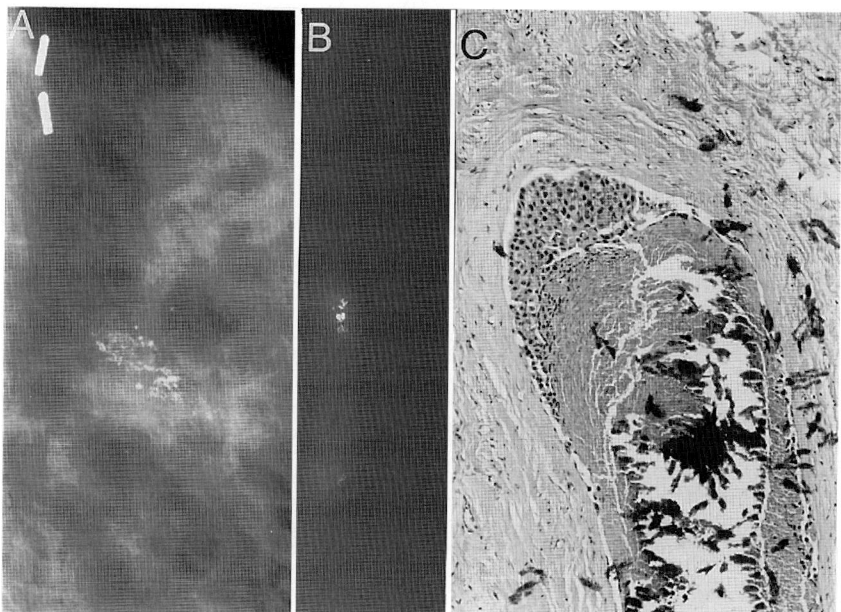

FIGURE 1.—**A,** magnified (original magnification, × 1.5) collimated mammogram of the right breast in the mediolateral oblique view in a 54-year-old woman who underwent lumpectomy and irradiation of ILC in the right axillary tail 4 years previously. Surgical clips mark the lumpectomy site. Image reveals highly suspicious pleomorphic microcalcifications remote from the surgical bed, extending over a length of 2.5 cm. **B,** radiograph of an SCB specimen demonstrates that the calcifications have been sampled. **C,** histopathologic section of core biopsy material reveals DCIS with comedo necrosis and calcification (hematoxylin-eosin stain; original magnification, ×40). *Abbreviations: ILC,* infiltrating lobular carcinoma; *SCB,* stereotaxic core biopsy; *DCIS,* ductal carcinoma in situ. (Courtesy of Liberman L, Dershaw DD, Durfee S, et al: Recurrent carcinoma after breast conservation: Diagnosis with stereotaxic core biopsy. *Radiology* 197:735–738, 1995.)

► Certainly, stereotaxic core needle biopsy (SCNB) has taken off as the "hot" new breast imaging modality. However, as with any new technique, scientific studies must be performed to analyze what lesions are best suited for this procedure. Dr. Liberman and her colleagues at Memorial Sloan-Kettering have done an admirable job, publishing numerous studies that have helped to clarify some of the problems with SCB. This paper focuses on patients who have undergone breast conservation, but who have non-palpable lesions that were suspicious for tumor recurrence. In their limited series of 14 patients, the authors noted that carcinoma was detected in 11. In 2 other patients with atypical ductal hyperplasia, excisional biopsy revealed DCIS. One patient had fat necrosis diagnosed with SCNB and surgical biopsy.

With more emphasis being placed on BCT, it is comforting to know that a less invasive procedure exists to diagnose recurrent carcinoma in the breast. However, as the authors note, this study was somewhat limited in that all the lesions were malignant. Presumably, the accuracy of SCNB for benign lesions in the treated breast should not differ considerably from SCNB in the nontreated breast. What remains to be determined is what mammographic abnormalities might be better served with excisional biopsy compared with SCB.

M. Rebner, M.D.

Automated Large-Core Needle Biopsy of Surgically Removed Breast Lesions: Comparison of Samples Obtained With 14-, 16-, and 18-Gauge Needles

Nath ME, Robinson TM, Tobon H, et al (Univ of Pittsburgh, Pa)

Radiology 197:739–742, 1995 1–10

Objective.—A wide range of needles have been used to obtain core biopsy samples of breast tissue with an automated biopsy device. Fifty-seven surgical biopsy and mastectomy specimens were sampled with a short-throw automated biopsy gun in an attempt to determine the optimal needle size.

Methods.—The samples were initially sampled with an 18-gauge needle and subsequently by 16- and 14-gauge needles. They were assessed independently by 3 pathologists, and the findings were compared to the final diagnosis from excisional biopsy.

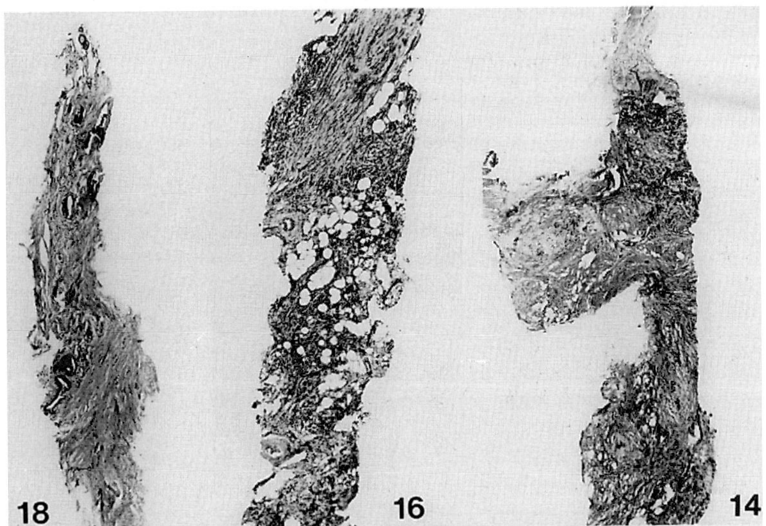

FIGURE 1.—Hematoxylin-eosin stain; original magnification ×390. Biopsy specimens of infiltrating ductal carcinoma. Samples obtained with 14- (*14*) and 16-gauge (*16*) needles show infiltrating malignant ductal cells in a fibrous stroma (*arrows*), which is indicative of an infiltrating carcinoma. The 18-gauge biopsy specimen (*18*) shows dense fibrous stroma without malignant ductal cells and was interpreted as benign, which produced a false negative result. (Courtesy of Nath ME, Robinson TM, Tobon H, et al: Automated large-core needle biopsy of surgically removed breast lesions: Comparison of samples obtained with 14-, 16-, and 18-gauge needles. *Radiology* 197:739–742, 1995. Radiological Society of North America.)

Results.—All 26 malignant lesions were correctly diagnosed by using the 14-gauge biopsy needle; 2 were undetected with the 16-gauge needle and 9 with the 18-gauge needle. The 14-gauge needle was most reliable in assessing infiltrating ductal carcinomas (Fig 1). All but 2 of 31 benign lesions were correctly diagnosed using all 3 needles. The larger needles provided wider and longer tissue samples.

Conclusion.—Larger core biopsy needles provide more breast tissue and therefore are best suited for making an accurate diagnosis.

► Stereotaxic large core needle biopsy has become more popular for the diagnosis of nonpalpable breast lesions. As the demand for the technique increases, so will the availability of different needles. "Bigger is better" is not a new slogan. It is not surprising that the pathologist can make a more definitive diagnosis when given more of the lesion to study. The question is, how far will we go with this technique? Currently, some centers are performing initial clinical trials whose purpose it is to evaluate the potential for percutaneous *excisional* breast biopsies using 1 and 2-cm core needles. The lack of access to control bleeding would certainly scare me. Nevertheless, it seems likely that this cheaper technique will continue to be scrutinized.

M. Rebner, M.D.

Breast Cancer: Prediction With Artificial Neural Network Based on BI-RADS Standardized Lexicon

Baker JA, Kornguth PJ, Lo JY, et al (Duke Univ, Durham, NC)

Radiology 196:817–822, 1995 1–11

Rationale.—Mammography, although a sensitive means of detecting breast cancers, always has had a relatively low positive predictive value (PPV). Both a conservative approach on the part of physicians and overlap with benign lesions account for this. An artificial neural network (ANN) has been contrived to help radiologists distinguish between benign and malignant breast lesions, thereby improving the specificity and PPV of screen-film mammography.

The Method.—An ANN is a set of processing units, or nodes, arranged in rows (Fig 1) that simulate the neuronal units in "learning" essential information. The input nodes are connected by relatively simple calculations with an internal layer of hidden nodes and a single output node. In place of a fixed algorithmic classification scheme, the ANN is presented with a sequence of supervised training cases as input data. It becomes "trained" by altering the strength or "weight" of its connections until its output corresponds to what is known to be correct. The "learned" information is stored as weighted connections between nodes. The ANN is relatively insensitive to minor variations within data. It is able to generalize from training cases when evaluating new cases not before seen. The network was constructed as a 3-layer feed-forward system with a back-propagation training algorithm.

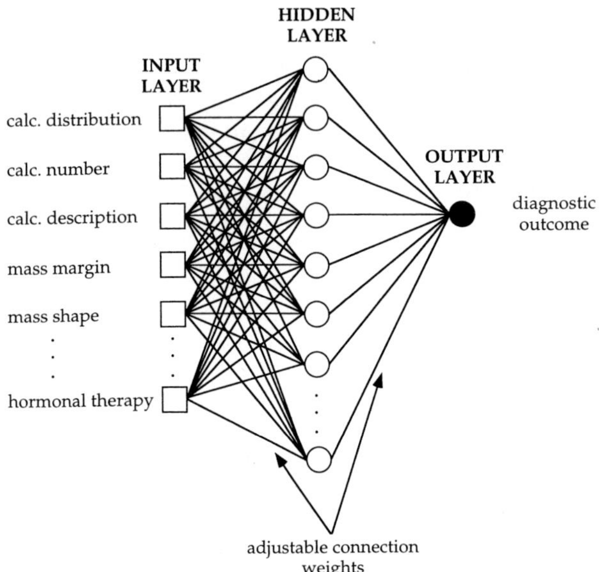

FIGURE 1.—Basic architecture of an ANN for the differentiation of benign from malignant breast lesions. The network used 18 input features, 10 nodes in the hidden layer, and 1 output node to predict the results of breast biopsies. *Abbreviations: ANN,* artificial neural network; *calc,* calcification. (Courtesy of Baker JA, Kornguth PJ, Lo JY, et al: Breast cancer: Prediction with artificial neural network based on BI-RADS standardized lexicon *Radiology* 196:817–822, 1995. Radiological Society of North America.)

Evaluation.—Mammograms from 194 of 402 women having needle localization of impalpable breast lesions were randomly chosen to be prospectively assessed. A total of 206 lesions was obtained by open excisional biopsy. Thirty-five percent of lesions were found to be malignant. Training mammograms were examined prospectively by 1 of 2 radiologists using the lexicon of the Breast Imaging Recording and Data System (BI-RADS) of the American College of Radiology. Ten BI-RADS lesion descriptors and 8 input values from the medical history were entered into the network.

Results.—The overall performance of the ANN compared with the radiologists, measured by receiver operating characteristic (ROC) curves, was not significantly superior. However, when analysis was limited to the part of the curve including most true positives and a sensitivity of 95% was specified, the ANN was significantly more specific than the radiologists (62% vs. 30%). At the part of the ROC curve where most mammographers practice, the high-sensitivity/low-specificity region, the ANN remained very sensitive and at the same time improved specificity significantly.

Conclusion.—It is possible to significantly improve the specificity and PPV of screen-film mammography without sacrificing sensitivity by using computer-aided methods such as the ANN.

► I chose this paper because a standardized lexicon offers a vision of the future. I believe the computer will eventually enhance the breast imager's capability to detect breast cancer. In this model, the authors showed an increase in specificity from the radiologist's 30% PPV to the computer's 62% PPV with a fixed sensitivity of 95%. Lesion characteristics were depicted with the BI-RADS lexicon. Relative values were assigned to these mammographic features, as well as to elements of the patient's medical history (family history of breast cancer, menstrual history, age, etc.).

Obviously, great importance goes into assigning values to each BI-RADS and medical history parameter. In addition, one must also be able to perceive the lesion if one is to assign values to it. With full-field-of-view digital mammography on the horizon, it may not be long before the computer will routinely identify abnormalities in the breast, assign a relative risk of breast cancer to each lesion, and ultimately raise the PPV of breast biopsy. Decisions as to what relative risk warrants a biopsy will then have to be made (2%?, 5%?, etc.). Something to look forward to. In the meantime, we still have our jobs!

M. Rebner, M.D.

Breast Imaging Reporting and Data System Standardized Mammography Lexicon: Observer Variability in Lesion Description

Baker JA, Kornguth PJ, Floyd CE Jr (Duke Univ, Durham, NC)

AJR 166:773–778, 1996 1–12

Background.—The American College of Radiology (ACR) has developed the Breast Imaging Reporting and Data System (BI-RADS) in an ongoing effort to improve quality in mammography. The BI-RADS is a standardized technique for assessing the morphology of breast lesions and classifying results in an unambiguous report. However, there have been no studies of the uniformity of descriptions of mammographic abnormalities

TABLE 3.—Interobserver Variability in Choosing Descriptions of Mammographic Abnormalities

BI-RADS Category	Kappa Value
Calcifications	
Distribution	0.77±0.03
Number	0.77±0.03
Description	0.50±0.02
Masses	
Margin	0.63±0.02
Shape	0.65±0.03
Density	0.62±0.03
Other findings	
Associated	0.32±0.04
Special cases	0.16±0.03

Abbreviation: BI-RADS, Breast Imaging Reporting and Data System.

(Courtesy of Baker JA, Kornguth PJ, Floyd CE Jr: Breast Imaging Reporting and Data System standardized mammography lexicon: Observer variability in lesion description. *AJR* 166:773–778, 1996.)

using BI-RADS. Interobserver and intraobserver variability in radiologists' descriptions of mammographic lesions with the BI-RADS standardized lexicon was investigated.

Methods.—Five radiologists independently evaluated 60 abnormal mammographic studies. Lesions were classified using a single BI-RADS lexicon term for each of 8 morphologic categories: calcification distribution, number, and description; mass margin, shape, and density; associated findings; and special cases. Each reader also rated the significance of each lesion on a 5-point scale. One reader examined each case twice.

Findings.—The terms used to describe masses and calcifications were consistent among readers. For these categories, intraobserver agreement was comparable. There was substantial interobserver and intraobserver variability for the categories of associated findings and special cases, which partly reflected the small number of cases assigned to these categories. When an assessment classification similar to that of BI-RADS was used, interobserver variability was moderate and intraobserver variability was minimal in the interpretation of lesion significance. The terms that readers used to describe calcifications did not always conform to BI-RADS-defined levels of suspicion (Table 3).

Conclusions.—The BI-RADS lexicon generally succeeds in decreasing ambiguity in the description and evaluation of breast lesions. However, attempts to correlate radiologic and pathologic findings should be continued to improve the specificity of the terms used in a standardized lexicon.

▶ The authors note that considerable inter- and intraobserver variabilities were seen for the "associated findings" and "special cases" categories. There was relatively good agreement among readers choosing terms to describe masses and calcifications. The purpose of the BI-RADS lexicon was to help standardize language for physicians to describe breast lesion morphology. The system cannot be so complex that radiologists are reluctant to use it. On the other hand, we have unfortunately seen too many mammography reports that ramble on for more than 2 pages and do not tell the referring physician what he or she needs to know about the findings and management recommendations. In this writer's opinion, BI-RADS is clearly a start in the right direction to help standardize mammography reporting. Obviously, modifications will have to be made as the system is tried. For example, some types of calcifications may have more than 1 descriptor with respect to their morphology. Nevertheless, this paper shows that good agreement for determining the morphologic characteristics of masses and calcifications can be obtained with a standardized lexicon. We can hopefully say "bye" to those bad reports and "Hi" to BI-RADS.

M. Rebner, M.D.

The Sternalis Muscle: An Unusual Normal Finding Seen on Mammography

Bradley FM, Hoover HC Jr, Hulka CA, et al (Harvard Med School, Boston; Massachusetts Gen Hosp, Boston)

AJR 166:33–36, 1996 1–13

Introduction.—The sternalis muscle, an uncommon anatomic variant of chest wall musculature, can be confused with a malignant lesion on mammography. Records and imaging studies of 6 patients in whom this irregular structure was apparent were reviewed to establish a diagnostic approach in such cases.

Methods.—From 1992 to 1994, 4 women among the approximately 32,000 who underwent screening and diagnostic mammographic imaging at Massachusetts General Hospital were found to have an unusual structure seen medially on the craniocaudal projection. Two more women evaluated at a second hospital had similar findings. All 6 patients were subsequently evaluated with CT, and 1 underwent MRI and surgery as well.

Results.—All 6 of these unusual mammographic findings were confirmed to be the sternalis muscle. This muscle has not been described previously and is not included in many anatomy texts. The muscle was identified when needle localization and exploratory surgery were performed in the index case. With this information, the remaining 5 patients were able to be diagnosed on cross-sectional imaging alone. Although the mammographic appearance of the sternalis muscle was variable, it was seen as a single focal density in all 6 cases. The structure typically measured 1–2 cm in maximum dimension, had an ill-defined margin, and appeared at the edge of the film. It was seen with certainty only on the craniocaudal projection, but its inferior extent may have been visualized on mediolateral oblique images in 2 patients. Multiplanar MR and spiral CT afforded better depiction of the sternalis muscle.

Conclusion.—This is the first known report of the sternalis muscle as a mammographic finding. The muscle may be seen more frequently with improved mammographic positioning, and the radiologist should be aware of this variant to avoid confusion with a malignant lesion. Correct diagnosis is suggested by the muscle's location, its configuration, and its absence on lateral views. Confirmation is possible with CT or MRI.

▶ I love articles that have practical value for all breast imagers. This study described the appearance of the sternalis muscle on mammography, CT, and MRI. I too have observed this irregularly shaped density in the posteromedial aspect of the breast on the craniocaudal projection. I felt this was a benign finding and incorrectly attributed it to the medial insertion of the pectoralis muscle. Dr. Bradley and colleagues have noted that the sternalis muscle is present in approximately 8% of both males and females. With more breast tissue visible on the mammogram, it behooves the radiologist to be able to identify this normal variant and not subject the patient to an inappropriate work-up or biopsy. Of course, if there is any doubt as to whether the posteromedial density on the mammogram represents the sternalis muscle or a carcinoma, it is reassuring that this can be differentiated by either CT or MRI.

M. Rebner, M.D.

Breast Sparganosis: Mammographic and Ultrasound Features
Chung SY, Park KS, Lee Y, et al (Hallym Univ, Seoul, Korea)
J Clin Ultrasound 23:447–451, 1995 1–14

Background.—Sparganosis, a human infestation by a larval form of an animal tapeworm of the *Spirometra* genus, commonly occurs in subcuta-

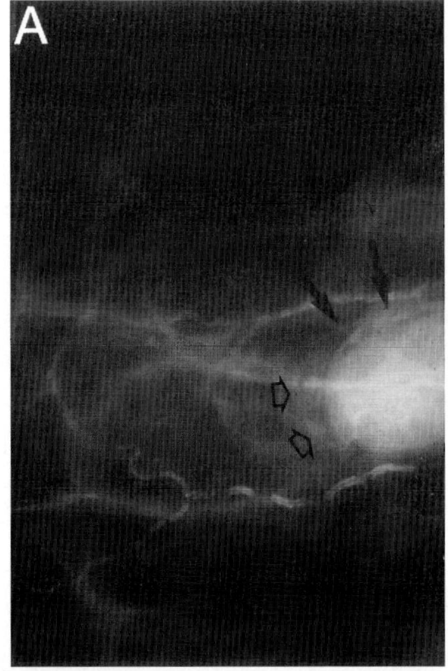

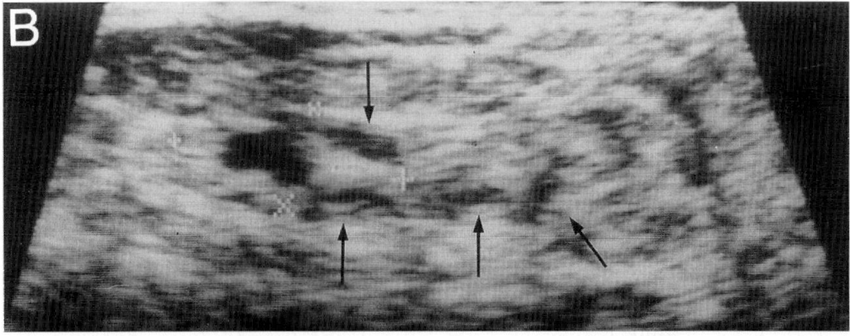

(*Continued*)

FIGURE 1 (cont.)

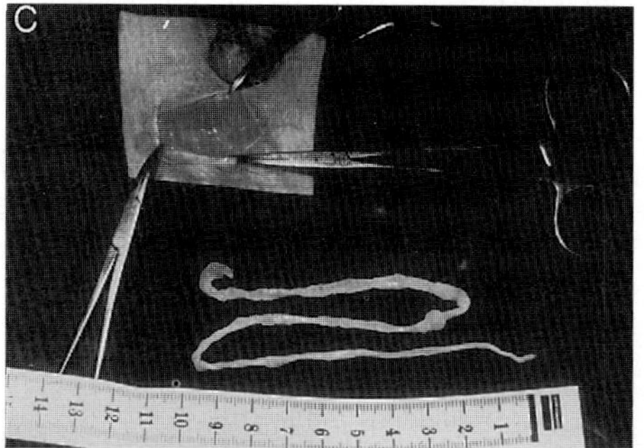

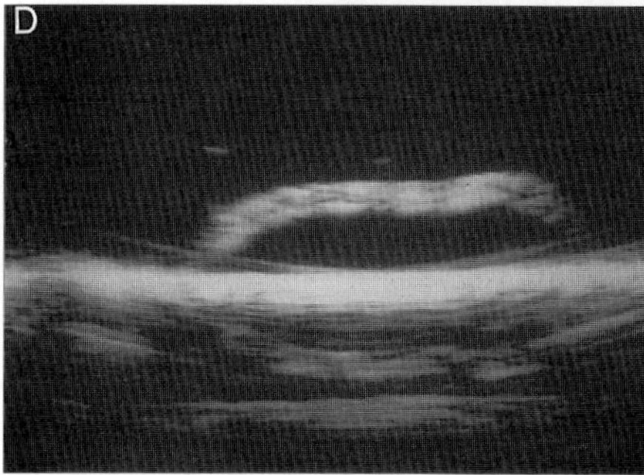

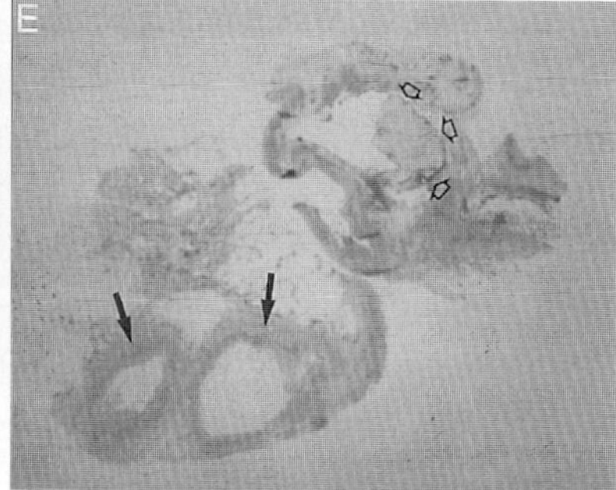

FIGURE 1.—Breast sparganosis. **A,** mammography shows an irregular, marginated, soft-tissue density mass (*arrows*) with adjacent smaller nodules (*open arrows*) in the breast. **B,** sonogram shows an ill-defined, heterogenous, hyperechoic mass with internal, folded band-like hypoechoic tracts (*arrows*). **C,** at operation, a living larval worm was extracted. **D,** sonogram of the extracted worm shows its hyperechoic nature. **E,** photomicrography shows empty tunnels (*arrows*) and sparganum in tunnel (*open arrows*). (Courtesy of Chung SY, Park KS, Lee Y, et al: Breast sparganosis: Mammographic and ultrasound features. *J Clin Ultrasound* 23:447–451, 1995. Reprinted by permission of John Wiley & Sons, Inc.)

neous tissue or skeletal muscle of the lower extremity, abdominal wall, abdominal viscera, chest, breast, scrotum, and brain. The mammographic and sonographic features of sparganosis of the breast in 1 patient were presented.

Case Report.—Woman, 76, was referred for evaluation of a nontender, softly palpable mass in the right upper quadrant of the breast. The mass had been present for 3 years. On mammography, the soft-tissue density measured 2 × 2 cm and was irregular, lobular, and marginated with adjacent smaller nodules (Fig 1). There was no calcification or subcutaneous thickening. The sonographic appearance was that of folded band-like hypoechoic structures in an ill-defined heterogenous hyperechoic mass in the parenchymal layer in the breast. At surgery, a living, ribbon-like larva, 30-cm long, was removed. Sonographically, the extracted larval worm in saline looked like a hyperechoic structure. Multiple empty tunnel-like tracts surrounded by palisading granulomatous lesions were noted microscopically.

Conclusions.—In this patient, sonography demonstrated elongated, folded band-like hypoechoic structures in a heterogenous hyperechoic mass. This proved to be the empty tunnel and the worm with surrounding granuloma. Hypoechoic band-like tracts in the mass suggested that tunnel. The extracted worm itself appeared as a hyperechoic structure on sonography. The hypoechoic tunnel in the heterogenous hyperechoic mass seems to be a reliable sonographic sign of breast sparganosis.

▶ I rarely choose case reports for the YEAR BOOK. Perhaps my fascination with tapeworms got the better of me. My mother always told me I ate like I had to feed one!

This human infestation is endemic to Southeast Asia, Japan, Korea and rarely the United States. For the disease to manifest as a palpable mass in the breast is very rare. The mammographic differential diagnosis is lengthy and includes the usual entities such as carcinoma, cyst, fibroadenoma, papilloma, etc. The authors provide a good differential diagnosis for the sonographic features of a heterogeneous hyperechoic mass with internal tracts (superficial thrombophlebitis and cysticercosis). The diagnosis is made microscopically by the identification of the worm in tunnels with surrounding inflammatory tissue. Because the source of this disease is drinking water, this might strengthen the case for bottled "aqua pura."

M. Rebner, M.D.

Paraffinomas of the Breast: Mammographic, Ultrasonographic and Radiographic Appearances With Clinical and Histopathological Correlation

Yang WT, Suen M, Ho WS, et al (Chinese Univ of Hong Kong)
Clin Radiol 51:130–133, 1996 1–15

Background.—In Hong Kong and other Asian countries such as Taiwan and Japan, unqualified practitioners use liquefied paraffin wax or beeswax injections—frequently administered under aseptic conditions—as a means to augment the size of the female breast. Women who have undergone paraffin injections may present with hard, nodular breast masses (paraffinomas) in later years, as demonstrated in the present case report.

Case Report.—Woman, 61, had received paraffin injection to the right breast 30 years ago because of breast asymmetry resulting from incision and drainage of a right breast abscess in childhood. Twenty-four years later, a hard breast mass without mastalgia or nipple discharge was noted. On physical examination, a large, firm, mobile, and nontender mass was observed on the incision and

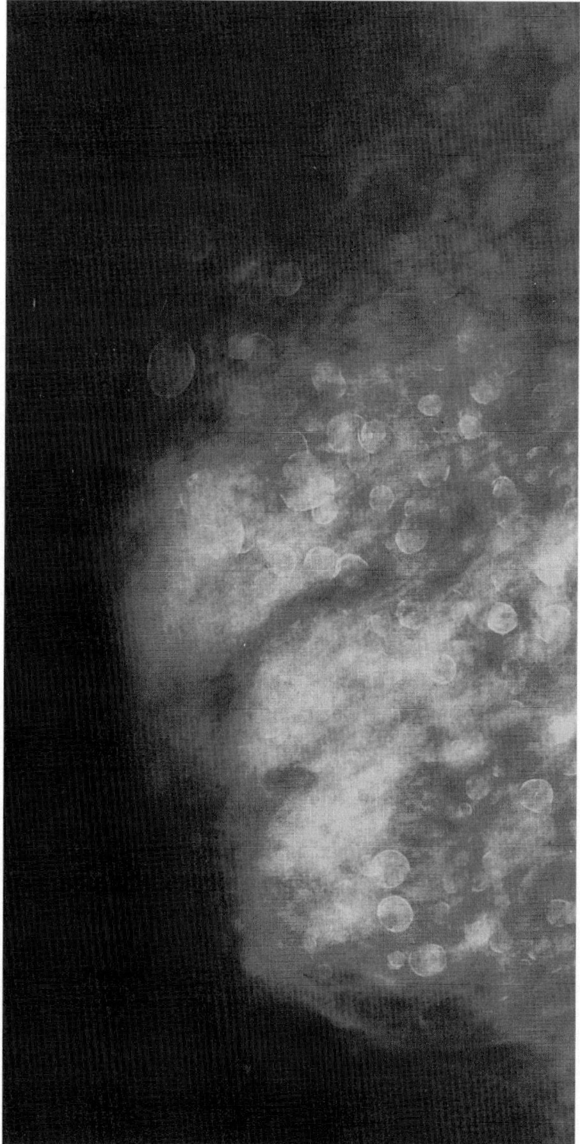

FIGURE 2.—Right mammogram shows abnormal lobulated densities replacing much of the normal breast parenchyma, with associated ring calcification in the rest of the breast. (Courtesy of Yang WT, Suen M, Ho WS, et al: Paraffinomas of the breast: Mammographic, ultrasonographic, and radiographic appearances with clinical and histopathological correlation. *Clin Radiol* 51:130–133, 1996.)

draining scar site. No overlying skin alterations were seen. Dense, lobulated masses, which replaced a large amount of the right breast, were demonstrated on mammography, and were accompanied by considerable and widely distributed flocculent ring calcifications (Fig 2).

Discussion.—The injection of paraffin, a hydrocarbon not absorbed by the body, causes a reaction in the breast tissue that triggers the gradual formation of fibrous tissue around the paraffin. Over time, this process results in a hard, fibrous mass. On mammography, diagnosis of paraffinomas is suggested by dense fibrosis, especially in the retroglandular midbreast area, causing streaky opacities and unusual architectural distortion. Flocculent, amorphous rings or rounded calcifications also may be observed in the breast and axilla. In some patients, paraffin migration through the soft tissue planes may occur, resulting in diffuse, conglomerate calcification in the chest and abdominal walls. Pathologic studies demonstrate grayish-white, rounded or flattened, plaque-like, homogenous, hard fibrous masses, with pockets of liquid wax contained within, and microscopy shows cystic spaces separated by hyalinized fibrous tissue. Microcalcifications may be found in granulomatous area, and axillary lymph nodes also may demonstrate reactive hyperplasia with aggregates of foamy histiocytes and occasional foreign body giant cells.

Conclusions.—Paraffinomas of the breast may be mistaken for breast cancer, given that both share similar clinical characteristics. Knowledge of the clinical, mammographic, and histologic features of paraffinomas will help reduce undue concern and avoid unnecessary biopsies and other unwarranted interventions.

► From a historic perspective, this article appealed to me. With all the focus on silicone breast implants, I thought it might be of interest to our readers to know what material was used before the advent of silicone. I never underestimate what people will do to themselves for the sake of their physical appearance.

As the authors note, in Asia, liquefied paraffin used to be injected into breasts, often without aseptic technique. The body attempts to ward off this foreign substance by forming granulomas and encasing the paraffin with fibrous tissue. The mammographic and sonographic appearances are striking. Rarely, the paraffin can migrate to the soft tissue planes of the chest and abdomen and result in diffuse, conglomerate calcification. Breast imagers need to be aware of this entity in order to avoid unnecessary biopsy.

M. Rebner, M.D.

Mammographic Features of Unilateral Breastfeeding

van Gelderen WFC, Goosen A (Univ of Stellenbosch Cape Town, South Africa)

Clin Radiol 51:134–135, 1996 1–16

Background.—The number of women who have breast-fed with only 1 breast for extended periods has not been established, and mammographic appearances in such women have never before been documented in the literature. This report describes the mammographic appearance in 2 women with long-term histories of breast-feeding, using only 1 breast.

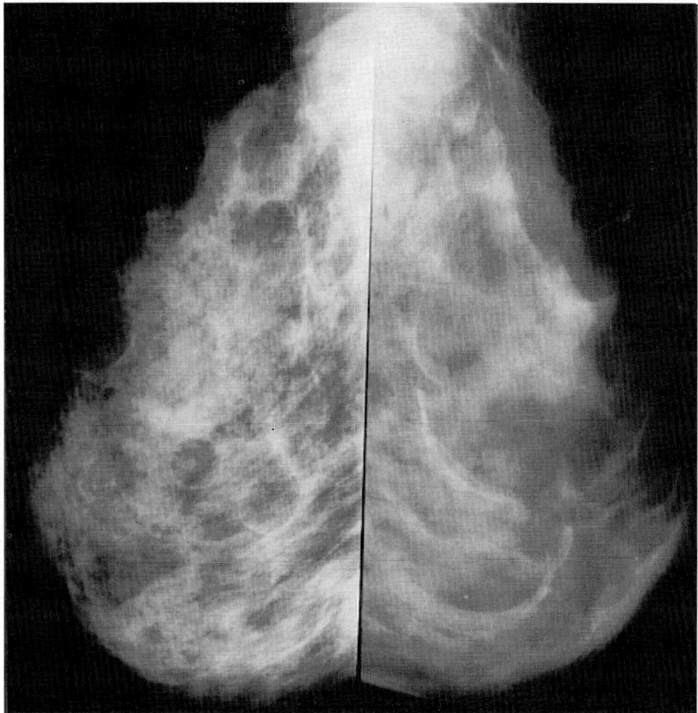

FIGURE 2.—Case 2. Bilateral mammography, mediolateral oblique projections. The left breast has involuted after recent breast-feeding and the right breast still has the appearance of a lactating breast. (Courtesy of van Gelderen WFC, Goosen A: Mammographic features of unilateral breastfeeding. *Clin Radiol* 51:134–135, 1996.)

Case Report.—Patient 1. Woman, 41, received a diagnosis of stage IIIb cervical carcinoma, for which prompt radiotherapy was initiated. A mass in the upper outer quadrant of the left breast, measuring 3 × 4 cm, was noted at presentation, and a referral for mammography was given. The woman was still breast-feeding her 18-month-old child, the youngest of her 7 children, using the left breast only. All 7 of her children had been fed on the left breast because of a breast abscess in the right side that occurred soon after delivery of her first child. On palpation, the left breast was enlarged, with a varicoid texture. The separate mass for which she had been referred was no longer evident. Mediolateral oblique and craniocaudal bilateral mammographic views were obtained. The left breast was considerably larger than the right. Numerous dilated ducts associated with a fibrocystic pattern also were seen on the left. The appearance of the right breast was grossly normal, and no dominant mass or indications of malignancy were seen in either breast.

Patient 2. Woman, 27, underwent aspiration of 3 cysts in the right breast, after which she was referred for mammographic study.

The patient had been breast-feeding her second child using only the left breast for 2 years. Her first child also had been breast-fed solely on the left breast because of a previous biopsy of the superolateral quadrant of the right breast. Biopsy findings were unknown. Immediately before mammography, the patient had breast-fed on the left breast. Mammography did not reveal any specific irregularities on this side, although the right breast showed increased density with numerous round, dense areas. The right breast had a congested appearance and was somewhat larger than the left (Fig 2).

Conclusions.—When milk is not extracted from the breast, glands will become markedly distended, resulting in compression of vessels and subsequent diminished milk flow. The secretion remaining in the alveolar spaces and ducts is absorbed, which results in gradual collapse of the alveoli. Consequently, the granular components steadily return to the resting state, and an increase in adipose tissue takes place. This course of events occurred in the right breast of both patients described in this report. In patient 2, however, the right breast still had the appearance of a lactating breast. It is believed, in the first patient's case, that breast-feeding 7 children solely on the left breast led to complete cessation of function in the contralateral breast, contributing to the lack of radiologic features associated with a lactating breast. These 2 patients have had the most unusual mammographic appearances documented during a 15-year period. It is concluded that atypical patterns of breast-feeding may result in asymmetrical-appearing breasts in later years.

▶ Different customs among various people fascinate me. When 1 such practice affects the mammographic appearance of the breasts in such a dramatic fashion, I choose its descriptive article for the YEAR BOOK. Marked asymmetry can be seen in the breasts secondary to postsurgical change, developmental causes such as Poland's syndrome, and also secondary to unilateral edema from congestive heart failure or tumor. Breast-feeding from only 1 breast may occur if there has been surgery or infection in the other breast. Interestingly, as the authors note, the Chinese Tanka (Boat People) women traditionally feed their infants with the right breast since the opening to their clothing is on the right side. On the negative side, these women have a three- to fourfold increased risk of having breast cancer develop in the unsuckled breast. For these children, unfortunately, "one good turn does not deserve another."

M. Rebner, M.D.

The Pleura

Comparison of Upright Inspiratory and Expiratory Chest Radiographs for Detecting Pneumothoraces

Seow A, Kazerooni EA, Cascade PN, et al (Univ of Michigan, Ann Arbor)

AJR 166:313–316, 1996 1–17

Objective.—A comparison of the effectiveness of expiratory upright and inspiratory upright chest radiographs in detecting pneumothoraces was carried out.

Background.—It is essential to diagnose pneumothorax early to prevent respiratory compromise and possible death. The most accurate technique for detecting pneumothoraces continues to be debated, and both inspiratory and expiratory upright chest radiographs are recommended. A precise technique is vital when evaluating for other conditions with symptoms that may mimic pneumothorax, such as pneumonia and pulmonary embolism.

Methods.—Three expert radiologists reviewed 86 pairs of inspiratory and expiratory radiographs showing pneumothoraces, and 93 pairs of inspiratory and expiratory radiographs without pneumothoraces. Radiographs were randomly arranged and rated on a 5-point scale for the presence or absence of a pneumothorax. Results were compared using receiver operating characteristic (ROC) analysis.

Results.—The difference in areas under the (ROC) curves for inspiratory and expiratory techniques was insignificant. There was no difference in sensitivity and specificity between the 2 techniques. Of the 86 cases of pneumothorax, 4 were rated by all readers as definitely pneumothorax on inspiratory radiographs and as definitely not pneumothorax on expiratory radiographs, and 3 were rated by all readers as definitely pneumothorax on expiratory radiographs and as definitely not pneumothorax on inspiratory radiographs.

Conclusions.—There was no significant difference in the sensitivity of inspiratory and expiratory radiographs in demonstrating pneumothorax. Both techniques are highly sensitive. Obtaining both inspiratory and expiratory radiographs doubles the radiation exposure and increases the time and cost of examination. Interpretation of the remainder of the chest can be hindered by using expiratory radiographs alone. Inspiratory upright chest radiographs are recommended as an initial test to detect pneumothorax.

► There was a surprising amount of interest in the pleura this year, enough to justify a new section in this year's "Chest" chapter. I particularly like this article because I generally appreciate articles that challenge traditional assumptions. We have assumed that expiratory radiographs should be ordered to detect pneumothorax, and yet it is hard to find scientific proof that this is correct. The study abstracted here demonstrates no advantage for expiratory radiographs and makes the valid point that other important lung abnormalities will be poorly evaluated using expiratory radiographs. One important note: these were all upright radiographs. Positional views are critical, and in supine patients, ultrasound demonstration of lung sliding (to-and-fro movement with respiration at the lung-chest wall interface) has recently been suggested as a way to rule out anterior pneumothorax.[1]

B.H. Gross, M.D.

Reference

1. Lichtenstein DA, Menu Y: A bedside ultrasound sign ruling out pneumothorax in the critically ill: Lung sliding. *Chest* 108:1345–1348, 1995.

Quantification of Pneumothorax Size on Chest Radiographs Using Interpleural Distances: Regression Analysis Based on Volume Measurements From Helical CT

Collins CD, Lopez A, Mathie A, et al (Hammersmith Hosp, London; Christie Hosp NHS Trust, Manchester, England)

AJR 165:1127–1130, 1995 1–18

Purpose.—Helical CT measurements of percentage pneumothorax size were correlated with interpleural distance measurements on erect posteroanterior chest radiographs to obtain a mathematical relationship that could be used to calculate pneumothorax size from radiograph measurements.

Methods.—Nineteen patients, ranging in age from 16 to 66 years, and with documented pneumothoraces, underwent both helical CT and upright posteroanterior chest radiography. The interpleural distance on the radiographs was determined by measuring in centimeters at 3 locations. The percentage of pneumothorax volume was calculated by manually

TABLE 1.—Prediction of Percentage Pneumothorax Size From Sum of Interpleural Distance Measurements

Sum of Interpleural Distances (cm)	Percentage Pneumothorax Size
2.0	13.6
4.0	23.0
6.0	32.4
8.0	41.8
10.0	51.2
12.0	60.6
14.0	70.0
16.0	79.4
18.0	88.8
20.0	98.2

(Courtesy of Collins CD, Lopez A, Mathie A, et al: Quantification of pneumothorax size on chest radiographs using interpleural distances: Regression analysis based on volume measurements from helical CT. *AJR* 165:1127–1130, 1995.)

drawing around the edge of the collapsed lung and the inner edge of the ipsilateral hemothorax on 10-mm sections of regions of interest.

Results.—The pneumothorax size ranged from 2% to 92% as determined by helical CT. When the helical CT values were regressed on the interpleural distances, the slope was 4.74. The formula for estimating a true percentage pneumothorax size was determined to be $y = 4.2 + [4.7 \times (A + B + C)]$. With this formula, percentage pneumothorax size can be predicted from the sum of the interpleural distances on a chest radiograph (Table 1).

Conclusions.—The formula derived in this study will help identify patients requiring active intervention for pneumothoraces from chest radiograph results.

▶ This very interesting study developed a relatively simple formula for pneumothorax size based on erect frontal chest radiography; the formula was validated by helical CT. I find it interesting, but I won't use it. In a previous YEAR BOOK,[1] I noted my reluctance to estimate pneumothorax size and found an article to support my position.[2] The current article may be correct, but the formula is still too complicated for routine use. I'm also not convinced that this gives more useful information than serial assessment of the distance from visceral to parietal pleura at the apex; in fact, I think a rough guess of small, moderate, or large pneumothorax and an estimation of larger, smaller, or the same (with modifiers like minimally and moderately) will suffice for patient management in almost every case.

B.H. Gross, M.D.

References

1. 1994 YEAR BOOK of DIAGNOSTIC RADIOLOGY, p. 59.
2. Engdahl O, Toft T, Boe J: Chest radiograph: A poor method for determining the size of a pneumothorax. *Chest* 103:26–29, 1993.

Detection and Estimation of the Volume of Pneumothorax Using Real-Time Sonography: Efficacy Determined by Receiver Operating Characteristic Analysis

Sistrom CL, Reiheld CT, Gay SB, et al (Univ of Virginia, Charlottesville; Univ of South Carolina, Charleston)

AJR 166:317–321, 1996 1–19

Objective.—The receiver operating characteristics (ROC) of radiologists in interpreting real-time sonograms for the presence of pneumothorax were assessed.

Background.—Pneumothorax may result from pre-existing chest disease or trauma, or it may be a complication of diagnostic or therapeutic procedures. It may be possible to detect pneumothorax with sonography. It is important to know the accuracy of sonologists who perform thoracic sonographic examinations.

Methods.—In 27 patients who were between 35 and 90 years of age, 26 lung biopsies and 2 transcostal biopsies of lesions in the right lobe of the liver were performed. Chest radiographs were obtained, and 13 pneumothoraces were identified. Chest sonographic examinations were performed and recorded onto videotape. Five readers blindly reviewed the videotape and scored each hemithorax for the presence and size of pneumothorax. Receiver operating characteristics were calculated.

Results.—The area under the ROC curves was 0.63 to 0.79 in detecting pneumothorax. After pooling readers and hemithoraces with the jackknife method, the area under the curve was 0.73. For the 5 readers, the average sensitivity was 73%, and the average specificity was 68%. The negative predictive value was 89%; the positive predictive value was 40%. There was no significant association between the estimates of pneumothorax size based on sonograms and actual pneumothorax size seen on chest radiographs.

Discussion.—In these patients, real-time sonography had a low sensitivity and specificity in screening for pneumothorax. Sonography is useful for confirming known pneumothorax, but it cannot exclude the diagnosis. Also, these readers were unable to determine the size of pleural air collections. Chest radiography may remain the method of choice in the diagnosis of pneumothorax. Caution is advised when interpreting the positive results of other studies.

▶ Although lung sliding was considered a helpful sign in excluding anterior pneumothorax in a previously referenced study,[1] the current study suggests that ultrasound is not sufficiently accurate to exclude pneumothorax or to estimate pneumothorax volume, and the authors noted a significant false positive rate. They "urge investigators to interpret the optimistic results reported elsewhere with some caution." It is difficult to report poorer results with an operator-dependent modality, but I believe that these authors do the field of radiology the same service that I attempt to do when I indicate my lukewarm enthusiasm for high-resolution chest CT. I readily admit that others have done it better than I do, but I believe I speak for a vast "silent majority" who can never achieve the glowing results that some report. (*N.B*: This is not the same silent majority championed by Richard Nixon, thank you!)

B.H. Gross, M.D.

Reference

1. Lichtenstein DA, Menu Y: A bedside ultrasound sign ruling out pneumothorax in the critically ill: Lung sliding. *Chest* 108:1345–1348, 1995.

"Fluid Color" Sign: A Useful Indicator For Discrimination Between Pleural Thickening and Pleural Effusion

Wu R-G, Yang P-C, Kuo S-H, et al (Lotung Poh-Ai Hosp, Taipei, Taiwan, Republic of China; Natl Taiwan Univ Hosp, Taipei, Republic of China)

J Ultrasound Med 14:767–769, 1995 1–20

Introduction.—Gray-scale ultrasonography is commonly used in investigating pleural opacities to evaluate the aspirability of pleural effusions, but findings are not always reliable. During color Doppler imaging, a color signal (fluid color sign) has been observed in the fluid in the pleural space. The applicability of this sign in the detection of pleural fluid capable of being removed by needle aspiration was assessed.

Methods.—A total of 76 patients with suspected pleural effusions underwent sonography in a blind study. A pleural lesion was classified as containing fluid if color Doppler signal related to respiratory movement appeared between the visceral and parietal pleurae (Fig 1) or near the costophrenic angle. A colorless pleural lesion was interpreted as negative (Fig 2).

Results.—Of the 65 patients with true fluid, 58 had a positive color signal (sensitivity 89.2%); none of the 11 with pleural thickening had a fluid color sign (sensitivity 100%).

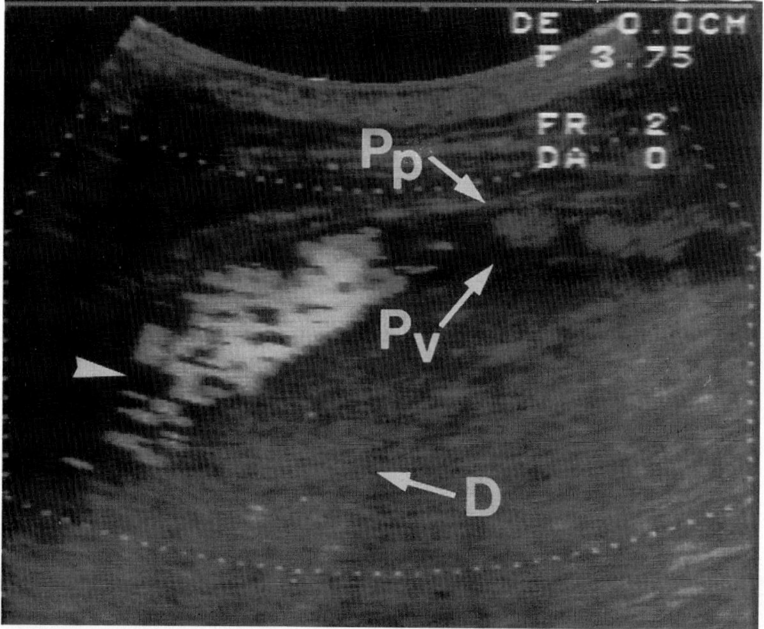

FIGURE 1.—True pleural effusion appears as a linear color band (*arrow*) between the visceral and parietal pleurae. *Abbreviations: Pp*, parietal pleura; *Pv*, visceral pleura; *D*, diaphragm. (Courtesy of Wu R-G, Yang P-C, Kuo S-H, et al: "Fluid color" sign: A useful indicator for discrimination between pleural thickening and pleural effusion. *J Ultrasound Med* 14:767–769, 1995.)

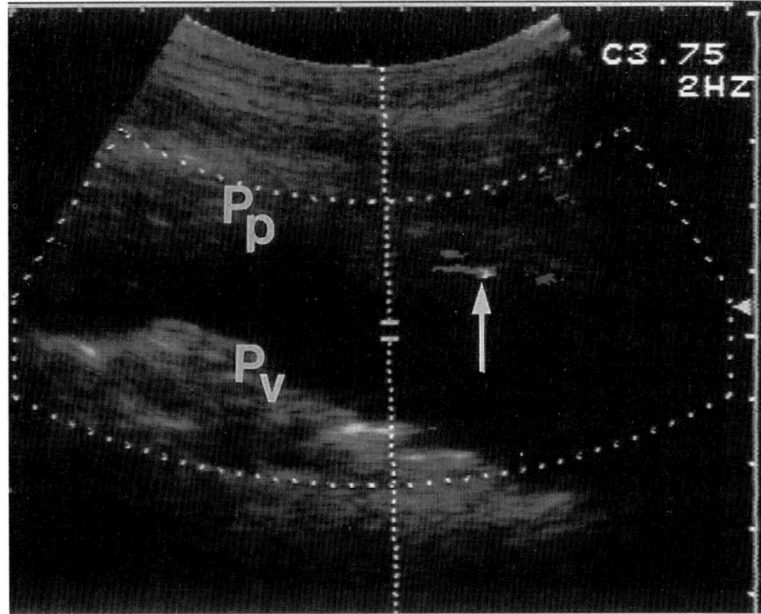

FIGURE 2.—The pleural thickening appears as a colorless pleural lesion on color Doppler ultrasonography. Some pleural vessels are also seen (*arrow*). *Abbreviations: Pp*, parietal pleura; *Pv*, visceral pleura. (Courtesy of Wu R-G, Yang P-C, Kuo S-H, et al: "Fluid color" sign: A useful indicator for discrimination between pleural thickening and pleural effusion. *J Ultrasound Med* 14:767–769, 1995.)

Conclusion.—The study demonstrates that the color Doppler signal is very useful for detecting minimal or loculated pleural effusions that can be aspirated.

► Now let's turn to a pleural application where ultrasound can contribute. When I was an ultrasound fellow in 1981 (revealing yet another closely guarded personal secret), I was taught that distinguishing pleural fluid from pleural thickening could be difficult. Floating strands or septations indicated fluid, as did change in shape with respiration (probably analogous to the "lung sliding" sign of pneumothorax). Applying color Doppler sonography to this distinction resulted in high sensitivity (89%) and very high specificity (100%) for aspiratable fluid in 76 patients. Interestingly, color signal ("fluid color" sign) appeared in the fluid during both respiratory and cardiac cycles. I believe that this is a real step forward.

B.H. Gross, M.D.

Peripheral Bronchopleural Fistula: CT Evaluation in 20 Patients With Pneumonia, Empyema, or Postoperative Air Leak

Westcott JL, Volpe JP (Hosp of Saint Raphael, New Haven, Conn)

Radiology 196:175–181, 1995 1–21

Introduction.—Bronchopleural fistulas (BPFs) can have many causes. Their treatment is optimized if their cause, location, and size can be identified. Although central BPFs can usually be diagnosed with bronchoscopy, peripheral BPFs are usually not visualized with bronchoscopy. The value of CT in visualizing the sites and causes of BPFs was evaluated.

Methods.—Twenty patients with known or potential BPFs were examined with standard CT, and 14 also underwent thin-section CT. All patients had clinical and/or radiographic evidence of either air and fluid collections (12 patients) or persistent air leaks (8 patients).

Results.—The BPFs could be directly visualized in 10 of the 20 patients with standard or thin-section CT. Of these 10, the BPFs were caused by necrotizing pneumonia in 5 (Fig 1), bronchiectasis in 4, and bronchoalveolar carcinoma in 1 (Fig 3). In 4 patients in whom the BPF was not directly visualized, bronchiectasis was identified just adjacent to the pleural collection. Of these 14 patients, 10 had empyemas, 2 had air or air and fluid collections without empyema, and 2 had persistent air leaks. Radiographs had not shown either the BPF or its cause in any of these patients, although the peripheral air and fluid collections were evident. In the remaining 6 patients, CT showed mild-to-moderate empyema in all, but

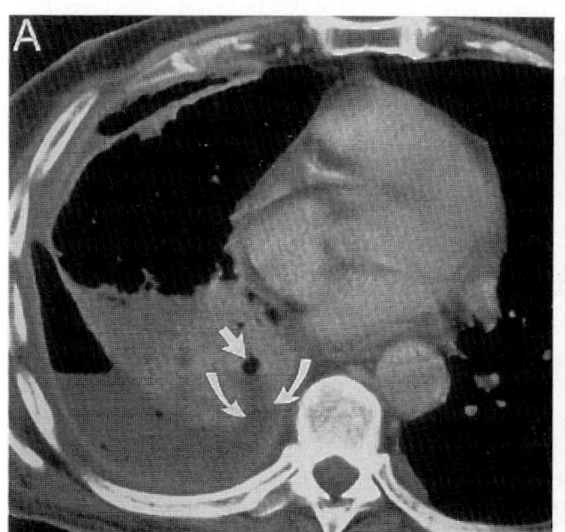

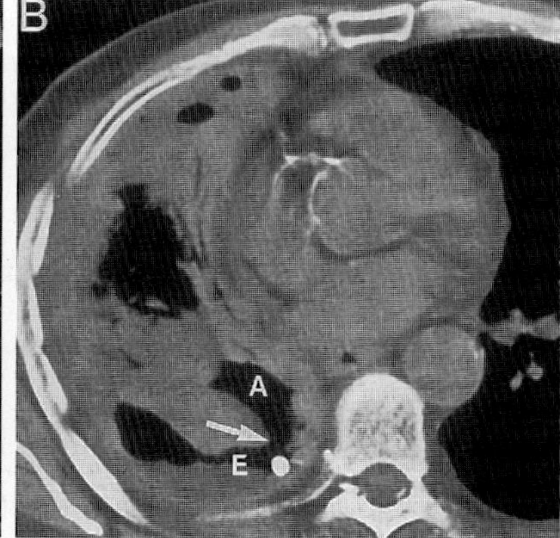

FIGURE 1.—Computed tomography scans obtained in a 72-year-old man who had undergone radiation therapy for squamous cell carcinoma of the right lower lobe bronchus and who had recurrent obstruction, postobstructive pneumonia, and an empyema on the right side. **A**, standard contrast-enhanced CT scan demonstrates a low-attenuation area that contains air and fluid in the enhanced atelectatic right lower lobe (*straight arrow*). It communicates directly (*curved arrows*) with an air and fluid collection in the right pleural space (*E*). Other low-attenuation areas are also demonstrated. **B**, follow-up non–contrast-enhanced standard CT scan obtained 3 months later demonstrates a large air-containing abscess (*A*) with a wide open communication (*straight arrow*) between the abscess and the pleural space (*E*). Scan also demonstrates chest tube (*curved arrow*). (Courtesy of Westcott JL, Volpe JP: Peripheral bronchopleural fistula: CT evaluation in 20 patients with pneumonia, empyema, or postoperative air leak. *Radiology* 196:175–181, 1995. Radiological Society of North America.)

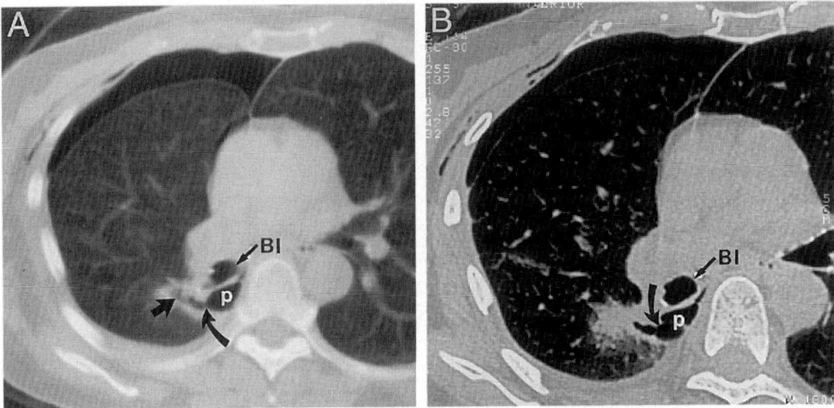

FIGURE 3.—Computed tomography scans obtained in a 55-year-old woman with cough and consolidation in the superior segment of the right lower lobe and a large persistent postoperative air leak. Exploratory thoracotomy findings revealed alveloar cell carcinoma. **A**, standard and **B** thin-section CT scans with 2-mm collimation were obtained in the area of consolidation. Multiple air-containing "cystic" spaces in the neoplasm are demonstrated (*straight arrow*). The bronchopleural fistula (*curved arrow*) is much better demonstrated with thin-section CT. The fistula was occluded successfully by means of transbronchial placement of several Gianturco coils. *Abbreviations*: *BI*, broncus intermedius; *P*, pneumothorax. (Courtesy of Westcott JL, Volpe JP: Peripheral bronchopleural fistula: CT evaluation in 20 patients with pneumonia, empyema, or postoperative air leak. *Radiology* 196:175–181, 1995. Radiological Society of North America.)

the BPF was not visualized. All 6 had postoperative air leaks and normal fiberoptic bronchoscopy findings. In 6 of 8 patients with evaluation of the BPF or its cause with both standard and thin-section CT, thin-section CT was considered superior, and the 2 methods were equally effective in the other 2 patients.

Conclusions.—Standard and thin-section CT scans have clinical value in the evaluation of known or suspected BPFs, particularly when they are caused by infection.

► I have generally been satisfied simply to suggest the presence of a BPF. The elegant illustrations in this article provide incentive for me to hone my technique in an effort to demonstrate the fistulas directly.

B.H. Gross, M.D.

Complications After Emergency Tube Thoracostomy: Assessment With CT

Baldt MM, Bankier AA, Germann PS, et al (Univ of Vienna, Austria)
Radiology 195:539–543, 1995 1–22

Introduction.—Increasingly, emergency tube thoracostomy (TT) is being performed before the patient arrives at the hospital. Critical injuries, such as a tension pneumothorax or hemopneumothorax, justify perform-

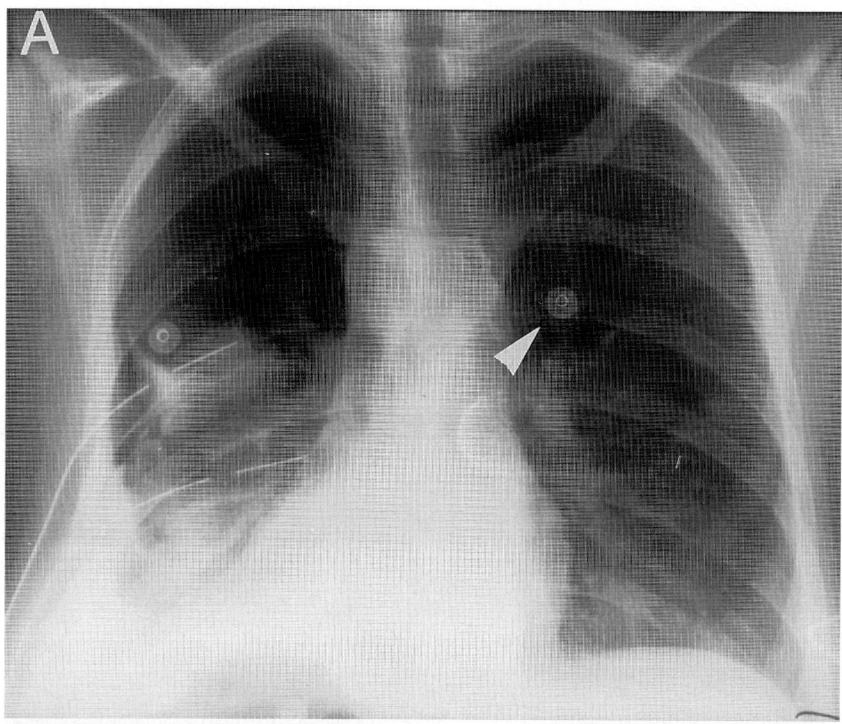

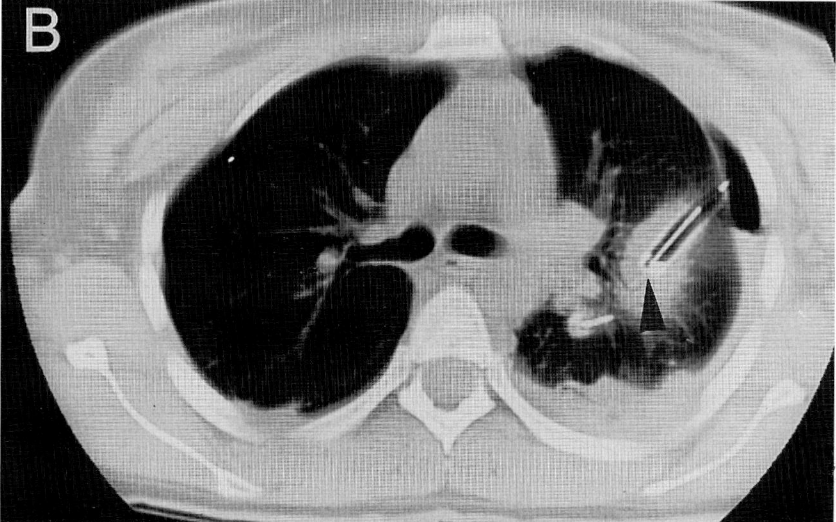

FIGURE 2.—A, chest radiography and **B**, CT scan show an intraparenchymal chest tube malposition (*arrowhead*) in the left lung of a 40-year-old man after an automobile accident. The tube tip is surrounded by a hematoma. The CT scan also shows a second tube tip in the area of the left major fissure; the exact position of the fissure is seen with use of caudal and cranial imaging planes. The exact position of the second tube tip cannot be defined on a chest radiograph. Both images show a small, persistent hemothorax. (Courtesy of Baldt MM, Bankier AA, Germann PS, et al: Complications after emergency tube thoracostomy: Assessment with CT. *Radiology* 195:539–543, 1995. Radiological Society of North America.)

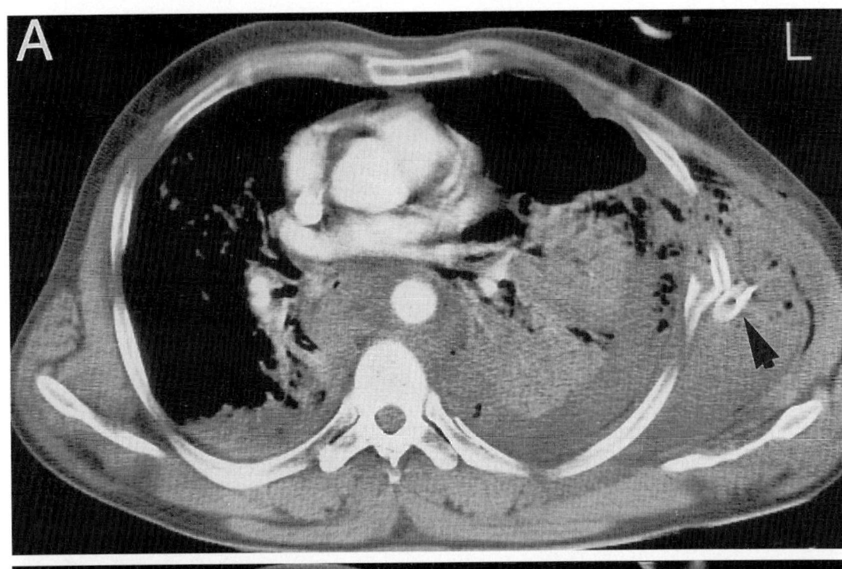

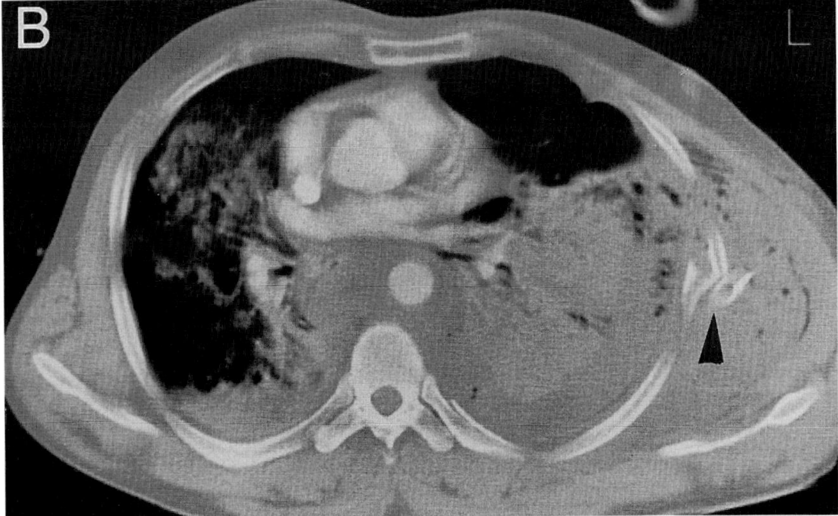

FIGURE 3.—A functioning tube in a 32-year-old man. Computed tomography scans show an extrathoracic tube malposition (*arrowhead*). **A**, soft-tissue window shows the tube tip adjacent to fractured ribs and surrounded by a large hematoma. **B**, parenchymal window better displays a severe, persistent pneumothorax and hemothorax. In addition there is a para-aortic hematoma due to a thoracic spine fracture at a lower level (not visible on this image). (Courtesy of Baldt MM, Bankier AA, Germann PS, et al: Complications after emergency tube thoracostomy: Assessment with CT. *Radiology* 195:539–543, 1995. Radiological Society of North America.)

ing TT without obtaining a chest radiograph at the trauma site. However, these patients are at increased risk for complications, such as chest tube malpositions (CTM). The spectrum and frequency of complications and the role of CT in their detection were investigated retrospectively.

Methods.—The chest radiographs, CT scans, and clinical charts were reviewed of 51 patients who had received an emergency TT, with placement of 77 chest tubes before arriving at the hospital. The radiographs and CT images were analyzed for chest tube positioning and for persistent pneumothoraces or hemothoraces.

Results.—Twenty of the 77 inserted tubes (26%) were malpositioned on CT. Of the 20 CTMs, 2 tubes had an extrathoracic location and 18 had an intrathoracic location. Of the 18 intrathoracic CTMs, 5 were intraparenchymal, 9 were intrafissural, and the position of 4 could not be determined. Chest radiographs revealed only 7 CTMs: 2 extrathoracic and 5 intrathoracic CTMs. Plain radiography could only identify 4 of the 9 intrafissural CTMs (Fig 2), and 1 of the 5 parenchymal CTMs were identified with CT. Computed tomography showed severe, persistent hemothoraces or pneumothoraces associated with 80% of the CTMs (Fig 3), whereas chest radiography showed severe, persistent hemothoraces or pneumothoraces associated with 60% of the CTMs. There were chest tube malfunctions in 32% of the 77 tubes, including 80% of the malpositioned tubes.

Conclusions.—There is a substantial risk of complications among patients who undergo emergency TT. Chest tube malpositioning is the most common complication and can be associated with further serious complications, such as persistent pneumo- or hemothoraces, intraparenchymal hematomas, or infections. Computed tomographic scanning is superior to plain chest radiography in the prompt diagnosis of CTM and is therefore recommended for all patients who undergo emergency TT without radiologic examination.

► It is not surprising that there were more complications in this series of emergent chest tube placements than in earlier series of nonemergent chest tube placements. However, I am uncertain how to use CT in the future, in part because of the retrospective nature of this study and because of an article abstracted in the 1996 YEAR BOOK that demonstrated no decrement in chest tube function when the tube was in a fissure.[1] Chest tube malposition was the most frequent complication found in the current study, and anywhere from 9 to 13 of the 18 malpositioned intrathoracic chest tubes may have been intrafissural; this should not have affected tube performance. The indication for chest CT in the current group of patients was simply blunt chest injury, so there is no clear evidence that the intrafissural tubes were causing clinical problems. Perhaps we can compromise and say that chest CT might be helpful in patients with pleural air or fluid that is not responding appropriately to chest tube drainage.

B.H. Gross, M.D.

Reference

1. 1996 YEAR BOOK of DIAGNOSTIC RADIOLOGY, pp 31–32.

Treatment of Complicated Pleural Fluid Collections With Image-Guided Drainage and Intracavitary Urokinase

Moulton JS, Benkert RE, Weisiger KH, et al (St Anthony Hosp, Denver)
Chest 108:1252–1259, 1995 1–23

Introduction.—To control pleural sepsis, restore pulmonary function, and prevent long-term sequelae of pleural fibrosis and entrapment, complete drainage is important in complicated exudative pleural fluid collections and clotted hemothoraces. Closed drainage is the most commonly used modality, moreso than open surgical drainage, and efforts to improve its efficacy have included combined image-guided thoracostomy and intracavitary fibrinolytic therapy, which helps drainage of gelatinous pleural fluid and allows enzymatic debridement of the restrictive fibrinous sheets covering the pleural surface. In the treatment of empyemas and other complicated pleural fluid collections, the results of image-guided catheter drainage with adjunctive enzymatic pleural debridement are reported.

Methods.—Image-guided drainage using 1 or more 12F to 16F chest drains was conducted on 118 patients with complicated pleural fluid collections. For 98 patients, adjunctive urokinase instillation was used with 100,000–250,000 U/mL of urokinase in 20- to 240-mL aliquots that were reaspirated in 1 to 4 hours. Seventy-nine patients had empyemas, 27 had sterile loculated parapneumonic effusions, 10 had sterile hemothoraces, and 2 had sterile postoperative exudative effusions. Large-bore thoracostomy drainage had failed in 41 patients. There was a mean estimated age of 13 days for effusions at the time of image-guided drainage, with a range of 1–175 days.

Results.—For 111 patients, or 94%, drainage was successful. Two patients had incomplete drainage and died of sepsis. Five patients had decortication, in which 3 recovered and 2 died after surgery. Placement of more than 1 drain was required in 53 patients, or 45%, and the mean duration of drainage was 6.3 days. A mean of 5 instillations of urokinase was required for patients treated with pleurolysis, and the mean total dose of urokinase was 466,000 U. No complications were seen.

Conclusion.—For complicated pleural fluid collections, image-guided drainage with adjunctive pleural urokinase therapy is an effective and safe method, and in most cases, surgery can be avoided (Fig 1). If treatment is begun early in the course of the disease, this method of treatment will be

FIGURE 1.—Stage 2 parapneumonic empyema in an 18-year-old woman. The effusion had been present for 5 days at the time of drainage. Treatment included image-guided drainage and intrapleural urokinase therapy. **A**, CT scan obtained on the day of chest tube removal shows moderate pleural thickening and significant residual parenchymal consolidation. These abnormalities represent the residual inflammatory changes of a stage 2 fibrinopurulent exudate. **B**, CT scan obtained 2 months after tube removal shows complete resolution of the inflammatory changes. (Courtesy of Moulton JS, Benkert RE, Weisiger KH, et al: Treatment of complicated pleural fluid collections with image-guided drainage and intracavitary urokinase. *Chest* 108:1252–1259, 1995.)

(*Continued*)

FIGURE 1 (cont.)

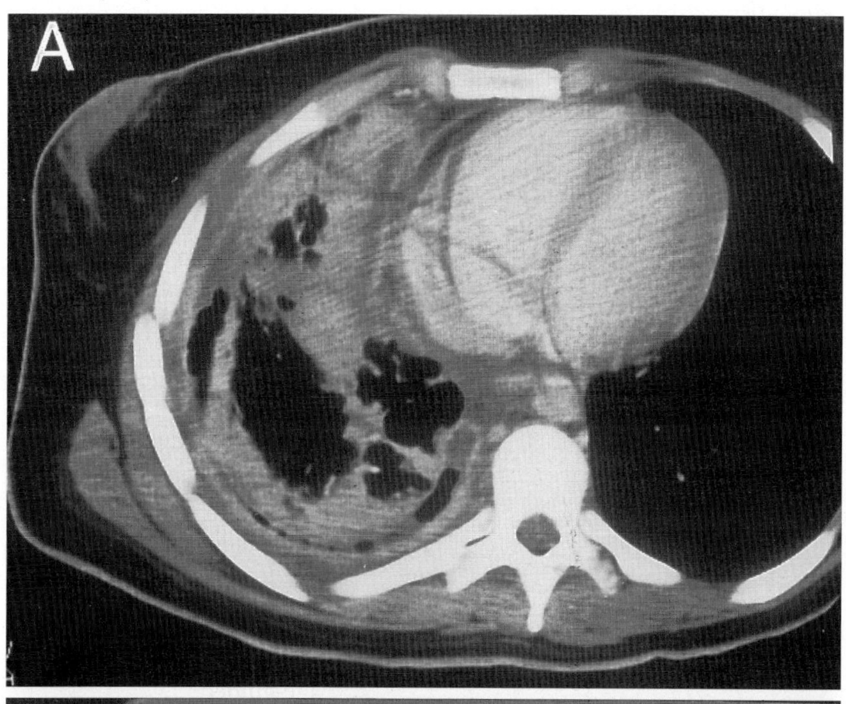

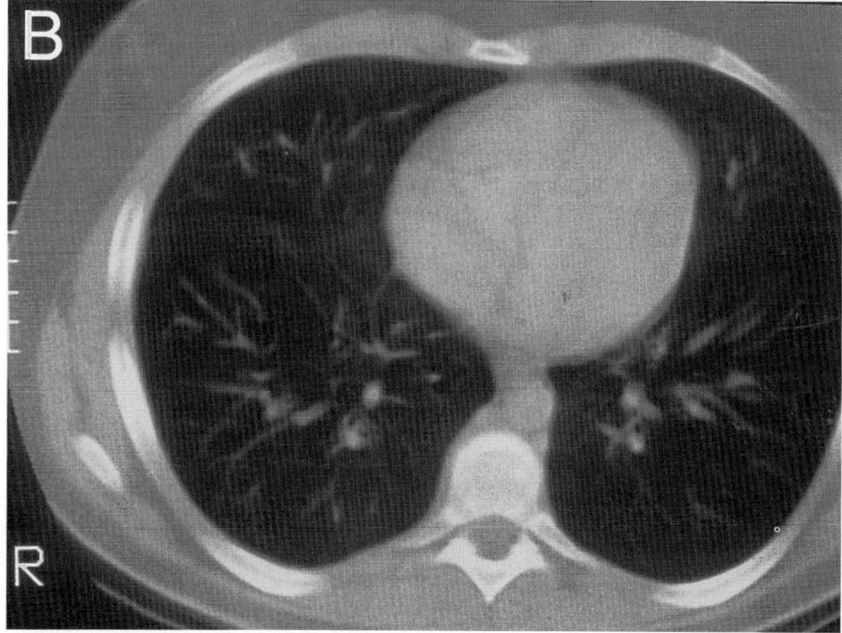

successful in most cases; however, the technique is time-intensive for the radiologist, requiring several patient rounds per day.

► Let me begin by pointing out that some radiologists could instead have been surgeons, and that many of these radiologists like to insert needles, tubes, and catheters into patients and find it especially rewarding when certain fluids are thereby extracted from patients. I, on the other hand, would certainly have been an internist, and I was initially gravitating toward a subspecialty (rheumatology) with hardly any invasive procedures. Let's face it: some radiologists have needles and catheters named for them; I hope to have several great-grandchildren named after me (or maybe I'll aim higher; my late father not only has 2 grandsons whose names honor his, he also has a bowling league named for him!)

I did my share of CT-guided aspirations and abscess drainages in the early 1980s and was interested to read about the potential application of N-acetylcysteine to loculated abdominal abscesses.[1] Subsequently, a note of caution was raised,[2] and I haven't heard much about it lately. We are not using it at all in our institution. I don't know if urokinase instillation into complicated pleural fluid collections will meet a similar fate; I only know that I won't be the instiller (and I hope I won't be the instillee, either).

B.H. Gross, M.D.

References

1. vanWaes PFGM, Feldberg MAM, Mali WPTW, et al: Management of abscesses that are difficult to drain: A new approach. *Radiology* 147:57–63, 1983.
2. Dawson SL, Mueller PR, Ferrucci JT Jr: Mucomyst for abscesses: A clinical comment. *Radiology* 151:342, 1984.

Nuclear Medicine

Thoracic Nodal Staging With PET Imaging With ^{18}FDG in Patients With Bronchogenic Carcinoma

Patz EF Jr, Lowe VJ, Goodman PC, et al (Duke Univ, Durham, NC)
Chest 108:1617–1621, 1995 1–24

Background.—Computed tomography is only 60% sensitive in the detection of nodal metastases of bronchogenic carcinoma, and it is not very specific. In addition, CT does not reliably help predict the histologic type of cancer. Positron emission tomography (PET) using 18-fluoro-2-deoxyglycose (^{18}FDG) provides both anatomical and physiologic information (Figs 1 and 2).

Patients.—Positron emission tomography was performed in 42 adult patients with newly diagnosed bronchogenic carcinoma before planned sampling of the thoracic nodes. Adenocarcinomas were most prevalent. A total of 62 node stations, 40 in the hilar/lobar region and 22 mediastinal sites, were sampled. Thoracic CT scanning also was performed, in 14 cases with IV contrast enhancement.

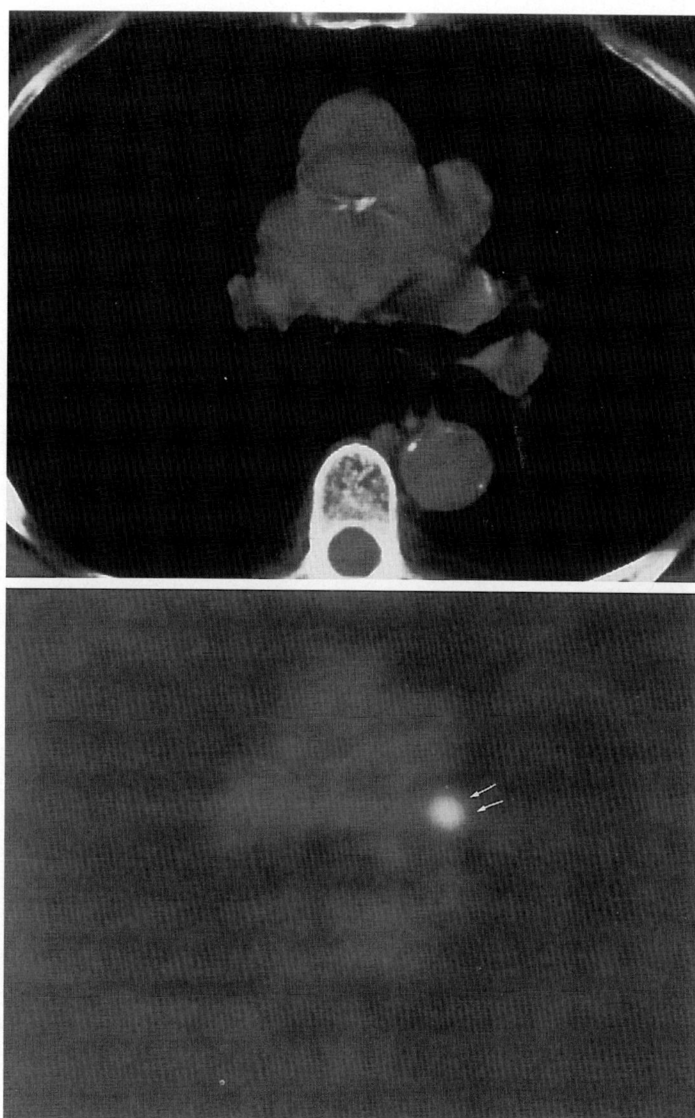

FIGURE 1.—Seventy-two-year-old woman with a 1.6-cm left upper lobe nodule. Surgery demonstrated stage II (T1N1) adenocarcinoma. **Top,** CT at the level of the left hilum is normal. **Bottom,** axial ^{18}FDG-PET image at the same level demonstrates a focal area of increased uptake in the left hilum (*arrow*). At surgery, there was metastatic adenocarcinoma in a hilar lymph node. *Abbreviations: ^{18}FDG,* 18-fluoro-2-deoxyglycose; *PET,* positron emission tomography. (Courtesy of Patz EF Jr, Lowe VJ, Goodman PC, et al: Thoracic nodal staging with PET imaging with ^{18}FDG in patients with bronchogenic carcinoma. *Chest* 108:1617–1621, 1995.)

Findings.—Imaging with PET was 83% sensitive and 82% specific in the detection of thoracic node metastases. The respective figures for CT were 43% and 85%. Imaging with PET helped to accurately predict the presence or absence of metastases in 75% of hilar/lobar node stations.

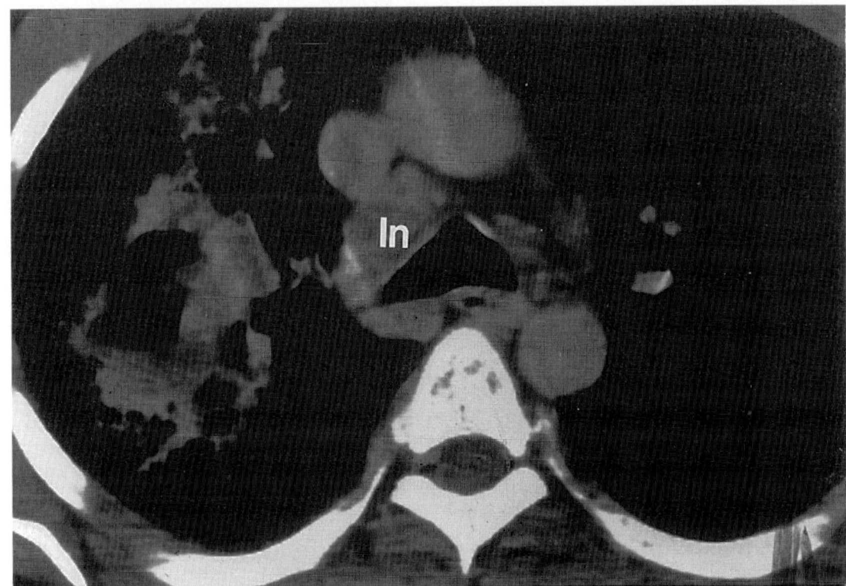

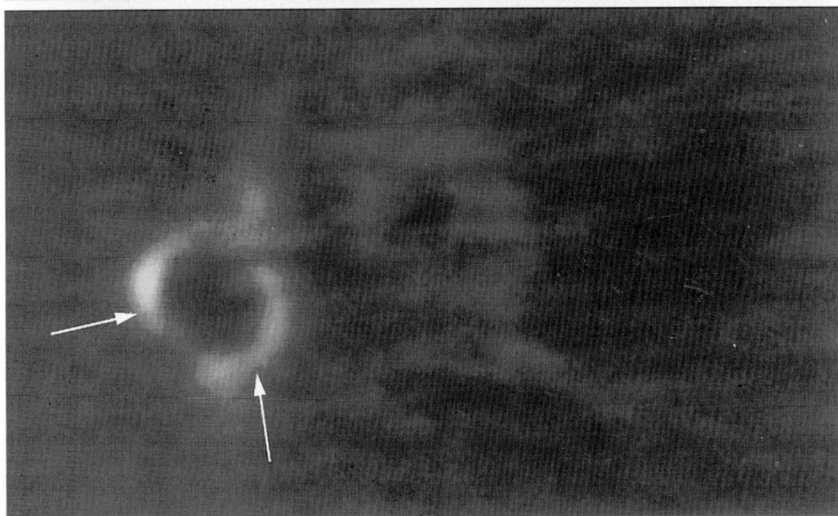

FIGURE 2.—A 44-year-old-man with a 4-cm right upper lobe cavitary mass. Surgery demonstrated stage I (T2N0) adenocarcinoma. **Top,** CT at the level of the aortic-pulmonic window shows the inferior aspect of the mass and a 1.8-cm right paratracheal lymph node (*1n*). **Bottom,** axial ^{18}FDG-PET image at the same level shows an area of increased ^{18}FDG uptake in the periphery of the mass (*arrows*) but no significant mediastinal activity. At thoracotomy, all nodes were reactive. *Abbreviations:* ^{18}*FDG*, 18-fluoro-2-deoxyglucose; *PET,* positron emission tomography. (Courtesy of Patz EF Jr, Lowe VJ, Goodman PC, et al: Thoracic nodal staging with PET imaging with ^{18}FDG in patients with bronchogenic carcinoma. *Chest* 108:1617–1621, 1995.)

There were 7 false positive node stations, 3 of which were normal on CT scanning. None of the 3 false negative stations were positive on CT. There was only 1 false negative PET study of the mediastinal nodes. In contrast, CT was only 58% sensitive in depicting mediastinal metastases.

Conclusions.—A normal ^{18}FDG-PET study nearly eliminates the need to sample the mediastinal nodes preoperatively. An abnormal study probably represents the spread of bronchogenic cancer to the mediastinum.

► Second section, second *new* section. I had never really considered the possibility of a whole section devoted to thoracic nuclear medicine, but when I spread this year's selections out on my desk I was amazed to find that such a section had been created. This also allows me the opportunity to review a paper on lung cancer staging without establishing a formal lung cancer section (and after carefully considering that topic in every YEAR BOOK from 1992 to 1995, I remain burned out).

Last year this group of authors showed that ^{18}FDG PET imaging could help distinguish persistent or recurrent bronchogenic carcinoma from fibrosis after therapy,[1] whereas another group found good specificity (80%) and fair sensitivity (67%) for PET evaluation of mediastinal lymph node metastases from lung cancer.[2] The latter article included only 25 patients in all, and only 3 of these had positive mediastinal lymph nodes—a surprisingly low percentage. The article's conclusion was that clinical application of PET in this patient population awaits the results of ongoing prospective studies.

Here is such a study. For hilar nodes, PET was 73% sensitive and 76% specific; for CT, 27% (!) and 86%, respectively. More importantly, for mediastinal lymph nodes, PET achieved a sensitivity of 92% with a specificity of 100%, as compared with 58% and 80% with CT. In yet another article this year, PET was 100% accurate at predicting mediastinal involvement in patients with lung cancer, and was 100% sensitive and 52% specific in predicting the malignant nature of intrathoracic abnormality.[3] It appears that ^{18}FDG PET imaging will prove superior to CT for staging lung cancer; it is unclear whether PET will actually supplant CT in the current socioeconomic environment.

B.H. Gross, M.D.

References

1. Patz EF Jr, Lowe VJ, Hoffman JM, et al: Persistent or recurrent bronchogenic carcinoma: Detection with PET and 2-(F-18)-2-deoxy-D-glucose. *Radiology* 191:379–382, 1994.
2. Scott WJ, Schwabe JL, Gupta NC, et al: Positron emission tomography of lung tumors and mediastinal lymph nodes using (18F) fluorodeoxyglucose. *Ann Thorac Surg* 58:698–703, 1994.
3. Sazon DAD, Santiago SM, Soo Hoo GW, et al: Fluorodeoxyglucose-positron emission tomography in the detection and staging of lung cancer. *Am J Respir Crit Care Med* 153:417–421, 1996.

Characterization of Chest Masses by FDG Positron Emission Tomography

Hübner KF, Buonocore E, Singh SK, et al (Univ of Tennessee, Knoxville)
Clin Nucl Med 20:293–298, 1995 1–25

Background.—Although the sensitivity of CT in evaluating chest masses is higher than that of plain film, its specificity is not improved. Scintigraphic techniques with single photon emitting agents have shown only marginally improved sensitivity and accuracy. Because malignant neoplasms demonstrate enhanced glucose uptake, high-resolution positron emission tomography (PET) with [F-18]-2-fluoro-2-D-deoxyglucose (FDG) may be useful in the evaluation of chest masses. The accuracy of dynamic PET scanning in the detection of primary or metastatic lung tumors was evaluated retrospectively.

Methods.—Fifty-four patients were identified who underwent PET lung studies, followed by either biopsy or at least 12 months' survival. These study patients were in 3 categories: those with unknown primary lung masses (23 patients), those with a suspected recurrence of lung carcinoma or lymphoma (13 patients), or those with a metastatic chest mass and an extrapulmonary primary malignancy (18 patients). The sensitivity and specificity of PET were calculated by comparing the imaging findings with histologic findings (for 45 patients who underwent biopsy), survival of at least 12 months, or the DNA proliferation index (in 5 patients).

Results.—The glucose uptake in normal tissue varied substantially, but normal lung parenchyma demonstrated low glucose uptake. Among patients with unknown primary lung masses, dynamic FDG PET had a sensitivity of 100% and a specificity of 67% in differentiating between benign and malignant tumors. Among patients with suspected recurrences, PET had an 83% sensitivity and an 80% specificity. Among the patients with suspected lung metastases, PET demonstrated a sensitivity of 87% and a specificity of 83%. However, in patients with lung metastases secondary to breast carcinoma, the sensitivity of PET increased to 100% and the specificity was 83% (Table 4).

Conclusions.—Dynamic FDG PET has clinical utility in the differentiation of benign from malignant primary lung masses, the confirmation of recurrent malignancy, and in the detection of pulmonary metastases. It has a high negative predictive value, which may obviate the need for follow-up invasive methods of evaluating benign lesions.

▶ Similarly, PET may be the best tool we have for characterizing various chest masses (solitary nodules, fibrosis vs, residual/recurrent lung cancer and lymphoma, suspected chest metastases from extrathoracic malignancies). And it may not matter because of its expense, particularly because PET is highly sensitive and specific, but not 100% sensitive and specific. In other words, if biopsy will remain necessary, why add the expensive imaging test?

TABLE 4.—Positron Emission Testing Results

Type of Lesion		True Positives	True Negatives	False Positives	False Negatives	Sensitivity	Specificity	Positive Predictive Value	Negative Predictive Value
Primary Lung Cancer		18*	4	2	0	100%	67%	90%	100%
Recurrent Tumor	Lung	3	4	1	1	75%	80%		
	Lymph.	2	6	2	0	100%	75%		
	Totals	5	10	3	1	83%	80%	62.5%	91%
Possible Metastasis	(other)	13	5	1	2	87%	83%	93%	71%
Breast Cancer	metastases	5	5	1	0	100%	83%	83%	100%

* The number represents the number of lesions analyzed on the PET images.
Abbreviation: PET, positron emission testing.
(Courtesy of Hübner KF, Buonocore E, Singh SK, et al: Characterization of chest masses by FDG positron emission tomography. *Clin Nucl Med* 20:293–298, 1995.)

Another nuclear medicine article looked at imaging of small-cell lung cancer.[1] A patient whose tumor took up indium-111 octreotide but not technetium-^{99}m MIBI failed to respond to chemotherapy. This case suggests that functional imaging may allow a prediction of whether tumor will respond to chemotherapy. Radiolabeled monoclonal antibody was also applied to squamous cell lung cancer; there is potential here for improved imaging and even therapy of these tumors.[2]

B.H. Gross, M.D.

References

1. Moretti JL, Caglar M, Boaziz C, et al: Sequential functional imaging with technetium-99m hexakis-2-methylisobutylisonitrile and indium-111 octreotide: Can we predict the response to chemotherapy in small cell lung cancer? *Eur J Nucl Med* 25:177–180, 1995.
2. Cuartero-Plaza A, Martinez-Miralles E, Rosell R, et al: Radiolocalization of squamous lung carcinoma with ^{131}I-labeled epidermal growth factor. *Clin Cancer Res* 2:13-20, 1996.

Crack Cocaine Mimicking Pulmonary Embolism on Pulmonary Ventilation/Perfusion Lung Scan: A Case Report

Smith GT, McClaughry PL, Purkey J, et al (Univ of Tennessee, Knoxville)
Clin Nucl Med 20:65–68, 1995 1–26

Introduction.—Several pulmonary complications are associated with the use of crack cocaine, including some that have not previously been associated with intravenous drug use. The pulmonary manifestations resembling pulmonary embolism that were seen in association with a patient's inhalational cocaine abuse are described.

Case Report.—Woman, 28, experienced dyspnea, cough, and vague chest discomfort after a week of heavy crack cocaine smoking. Diffuse bilateral wheezing was detected, but there was no accessory respiratory muscle use and no other abnormal findings on chest examination. The chest x-ray was normal. There were only matching ventilation and perfusion defects in both bases on radionuclide ventilation/perfusion (V/Q) lung scan (Fig 1). A peripheral Doppler examination showed deep venous incompetence

FIGURE 1.—Radionuclide ventilation/perfusion scan at the time of admission. **A**, posterior Xe-133 images obtained during 90-second washin and 2½ -minute washout. **B**, TC-99m macroaggregated albumin perfusion images in multiple projections. The scan shows multiple bilateral large, matched, segmental and subsegmental defects with diffuse air trapping. Chest radiograph was normal. This is intermediate probability for pulmonary embolism by PIOPED criteria. *Abbreviations: LAO*, left anterior oblique; *LL*, left lateral; *LPO*, left posterior oblique; *RPO*, right posterior oblique; *RL*, right lateral; *RAO*, right anterior oblique. (Courtesy of Smith GT, McClaughry PL, Purkey J, et al: Crack cocaine mimicking pulmonary embolism on pulmonary ventilation/perfusion lung scan: A case report. *Clin Nucl Med* 20:65–68, 1995.)

(*Continued*)

FIGURE 1 (cont.)

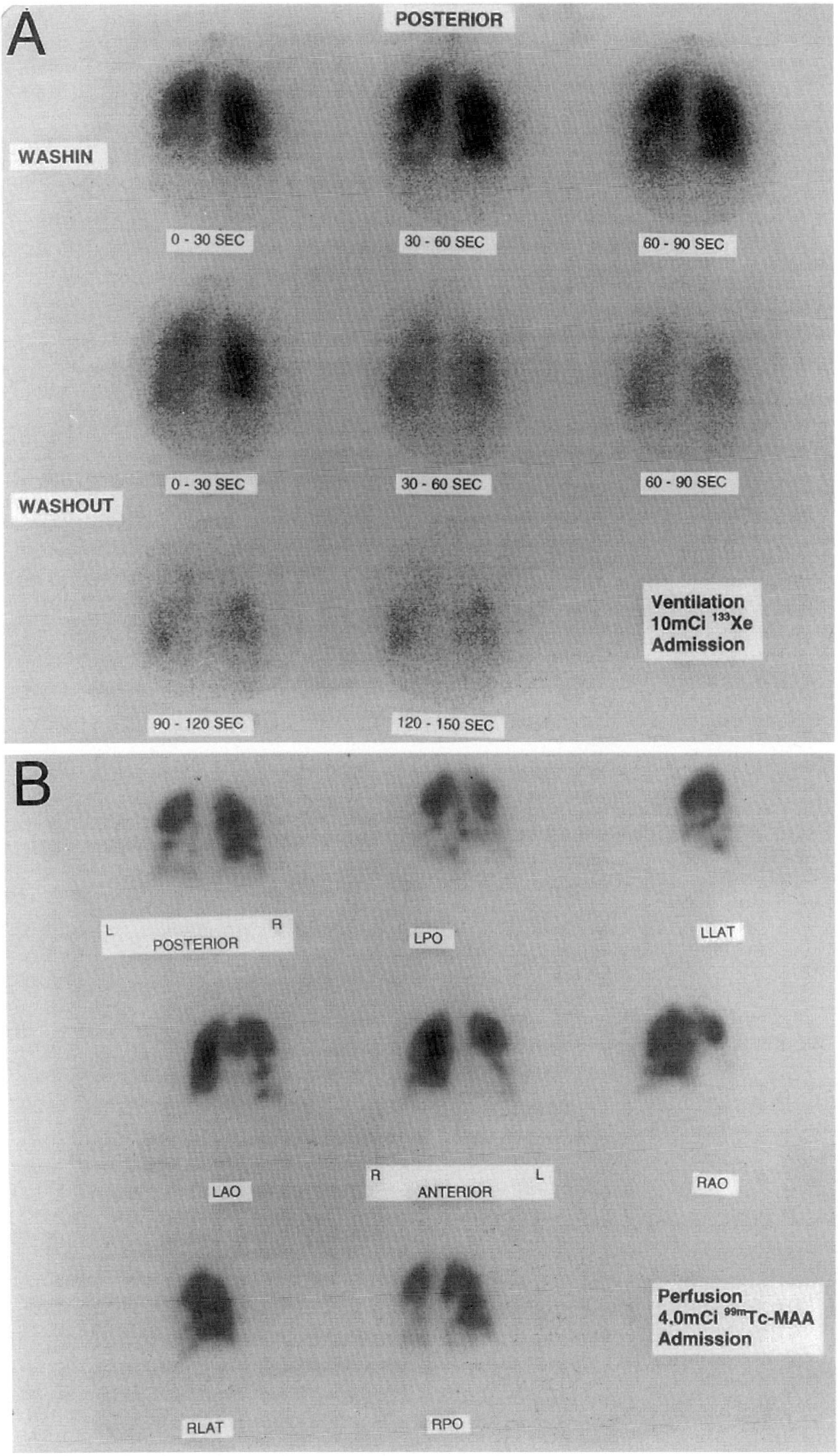

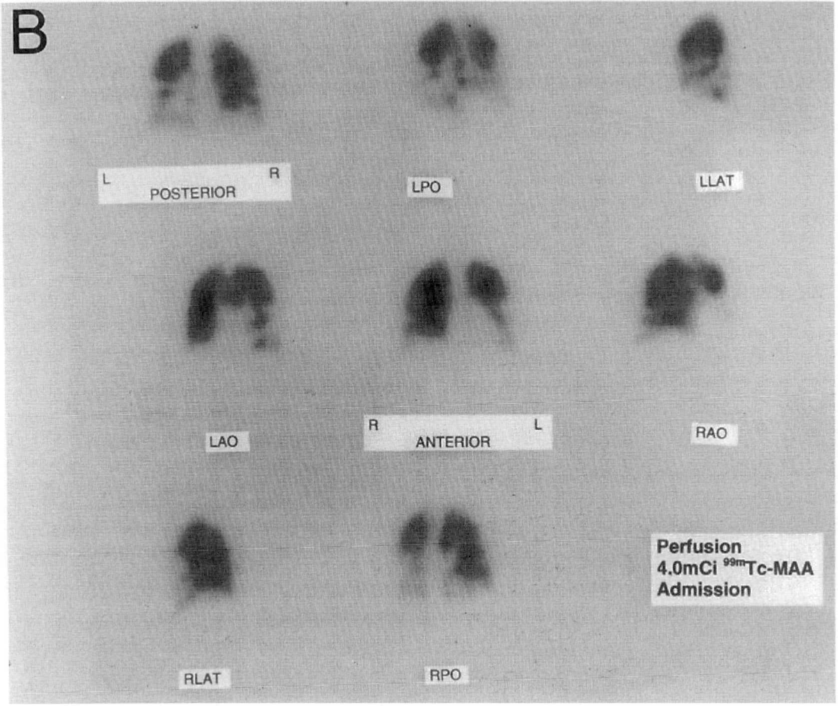

unassociated with occlusive disease in both lower extremities. Pulmonary function tests suggested moderate restrictive and diffusion impairment. Another V/Q scan 4 days after the first showed the same air trapping with improved perfusion, consistent with resolving pulmonary emboli (Fig 2). The patient showed improvement with anticoagulation and bronchodilator therapy. She was readmitted 2 weeks after discharge with pleuritic chest pain, hemoptysis, and dyspnea. She reported smoking cocaine again. Another V/Q scan revealed diffuse air trapping and multiple perfusion defects in a different distribution than had appeared in the 2 previous scans (Fig 3), which suggested recurrent pulmonary emboli. There was no evidence of pulmonary embolism on a pulmonary angiogram, and so anticoagulant therapy was discontinued. After gradual improvement of respiratory status during a period of 3 days, the patient was discharged.

Discussion.—Pulmonary manifestations of cocaine inhalation can mimic pulmonary embolism both clinically and on radionuclide testing. The changes in the radionuclide perfusion abnormalities suggest that pulmonary vasospasm may play a role in respiratory complications.

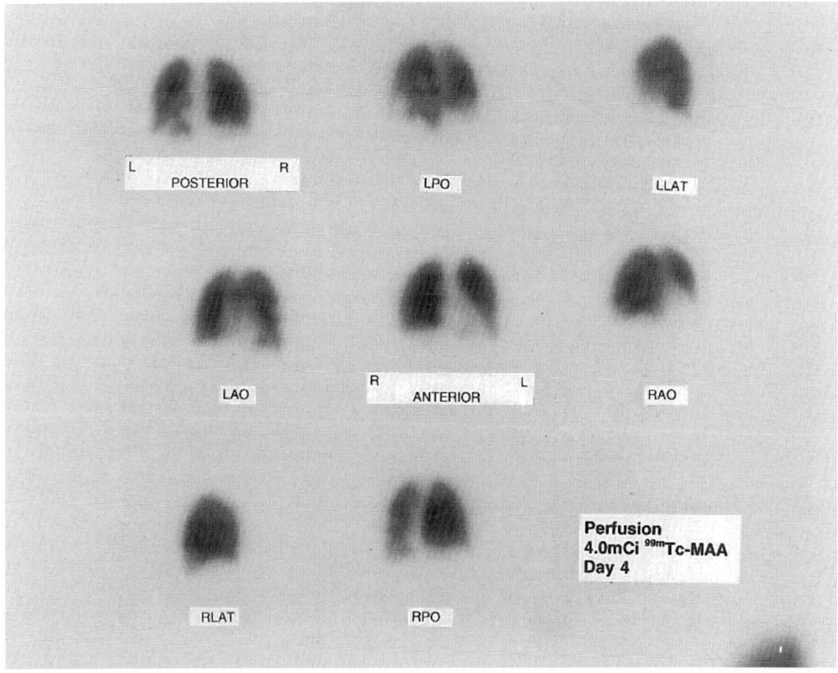

FIGURE 2.—Follow-up TC-99m macroaggregated albumin perfusion scan on day 4, showing near-complete resolution of perfusion to both lung fields in comparison with the initial scan. A repeat X-133 ventilation scan was unchanged from admission (see Fig 1, A). View labels are the same as in Figure 1, B. (Courtesy of Smith GT, McClaughry PL, Purkey J, et al: Crack cocaine mimicking pulmonary embolism on pulmonary ventilation/perfusion lung scan: A case report. *Clin Nucl Med* 20:65–68, 1995.)

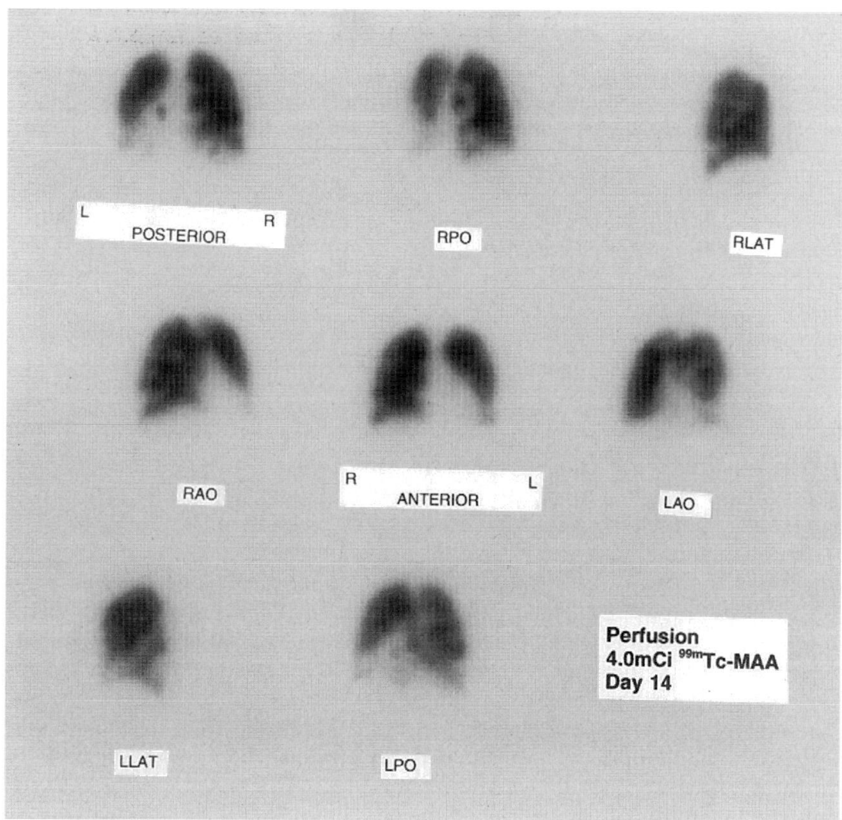

FIGURE 3.—Repeat perfusion scan at the time of the second admission, 3 weeks after the initial scan, showing multiple new perfusion defects compared with the previous scan, suggesting recurrent pulmonary embolism. An Xe-133 ventilation scan (not shown) was again unchanged from admission (see Figure 1, A). Projection labels are the same as in Figure 1, B. (Courtesy of Smith GT, McClaughry PL, Purkey J, et al: Crack cocaine mimicking pulmonary embolism on pulmonary ventilation/perfusion lung scan: A case report. *Clin Nucl Med* 20:65–68, 1995.)

► Given the magnitude of the crack cocaine epidemic and the similarity of its signs and symptoms to pulmonary emboli, it's surprising that there isn't more literature on ventilation-perfusion lung scanning in crack smokers. The resultant false positive nuclear scans are a hazard to these patients and their treating physicians because of the likelihood of subsequent unnecessary anticoagulation.

Another application of lung scanning this year was in the assessment of asthma response to therapy.[1] After 1 week of inhaled beclomethasone, there was more homogeneous distribution of Tc-99m human serum albumin radioaerosol, correlating with improvement in bronchial obstruction.

B.H. Gross, M.D.

Reference

1. Changlai S-P, Kao C-H, Wang S-J, et al: The change in the distribution of Tc-99m human serum albumin radioaerosols in asthma after a 1-week course of corticosteroid inhalation treatment. *Clin Nucl Med* 20:626-629, 1995.

Pulmonary Scintigraphy at the Bedside in Intensive Care Patients With Suspected Pulmonary Embolism

Jolliet P, Slosman DO, Ricou B, et al (Hôpital Cantonal Universitaire, Geneva; Univ Hosp, Geneva)

Intensive Care Med 21:723–728, 1995 1–27

Purpose.—The feasibility of performing pulmonary scintigraphy (PS) for suspected pulmonary embolism (PE) at the bedside of patients in the ICU was studied retrospectively. This procedure eliminates the risk of transporting patients to the nuclear medicine unit, especially when the patient is experiencing hemodynamic or gas-exchange instability.

Methods.—The files of 45 patients, with an average age of 59.6 years, who were in the ICU for suspected PE, were studied. The PS was performed with a mobile gamma camera at the bedside of patients who were in a supine position. The perfusion tracer was ^{99m}Tc-labeled albumin macroaggregates, and the ventilation tracers were gasified ^{99m}Tc or krypton. The probability of PE was determined according to several criteria (Table 3), such as segmental mismatches on V/Q scans.

Results.—Of the 45 patients studied, 29 were intubated and 21 were in shock. The presence of PE was confirmed (12 patients) or excluded (10 patients) in 49% of the patients by PS. Pulmonary angiography was performed to assess the presence of PE in 4 patients with low, very low, or intermediate probability of PE as predicted by PS. The remaining patients had low clinical and low or very low PS probabilities of PE, and no PE was noted in follow-up examinations of these patients. A drawback of this procedure is that not all incidences of image acquisition can be used.

Conclusions.—The use of a mobile gamma-camera to perform PS at the bedside of patients in the ICU avoids the risk of transporting unstable

TABLE 3.—Type and Result of Pulmonary Scintigraphies Performed in 45 Patients

Procedure	Scintigraphic probability of PE				
	Normal	High	Intermediate	Low	Very Low
V/Q	1*	2*	1	4	1
Q only	9*	10*	0	11	6
Total	10	12	1	15	7

V/Q is ventilation-perfusion scintigraphy; *Q only* is perfusion scintigraphy only.
* Difference = NS between V/Q and Q only for high and normal scans (χ^2 test). (*Intensive Care Med*, Pulmonary scintigraphy at the bedside in intensive care patients with suspected pulmonary embolism, Jolliet P, Slosman DO, Ricou B, et al, vol 21:723–728, table 3, 1995, copyright notice of Springer-Verlag.)

patients and predicts PE with an accuracy comparable to that of PS performed in the nuclear medicine unit.

► This is a very important technique. Intensive care unit patients are susceptible to frequent variability in blood pressure, oxygen saturation, and other parameters. In particularly unstable patients, the point comes when someone considers the diagnosis of PE. It is perfectly reasonable to entertain this thought but it creates a major management problem. Such patients are generally so ill that transporting them to angiography or nuclear medicine is in itself life-threatening. Simply treating is not always an option because some of these patients already are thrombocytopenic or have marginal coagulopathy. Yet the diagnosis of PE, once considered, will not be dismissed without further tests. In this article, a mobile scintigraphic camera allowed the performance of bedside scintigraphy in 45 patients; although it was a small group, accuracy (judged by the subsequent clinical course in most patients) seemed to be good.

B.H. Gross, M.D.

Fe-52 Imaging of Intrathoracic Extramedullary Hematopoiesis in a Patient With β-Thalassemia

Adams BK, Jacobs P, Byrne MJ, et al (Univ of Cape Town, South Africa; Groote Schuur Hosp, South Africa)

Clin Nucl Med 20:619–622, 1995 1–28

Introduction.—β-thalassemia, characterized by the doubly heterozygous state for hemoglobin, is more common in the Far East, and is accompanied by moderate-to-severe hypochromic, microcytic anemia. It can be similar to homozygous β-thalassemia with severe symptomatic anemia, accompanied by hepatosplenomegaly, small stature, and typical skeletal deformities seen with the medullary expansion associated with severe chronic hemolysis and ineffective erythropoiesis. Patients can remain stunted in growth unless they have frequent transfusions.

Methods.—A patient with clinically mild hemoglobin E/β-thalassemia is reported who had an asymptomatic posterior mediastinal mass documented as extramedullary hematopoiesis, which was confirmed with Fe-52 scintigraphy.

> *Case Report.*—Man, 51, with hemoglobin varying between 7 and 9 g/dL required red blood cell transfusions about 3 to 4 times a year. A paravertebral mass was demonstrated in his posterior mediastinum with a chest radiograph. Bilateral extrapleural masses were seen on CT, with the right mass being larger than the left (Fig 2). He underwent radionuclide scintigraphy to diagnose extramedullary hematopoiesis, which was followed by Fe-52 scintigraphy using Fe-52 ferric citrate. No abnormal uptake was revealed in radiocolloid scintigraphy. No uptake in masses was revealed with

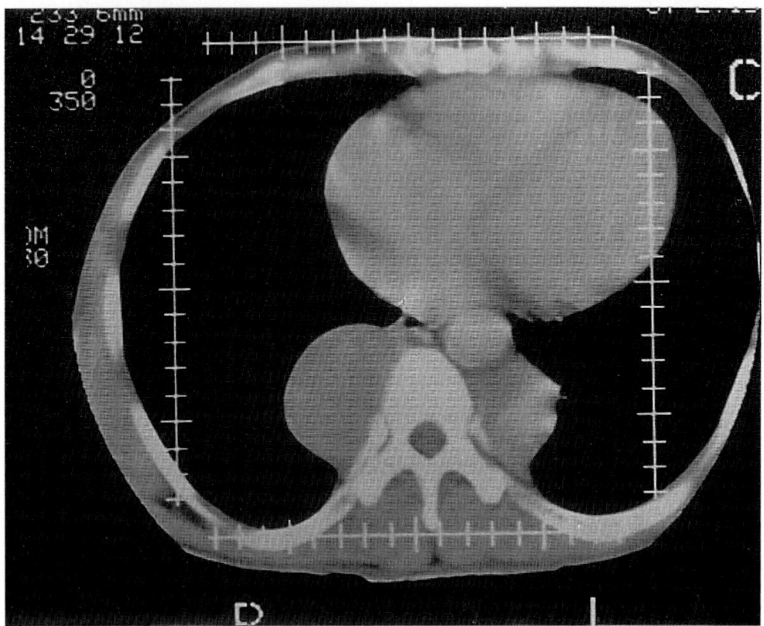

FIGURE 2.—Computed tomography showing bilateral paraspinal masses. (Courtesy of Adams BK, Jacobs P, Byrne MJ, et al: Fe-52 imaging of intrathoracic extramedullary hematopoiesis in a patient with β-thalassemia. *Clin Nucl Med* 20:619–622, 1995.)

In-111 chloride images. However, marked concentration of radioiron in the paraspinal masses was seen with Fe-52 scintigraphy (Fig 6).

Conclusion.—For diagnosing extramedullary hematopoiesis in mass lesions, Fe-52 ferric citrate may be perhaps the only reliable noninvasive

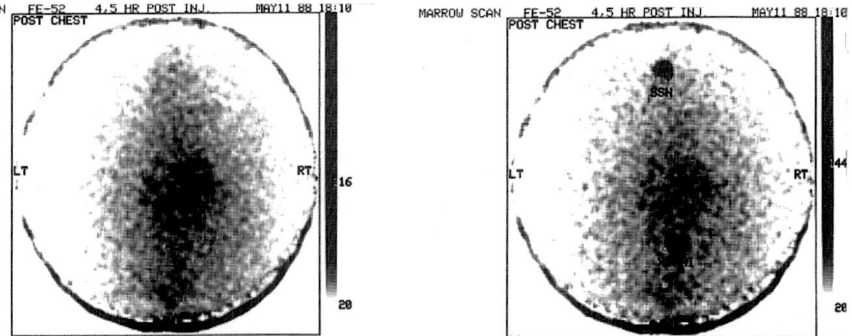

FIGURE 6.—Posterior chest gamma camera image showing accumulation of Fe-52 in paraspinal masses. (Courtesy of Adams BK, Jacobs P, Byrne MJ, et al: Fe-52 imaging of intrathoracic extramedullary hematopoiesis in a patient with β-thalassemia. *Clin Nucl Med* 20:619–622, 1995.)

method. Diagnostically, adequate images were obtained with a standard gamma camera system fitted with a high-energy collimator.

► Extramedullary hematopoiesis is an uncommon disorder seen mainly in oral board examinations and film panels. However, in patients with inherited anemias such as thalassemia, extramedullary hematopoiesis becomes a credible diagnosis. Previously, radionuclide imaging of extramedullary hematopoiesis has relied on colloids (such as sulfur colloid) and on In-111 chloride. However, there have been reports of false negative scan results with these agents, and in the patient reported in this article, they were similarly negative. Fe-52 accumulates in erythropoietically active tissue, and it was able to establish the correct diagnosis noninvasively. It is more easily imaged with positron emission testing, but in this report, a standard gamma camera with a high-energy collimator was an acceptable substitute.

B.H. Gross, M.D.

Topics in Computed Tomography

Excessive Thoracic Computed Tomographic Scanning in Sarcoidosis
Maña J, Teirstein AS, Mendelson DS, et al (Hosp de Bellvitge, Barcelona; Mount Sinai Md Ctr, New York)
Thorax 50:1264–1266, 1995 1–29

Objective.—The frequency and value of CT scanning in the diagnosis and treatment of sarcoidosis were investigated.

Background.—There have been various reports in the past 10 years of the value of CT scanning of the chest in interstitial lung disease, especially sarcoidosis. Better sensitivity for detecting mediastinal adenopathy and parenchymal infiltrations has been described for CT than for standard radiography. Various patterns of abnormalities on CT scans have been suggested in the diagnosis of sarcoidosis, and more and more CT scans are being obtained in patients with presumed sarcoidosis.

Methods.—Chest radiographs from 100 patients with presumed sarcoidosis, and CT scans from 35 of the 100 patients, were reviewed. Sarcoidosis was diagnosed with tissue biopsy. Chest radiographs were categorized by stage of sarcoidosis. Computed tomography scans were compared with clinical data and radiographs to determine if they provided additional useful information.

Results.—In the 35 patients with scans, the CT scans provided no additional useful information compared with chest radiographs. In 2 patients, mediastinal adenopathy was seen on CT scans but not on radiographs. In 2 patients, hilar adenopathy and pulmonary infiltrations were seen on radiographs, but no parenchymal disease was seen on CT scans. One patient had bilateral parenchymal infiltrates that were interpreted as unilateral infiltrates on standard radiographs.

Conclusions.—Computed tomography adds no clinically useful information to the information provided by standard radiographs in the initial assessment of sarcoidosis. However, thoracic high-resolution CT scanning of the thorax is proposed in patients with suspected or proven sarcoidosis when standard chest radiographs are normal or atypical for sarcoidosis; in patients with hemoptysis and proven sarcoidosis; in patients with a suspected second complicating disease; and in patients who are candidates for lung transplantation.

▶ I am often amazed by the requisitions I preview for CT scans. It is depressing to see the thinking that takes place (or more accurately, that doesn't take place) as clinical house officers evaluate patients. The worst such requisitions are for conditions in which it is well known that CT plays no role, such as cholelithiasis. Come to think of it, those are sufficiently uncommon that the worst are really for applications in which CT is almost never helpful, such as chronic abdominal pain! No, I changed my mind, even worse are indications for which CT is seldom helpful and there are better, easier alternatives that are generally ignored, such as large pleural effusion (decubitus views and thoracentesis about cover it, don't they?). Wait, it's even more aggravating when CT might be helpful, but not at the intervals obtained, such as in following up a metastatic tumor only a few weeks after the last scan! I just remembered, what really gets me going is CT for evaluation of a plain film abnormality that is only imagined by the clinician, and the radiologic expert has correctly reported no such abnormality (why didn't you read the report?!?!).

I guess breathing into a paper bag really is helpful. The point is that many requisitions set me off, but it always comes back to this issue: what question are you (the clinician) asking, and how will this test help you to answer it? I've seen several recent requisitions for standard chest CT with a diagnosis of possible sarcoidosis. We never used to scan such patients; experienced pulmonologists evaluated them based on chest radiographs, age, gender, clinical symptoms (or lack thereof), and pulmonary function tests. One patient last week had his second scan in 3 months. It showed bilateral hilar and right paratracheal lymph node enlargement, but so what? The chest radiograph showed the same findings. I asked the medicine resident why he ordered CT, and he replied that he wanted to exclude lymphoma. I want to exclude lymphoma, too, but I don't see how another CT (or even the first CT) will help as much as a good clinical evaluation and possibly a transbronchial biopsy.

The authors of this article apparently have had similar experience in several ways. First, they must be performing more CT in sarcoid patients than in the past (35 of 100 consecutive patients with sarcoid had CT). Second, they are not finding any clinical value—not even in 1 patient did CT alter management. They conclude that CT is not helpful in patients with typical radiologic features of sarcoid, but that it might be useful when the chest radiograph is normal or atypical, when upper airway obstruction is suspected, if there is hemoptysis, if there might be a concurrent illness with sarcoid, or before lung transplantation.

Speaking of lung transplantation, another article this year focused on chest CT as a tool for finding unsuspected lung cancers in the pre–lung-transplant population.[1]

B.H. Gross, M.D.

Reference

1. Kazerooni EA, Chow LC, Whyte RI, et al: Preoperative examination of lung transplant candidates: Value of chest CT compared with chest radiography. *AJR* 165:1343–1348, 1995.

Can CT Distinguish Hypersensitivity Pneumonitis From Idiopathic Pulmonary Fibrosis?

Lynch DA, Newell JD, Logan PM, et al (Univ of Colorado Health Sciences Ctr, Denver; Univ of British Columbia, Vancouver, Canada)
AJR 165:807–811, 1995 1–30

Purpose.—The clinical distinction between idiopathic pulmonary fibrosis (IPF) and hypersensitivity pneumonitis (HP) can be difficult to make. It is important, however, because the management of the 2 conditions is much different. The ability of CT to differentiate between HP and IPF was assessed.

Methods.—The study sample comprised 36 patients with IPF and 27 with HP. In each patient, the diagnosis was established with the help of open lung biopsy. Most of the patients with IPF had usual interstitial pneumonia, although 3 had desquamative interstitial pneumonia. Nineteen of 27 patients with HP had chronic symptoms lasting more than 1 year; the rest had acute or subacute HP. Computed tomography scans from each patient were reviewed in blinded fashion by 2 radiologists. The reviewers made a CT diagnosis by consensus for each patient and recorded their level of diagnostic confidence.

Results.—The recorded level of confidence was high in 62% of patients. Of these cases, the correct diagnosis was made in 90%. The correct CT diagnosis was made in 23 of 26 patients with IPF and 12 of 13 with HP. The 3 patients with desquamative interstitial pneumonitis all received a CT diagnosis of probable or definite HP. Just 7 of 19 patients with chronic HP received a CT diagnosis of definite HP. Three received a diagnosis of definite IPF.

The CT features of honeycombing and peripheral or lower lung zone predominance were more likely to be noted in patients with IPF and usual interstitial pneumonia, whereas micronodules were more likely to be noted in patients with chronic HP. Widespread ground-glass opacity, sometimes indistinguishable from that seen in patients with acute or subacute HP, was noted in patients with IPF and desquamative interstitial pneumonitis (Figs 3–5).

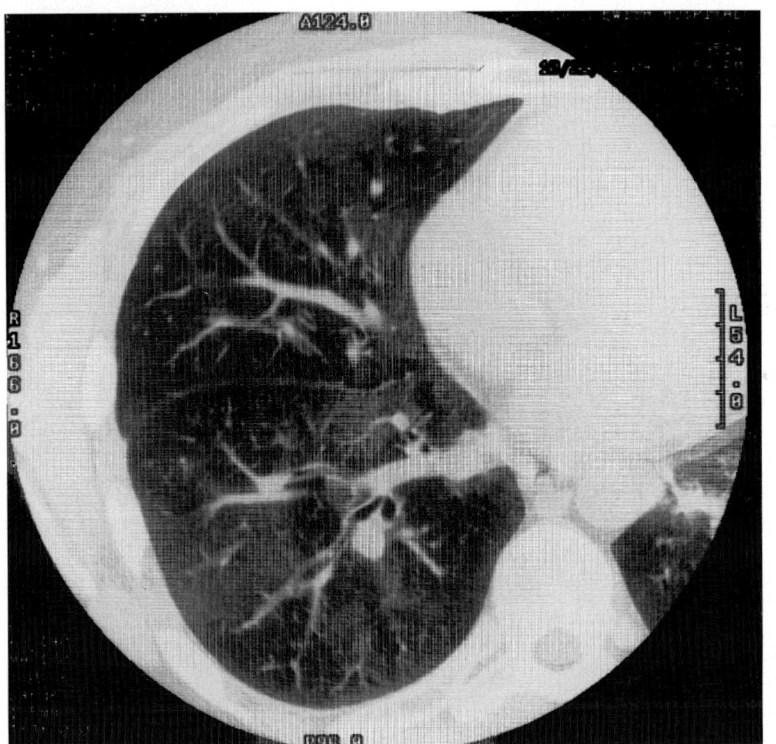

FIGURE 3.—Desquamative interstitial pneumonia. A 28-year-old man with biopsy-proven desquamative interstitial pneumonia. Computed tomography scan shows diffuse ground-glass attenuation. (Courtesy of Lynch DA, Newell JD, Logan PM, et al: Can CT distinguish hypersensitivity pneumonitis from idiopathic pulmonry fibrosis? *AJR* 165:807–811, 1995.)

Conclusions.—In most patients, CT can differentiate between IPF and HP. However, it cannot always tell desquamative interstitial pneumonia from acute or subacute HP, and the CT findings of chronic HP may be identical to those of usual interstitial pneumonia. Thus, lung biopsy is still needed to establish the correct diagnosis in patients with interstitial lung disease.

► Articles about a new radiologic modality tend to follow a well-established cycle. In phase 1, there is initial great enthusiasm about the new modality for diagnosing a potpourri of diseases. In phase 2, the new modality is applied to small groups of patients with specific diseases, still with excellent results. In phase 3, different investigators publish their inability to reproduce the initial glowing results. Phase 4 finds the early investigators retrenching somewhat, with the new modality still far better than its predecessors, but not as good as initially thought. In phase 5, everyone gives up and tries something else. This is a phase-4 article on high-resolution CT.

B.H. Gross, M.D.

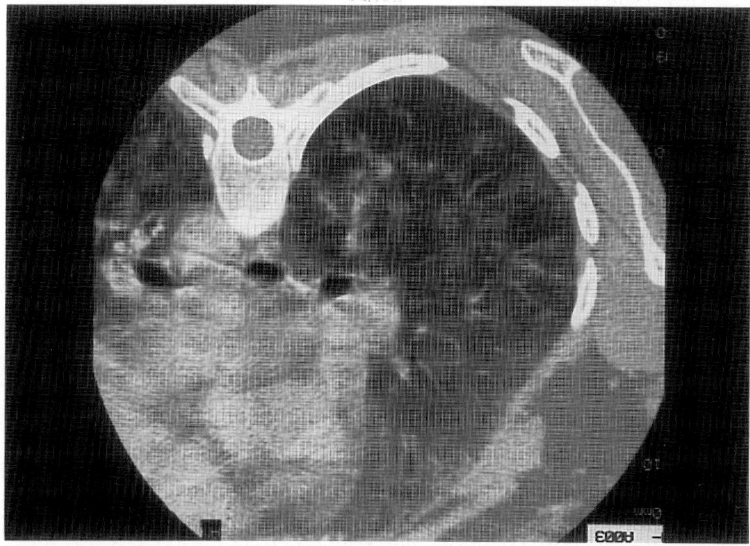

FIGURE 4.—Acute hypersensitivity pneumonitis, identical to desquamative interstitial pneumonia. A 49-year-old woman with biopsy-proven acute hypersensitivity pneumonitis (bird-fancier's lung) was elevated. A CT scan with patient in prone position shows widespread ground-glass attenuation indistinguishable from that seen in desquamative interstitial pneumonia. No micronodules are seen. (Courtesy of Lynch DA, Newell JD, Logan PM, et al: Can CT distinguish hypersensitivity pneumonitis from idiopathic pulmonry fibrosis? *AJR* 165:807–811, 1995.)

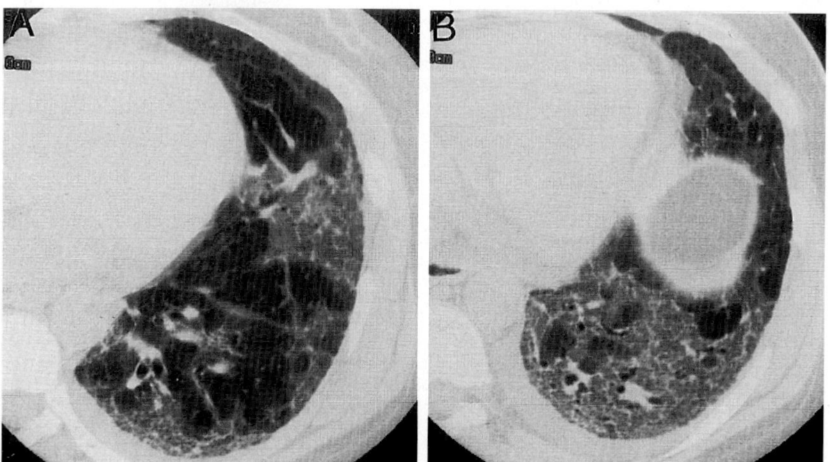

FIGURE 5.—Chronic hypersensitivity pneumonitis, identical to usual interstitial pneumonia. A 48-year-old woman with biopsy-proven chronic hypersensitivity pneumonitis (tobacco-stripper's lung). **A** and **B**, CT scans at 2 levels show patchy basal lung fibrosis with ground-glass attenuation, honeycombing, and traction bronchiectasis, indistinguishable from idiopathic pulmonary fibrosis. (Courtesy of Lynch DA, Newell JD, Logan PM, et al: Can CT distinguish hypersensitivity pneumonitis from idiopathic pulmonary fibrosis? *AJR* 165:807–811, 1995.)

Discrete Lung Involvement in Systemic Lupus Erythematosus: CT Assessment

Bankier AA, Kiener HP, Wiesmayr MN, et al (Univ of Vienna)
Radiology 196:835–840, 1995 1–31

Objective.—In systemic lupus erythematosus (SLE), lung disease is the predominant manifestation of the illness and a primary indicator of overall prognosis. The frequency and nature of early pulmonary manifestations of SLE as seen on CT were evaluated.

Methods.—In a prospective study, 48 patients with serologically confirmed SLE but no previous clinical evidence of lung involvement underwent chest radiography, CT, and spirometry. The CT scans were reviewed for signs of parenchymal and pleural disease, as well as the extent and distribution of disease. The CT scans were correlated with radiographic, clinical, and functional data.

Findings.—Forty-five patients had normal chest radiographs. Of these, 38% had pathologic findings at CT, including interlobular septal thickening in 33%, intralobular interstitial thickening in 33%, air-space nodules in 22%, architectural distortion in 22%, bronchial wall thickening in 20%, bronchial dilatation in 18%, pleural irregularities in 13%, ground-glass attenuation in 13%, and air-space consolidation in 7% (Fig 4).

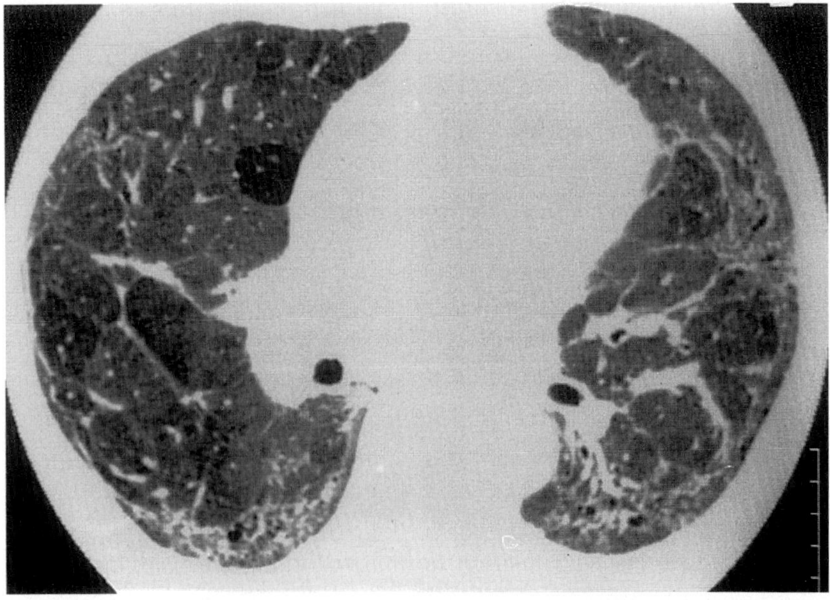

FIGURE 4.—A CT scan obtained at the level of the lower lobes depicts extensive parenchymal involvement with honeycombing, areas of ground-glass attenuation, traction bronchiectasis, bronchial wall thickening, and architectural distortion. Prospectively, the chest radiograph in this patient was interpreted as normal; retrospectively, however, subtle abnormalities could be detected in both lower lobes. (Courtesy of Bankier AA, Kiener HP, Wiesmayr MN, et al: Discrete lung involvement in systemic lupus erythematosus: CT assessment. *Radiology* 196:835–840, 1995. Radiological Society of North America.)

Despite the relatively short clinical duration of SLE (mean, 28.3 months), interlobular septal and intralobular interstitial thickening combined with architectural distortion that resulted in traction bronchiectasis and pleural irregularities developed in one third of the patients. The extent of the disease seen with CT correlated significantly with the duration of clinical history, ratio of forced expiratory volume in 1 second to forced vital capacity, and decreased single-breath diffusing capacity for carbon monoxide.

Conclusions.—A relatively high percentage of pathologic findings at CT occur in patients with SLE with normal chest radiographs. Although the changes in lung parenchyma on CT scans are discrete, they correlate significantly with the duration of clinical history and functional impairment. Furthermore, the early occurrence of fibrotic and, thus, irreversible parenchymal changes, emphasizes the importance of early CT, even in patients with no clinical symptoms and normal chest radiographs. These findings suggest that CT is superior to radiography for the depiction of functionally relevant pulmonary disease and is an important adjunct in the early assessment of SLE.

High-Resolution Chest CT in Systemic Lupus Erythematosus

Fenlon HM, Doran M, Sant SM, et al (Mater Misericordiae Hosp, Dublin)

AJR 166:301–307, 1996 1–32

Introduction.—The reported incidence of pulmonary and pleural involvement in patients with systemic lupus erthythematosus (SLE) ranges from 7% to 100%. Thoracic involvement in patients with SLE has typically been detected with clinical findings, chest radiography, pulmonary function testing, and lung biopsy. High-resolution CT (HRCT) findings in 34 patients with SLE are reported and correlated with clinical and diagnostic evaluations.

Methods.—The mean age of 32 women and 2 men was 41 years. Eleven patients were current smokers, 4 were exsmokers, and 19 never smoked. Twenty-six patients had no respiratory symptoms and 6 complained of dyspnea on exertion. Five patients had abnormal chest examination findings. At disease onset, 3 patients had pulmonary involvement. Respiratory symptoms developed in 1 patient 6 years after SLE was diagnosed. All patients underwent chest radiography on the same days as the CT examination. Pulmonary function studies were completed within 48 hours of imaging. Chest radiographs and CT examinations were read by 2 radiologists, who had no knowledge of the clinical or functional status of the patients.

Results.—Abnormalities were detected in 24 HRCT examinations, compared with 8 in chest radiographs. It was determined by HRCT that 11 patients had interstitial lung disease. Of these 11 patients, 7 had no abnormal radiographic findings. Two patients with normal radiographs had ground glass opacification on HRCT. Bronchiectasis was observed in

7 HRCT and 1 radiograph examinations. Other HRCT findings included 7 minor interstitial abnormalities that were considered neither severe nor extensive enough to justify a diagnosis of interstitial lung disease, 6 mediastinal or axillary lymphadenopathy, and 5 pleuropericardial disease. Abnormal pulmonary function test findings were 6 restrictive pattern, 3 obstructive physiology, and 4 isolated reduction in a gas transfer measurement (DLCO). Normal pulmonary function test findings were determined in 4 of 11 patients with interstitial lung disease and in all 7 patients with bronchiectasis on HRCT. There was no correlation between disease activity, disease duration, chest symptoms, drug treatments, or smoking history and the presence of abnormal pulmonary physiology.

Conclusion.—This investigation is the first to address HRCT findings in SLE. Pleural abnormalities were less common than previously reported. Airway disease, lymphadenopathy, and interstitial lung disease were common HRCT findings. Findings of interstitial lung disease were definitive on HRCT in 21% of patients, despite normal chest radiographs and uncertain pulmonary function results. Patients with SLE with equivocal clinical, pulmonary function, or chest radiographic findings should be offered HRCT.

▶ As I pointed out in an earlier comment, I once considered myself a budding rheumatologist; fascinating diseases like lupus sparked my interest. I was taught that chronic lung disease almost never occurred in SLE; instead, I was told that such patients usually had no lung abnormality or else had a fleeting airspace disease that represented either lupus pneumonitis or pulmonary hemorrhage. The rheumatologists use a great example of circular reasoning to ensure that this holds true. They call it "mixed connective tissue disease" (MCTD) if a rheumatologic disease includes unexpected manifestations; therefore, lupus with chronic lung disease gets the MCTD label.

Although I have used these pages for years to rail against HRCT, I have to admit that it sometimes (?10%) reveals abnormalities that were utterly unsuspected on plain radiographs. These 2 articles include 79 patients with SLE, 41 of whom had HRCT abnormality. In the series by Bankier et al., all 45 patients had normal chest radiographs, but 17 had HRCT abnormalities; in the series by Fenlon et al., 8 of 34 patients had abnormal chest radiographs, but 24 had abnormal HRCT.

This requires a major change in our preconceptions. It isn't just that chronic lung disease may occur in SLE; in the words of Fenlon et al. "... airways disease, lymphadenopathy, and interstitial lung disease are common thoracic manifestations of SLE." In the article by Bankier et al., HRCT abnormality was significantly correlated with pulmonary function test abnormalities, but in the article by Fenlon et al., pulmonary function tests were abnormal in only 14 patients (again, 24 had abnormal HRCT). Thus, 3 conclusions:

1. This may still partly be a definitional problem, inasmuch as the diagnosis of SLE is a clinical one and since there may be confusion with MCTD.

2. There is no gold standard for evaluating HRCT abnormalities; we don't really know if some of these cases aren't HRCT false positive results or else unrelated abnormalities.
3. Still and all, chronic lung disease in SLE is probably far more common than previously suspected.

Another HRCT study this year correlated preoperative HRCT assessment of bronchiectasis with the pathologic findings in subsequently resected specimens.[1]

B.H. Gross, M.D.

Reference

1. Kang EY, Müller RR, Müller NL: Bronchiectasis: Comparison of preoperative thin-section CT and pathologic findings in resected specimens. *Radiology* 195:649–654, 1995.

CT Reconstruction Algorithm Selection in the Evaluation of Solitary Pulmonary Nodules

Swensen SJ, Morin RL, Aughenbaugh GL, et al (Mayo Clinic and Mayo Found, Rochester, Minn; Mayo Clinic Jacksonville, Fla)

J Comput Assist Tomogr 19:932–935, 1995 1–33

Introduction.—Computed tomography reconstruction artifacts can lead to image misinterpretation. There is particular concern with the use of high–spatial-frequency reconstruction algorithms and the occasional resultant false positive diagnosis of calcification (Figs 1 and 2). The various effects of several reconstruction algorithms are reviewed by using 4 different scanners.

Methods.—Standardized Computerized Imaging Reference Systems 6- and 10-mm phantoms were scanned using high–spatial-frequency, smoothing, and intermediate reconstruction algorithms. The mean pixel value of the cylinders was computed for the 3 reconstruction algorithms. The scanners were the GE 9800 Quick, U C-100, GE HiSpeed Advantage, and Picker 1200 SX. Uncalcified lung nodules, ranging in size from 8 to 16 mm in diameter, were also imaged in 8 patients. All nodules were resected and subjected to histologic examination.

Results.—Peripheral edge enhancement artifact was observed on phantom cylinders of some CT images. These findings were most marked on the 6-mm cylinder. None of the 8 lung nodules showed histologic evidence of calcification. Seven malignancies were classified: 3 adenocarcinomas, 2 squamous cell carcinomas, 1 bronchioloalveolar carcinoma, and 1 metastatic melanoma. One nodule was a granuloma. Peripheral calcification was not observed in any nodules with CT edge enhancement artifact. With the use of high–spatial-frequency algorithms, the nodule images with edge enhancement artifact were acquired using the Picker 1200 SX and GE HiSpeed Advantage, but not the GE 9800 Quick or the C-100 scanners.

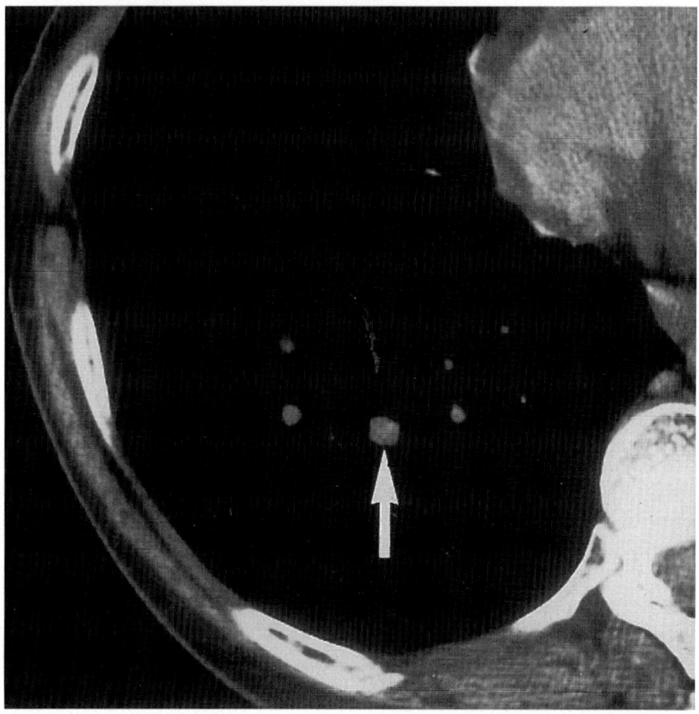

FIGURE 1.—Computed tomography scan (Picker 1200 SX, 2mm collimation, smooth reconstruction algorithm 3) of 69-year-old woman with a metastatic melanoma nodule (*arrow*). (Courtesy of Swensen SJ, Morin RL, Aughenbaugh GL, et al: CT reconstruction algorithm selection in the evaluation of solitary pulmonary nodules. *J Comput Assist Tomogr* 19:932–935, 1995.)

Conclusion.—Care must be used in the evaluation of pulmonary nodule attenuation using high–spatial-frequency reconstruction algorithms. There is potential for an erroneous diagnosis of calcification with edge enhancement artifact.

► The Mayo group made several more contributions to the important literature on CT evaluation of the solitary pulmonary nodule (SPN). Their recent promising work[1] suggests that evaluation of lesion enhancement may play an important role in separating benign and malignant nodules, but first we will generally look for nodule calcification. In any noninvasive evaluation of the SPN we must avoid falsely benign diagnoses at all costs; a falsely indeterminate diagnosis means that the work-up will proceed as though that test had not been invented, but a falsely benign diagnosis stops the work-up, and probably leads to a worse outcome when the error is subsequently discovered. Thus, the artifact of false positive nodule calcification that occurs with high–spatial-frequency reconstruction algorithms is dangerous. Please note that this is an edge-enhancement artifact; the false positive calcification is peripheral, not central.

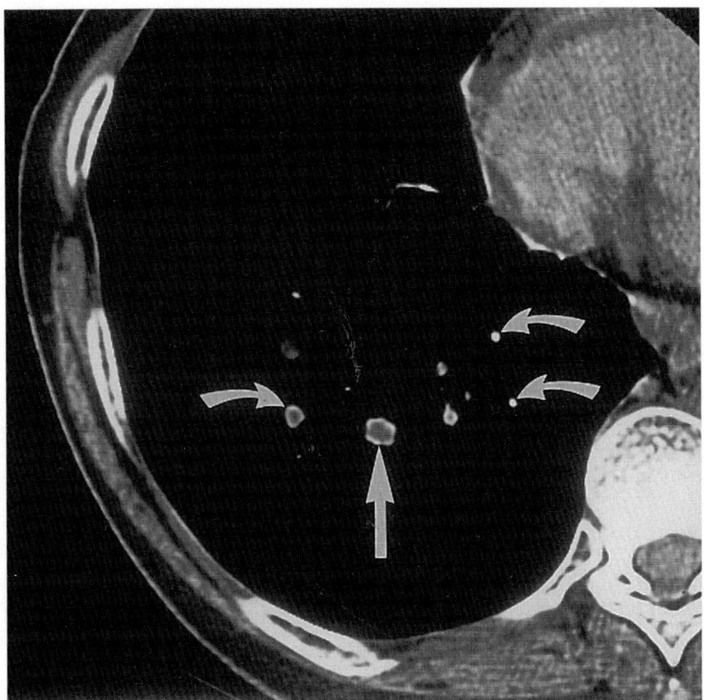

FIGURE 2.—Retrospectively constructed image (sharp reconstruction algorithm 1) of the scan from Fig 1 shows an edge-enhancement artifact of the nodule (*straight arrow*) and pulmonary vessels (*curved arrows*). Note that small vessels and the periphery of the nodule appear calcified on this non–contrast-enhanced image. (Courtesy of Swensen SJ, Morin RL, Aughenbaugh GL, et al: CT reconstruction algorithm selection in the evaluation of solitary pulmonary nodules. *J Comput Assist Tomogr* 19:932–935, 1995.)

Another Mayo contribution was Steve Swensen's collaboration with Jud Gurney on neural network analysis in determining the likelihood of malignancy in SPNs.[2] This continues Jud's previous work on Bayesian analysis in determining the same likelihood.[3, 4] Detection of pulmonary nodules was also addressed this year in an article on spiral CT.[5] Vascular segmentation and extraction resulted in improved nodule detection. Finally, the role of percutaneous biopsy of SPNs vs. thoracoscopic biopsy was studied.[6] The authors found that CT-guided biopsy was accurate when a malignant or specific benign diagnosis was obtained. However, 32 of 47 patients with nonspecific benign diagnoses were found to have malignant lesions. The authors suggest that CT-guided biopsy be reserved for unresectable lesions and for highly suspicious nodules in patients with severe physiologic impairment.

B.H. Gross, M.D.

References

1. Swensen SJ, Brown LR, Colby TV, et al: Pulmonary nodules: CT evaluation of enhancement with iodinated contrast material. *Radiology* 194:393–398, 1995.

2. Gurney JW, Swensen SJ: Solitary pulmonary nodules: Determining the likelihood of malignancy with neural network analysis. *Radiology* 196:823–829, 1995.
3. Gurney JW: Determining the likelihood of malignancy in solitary pulmonary nodules with Bayesian analysis. I. Theory. *Radiology* 186:405–412, 1993.
4. Gurney JW, Lyddon DM, McKay JA: Determining the likelihood of malignancy in solitary pulmonary nodules with Bayesian analysis. II. Application. *Radiology* 186:415–422, 1993.
5. Croisille P, Souto M, Cova M, et al: Pulmonary nodules: Improved detection with vascular segmentation and extraction with spiral CT. Work in progress. *Radiology* 197:397–401, 1995.
6. Mitruka S, Landreneau RJ, Mack MJ, et al: Diagnosing the indeterminate pulmonary nodule: Percutaneous biopsy versus thoracoscopy. *Surgery* 118:676–684, 1995.

Traumatic Chest Lesions in Patients With Severe Head Trauma: A Comparative Study With Computed Tomography and Conventional Chest Roentgenograms

Karaaslan T, Meuli R, Androux R, et al (Univ Hosp, Lausanne, Switzerland)
J Trauma: Injury Infect Crit Care 39:1081–1086, 1995 1–34

Introduction.—Computed tomographic scanning has been accepted as the standard diagnostic examination in evaluating craniocerebral injuries. Conventional supine chest radiographs are usually used in the identification of associated thoracic injuries in these patients. Pulmonary and mediastinal traumatic lesions, particularly pneumothorax, could alter management in those patients who need continuous positive-pressure breathing. Limited CT examination of the chest was performed in 47 consecutive patients with severe craniocerebral trauma on mechanical ventilation support to prospectively evaluate the incidence of overlooked or underestimated traumatic pulmonary or mediastinal lesions with conventional chest radiography and the utility of a limited CT examination.

Methods.—The mean age of 38 males and 9 females was 35 years. Supine chest radiography with transportable apparatus was performed on all patients upon admission. Immediately after head CT, a limited chest CT scan was performed. Four blinded radiologists read radiographic and CT examinations in 2 separate sessions.

Results.—Nine of 47 patients had a pneumothorax; this lesion was bilateral in 1 patient. Six pneumothoraces were identified on chest radiography and CT. In 4 patients, the lesion was only detectable on CT. Thirty-one areas of pulmonary parenchymal contusions were observed in 19 patients with CT. With conventional radiography, 17 areas were identified in 11 patients. Clinical management was not altered in any patients with pulmonary parenchymal contusions. Mediastinal injury was not suspected on conventional chest radiography (Fig 3, A) in 1 patient with minor cerebral frontal lobe contusion. However, limited CT examination (Fig 3, B) showed mediastinal hemorrhage and a traumatic rupture at the origin of the descending thoracic aorta. Findings of aortic rupture were confirmed with angiography (Fig 3, C) and surgery. There was a high

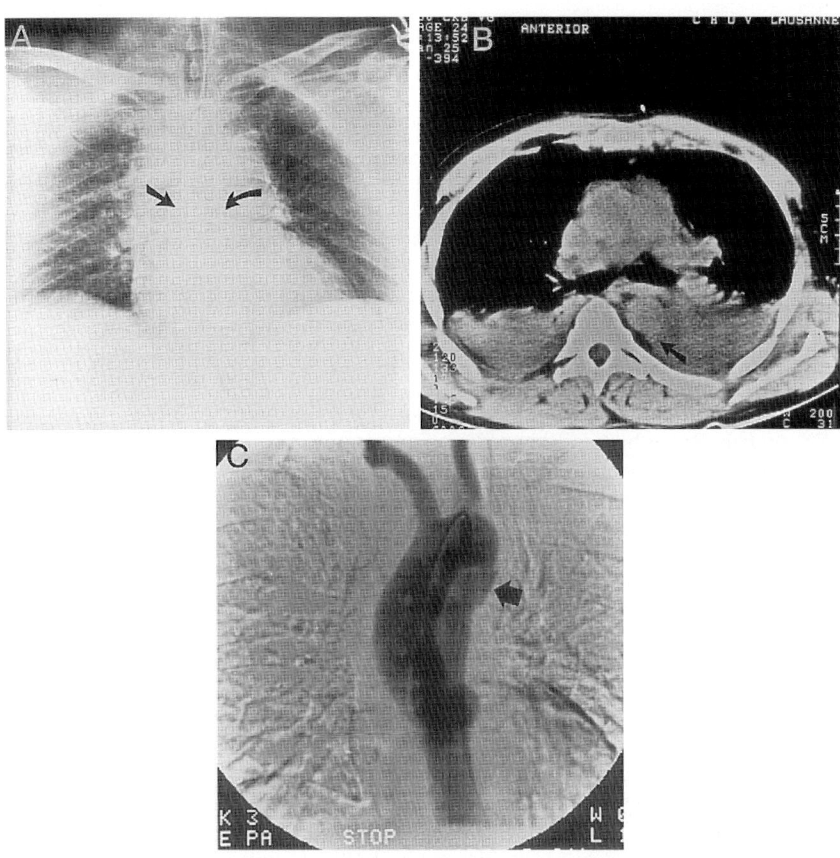

FIGURE 3.—**A**, initial supine conventional chest roentgenogram of a male victim of a motor vehicle crash. On this underexposed roentgenogram taken at the emergency department, it is difficult to evaluate the mediastinum. Note the discrete right deviation of the nasogastric tube (*straight arrows*) and slight depression of the left main bronchus (*curved arrows*). **B**, limited, unenhanced CT study showed an irregularity of the posterior wall of proximal descending thoracic aorta (*arrow*), suggesting rupture, **C**, because the limited CT study strongly suggested aortic rupture, angiography was performed. Diagnosis was confirmed (*arrow*) and repaired surgically. (Courtesy of Karaaslan T, Meuli R, Androux R, et al: Traumatic chest lesions in patients with severe head trauma: A comparative study with computed tomography and conventional chest roentgenograms. *J Trauma: Injury Infect Crit Care* 39:1081–1086, 1995.)

suspicion of right diaphragmatic rupture on chest radiography in 1 patient, confirmed with CT examination and surgically repaired. Limited CT examinations supplied additional information in 14 patients (30%) that was not detected on a conventional chest radiograph. The added information was significant enough in 6 patients (12.7%) to alter management.

Conclusion.—A limited chest CT examination allows a more precise evaluation of the mediastinum and pulmonary lesions, particularly pneumothorax, compared with conventional chest radiography. In this cohort, CT findings altered clinical management in 12.7% of patients. Computed tomography is useful in confirming or showing diaphragmatic ruptures that are suspected or overlooked on conventional radiography, but it is not the method of choice for the diagnosis of this serious lesion.

▶ I'll go along with the authors' premise that thoracic traumatic lesions may be associated with severe craniocerebral trauma. I'll agree that the detection of thoracic trauma is important because the patients may require positive-pressure ventilation. I'll accept that CT proved superior in detection of pneumothoraces and parenchymal contusions. But I advise caution when they add that they detected an aortic laceration. Their limited chest CT technique used noncontrast 1-cm-thick sections at 3-cm intervals. I don't want anyone to believe that this is a valid screening tool for aortic injury.

B.H. Gross, M.D.

CT of the Bronchus Intermedius: Frequency and Cause of a Nodule in the Posterior Wall on Normal Scans

Kim JS, Choi D, Lee KS (Samsung Med Ctr, Seoul, Korea)

AJR 165:1349–1352, 1995 1–35

Introduction.—A focal nodule in the posterior wall of the bronchus intermedius (PWBI) or a round elevation occupying part of the posterior wall is an occasional finding on normal chest CT scans. Some reports suggest that this nodularity is caused by a branch of the draining vein from the posterior segment of the right upper lobe that passes in close contact with the PWBI and drains into the right inferior pulmonary vein. Helical CT scans of 280 consecutive patients were prospectively analyzed to evaluate the frequency of nodularity in the posterior wall of the bronchus intermedius.

Methods.—Parameters for the helical CT scans were 10-mm collimation, 10-mm/sec table speed, 120 kVp, and 250 mA. The scans were taken from the level of the distal trachea to the level of the inferior pulmonary vein. The presence or absence of nodularity was determined by agreement of 2 chest radiologists.

Results.—By using 10-mm collimation CT scans, nodularity was observed in 14 of 280 patients. Nodularity was observed in 10 men and 4 women with a mean age of 49 years. Using narrower collimation (1- to 5-mm) CT scans, the draining pulmonary vein was found to be the cause of nodularity in the PWBI in all 14 patients. In 10 of 14 patients, this vein originated from a branch of the vein from the posterior segment of the right upper lobe (Fig 2). It originated from a branch of the vein in the superior segment of the right lower lobe in the remaining 4 patients. The vein from the upper lobe that caused nodularity in the posterior wall of the bronchus intermedius drained into the inferior pulmonary vein in 7 of 10 patients and into the superior pulmonary vein in 3 of 10 patients. The vein drained into the inferior pulmonary vein in all patients whose nodularity was caused by the vein from the superior segment of the right lower lobe.

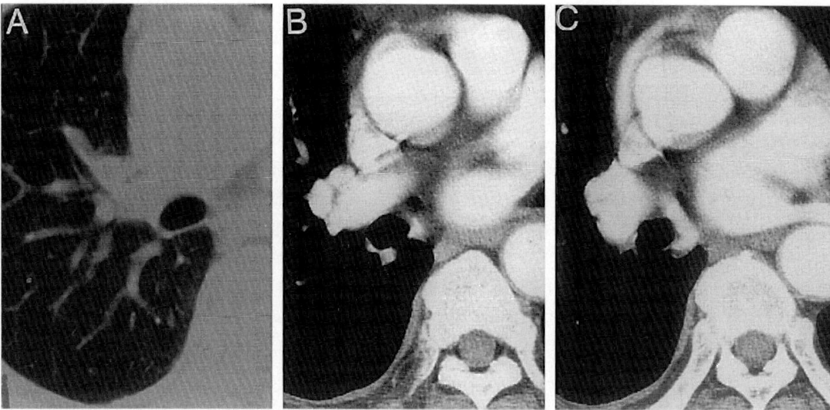

FIGURE 2.—Normal nodularity in posterior wall of bronchus intermedius caused by draining vein in 67-year-old man in whom CT scans were performed for suspicion of pulmonary metastases. **A**, CT scan (5-mm collimation) obtained at subcranial level shows posterior segmental vein in right upper lobe of lung (*arrow*), located lateral to bronchus intermedius. Right major fissure was located posterior to vein (not shown). **B**, mediastinal window of enhanced CT scan obtained 10 mm caudal to **A** shows vein (*arrow*) causing nodularity in posterior wall of bronchus intermedius. **C**, CT scan obtained 5 mm caudal to **B** shows vein (*arrow*) draining into superior pulmonary vein. Vein still causes nodularity behind posteromedial wall of bronchus intermedius. (Courtesy of Kim JS, Choi D, Lee KS: CT of the bronchus intermedius: Frequency and cause of a nodule in the posterior wall on normal scans. *AJR* 165:1349–1352, 1995.)

Conclusion.—In normal chest CT scans, focal nodularity caused by a draining pulmonary vein can be observed occasionally. This normal nodularity needs to be differentiated from uniform or lobulated irregular thickening associated with an abnormality in the bronchus intermedius.

► I suppose I should be embarrassed by this article. I teach residents that the back wall of the bronchus intermedius should be thin and smooth on CT. It would be bad enough to have noticed this variant and simply to have been uncertain of its etiology. But to tell the truth, I haven't noticed it before! I am fond of teaching residents the general principle of being unable to see the forest for the trees at chest radiography by constantly telling them that they are too close to the radiograph to see the abnormality. (I'll sometimes repeat this litany until the resident gets up and crosses the room.) Maybe as a result I'm too far from the CT image ...

Another CT vascular application is to the diagnosis of pulmonary emboli. Two-dimensional multiplanar reformations improved the ability of helical CT to exclude central pulmonary emboli.[1]

B.H. Gross, M.D.

Reference

1. Remy-Jardin M, Remy J, Cauvain O, et al: Diagnosis of central pulmonary embolism with helical CT: Role of two-dimensional multiplanar reformations. *AJR* 165:1131–1138, 1995.

Uncommon Pneumoconioses: CT and Pathologic Findings

Akira M (Natl Kinki Chuo Hosp, Osaka, Japan)
Radiology 197:403–409, 1995 1–36

Purpose.—Computed tomography scans obtained in patients with a history of occupational exposure to dust were reviewed retrospectively to correlate the CT features of pneumoconioses with histologic findings.

Methods.—Thin-section CT scans were obtained in 48 male patients (21 arc welders, and 19 graphite, 6 aluminum, and 2 hard metal workers) with an average age of 59 years and a history of an average of 20.3 years of occupational exposure to dust. The scans were assessed for the presence or absence of various features of pneumoconioses. Histologic material from 22 patients was assessed for the presence of pneumoconioses.

Results.—In arc welders, the most prominent radiographic (Fig 1, A) and CT (Fig 1, B) findings were ill-defined micronodules. Other CT features in the arc welders were emphysema, decreased attenuation, honeycombing, reticulation, pleural irregularity, bronchiectasis, and conglom-

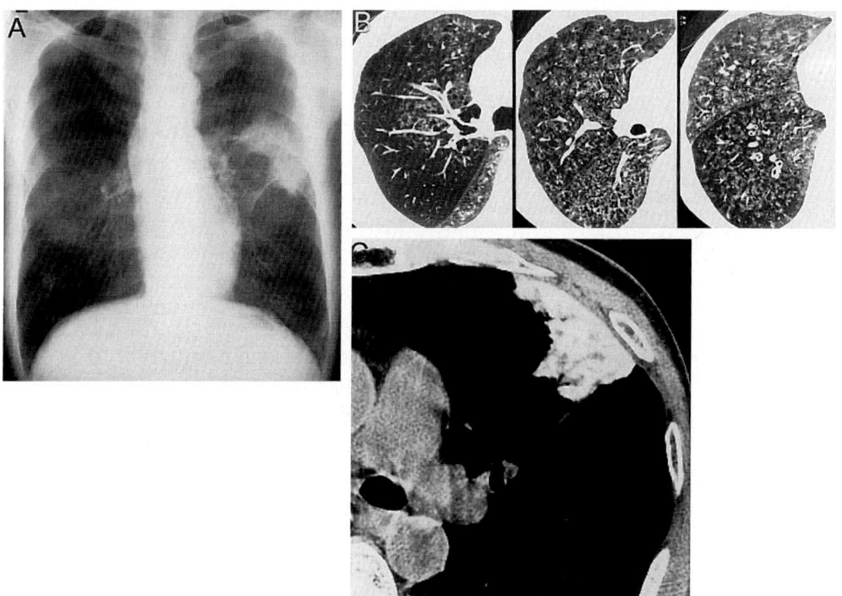

FIGURE 1.—Images were obtained in a 60-year-old man employed as an arc welder for 30 years, who had never smoked. **A**, chest radiograph reveals ill-defined micronodules, most prominent in the middle third of each lung about the hilar regions. Hyperlucency is seen in the right upper and right lower lung zone. Irregularly shaped mass lesion is found in the left middle lung zone. **B**, thin-section CT scans show numerous ill-defined micronodules concentrated in the centrilobular regions (*arrows*). In more affected lung, gathering of micronodules and fine branching areas of increased attenuation create a fine network pattern. Focal decreased attenuation is found in the peripheral half of the right upper lobe. C, when viewed at mediastinal windows (level, 35 HU; width, 400 HU), the pulmonary and peripheral mass in the left middle lung zone is seen to contain high-attenuation material. (Hematoxylin-eosin stain; original magnification ×64.) (Courtesy of Akira M: Uncommon pneumoconioses: CT and pathologic findings. *Radiology* 197:403–409, 1995. Radiological Society of North America.)

erate masses with areas of high attenuation (Fig 1, C). The pathologic specimens from 6 of the 21 arc welders showed marked interstitial accumulation of opaque particles in the perivascular and peribronchiolar regions. In graphite workers, the most prominent radiographic (Fig 2, A) and CT (Fig 2, B) features were small nodular hyperattenuating areas, interlobular septal thickening, and prevalence of large hyperattenuated

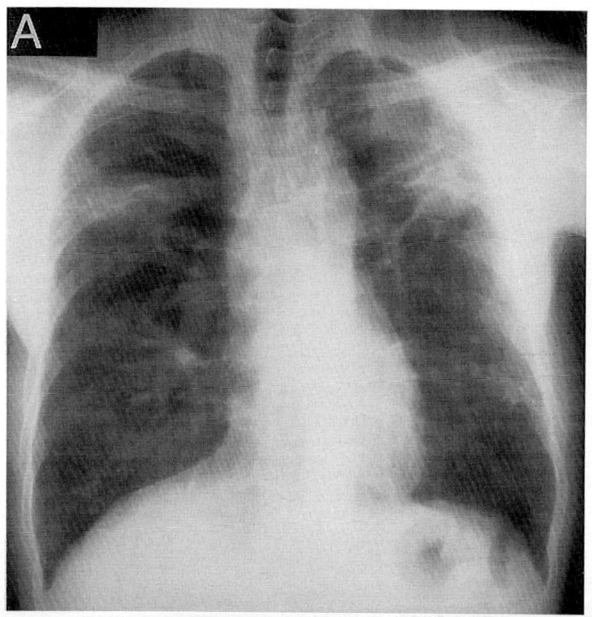

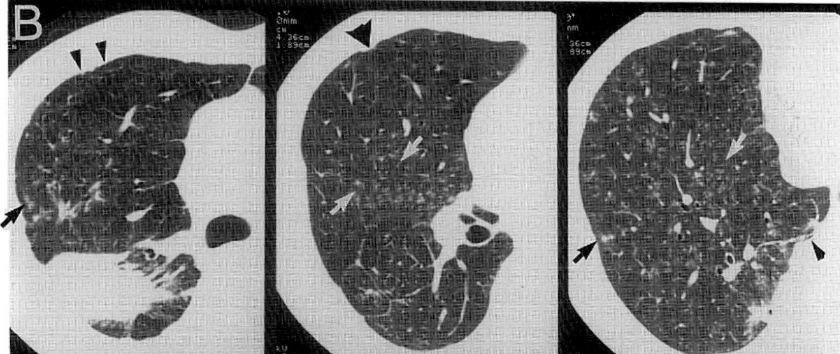

FIGURE 2.—A, images were obtained in a 53-year-old man employed in the graphite industry for 12 years. Chest radiograph in **A** reveals areas of hyperattenuation in upper zones and disseminated small nodules. Thin section CT scans in **B** show small nodular areas of hyperattenuation, interlobular septal thickening, and conglomerate masses. Note 2 types of small nodules: ill-defined tiny areas of hyperattenuation (some of which appear as fine branching areas of increased attenuation or clusters of a few dots [*white arrows*]) and well-defined small nodules (*black arrows*). Some subpleural nodules (*small arrowhead on left*) and confluent subpleural nodules or pseudoplaque (*arrowhead in middle and at right*) are also seen. (Courtesy of Akira M: Uncommon pneumoconioses: CT and pathologic findings. *Radiology* 197:403–409, 1995. Radiological Society of North America.)

areas. Correlation of these findings with pathologic specimens from 12 of the 19 graphite workers showed correspondences between ill-defined hyperattenuated areas and macular lesions along the walls of the bronchioles and between discrete nodules and larger macular or nodular lesions. Reticulonodular opacity was evident in the chest radiographs of aluminum workers (Fig 3, A). The CT scans revealed reticular, nodular, and upper lobe fibrosis, and honeycombing (Fig 3, B). Lung biopsies from 2 alumi-

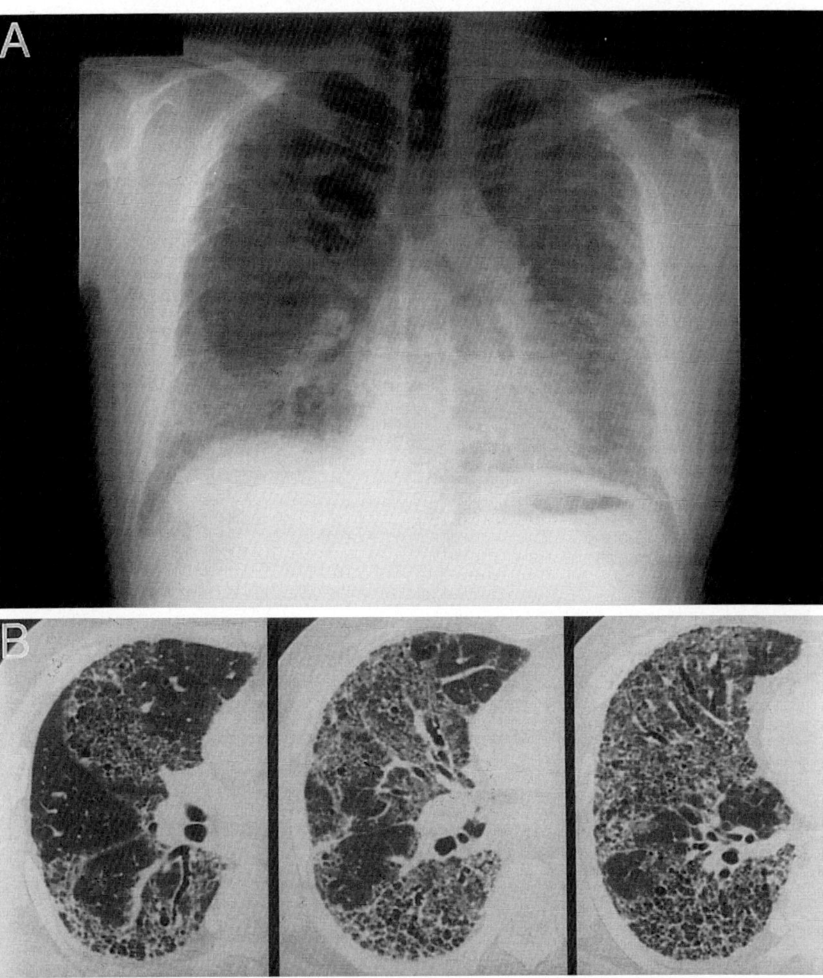

FIGURE 3.—**A**, images were obtained in a 52-year-old man with a history of exposure to aluminum for 7 years. Chest radiograph in **A** reveals reticulonodular opacity, predominantly distributed in the lower lung zones. Thin-section CT scans in **B** show diffusely distributed reticular hyperattenuation. Honeycomb formation is seen. In the intralobular interstitial thickening, dilated air bronchiolograms are present. The thin-section CT appearance is similar to that of idiopathic pulmonary fibrosis. However, unlike findings in idiopathic pulmonary fibrosis, the lesions are marked in both the central and peripheral portions. (Courtesy of Akira M: Uncommon pneumoconioses: CT and pathologic findings. *Radiology* 197:403–409, 1995. Radiological Society of North America.)

num workers showed interstitial fibrosis with honeycombing. Coarse reticular opacity was also noted in the chest radiographs of hard metal workers (Fig 4, A). Thin-section CT scans in these patients showed bilateral air space consolidations and ground-glass attenuation (Fig 4, B). Histologic specimens from 2 hard metal workers showed interstitial pneumonia and fibrosis with unusual multinucleate giant cells.

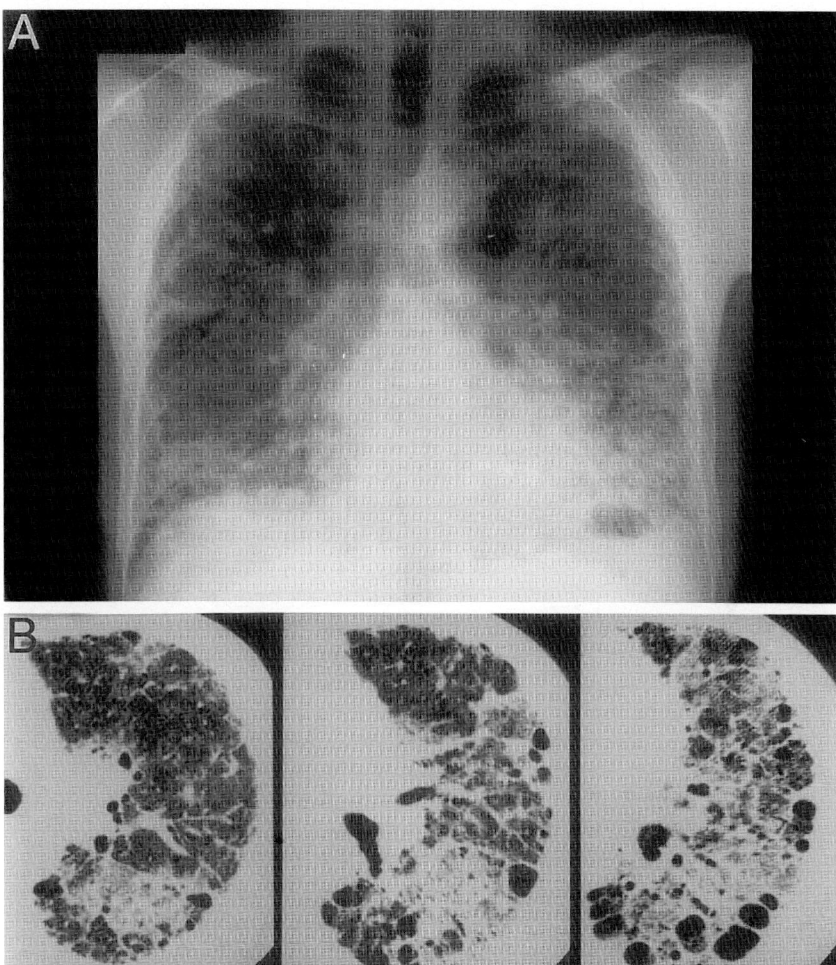

FIGURE 4.—**A**, images were obtained in a 45-year-old man with a history of exposure to hard metal for 5 years. Chest radiograph in **A** reveals coarse reticular opacity with peripheral patchy areas of dense opacity, predominantly in the lower lung zones. Thin-section CT scans in **B** show air space consolidation and ground-glass attenuation with traction bronchiectasis and dilated air bronchiolograms, predominantly distributed in the lower lung zones. Multiple bullae are seen. Small branching areas of increased attenuation are present to some degree, corresponding to peribronchiolar fibrosis histologically (*arrows*). (Courtesy of Akira M: Uncommon pneumoconioses: CT and pathologic findings. *Radiology* 197:403–409, 1995. Radiological Society of North America.)

Conclusions.—Thin-section CT features of pneumoconioses are characteristic and reflect underlying pathologic findings for each type of pneumoconiosis.

► This article serves as an important high-resolution reference tool for patients with uncommon pneumoconioses. The CT features found in arc welders, graphite workers, aluminum workers, and hard metal workers are catalogued and illustrated. Distinctive features are emphasized.

B.H. Gross, M.D.

Recent Advances in Diagnosis and Therapy

Reduction Pneumonoplasty for Emphysema: Early Results

Little AG, Swain JA, Nino JJ, et al (Univ of Nevada, Las Vegas)

Ann Surg 222:365–374, 1995 1–37

Background.—There is new interest in the use of surgical treatment for patients with diffuse, bullous emphysema. Thirty years ago, Brantigan suggested that excising "localized emphysematous areas" could be of benefit. More recent studies have found that lung reduction surgery can improve symptomatic breathlessness and pulmonary function measures in selected patients with emphysema. A minimally invasive approach could enhance the clinical results of such operations while reducing surgical morbidity. The results of neodymium:yttrium aluminum garnet (Nd:YAG) laser reduction pneumonoplasty for selected patients with diffuse emphysema are reported.

Methods.—The study group consisted of 55 patients with advanced symptomatic emphysema. All underwent unilateral Nd:YAG laser reduction pneumonoplasty to reduce lung volume. Patients selected for the operation had CT scans showing large spaces, or "black holes" between vascular markings, which represented the localized emphysematous areas in which bullous disease is found. The operation was performed under thoracoscopic vision. Patients with major adhesions received a lung-shaving approach via median sternotomy during the same anesthesia. Radiation was applied to the lung surface with a Laser Sonics G56 YAG laser fiber by free-beam technique. After laser treatment, talcum powder was

TABLE 4.—Pulmonary Function Analysis

	FEV_1 (n = 28) (L)	FVC (n = 28) (L)	DLCO (n = 10) (mL/min/mmHg)	Po_2 (n = 22) (mmHg)
Before operation	0.74 ± 0.07	1.82 ± 0.13	10.3 ± 2.3	59.3 ± 1.7
After operation	0.85 ± 0.06	2.21 ± 0.15	13.7 ± 2.4	63.3 ± 2.3
% Change	18.1 ± 5.5	29.6 ± 7.9	42.3 ± 18.6	11.3 ± 1.1
p Value	0.009	0.003	0.005	0.036

(Courtesy of Little AG, Swain JA, Nino JJ, et al: Reduction pneumonoplasty for emphysema: Early results. *Ann Surg* 222:365–374, 1995.)

instilled through the chest trocars in most patients. Thirty-two patients were evaluated 3 months after the procedure, and 17 patients were evaluated at 6 months.

Results.—Patients showed significant symptomatic improvement at 3 months, with a trend toward continued improvement at 6 months. There was also significant improvement in the results of pulmonary function testing (Table 4). Radiographs and spirometry both showed a significant reduction in lung volume. There was significant hospital morbidity, with 11 patients requiring a new chest tube for late pneumothorax, 9 having urinary complications, and 25 having moderate-to-severe subcutaneous emphysema. Three patients died in the hospital, for a 30-day mortality of 5.5%.

Conclusions.—Encouraging results are reported with unilateral laser reduction pneumonoplasty for selected patients with diffuse bullous emphysema. Significant objective and subjective improvements have been noted with short-term follow-up. The authors plan future reports of the results of sequential treatment of both lungs and are examining the possibility of performing simultaneous, bilateral reduction pneumonoplasty.

Thoracoscopic Laser Pneumoplasty in the Treatment of Diffuse Bullous Emphysema

Wakabayashi A (Wakabayashi Inst, Irvine, California)
Ann Thorac Surg 60:936–942, 1995 1–38

Background.—A retrospective study of 443 patients with diffuse bullous emphysema was undertaken to assess the effectiveness of thoracoscopic laser pneumoplasty (TLP) with a contact neodymium:yttrium-aluminum garnet laser.

Methods.—A group of 443 patients with an average age of 66.95 years underwent 500 TLP procedures. The TLP was carried out with 1-lung ventilation, and the patient was given general anesthesia. More than half of the 500 procedures (381) were for type 3 bullae, which were contracted by touching them with a contact neodymium:yttrium-aluminum garnet laser, and the remainder (119) were for type 4 bullae, which were opened widely and detached with a contact laser scalpel.

Results.—The mortality rate within 3 months of the TLP was 4.8%, due primarily to pneumonia and acute respiratory failure. Nonfatal complications included persistent air leaks and subcutaneous emphysema. Follow-up pulmonary function tests, available in 229 patients, showed improved breathing and physical capacity in 87.4% of the patients. The treadmill test, forced vital capacity, forced expiratory volume for 1 second (FEV_1), airway resistance, residual volume, and total lung capacity showed significant improvement.

Conclusions.—Thoracoscopic laser pneumoplasty is an effective treatment for diffuse bullous emphysema with acceptable risk and mortality and morbidity rates.

▶ Reduction pneumonoplasty is a potentially important therapy for the many cigarette smokers who have had emphysema develop. It is particularly appealing to think of a surgical therapy that doesn't reqiure implanting someone else's healthy lung. The pitfall with this surgery has been air leak, and that remains a problem in the experience our institution has accumulated thus far with this procedure. Little, et al. (Abstract 1–37) used Nd:YAG laser in the hope that less invasive pneumonoplasty would result in reduced morbidity and mortality. They also treated only 1 lung in each patient. In 55 patients undergoing this procedure, there was a significant decrease in breathlessness, with relatively low rates of morbidity and mortality. Prolonged air leak was seen in 20%, which is better than in many surgical series. The authors plan to extend their protocol to sequential lung and simultaneous bilateral lung reduction procedures.

Wakabayashi reports a larger series of 500 procedures in 443 patients with similar functional improvement and morbidity, and with a mortality rate of 4.8%. Of particular note in this large series was the author's recommendation of limited noncontrast CT when occult pneumothorax was suspected. The author also makes some very good points in analyzing recent reports of surgical pneumonoplasty with stapling. He notes the small size of most such series and points out that there were no deaths among his first 31 patients, either. He also emphasizes the need for a long follow-up period; his series has been in progress since 1991.

B.H. Gross, M.D.

Study of Endoscopic Staple Formation by Specimen Radiography on Pulmonary Wedges

Yim APC, Leung CMY (Chinese Univ of Hong Kong; Prince of Wales Hosp, Hong Kong)

Chest 108:1728–1730, 1995 1–39

Introduction.—The use of mechanical staplers during video-assisted thoracic surgery (VATS) has been shown to be safe and reliable. There is concern about the outcome of malfunction, particularly when using a vascular staple cutter. Staple formation was prospectively analyzed on resected lung specimens by radiography. Radiographs were correlated with clinical findings.

Methods.—Thirty-six consecutive pulmonary wedges from 31 patients who had undergone endoscopic staple-cutter resection included 23 apical bullae, 12 pulmonary metastases, and 1 tuberculoma. Fresh specimens underwent 2-plane specimen radiography. The dimensions and volume of each specimen were determined. An irregular or incompletely closed staple was considered imperfect (Fig 1). Patients' hospital courses were closely

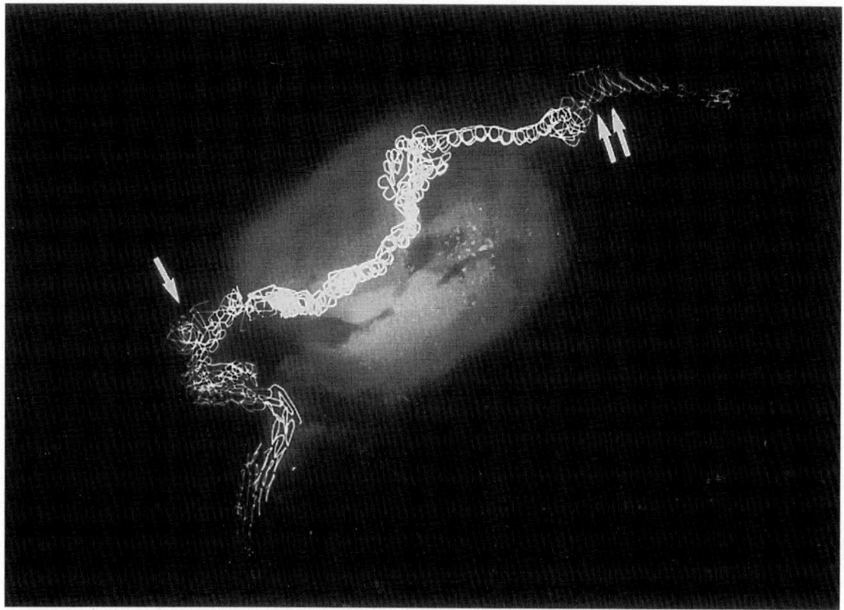

FIGURE 1.—Specimen radiograph showing grade 2 irregular (*single arrow*) and grade 2 incompletely closed (*double arrows*) staples. (Courtesy of Yim APC, Leung CMY: Study of endoscopic staple formation by specimen radiography on pulmonary wedges. *Chest* 108:1728–1730, 1995.)

followed, particularly for persistent air leak or other complications. Staple formation and clinical outcome were stratified according to type of specimen, either bullectomy (group B) metastases or tuberculoma (group M).

Results.—The median volume of group B and group M specimens were 4.2 mL and 36.0 mL, respectively. The incidence of imperfect staple formation was 58% (21 of 36 specimens). In group B and group M specimens, the incidence of imperfect staple formation was 77% (10 of 13) and 57% (13 of 23), respectively. The median postoperative chest drainage and median hospital stay for patients in both groups were comparable. A man, 17 years of age, with recurrent spontaneous pneumothorax and prolonged air leak, had chest drainage for 12 days after VATS for bullectomy and pleurodesis. The resected specimen had only minor staple irregularities and perfect staple closures. The complication may have been caused by an error in surgical technique or because a ruptured bleb was missed, rather than stapler failure. There were no delayed complications.

Conclusion.—There is a high incidence of imperfect staple formation, particularly when resecting large specimens. The current endoscopic equipment and staplers were originally meant for laparoscopic work. Findings indicate the continued need for improvements in endoscopic stapler design for VATS.

► Because air leak has been a problem with pneumoplasties, it pays to examine the work of endoscopic staplers. The authors conclude that in most resections, there is imperfect stapling, although this does not necessarily result in increased patient morbidity. Nevertheless, they advocate a continued quest for improvements in endoscopic stapler design.

A review article this year looked at the current state of the art for VATS.[1]

B.H. Gross, M.D.

Reference

1. Kaiser LR, Shrager JB: Video-assisted thoracic surgery: The current state of the art. *AJR* 165:1111–1117, 1995.

Unsuspected Lung Cancer Found in Work-Up for Lung Reduction Operation

Pigula FA, Keenan RJ, Ferson PF, et al (Univ of Pittsburgh, Pa)
Ann Thorac Surg 61:174–176, 1996 1–40

Background.—Lung reduction surgery is a relatively new treatment for patients with severe diffuse emphysema. Primary lung neoplasms were identified in patients who were evaluated for this procedure. A significant risk for these lesions in these patients is identified.

Methods.—Extensive screening for lung reduction operation was performed in 210 patients; 128 underwent the lung reduction procedure. Preoperative assessment included chest CT, chest radiography, echocardiography, fiberoptic bronchoscopic examination of the airway (in the operating room), pulmonary function and arterial blood gases, and ventilation scan with tomographic perfusion scan.

Results.—Of the 210 patients, 10 had previously unsuspected neoplastic lesions. The average age of these 10 patients was 67 years. All were heavy cigarette smokers with an average of 72 pack/years. The pulmonary function of these patients was severely impaired. Of the 10 patients, 6 had primary lung cancers and 4 had various other neoplastic lesions.

Discussion.—Patients who are candidates for lung reduction operation are at high risk for underlying lung pathology. It is essential to conduct thorough preoperative radiographic and bronchoscopic evaluations.

▶ To continue with the theme for 1 more article, it is no surprise that lung cancers could be present in the heavy smokers who comprise the population of reduction pneumoplasty candidates. What is surprising is that only 4 of the 10 neoplasms (6 bronchogenic carcinomas, 2 carcinoid tumorlets, 1 squamous dysplasia, 1 chemodectoma) were discovered by preoperative radiographic evaluation, which includes chest radiographs and chest CT in all patients. Two of the 6 lesions undetected by radiographic evaluation were lung cancers: 1 endobronchial and 1 "a microscopic focus of invasive adenocarcinoma...identified on routine pathologic examination of one of the tissue strips after lung reduction operation." The other 4 missed lesions ranged from 2 to 5 mm. The 4 patients with lesions that were detected preoperatively underwent wedge rather than anatomic resection because of physiologic impairment and did not undergo reduction pneumoplasty.

An important take-home message here is that candidates for reduction pneumoplasty may comprise an especially high-risk population for lung cancer. This necessitates careful evaluation of preoperative radiographs and CTs, as well as careful pathologic inspection of resected material in those who undergo pneumoplasty.

B.H. Gross, M.D.

Selenium-Based Digital Radiography of the Chest: Radiologists' Preference Compared With Film-Screen Radiographs

Floyd CE Jr, Baker JA, Chotas HG, et al (Duke Univ, Durham, NC)
AJR 165:1353–1358, 1995 1–41

Objective.—The results of a digital thoracic radiography system that uses an amorphous selenium detector were compared to results of a conventional film-screen system.

Background.—It has been reported that the detective quantum efficiency of this selenium-based digital radiography system is significantly higher than that of film-screen systems. The detective quantum efficiency is a measure of the signal-to-noise ratio and is related to the spatial resolution. A system with a higher detective quantum efficiency might provide superior detection of faint lesions. The hypothesis that images produced by the digital system would be equal or superior to those of a conventional system was tested.

Methods.—Imaging with the selenium-based digital and film-screen systems was performed in 53 patients. Posteroanterior and lateral radiographic images were obtained with both systems. Images were evaluated and compared by 3 chest radiologists trained in thoracic imaging and 3 general radiologists. Normal radiographs and radiographs with abnormal findings were included. Images were rated for 17 features and for observer preference of technique.

Results.—For all 17 features, the chest radiologists significantly preferred the selenium-based system. For 10 of 17 features, the general radiologists significantly preferred the selenium-based system. There was no significant preference for the conventional system in either group.

Discussion.—The images produced by the selenium-based digital radiography system were preferred by all radiologists and were rated as equal or superior to those from conventional film-screen systems. Digital radiography images can be processed to meet the requirements of individual radiologists. The image is stored in a digital format and can be reprinted to enhance its appearance for different anatomical regions.

► The search continues for the optimal imaging system for conventional radiography. A new digital radiographic system that uses selenium as a detector was preferred over an asymmetric film-screen system developed specifically for chest radiology. It was especially preferred by the 3 chest radiologists who reviewed the images, but 3 general radiologists also found the selenium-based system preferable for the majority of evaluated features. The authors note the possibility of bias because the film appearance was sufficiently different to allow observers to differentiate. Similar results were published by a second group.[1]

Related articles this year included a comparison of conventional film-screen radiographs and storage phosphor radiographs for detecting simulated miliary nodules[2] (no significant difference for the group as a whole), a comparison of conventional and AMBER chest radiographs for interstitial lung disease[3] (AMBER statistically significantly better), and a comparison of conventional and asymmetric film-screen combinations for imaging pulmonary nodules[4] (asymmetric statistically significantly better).

B.H. Gross, M.D.

References

1. van Heesewijk HPM, Neitzel U, van der Graaf Y, et al: Digital chest imaging with a selenium detector: Comparison with conventional radiography for visualization of specific anatomic regions of the chest. *AJR* 165:535–540, 1995.
2. Mosser H, Pèrtan G, Urban M, et al: Conventional film-screen versus computed storage phosphor radiography: Simulated miliary lung disease in an anthropomorphic phantom. *Invest Radiol* 30:186–191, 1995.
3. Dammann VF, Sokiranski R, Schèfer C, et al: Wertigkeit des AMBER-systems bei interstitiellen lungenverènderungen. *Fortschr Rüntgenstr* 163:99–103, 1995.
4. Müller VR-D, Wèhling S, Hirche H, et al: Einsatz einer asymmetrischen film-folien-kombination zur abbildung pulmonaler rundherde. *Fortschr Rüntgenstr* 163:290–296, 1995.

Multi-Slice, Breathhold Imaging of the Lung With Submillisecond Echo Times

Alsop DC, Hatabu H, Bonnet M, et al (Univ of Pennsylvania, Philadelphia)
Magn Reson Med 33:678–682, 1995 1–42

Introduction.—Magnetic resonance imaging of the lung parenchyma requires echo times shorter than those achieved with T_2 and T_2*. However, with standard MR imaging, the field strength corresponding to short echo times requires long scans, causing signal decay from respiratory motion. However, improved hardware and nonstandard techniques can achieve submillisecond echo times to produce multislice images of lung tissue within a single breath-hold.

Methods.—A prototype enhanced gradient system was used with a GE SIGNA scanner to perform imaging at 1.5 T with dramatically shorter echo times. The data were acquired with a sampling rate of 125 kHz with asymmetrical gradient echo sampling (16 samples before and 128 samples after the echo and a very narrow RF pulse width [480 μs]). The lungs of 4 normal volunteers were imaged in 10-mm slices, using a 40-cm field of

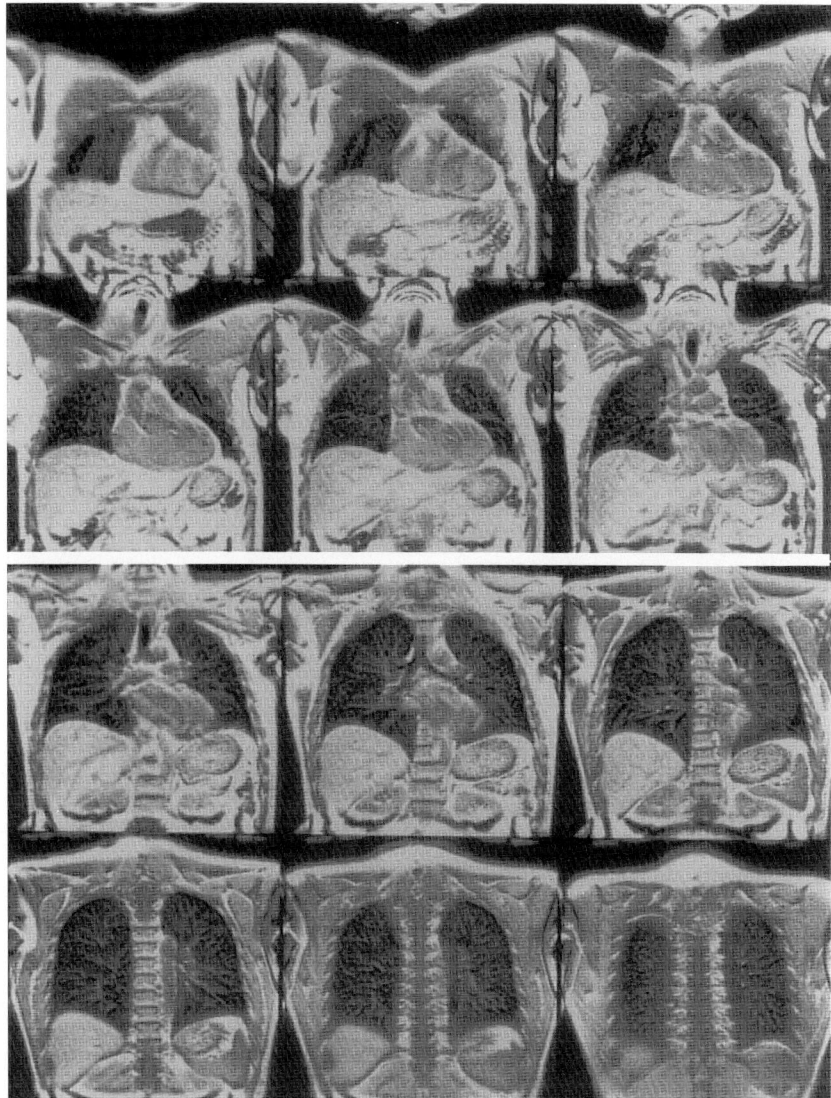

FIGURE 4.—Twelve coronal images through the thorax of a normal volunteer acquired with an echo time of 0.7 msec. The images were all acquired in a single breath-hold, normal inspiration. (Courtesy of Alsop DC, Hatabu H, Bonnet M, et al: Multi-slice, breathhold imaging of the lung with submillisecond echo times. *Magn Reson Med* 33:678–682, 1995.)

view, a 100-ms TR, and a 128 × 256 image matrix. The images were acquired during a single, 16-second breath-hold.

Results.—The average echo time was 0.7 msec. Lung parenchyma were clearly visualized on axial images, which were without respiratory motion artifact and had minimal cardiac motion artifact. The signal-to-noise ratio could be optimized by averaging images obtained during different breath-holds acquired at similar echo times. Doubling the signal-to-noise ratio produced better visualization of the parenchyma, but worse visualization of the vessels. Cardiac artifact was greatest with longer echo times. Coronal images of both entire lungs could be obtained in 16 seconds, with single slice images and interleaved multislice images having similar quality (Fig 4). There was significant chemical shift between fat and muscle and lung parenchyma and pleura.

Discussion.—The use of enhanced gradient hardware enables the detection of parenchymal signal with submillisecond echo times during a single breath-hold, which cannot be achieved with longer echo times. However, the images contain significant chemical shift, possibly caused by the phase offset at the echo time.

► I don't know where (if anywhere) thoracic MR is headed, but it keeps getting to places that I don't think it can reach. With an echo time of 0.7 msec, images can be acquired in a single breath-hold, eliminating respiratory motion artifacts. The resultant parenchymal detail is surprisingly good!

Although I am not expecting MR to wrest the parenchymal lung evaluation title from CT, it has a better shot at the pleural and chest wall championship.[1]

B.H. Gross, M.D.

Reference

1. Bittner VRC, Schnoy N, Schönfeld N, et al: Hochauflösende magnetresonanztomographie (HR-MRT) von pleura und thoraxwand Normalbefund und pathologische veränderungen. *Fortschr Röntgenstr* 162:296–303, 1995.

Evaluation of Solitary Pulmonary Nodules With Dynamic Contrast-Enhanced MR Imaging—A Promising Technique?

Hittmair K, Eckersberger F, Klepetko W, et al (MR Inst, Vienna; Univ of Vienna)

Magn Reson Imaging 13:923–933, 1995 1–43

Background.—Solitary pulmonary nodules (SPNs) are a common radiologic finding. Although frequently benign in nature, SPNs also are the most common manifestation of asymptomatic bronchogenic carcinoma. Differentiation between benign and malignant disease poses a difficult diagnostic challenge; however, dynamic contrast-enhanced MRI may potentially improve the characterization of SPNs. A prospective study was done to determine whether dynamic contrast-enhanced MRI can adequately evaluate the degree and kinetics of MR contrast enhancement and whether it could facilitate the noninvasive characterization of SPNs.

Patients and Methods.—Twenty-one patients (mean age, 58 years) with SPNs were included. All patients underwent MR examinations, with T1-weighted and proton image density-weighted spoiled gradient-echo-breath-hold images (two-dimensional FLASH) obtained before and after

Gd-DTPA was given (standard dosage of 0.1 mmol/kg body weight). Biopsies or resections were performed within 1 week after MRI. Correlations between pathologic findings and maximum enhancement and initial velocity of contrast uptake were evaluated. The relative signal intensity increase, enhancement factor, and contrast equivalent were used to quantify contrast enhancement.

Results.—There were 6 benign and 15 malignant lesions identified on pathohistologic assessment. Nodule size ranged from 0.5 to 3.6 cm. With the exception of 1 SPN (diameter of 0.5 cm), all other SPNs were reliably assessed on MRI. Significant differences in the degree and kinetics of contrast enhancement were noted for the specific SPN types. The strongest and fastest contrast enhancement was noted in the 2 benign inflammatory fibrous lesions. Benign neoplastic lesions had the weakest and slowest contrast uptake, whereas values for primary and secondary malignant neoplastic nodules were between the 2 benign pathologic groups for maximal enhancement and the initial slope of contrast uptake. When enhancement factor and contrast uptake equivalent were used for quantification of contrast enhancement, differences between the various pathologic groups proved to be more significant than when signal intensity increase was used.

Conclusions.—Dynamic contrast-enhanced MRI, using enhancement factor and contrast uptake equivalent as contrast uptake evaluation parameters, appears to have a potential role in the preoperative noninvasive assessment of SPNs. Preliminary findings suggest that weak contrast agent uptake is indicative of benign lesions, and this could help reduce the number of patients undergoing unnecessary surgical resection. Definitive threshold values for the differentiation between benign and malignant SPNs, and the sensitivity, specificity, and accuracy of dynamic contrast-enhanced MRI for evaluation of SPNs must still be determined.

► Who would have thought that MR could be used to evaluate SPNs? It becomes feasible and even logical (given the advances in MR technology) when lesion enhancement is found to be an important marker of the benign or malignant nature of the lesion. In this series, malignant neoplasms enhanced to a greater extent and more quickly than benign neoplasms, but the greatest and fastest enhancement was seen in benign inflammatory/fibrous lesions.

B.H. Gross, M.D.

Pulmonary: General Topics

Bronchogenic Carcinoma: Incidence of Metastases to Normal Sized Lymph Nodes

Arita T, Kuramitsu T, Kawamura M, et al (Yamaguchi Univ, Japan)
Thorax 50:1267–1269, 1995 1–44

Objectives.—The incidence of metastases to normal-sized nodes in patients with non–small-cell lung cancer and the use of hilar lymph nodes in predicting mediastinal lymph node metastases were assessed.

Background.—The value of CT in staging bronchogenic carcinoma is debated. It has been reported that CT scanning has both a high and low sensitivity in depicting mediastinal lymph node metastases. The frequency of metastases to normal-sized mediastinal lymph nodes directly affects the sensitivity of CT scanning, but this frequency has not been determined.

Methods.—Computed tomography was performed in 90 patients who were between the ages of 40 and 79 years with primary lung cancer. All patients later underwent thoracotomy with dissection of the mediastinal lymph nodes.

Results.—In 19 patients, mediastinal lymph node metastases were observed at thoracotomy. In 14 of these 19 patients, the lymph node metastases were misdiagnosed because they were of normal size on the scans. An N1 lymph node was enlarged in only 1 of the 19 patients with N2 nodes. In 4 of the 19 patients with N2 nodes, metastases to the mediastinal nodes were present without N1 disease.

Conclusions.—The status of hilar lymph nodes was not predictive of the presence or absence of metastases to mediastinal lymph nodes. A serious problem in staging was a number of metastases that were of normal size on CT scans. In assessing N3 nodes, mediastinoscopy is more helpful than CT scanning.

► This may look like a Lung Cancer section, but it's not; it's a Pulmonary: General Topics section. This article is particularly interesting to me because its results differ markedly from a previous article that I wrote.[1] This study concludes that metastases to normal-sized nodes occur frequently (14 of 90 patients), whereas we had concluded that only 7% of patients had metastases limited to normal-sized nodes.

When current work on lung cancer staging contradicts prior work, I am usually at a loss for how to explain the discrepancy. This time I think I have it figured out. I think there is a very strong selection bias in this article. The authors start with 243 patients undergoing primary lung cancer evaluation, but they only report 90 patients who get to thoracotomy. What happened to the other 153 patients? They were eliminated from consideration because of stage IIIB or stage IV disease. Because stage IIIB disease includes contralateral mediastinal lymph node enlargement and stage IV disease includes distant metastases, many of these 153 patients were eliminated from consideration for thoracotomy because of accurate CT depiction of disease. Simply to discard them from further consideration is an error of the first magnitude.

I may not have all of the facts here, but from where I sit it looks as though 243 patients were evaluated, and in only 14 were metastases to normal-sized nodes a problem. That comes to 5.8%, similar to the 7% we reported, and I still don't consider it a major problem!

B.H. Gross, M.D.

Reference

1. Gross BH, Glazer GM, Orringer MB, et al: Bronchogenic carcinoma metastatic to normal-sized lymph nodes: Frequency and significance. *Radiology* 166:71–74, 1988.

Survival of Patients After Resection for Lung Cancer: Predictive Value of Staging by CT vs Thoracotomy

Lähde S, Rainio P, Bloigu R (Univ Central Hosp, Oulu, Finland; Univ of Oulu, Finland)

Acta Radiol 36:515–519, 1995 1–45

Introduction.—In patients with lung cancer, the results of staging CT commonly disagree with those of surgical staging. Although surgical staging is generally regarded as the gold standard, there is evidence that the staging information provided by CT is actually more reliable. The ability of staging CT and thoracotomy to predict long-term outcome after resection of lung cancer was assessed.

Methods.—The study included 151 patients with primary non–small-cell lung cancer. All underwent preoperative physical examination, chest radiograph, and bronchoscopy, followed by staging CT. Both CT and thoracotomy staging were performed according to the new international staging system. For patients in whom no definite classification could be assigned by CT, an additional indeterminate stage was used. The 2 staging techniques were compared for their ability to predict survival.

Results.—Staging CT was insufficient for the detection of hilar lymph node metastases. The CT staging score was "indeterminate" in 22% of patients. In 48% of cases, surgical and CT staging agreed completely in terms of TN classification. Thirty-six month survival according to surgical stage was 71% for stage I, 55% for stage II, 30% for stage IIIa, and 9% for stage IIIb. For CT staging, survival was 71% for stage I, 35% for "indeterminate," and 33% for stage IIIa. These figures showed moderate-to-good parallelism. Survival was worse for patients with tumor stage I at thoracotomy but "indeterminate" or stage IIIa at CT compared to patients with tumor stage I by both methods.

Conclusions.—For patients with lung cancer, the results of CT and surgical staging provide complementary prognostic information. By either technique, the more deleterious the sign, the greater its prognostic reliability. A sign of tumor spread at either CT or surgical staging should lead to an active approach: either performance of more radical surgery or omission of noncurative operations.

▶ What's the matter with you? Didn't you hear me the first time? I said, this is not a Lung Cancer section! Don't ask again.

These authors are asking the right question. The CT assessment of resectability is important, but the real goal is to assess outcome. Interestingly, CT is sometimes more reliable than surgical staging in assessing the stage of disease. The survival rate curves for CT and surgical staging were reasonably parallel. Most importantly, if *either* staging tool showed a sign of tumor spread it was felt that active investigation (and possibly more radical surgery) was indicated.

One final word on lung cancer. Another article[1] asks whether there is increased risk of lung cancer with a history of asbestos exposure but without small opacities on chest radiographs. The final word: Yes.

B.H. Gross, M.D.

Reference

1. Wilkinson P, Hansell DM, Janssens J, et al: Is lung cancer associated with asbestos exposure when there are no small opacities on the chest radiograph? *Lancet* 345:1074–1078, 1995.

Artificial Widening of the Mediastinum to Gain Access for Extrapleural Biopsy: Clinical Results

Langen H-J, Klose K-C, Keulers P, et al (Technical Univ of Aachen, Germany)
Radiology 196:703–706, 1995 1–46

Background.—Pneumothorax is a common complication of transpulmonary biopsy. The authors have developed a technique of dilating the mediastinum by injection of a physiologic saline solution from a dorsal paravertebral or ventral parasternal approach. This permits mediastinal biopsy with an extrapleural access route to the anterior and posterior mediastinum (Fig 2). The value of this technique of artificial mediastinal widening was assessed in a clinical series.

Methods.—The retrospective analysis included 20 patients, 5 to 78 years of age, undergoing biopsy of mediastinal masses. In each patient, the extrapleural space was dilated by injection of about 20 mL of physiologic saline solution. A dorsal approach was used in 14 patients and a ventral parasternal approach in 6. All mediastinal biopsies were performed under CT guidance.

Results.—In 11 of the 14 patients in whom a dorsal approach was attempted, right-sided paravertebral extrapleural access to the mediastinum was successfully achieved. Mean dilation of the paravertebral extra-

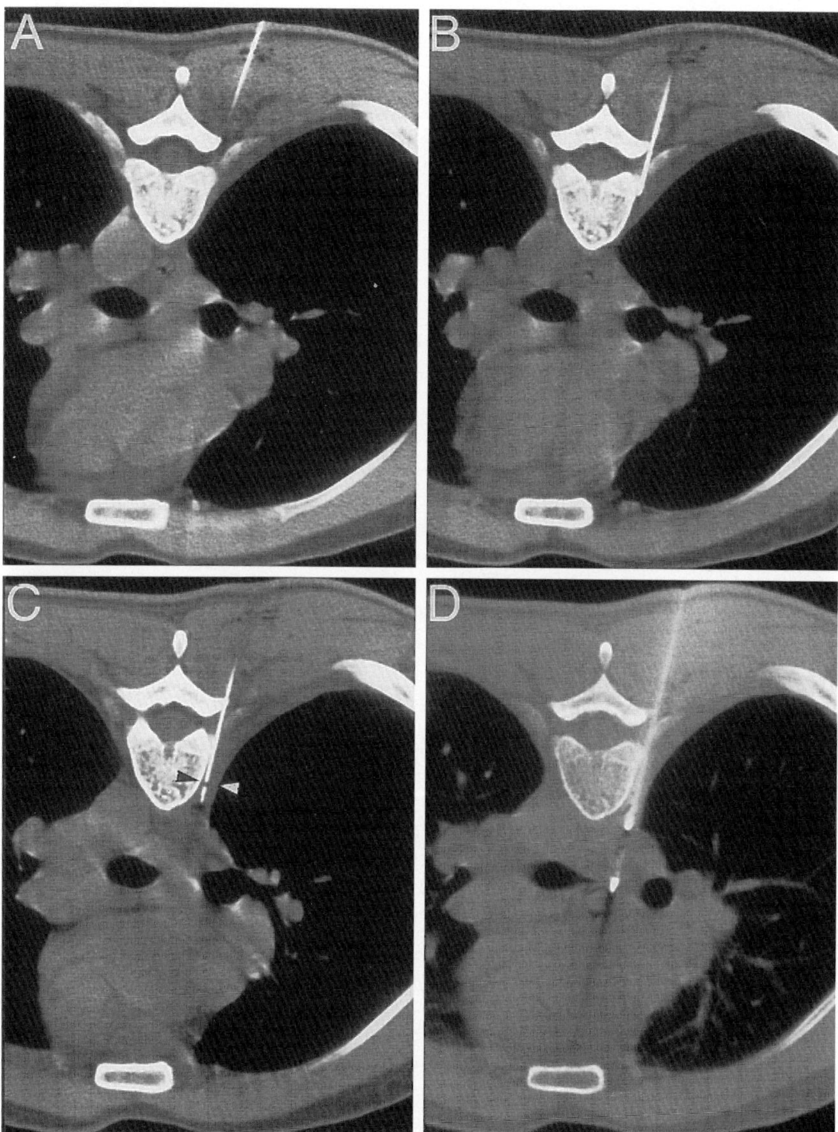

FIGURE 2.—Dilation of the extrapleural space with injection of physiologic saline solution by means of a right-sided dorsal approach. Patient is in a prone position. The CT scans obtained (**A**) before and (**B**) after injection of 10 mL of saline solution. C, the extrapleural space was not widened enough for biopsy, and the needle was pushed forward, and an additional 10 mL of saline solution was injected. **D**, extrapleural biopsy of the infracarinal mass in the mediastinum was performed with an 18-gauge needle. The width of the access route is indicated by the *arrowheads* in **C**. (Courtesy of Langen H-J, Klose K-C, Keulers P, et al: Artificial widening of the mediastinum to gain access for extrapleural biopsy: Clinical results. *Radiology* 196:703–706, 1995. Radiological Society of North America.)

pleural soft tissue was from 0.2 to 0.9 cm. Nine patients had extrapleural biopsy. The pleura was traversed, leading to pneumothorax in 2 of 4 patients.

The ventral approach led to successful creation of a parasternal access route in 6 of 6 patients. All patients underwent biopsy without complication. The minimal anterior mediastinal width in these patients increased from 2.8 cm before to 4.5 cm after dilation.

Conclusions.—The described technique of artificial widening of the mediastinum is a useful one. It can provide an extrapleural access route for large-bore biopsy of either the anterior or posterior mediastinum. Because of pleural fixation, the paravertebral mediastinum is much more difficult to dilate than the ventral mediastinum.

▶ It's not for me, but here is a nice technique that allows mediastinal biopsy with a reduced risk of pneumothorax.

B.H. Gross, M.D.

Clinical Profile, Laboratory Characteristics and Outcome in Miliary Tuberculosis

Sharma SK, Mohan A, Pande JN, et al (All India Inst of Med Sciences, New Delhi)

Q J Med 88:29–37, 1995 1–47

Introduction.—In miliary tuberculosis (MTB), there is massive hematogenous dissemination of tubercle bacilli resulting in tiny discrete foci distributed throughout the lungs and other viscera. The typical appearance is a miliary pattern on the chest radiograph; however, atypical presentations can occur. Disseminated tuberculosis in general and the cryptic form of MTB in particular are common in patients with AIDS. A large series of non–HIV-infected patients with MTB from India are reported.

Patients.—The patients—51 men and 49 women, mean age 35 years—were treated from 1983 to 1994 at a tertiary care center. All received 9 months of antituberculosis treatment. Thirty-four patients had predisposing conditions, most commonly steroid use, connective tissue disease, alcoholism, and diabetes mellitus. Chest radiographs showed shadows larger than miliary size, i.e., 2 mm, in 12 patients. The rest of the patients had the classic miliary pattern (Fig 1, A and B). The most common presenting symptom was fever, and 10 patients had meningitis. Five patients had adult respiratory distress syndrome (ARDS), and their chest radiographs showed air-space consolidation (Fig 2). Seventy percent of patients were hyponatremic.

Outcomes.—Twelve patients died. With early treatment, 4 of the 5 patients with ARDS survived. Independent predictors of death were temperature of 39.3° C or greater, hypoalbuminemia, hyponatremia, history of vomiting, and presence of crepitations on auscultation.

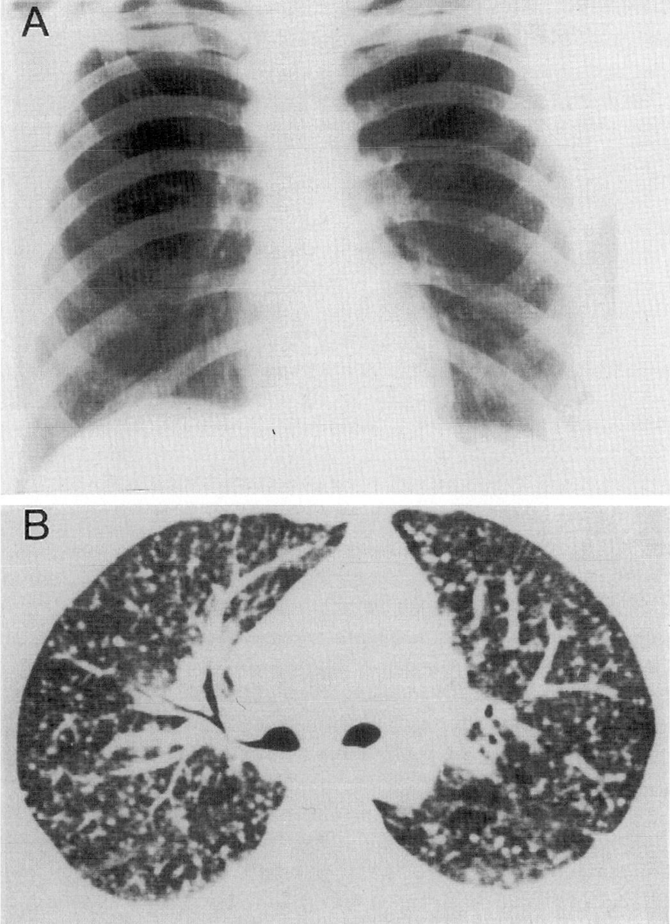

FIGURE 1.—**A,** chest x-ray film, posteroanterior view, showing subtle miliary shadows; **B,** CT-chest of the same patient, showing extensive miliary shadows. (Hematoxylin and eosin, ×80). (Courtesy of Sharma SK, Mohan A, Pande JN, et al: Clinical profile, laboratory characteristics and outcome in miliary tuberculosis. *Q J Med* 88:29–37, 1995, by permission of Oxford University Press.)

Conclusions.—Miliary tuberculosis can be difficult to diagnose, even in areas endemic for tuberculosis. The symptoms of MTB are nonspecific, and the classic miliary pattern is not always present on chest radiographs. It is essential to maintain a high level of clinical suspicion and to continue efforts to confirm the diagnosis by early demonstration of *Mycobacterium tuberculosis.* Newer techniques for early diagnosis of sputum smear-negative MTB warrant investigation, such as enzyme-linked immunosorbent assay and polymerase chain reaction.

► Infection marches on. It is surprising how many of us know of a young, previously healthy person who died unexpectedly of an infectious disease.

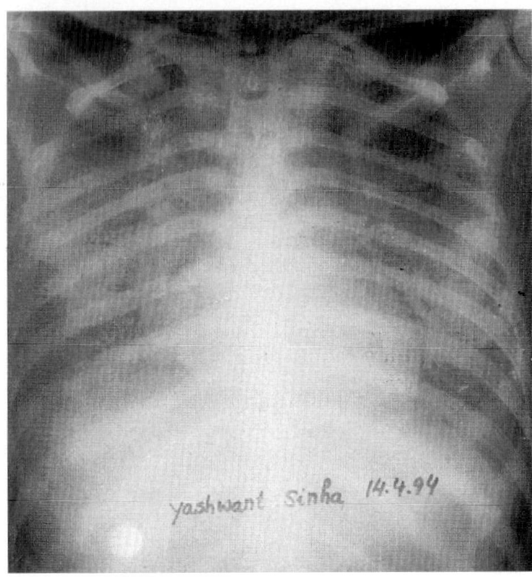

FIGURE 2.—Chest x-ray film (done bedside, with a portable machine) showing consolidation, with air-bronchogram. (Courtesy of Sharma SK, Mohan A, Pande JN, et al: Clinical profile, laboratory characteristics and outcome in miliary tuberculosis. *Q J Med* 88:29–37, 1995, by permission of Oxford University Press.)

As the authors point out, infections are sometimes difficult to diagnose even in a place where they are common. During an 11-year period, the authors accumulated 100 cases of non-HIV miliary TB. Twelve patients died, with independent predictors of mortality including temperature of 39.2° C or more, hypoalbuminemia, hyponatremia, vomiting, and crepitations on auscultation.

As usual, there were also a large number of articles on immunocompromised hosts. For acute lung disease in the immunocompromised host, chest radiography suggested a correct first-choice diagnosis in 90% of patients with AIDS patients and in 34% of non-AIDS patients.[1] A study of patients with AIDS concludes that imaging is unnecessary in the absence of pulmonary symptoms, but that high-resolution should be performed in symptomatic patients whether the chest x-ray film is normal or not.[2] Specific infections in AIDS that were the subject of articles included *Mycobacterium avium* complex[3] and cryptococcosis.[4] Two articles detailed the radiographic findings in AIDS-related Kaposi sarcoma,[5,6] and there was a report of unusual lymphoproliferative disorders in 9 patients with AIDS.[7]

B.H. Gross, M.D.

References

1. Logan PM, Primack SL, Staples C, et al: Acute lung disease in the immunocompromised host: Diagnostic accuracy of the chest radiograph. *Chest* 108:1283–1287, 1995.
2. Kauczor VH-U, Schnütgen M, Fischer B, et al: Pulmonale manifestationen bei HIV-patienten: Rolle von thoraxübersicht, CT und HRCT. *Fortschr Röntgenstr* 162:282–287, 1995.

3. Kalayjian RC, Toossi Z, Tomashefski JF Jr, et al: Pulmonary disease due to infection by *Mycobacterium avium* complex in patients with AIDS. *Clin Infect Dis* 20:1186–1194, 1995.
4. Meyohas M-C, Roux P, Bollens D, et al: Pulmonary cryptococcosis: Localized and disseminated infections in 27 patients with AIDS. *Clin Infect Dis* 21:628–633, 1995.
5. Gruden JF, Huang L, Webb WR, et al: AIDS-related Kaposi sarcoma of the lung: Radiographic findings and staging system with bronchoscopic correlation. *Radiology* 195:545–552, 1995.
6. Khalil AM, Carette MF, Cadranel JL, et al: Intrathoracic Kaposi's sarcoma: CT findings. *Chest* 108:1622–1626, 1995.
7. McGuinness G, Scholes JV, Jagirdar JS, et al: Unusual lymphoproliferative disorders in nine adults with HIV or AIDS: CT and pathologic findings. *Radiology* 197:59–65, 1995.

Giant Pericardial Cysts

Satur CMR, Hsin MKY, Dussek JE (Guy's Hosp, London)
Ann Thorac Surg 61:208–210, 1996 1–48

Introduction.—Pericardial cysts are uncommon, congenital abnormalities and are usually asymptomatic. They are often incidental findings on chest roentgenograms. Giant cysts are less common and, therefore, there is little information about them. The cases of 2 patients with giant cysts are reported.

> *Case 2.*—Man, 58, underwent a chest radiograph that showed a 7-cm spherical shadow in the right costophrenic angle. A pericardial cyst was diagnosed. The patient refused surgical excision by thoracotomy. During the next 20 years, the cyst enlarged progressively and dyspnea developed on exertion. A chest radiograph revealed a mass filling the lower two thirds of the right hemithorax. Computed tomography showed a large, thin-walled cystic structure in the lower anterior right hemithorax abutting the right border of the heart. The giant cyst contained 2.5 L of fluid and was resected. Chest radiography at 6 weeks showed a small residual stump. The patient reported no further symptoms. The features of the cyst were consistent with a benign mesothelial pericardial cyst.

Discussion.—In this patient, the thoracoscope was mainly a diagnostic tool at the time of initial examination, and treatment would have required a thoracotomy. Over time, the technology associated with thoracoscopy developed and allowed this giant pericardial cyst to be resected with minimal invasion. Large pericardial cysts should be included in the differential diagnosis of pleural effusion. Diagnosis of these cysts may be confirmed with two-dimensional echocardiography or CT.

► I imagine myself as a sort of Venus flytrap. I lie in wait, and occasionally when a stray article gets too close, I snap it up. This should have gone to the cardiovascular section, but fortunately it was mistakenly routed to me. These giant cysts contained 2 and 2.5 L of fluid, respectively. Both were resected with video-assisted thoracoscopy.

B.H. Gross, M.D.

Case Report: Mobile Fatty Globules in Benign Cystic Teratoma of the Mediastinum

Hession PR, Simpson W (Newcastle Gen Hosp, Newcastle Upon Tyne, England)

Br J Radiol 69:186–188, 1996 1–49

Introduction.—Benign cystic teratoma can cause an anterior mediastinal mass. The diagnosis is suggested by the presence of fat, which is found in 50% of patients. A new feature consisting of components of the tumor drifting upward, or anteriorly, during a CT examination is described, and the effect is compared to that seen in a popular decorative light.

> *Case Report.*—Woman, 37, had a 3-month history of increasing dyspnea and nonproductive cough. A CT scan showed a well-encapsulated mass in the anterior mediastinum with lumps of tissue with a low attenuation lying posteriorly within the mass (Fig 2, A). In scans obtained a few minutes later, the lumps of tissue had moved anteriorly within the main mass (Fig 2, B). Histopathologic examination revealed a benign cystic teratoma.

Discussion.—Benign cystic teratoma is the most common type of mediastinal germ cell tumor, and is more common in women than men. It is usually an incidental finding. The movement of the mobile lumps of low attenuation material resulted from their density being lower than the surrounding semifluid matrix. A similar effect is seen in the Astro lamp (Fig 3), which contains mobile globules of wax that float and sink as their specific gravity changes relative to the surrounding liquid.

► Two reasons why I chose this article:

1. One of my first published articles was on cavitary lesions in invasive aspergillosis.[1] To simulate these lesions (and to demonstrate their variable appearance depending on the radiographic projection), I created and radiographed a model using a L'eggs pantyhose container with a central lump of Play-Doh. I am thus favorably disposed to articles that relate disease states to commercially available products.
2. My son recently bought a lava lamp, and it will make me appear especially knowledgeable about the important issues in his life when I go home tonight and explain how his lava lamp really works!

B.H. Gross, M.D.

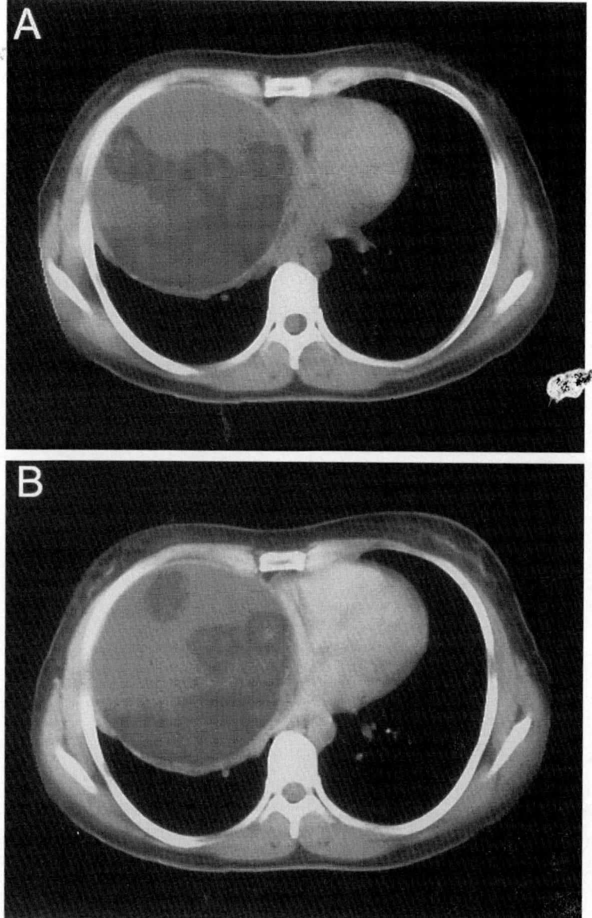

FIGURE 2.—A, contiguous 11-mm-thick sections (from a helical scan) through the mediastinum. There is a large cystic tumor containing globules of low attenuation material (fat); **B**, an image at the same level, 5 minutes later, shows that the fatty globules have risen to a more anterior (higher) position. (Courtesy of Hession PR, Simpson W: Case report: Mobile fatty globules in benign cystic teratoma of the mediastinum. *Br J Radiol* 69:186–188, 1996.)

Reference

1. Gross BH, Spitz HB, Felson B: The mural nodule in cavitary opportunistic pulmonary aspergillosis. *Radiology* 143:619–622, 1982.

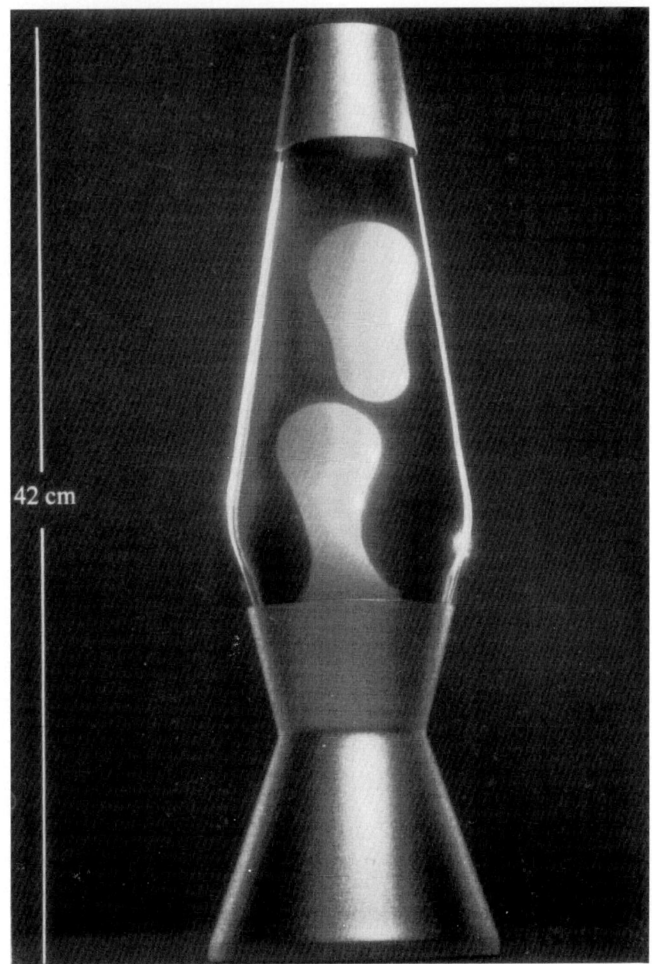

FIGURE 3.—The Astro (lava) lamp. The illustration and the technical details in the text were supplied by Crestworth Trading Ltd, Poole, Dorset. (Courtesy of Hession PR, Simpson W: Case report: Mobile fatty globules in benign cystic teratoma of the mediastinum. *Br J Radiol* 69:186–188, 1996.)

Bronchopleural-Subarachnoid Fistula Manifesting as Intracranial Gas on CT Scans

Smith DN, Munden RF, Schwartz RB, et al (Brigham and Women's Hosp, Boston)

AJR 165:1364–1365, 1995 1–50

Introduction.—Complications after thoracic surgery for lung carcinoma can occur. Imaging is important in evaluating and treating these complications. The case of a patient with a bronchopleural-subarachnoid fistula manifesting as intracranial gas on CT scans obtained after pneumonectomy is reported.

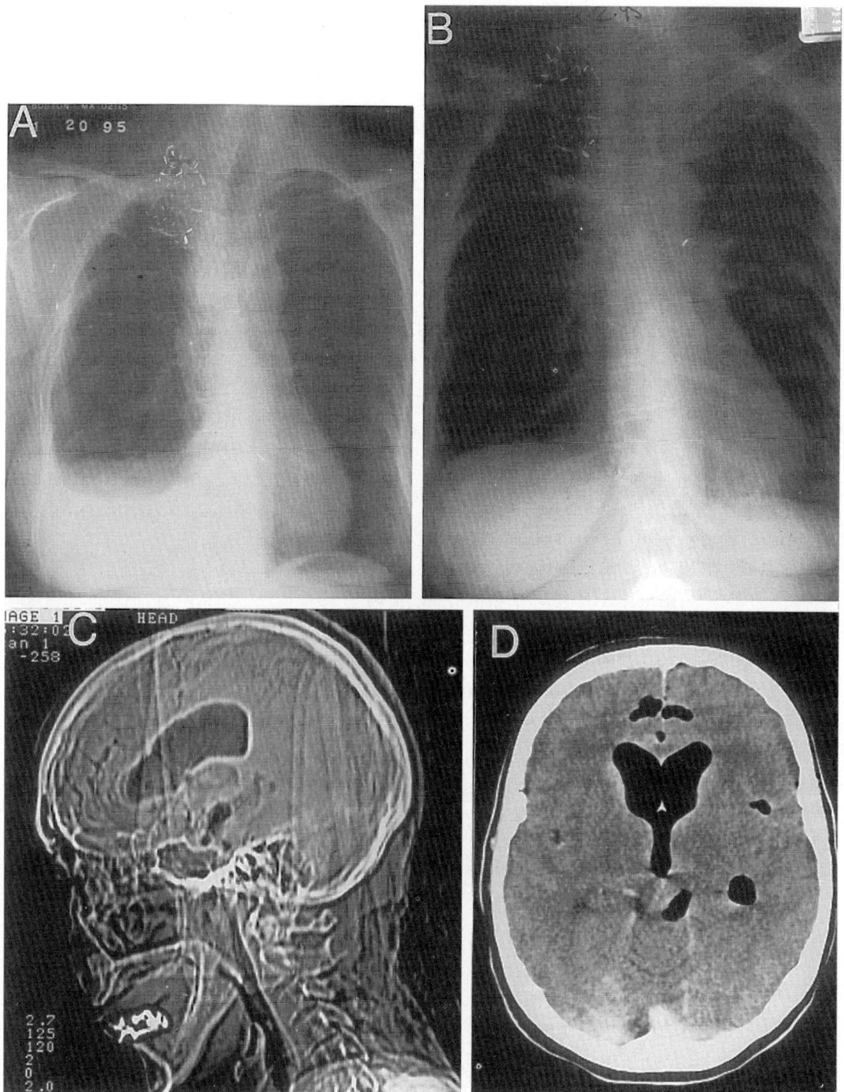

FIGURE 1.—A 65-year-old woman with bronchopleural-subarachnoid fistula. **A**, posteroanterior chest radiograph obtained before discharge on postoperative day 6 shows small postoperative pneumothorax at right apex and small pleural effusion; **B**, posteroanterior chest radiograph obtained 2 months later shows that the right apical pneumothorax has enlarged. No pleural effusion is apparent. **C**, lateral CT scan (patient supine) shows extensive gas collection in lateral ventricle, infundibular recess of third ventricle, and anterior subarachnoid space. **D**, axial enhanced CT scan shows gas within frontal horns, temporal horn of lateral ventricle, third ventricle, and subarachnoid spaces. (Courtesy of Smith DN, Munden RF, Schwartz RB, et al: Bronchopleural-subarachnoid fistula manifesting as intracranial gas on CT scans. *AJR* 165:1364–1365, 1995.)

Case Report.—Woman, 65, was treated for a right-sided Pancoast tumor. A leak of cerebrospinal fluid from the dural sleeve of the right T2 nerve root occurred. After a tear in the dura was overlaid by 2 fat grafts, there was no evidence of residual leak of cerebrospinal fluid. At discharge 6 days postoperatively, a small pneumothorax at the apex of the right lung was noted on a chest radiograph (Fig 1, A). Dizziness, malaise, and confusion developed 2 months later, and a chest radiograph showed an enlarged right apical gas collection and no pleural fluid (Fig 1, B). A bronchopleural fistula was considered, but a CT scan of the head was obtained to rule out metastatic disease because of the patient's change in mental status. The CT scan (Fig 1, C) showed gas within the ventricular system (Fig 1, D); subarachnoid gas was also present. Fluid consistent with cerebrospinal fluid was obtained by aspiration. The fistula was drained by a chest tube and treated, and a follow-up CT scan showed resolution of the ventricular and subarachnoid gas.

Discussion.—These bronchopleural fistulas are a rare complication of pulmonary resection. Current risk factors include residual tumor; extensive resection; preoperative or postoperative adjuvant therapy; comorbid diabetes mellitus, hypoalbuminemia, cirrhosis and other conditions; and use of steroids.

▶ Now for some fun! Bronchopleural fistula alone is well and good, but gas in the ventricular system adds effervescence. The first runner-up in this category is a colobronchial fistula in a patient with Crohn's disease.[1] I'm trying hard not to imagine what gets coughed up with that fistula.

B.H. Gross, M.D.

Reference

1. Karmy-Jones R, Chagpar A, Vallieres E, et al: Colobronchial fistula due to Crohn's disease. *Ann Thorac Surg* 60:446–448, 1995.

2 Abdomen

Introduction

There were a few new hot topics in abdominal imaging this year and some further refinements of perennial favorites. As helical CT scanning becomes the most prevalent mode, we are learning some important principles about optimal use of intravascular contrast medium and the importance of precise timing of scanning relative to the bolus (Abstracts 2–8, 2–9, and 2–10). The danger of missing hepatic lesions by using an inadequate volume or rate of contrast administration was emphasized. The prevalence and pathophysiology of focal fatty infiltration of the liver were clearly noted in Abstracts 2–13 and 2–14. As liver imaging improves, other benign lesions challenge our diagnostic abilities; 3 important abstracts (2–15, 2–16, and 2–17) should sharpen your skills.

The proper role of endoscopic retrograde cholangiopancreaticography (ERCP), ultrasound, and liver function tests prior to planned cholecystectomy remains a hot topic, and Abstracts 2–22, 2–23, and 2–24 should prove interesting and helpful. Magnetic resonance cholangiography (and pancreatography) is emerging as an important noninvasive alternative to ERCP (Abstract 2–27).

Helical CT also offers improved visualization and staging of pancreatic tumors (Abstracts 2–28 and 2–29). The competetive role of MR is addressed (Abstract 2–30), although no consensus is yet available.

Helical CT of the kidney can actually result in more missed lesions unless you pay careful attention to timing after the IV contrasts administration. Read Abstract 2–31 for an excellent discussion.

After several years of investigation of the role of MRI in distinguishing between adrenal adenomas and metastasis, the role of CT seems to have been rediscovered (Abstracts 2–37 and 2–38). Chemical shift MR is also valuable (Abstract 2–39), although its role relative to CT remains debatable.

Asymptomatic testicular masses are a fairly common cause of morbidity and great anxiety. The roles of ultrasound, surgical exploration, and biospy are discussed in Abstracts 2–41 and 2–42.

There have been hundreds of articles and case reports on in utero sonographic diagnosis of fetal anomalies. (As editor of this section, I know, because I have to read them all.) So, how are we doing in the "real world" of practice? Not as well as we might hope (see Abstracts 2–45 and 2–46)

I hope you find our selections and comments both interesting and informative.

Michael P. Federle, M.D.

General

CT in Patients With Blunt Abdominal Trauma: Clinical Significance of Intraperitoneal Fluid Detected on a Scan With Otherwise Normal Findings

Levine CD, Patel UJ, Wachsberg RH, et al (Univ Hosp, Newark, NJ)
AJR 164:1381–1385, 1995 2–1

Background.—In patients with blunt abdominal trauma, CT can aid in rapid diagnosis of internal injuries and detection of intraperitoneal fluid, which may result from hemoperitoneum. The scan will often show the source of the fluid, but fluid may be the only evidence of occult injury. To determine the significance of intraperitoneal fluid on CT scans in patients with blunt abdominal trauma whose scans are otherwise normal, CT scans were analyzed retrospectively.

Methods.—The CT scans of 60 patients with blunt abdominal trauma with intraperitoneal fluid as the only abnormality on the scans were reviewed. Patients were excluded if they had peritoneal lavage or surgery before CT scans, CT scans showing intra-abdominal organ injury or pelvic fractures, or scans showing a sentinel clot sign.

Results.—Laparotomy was required in 6 of the 60 patients. The intraperitoneal fluid accumulated primarily in the pouch of Douglas and Morison's pouch. Higher total fluid volumes and larger amounts of fluid in the upper abdomen were present in patients requiring laparotomy compared with patients managed conservatively. Of 44 patients with small total fluid volumes, only 1 required laparotomy, which revealed a periduodenal hematoma. Of 11 patients with moderate total fluid volumes, 3 required laparotomy, which revealed jejunal perforation in 1 patient and mesenteric lacerations in 2 patients. Of 5 patients with large total fluid volumes, 2 required laparotomy, which revealed ileal perforation and mesenteric hematoma in both patients. One patient had a small liver laceration not seen on CT scan.

Conclusions.—Peritoneal lavage or surgical exploration is not necessarily required in patients with small amounts of intraperitoneal fluid, unless there are other abnormal findings. Peritoneal lavage may be indicated in patients with mesenteric fluid, which may suggest bowel or mesenteric injury. Peritoneal lavage or surgery should be considered in patients whose CT scans show an intermediate amount of fluid.

▶ This is a valuable investigation, but careful attention must be paid to the details of the study and its recommendations. In the trauma setting it is important to analyze the location, amount, and character of any intraperitoneal fluid. Clotted blood accumulates near the site of hemorrhage and is an important clue in recognition of splenic, bowel, and mesenteric injuries (the sentinel clot). Lower than blood density fluid (less than 35 H) may reflect pre-existing ascites, bowel contents, urinary bladder rupture, or prior peritoneal lavage. Mesenteric collections of fluid are almost always due to bowel or mesenteric injuries in my experience, and I would favor surgical exploration in most cases, rather than peritoneal lavage for further evaluation.

M.P. Federle, M.D.

Diagnostic Accuracy of Ultrasound and Computed Tomography in the Staging of Hodgkin's Disease: Verification by Laparotomy in 100 Cases

Munker R, Stengel A, Stäbler A, et al (Ludwigs-Maximilians-Universität, München, Germany)

Cancer 76:1460–1466, 1995 2–2

Objective.—Staging laparotomy and splenectomy is still considered the gold standard for the detection of occult abdominal involvement in patients with Hodgkin's disease. In recent years, CT and ultrasound have become routinely available for diagnostic imaging. However, there have been no studies to define the precise contribution of ultrasound to the staging of Hodgkin's disease. The diagnostic accuracy of ultrasound in the staging of Hodgkin's disease was assessed.

Methods.—The study included 100 patients with biopsy-proven Hodgkin's disease. All underwent abdominal ultrasound, CT, and laparotomy, the diagnostic accuracy of which was compared. Each imaging study was performed without knowledge of the results of the other study. Separate evaluations were conducted to assess the liver, spleen, para-aortic, and iliac lymph nodes.

Results.—The disease stage was higher after surgery in 17% of patients. Of 79 patients without known abdominal disease, 18% had positive results on staging laparotomy. The sensitivity of ultrasound in detecting splenic involvement was 63%, compared with 37% for CT; specificity was 99% vs. 96%, respectively. Ultrasound was better at depicting structural inhomogeneities, small nodular infiltrates, and liver involvement. Sensitiv-

TABLE 4.—Histopathologic Correlations of CT and Ultrasound in Patients with Hodgkin's Disease (Liver and Splenic Involvement)

	No. of patients							
	Liver Involvement				*Splenic Involvement*			
Characteristic	CT	%	US	%	CT	%	US	%
Sensitivity	2/6	33	4/6	67	13/35	37	20/32	63
Specificity	90/92	98	79/79	100	55/57	96	46/47	98

Abbreviation: US, ultrasound.

(Courtesy of Munker R, Stengel A, Stäbler A, et al: Diagnostic accuracy of ultrasound and computed tomography in the staging of Hodgkin's disease: Verification by laparotomy in 100 cases. *Cancer* 76:1460–1466, 1995.)

ity in identifying lymph nodes at the splenic hilus was 64% with ultrasound and 62% with CT. Computed tomography was better at demonstrating para-aortic and iliac lymph nodes—sensitivities were 93% and 100%, respectively, compared with 77% and 67% with ultrasound.

Conclusions.—The combination of ultrasound and CT appears to be the best approach to the staging of Hodgkin's disease. Ultrasound is most accurate in depicting splenic involvement, but CT is more acurate in depicting para-aortic or iliac lymph node involvement (Table 4). Where CT is regarded as the standard, patients with negative CT results should undergo ultrasound, with special attention to splenic texture and size. Some patients may still need surgical staging to detect occult abdominal disease, however.

▶ This investigation confirms results from another recent study[1] that showed a higher sensitivity of ultrasound for the detection of splenic disease in comparison with CT. The technical details were not addressed in this article, but others have shown that a high frequency transducer can depict multifocal splenic (and hepatic) parenchymal lesions when lower frequency ultrasound transducers and CT show only nonspecific organomegaly. We rarely use lymphangiography or gallium scanning in the evaluation of Hodgkin's disease because of radiation exposure and often ambiguous findings. Staging laparotomy usually can be limited to cases in which no radiographic (CT or ultrasound) nor clinical risk factors (e.g., male gender or mixed cellularity histologic types) are present.

M.P. Federle, M.D.

Reference

1. Siniluoto T, Tikkakoski TA, Lahde ST, et al. Ultrasound or CT in splenic diseases? *Acta Radiol* 35:597–605, 1994.

Esophagus and Gut

Dysplasia in Ulcerative Colitis: Is Radiography Adequate for Diagnosis?

Matsumoto T, Iida M, Kuroki F, et al (Kyushu Univ, Fukuoka, Japan; Fukuoka Univ, Japan; Matsuyama Red Cross Hosp, Japan)

Radiology 199:85–90, 1996 2–3

Background.—Patients with long-term ulcerative colitis are at increased risk for colorectal cancer. Although surveillance colonoscopy is used to diagnose precancerous lesions (dysplasia) in such patients, these lesions nevertheless, frequently go unrecognized. An attempt was made to determine whether dysplasia can be identified at barium enema examination. Correlations between radiologic findings and grade of dysplasia also were examined.

Patients and Methods.—Ten patients, including 7 men and 3 women, aged 34 to 81 years at diagnosis of ulcerative colitis, were studied. All patients had undergone surveillance colonoscopy, with 22 areas of dys-

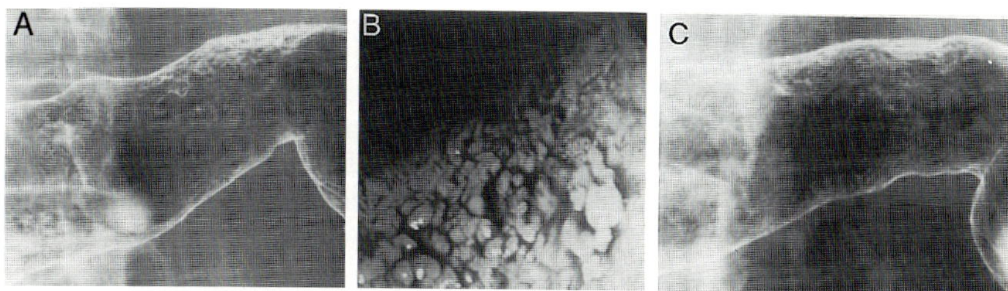

FIGURE 3.—Low-grade dysplasia in the splenic flexure. **A,** barium enema radiograph shows a 5 × 3–cm area (*white arrows*) of finely nodular mucosa that is sharply demarcated from the surrounding mucosa. A small focus of mucosal nodularity is also shown in the transverse colon (*black arrow*). **B,** colonoscopic image shows the dysplasia as a slightly elevated, nodular, plaquelike lesion. **C,** barium enema radiograph obtained 5 years earlier shows nodular mucosa in the transverse colon that is similar to the mucosa seen in **A.** However, the small focus of mucosal nodularity shown in **A** cannot be discerned. (Courtesy of Matsumoto T, Iida M, Kuroki F, et al. Dysplasia in ulcerative colitis: Is radiography adequate for diagnosis? *Radiology* 199:85–90, 1996. Radiological Society of North America.)

plasia identified. Double-contrast barium enema examinations were performed, and radiographic findings of these 22 areas of dysplasia were independently reviewed by 3 radiologists.

Findings.—Fourteen areas of dysplasia were depicted on radiographs. Compared with other segments of the colon, in the rectum and the sigmoid colon were noted to be less common sites of dysplasia. Radiographic traits were categorized as obvious nodular protrusions, irregular mucosa, or nodular protrusions with irregular mucosa. They were observed in 7, 5, and 2 lesions, respectively (Fig 3). Minute spiculations, found in the margins of the colonic lumen, were observed in 6 of the 7 areas of dysplasia classified as irregular mucosa. No correlation between radiologic features and histologic grade of dysplasia was identified (Fig 6). At histologic evaluation, each type of lesion, including evident protrusions and nodular mucosa, were found to consist of both carcinoma and dysplasia. Therefore, colonoscopy must be performed after radiography to obtain

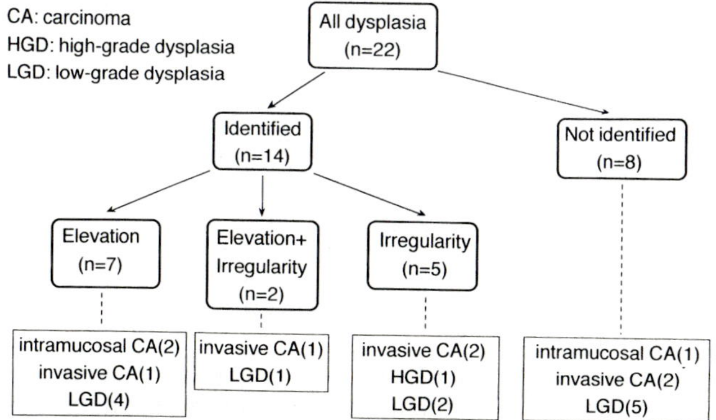

FIGURE 6.—Chart shows radiographic features and grades of dysplasia. (Courtesy of Matsumoto T, Iida M, Kuroki F, et al: Dysplasia in ulcerative colitis: Is radiography adequate for diagnosis? *Radiology* 199:85–90, 1996. Radiological Society of North America.)

TABLE.—Correlation of Mucosal Abnormalities in 699 Bowel Segments Depicted at Both Colonoscopy and DCBE

Abnormality	κ Value (%) CD (n = 51)	UC (n = 48)
Mucosal		
Normal	74	75
Fine granularity	0	91
Coarse granularity	100	86
Aphthoid erosions	83	0
Ulcers		
Superficial	75	87
Deep	62	74
Longitudinal	74	56
Serpiginous	78	65
Ulcerations		
Few scattered	33	51
Extensive	84	88
Complete	93	92
Abnormal surrounding mucosa	22	52
Cobblestones	60	0
Pseudopolyps	94	85
Structural		
Normal	93	85
Fold thickening	93	84
Loss of haustration	93	96
Tubular narrowing	99	94
Shortening	100	71
Stricture	87	77
Coarse scarring	68	0
Iliocecal valve		
Gaping	0	100
Narrowed	100	0
Distribution of lesions		
Asymmetric	83	0
Symmetric	0	77
Type of involvement		
Rectal	68	72
Continuous	96	88
Skip lesions	77	0

(Courtesy of Dijkstra J, Reeders JWAJ, Tytgat GNJ: Idiopathic inflammatory bowel disease: Endoscopic-radiologic correlation. *Radiology* 197:369–375, 1995. Radiological Society of North America.)

▶ The double-contrast BE retains an important complementary role to endoscopy in patients with inflammatory bowel disease (IBD), primarily because the entire colon and the terminal ileum can be assessed routinely with BE, whereas complete endoscopy is frequently impossible. The higher incidence of skip lesions, strictures, and carcinomas in IBD makes this feature especially pertinent. Although endoscopy undoubtedly reveals some cases of superficial erosions missed by BE, the DCBE remains the most accurate means of assessing fistulas, strictures, perforations, and the depth of ulceration.

M.P. Federle, M.D.

"Acute" Fat Deposition in Bowel Wall Submucosa: CT Appearance

Muldowney SM, Balfe DM, Hammerman A, et al (Washington Univ, St Louis, Mo; St Elizabeth's Hosp, Granite City, Ill)

J Comput Assist Tomogr 19:390–393, 1995 2–5

Background.—In patients with long-term chronic illnesses such as inflammatory bowel disease, the deposition of submucosal fat in small and large bowel can and does occur. Although this occurrence is believed to be indicative of long-standing disease duration, submucosal fat deposition has been observed in a short period of time, as described in the present report.

Patients and Findings.—Four patients, aged 44, 35, 31, and 23, respectively, with diagnoses of lymphoma or leukemia, were evaluated with serial CT examinations. Normal CT findings initially were documented in all 4 patients. All patients underwent cytoreductive chemotherapy for treatment of their diseases. Serial CT examinations showed subsequent fat-attenuation bowel wall thickening, which had occurred in a relatively short time period: 12, 36, 67, and 186 days, respectively. Hounsfield unit measurements confirmed the presence of fatty deposition in all patients. In 2 patients, pathologic examination of bowel specimens also showed lobules of mature fat confined to the submucosa, which consisted of morphologically bland adipocytes separated by narrow bands of fairly acellular fibrous tissue and stromal blood vessels. In 3 of the 4 patients, wall thickening was originally thought to have resulted from other causes, including intussusception or colitis.

Conclusions.—The occurrence of submucosal fat deposition in bowel wall is not restricted to patients with long-term, chronic illnesses. Fatty infiltration can occur in a fairly short time, and is likely to take place after cytoreductive treatment.

▶ Characterization of the nature of CT-detected bowel wall thickening can be helpful in narrowing the differential diagnosis. Soft-tissue density submucosal tissue may be neoplastic or inflammatory, whereas fat density submucosal thickening (the "halo" or "target" sign) has been associated with chronic inflammatory bowel disease. These authors have made a novel observation of acute submucosal fat deposition not related to bowel disease at all apparently, but rather due to prior cytoreductive drug therapy. The presumed mechanism is fatty metamorphosis due to stimulation of proliferation of adipocytes.

M.P. Federle, M.D.

Glutaraldehyde Colitis: Radiologic Findings

Birnbaum BA, Gordon RB, Jacobs JE (Univ of Pennsylvania, Philadelphia; New York VA Med Ctr; New York Univ Med Ctr)
Radiology 195:131–134, 1995 2–6

Introduction.—For high-level disinfection of flexible gastrointestinal endoscopes, glutaraldehyde (2% solution) is the most common chemical germicide used. Known to be toxic and an irritant, this aldehyde agent is allergenic to those handling endoscopes, and its vapors may cause nasal, ocular, and respiratory irritation. During endoscopic procedures, inadvertent contact of glutaraldehyde with colonic mucosa has lead to a self-limited syndrome of tenesmus and bloody diarrhea. The radiologic appearance of glutaraldehyde-induced toxic colitis was determined so that its features could be differentiated from those of colonic ischemia.

Methods.—During a 6-year period, 4 patients with glutaraldehyde-induced colitis were seen, and a retrospective review was performed with their clinical and imaging findings. One of the patients was a 65-year-old man with diverticulosis coli who had a sigmoidoscopy. On the endoscopy tray, glutaraldehyde in a light green container was included. A nurse may

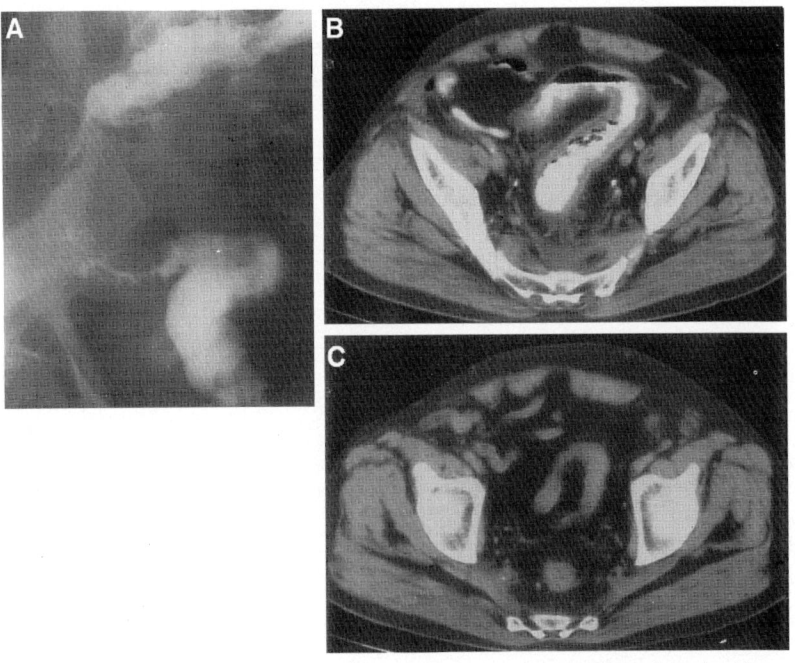

FIGURE 3.—**A**, anteroposterior image obtained during an enema study performed with use of diatrizoate meglumine (Hypaque 30%; Winthrop Pharmaceuticals, New York, NY) demonstrates an irritable rectosigmoid colon with thickened mucosal folds. **B**, contrast-enhanced CT scan shows corresponding mural thickening of the sigmoid colon and presacral fluid. **C**, follow-up CT scan demonstrates an appearance unremarkable for a collapsed rectosigmoid colon with resolution of presacral edematous changes. (Courtesy of Birnbaum BA, Gordon RB, Jacobs JE: Glutaraldehyde colitis: Radiologic findings. *Radiology* 195:131–134, 1995. Radiological Society of North America.)

have mistakenly assumed that the glutaraldehyde was water and inadvertently used it to check the patency of the endoscope channels and to flush the channels of the endoscope during the procedure. After sigmoidoscopy, several hours later the patient had bloody diarrhea, sudden nausea, and severe abdominal pain. Computed tomography showed homogenous, circumferential, mural thickening of the rectosigmoid colon (Fig 3).

Results.—All 4 patients had abdominal pain, cramps, and rectal bleeding within 48 hours of uncomplicated colonoscopy or sigmoidoscopy. The clinical presentation mimicked that of colonic ischemia. Enteric pathogens were excluded through sample cultures. In all patients, CT showed circumferential thickening of the colonic wall in a left-sided distribution. In 2 patients, heterogeneous mural enhancement (target-sign appearance) was noted. Mural wall thickening and conservative management was confirmed by follow-up CT studies.

Conclusion.—Colonic ischemia may be mimicked by the clinical and radiologic features of glutaraldehyde-induced toxic colitis. In patients in whom hemorrhagic colitis develops immediately after colonoscopy, this complication should be suspected.

► This article serves to make radiologists aware of another cause of acute colitis. "Postcolonoscopy colitis" should be preventable by following appropriate protocols for cleansing endoscopes, including thorough washing and forced air drying after disinfection with glutaraldehyde.

M.P. Federle, M.D.

Midgut Carcinoid Tumors: CT Findings and Biochemical Profiles

Woodard PK, Feldman JM, Paine SS, et al (Duke Univ, Durham, NC; Durham VA Med Ctr, Durham, NC)

J Comput Assist Tomogr 19:400–405, 1995 2–7

Introduction.—About 20% of gastrointestinal carcinoid tumors arise from the embryologic midgut, which is the most common origin for metastatic carcinoid in the abdomen. The abdominal CT findings of only midgut carcinoid tumors were described, and these findings were correlated with biochemical profiles.

Methods.—The abdominal CT findings of 52 patients with midgut carcinoid tumors were retrospectively reviewed for the presence of mesenteric and peritoneal disease, liver metastasis, lymphadenopathy, bowel changes, and the presence of the primary tumor. Primary tumor sites were the cecum for 1 patient, the jejunum for 1 patient, and the ileum for 43 patients. The association between these findings and the serum and platelet serotonin and urine 5-hydroxyindolacetic acid levels was evaluated using logistic regression models.

Results.—In 34 of 52 patients, liver metastases were seen. In 26 of 52 patients, nonspecific mesenteric soft tissue stranding was seen, and in 25 of 52 patients, a discrete mesenteric mass was seen. In 16 of 25 patients, these

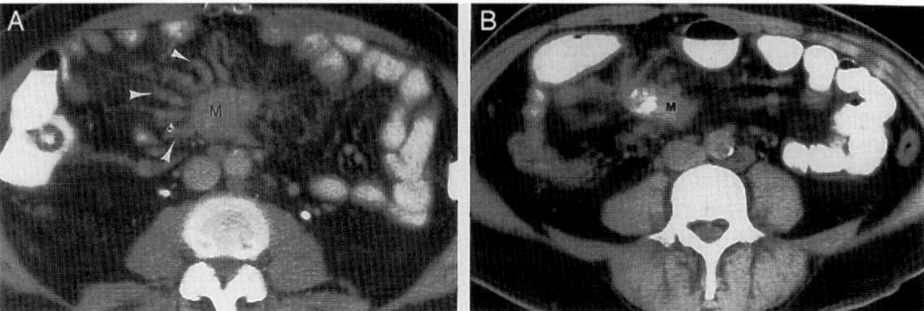

FIGURE 1.—Computed tomography in 2 separate patients demonstrating a mesenteric mass (*M*) with radiating soft tissue spokes (*arrowheads,* **A**) and a mass with bulky calcification (**B**). (Courtesy of Woodard PK, Feldman JM, Paine SS, et al: Midgut carcinoid tumors: CT findings and biochemical profiles. *J Comput Assist Tomogr* 19:400–405, 1995.)

masses had linear, radiating soft tissue spokes, and 10 of 25 patients had calcification in the masses (Fig 1). In 14 of 52 patients, retroperitoneal lymphadenopathy was present; in 11 of 52 patients, mesenteric lymphadenopathy was seen; in 11 of 52 patients, carcinomatosis was present; and in 9 of 52 patients, bowel wall thickening was seen. Bowel obstruction was present in 6 patients (Fig 5). The presence of liver metastases was significantly associated with elevated serum serotonin, platelet serotonin, and urine 5-hydroxyindolacetic acid levels. There was a significant association between elevated platelet serotonin levels and the presence of a mesenteric mass.

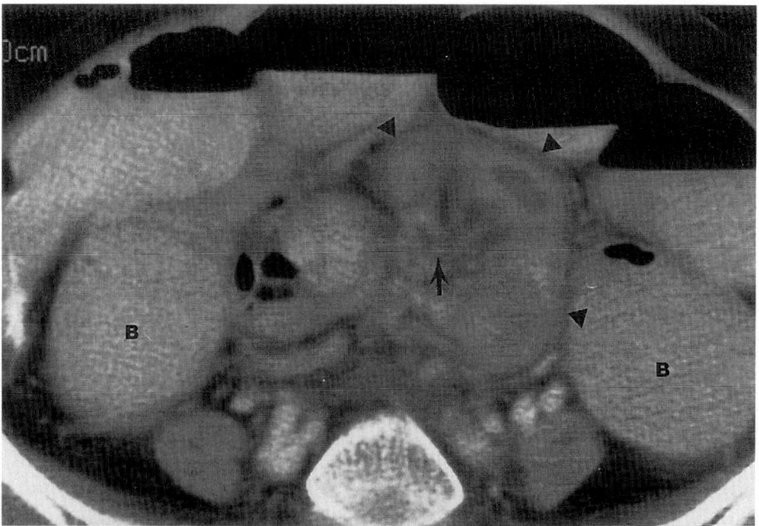

FIGURE 5.—Computed tomography showing thick-walled, narrowed loop of small bowel (*arrowheads*) causing a small bowel obstruction (note dilated, fluid-filled small bowel, *B*). The abnormal loop is associated with soft tissue strands in the mesentary (*arrow*). (Courtesy of Woodard PK, Feldman JM, Paine SS, et al: Midgut carcinoid tumors: CT findings and biochemical profiles. *J Comput Assist Tomogr* 19:400–405, 1995.)

Conclusion.—Liver metastases, nonspecific mesenteric soft tissue changes, a discrete mesenteric mass with radiating soft tissue spokes, often with calcification, and lymphadenopathy were the most common findings of a midgut carcinoid tumor. The presence of elevated biochemical levels are associated strongly with liver metastases. Mesenteric masses are associated with elevated platelet serotonin levels. Stromal cells may be stimulated by platelet serotonin to produce mass formation and mesenteric fibrosis.

► This is by far the largest series of carcinoid tumors with an extensive description of associated CT findings. Whereas these authors noted a much higher prevalence of certain findings (e.g., calcified mesenteric masses) than others have reported, their findings are consistent with our experience and should serve as a useful reference.

M.P. Federle, M.D.

Liver

Hepatic Enhancement During Helical CT: A Comparison of Moderate Rate Uniphasic and Biphasic Contrast Injection Protocols

Birnbaum BA, Jacobs JE, Yin D (Univ of Pennsylvania, Philadelphia)
AJR 165:853–858, 1995 2–8

Background.—Helical CT offers an improved scanning repetition rate, which permits pre-equilibrium hepatic scanning within a shorter temporal window. To make sure scanning takes place at the highest possible level of hepatic enhancement, it is essential to choose the proper scan delay time. Moderate-rate uniphasic and biphasic contrast injection protocols for hepatic enhancement were studied, including a determination of the optimal scan delay times for hepatic helical CT.

Methods.—The randomized study included 150 patients undergoing hepatic helical CT. They were assigned to receive 150 mL of iothalamate meglumine (42.3 g of iodine) using either a 3 mL/sec uniphasic technique; a 2 mL/sec uniphasic technique; or a biphasic technique, using 3 mL/sec

TABLE 3.—Hepatic Enhancement Data

Protocol	Peak Enhancement (H)*	Time to Peak (sec)†	Time to Equilibirum (sec)‡
3 ml/sec uniphasic	64 ± 15	73 ± 8	90 ± 10
2 ml/sec uniphasic	62 ± 15	96 ± 10	123 ± 12
3 ml/sec biphasic	52 ± 10	141 ± 9	159 ± 7

Note.—Values are mean ± 1 SD.
* Significant difference between biphasic protocol and both uniphasic protocols observed ($P < 0.001$).
† Significant differences between all 3 protocols observed ($P < 0.0001$).
‡ Significant differences between all 3 protocols observed ($P < 0.0001$).
(Courtesy of Birnbaum BA, Jacobs JE, Yin D: Hepatic enhancement during helical CT: A comparison of moderate rate uniphasic and biphasic contrast injection protocols. *AJR* 165:853–858, 1995.)

TABLE 4.—Contrast Enhancement Index Data

Protocol	Optimal Scan Delay (sec)*	Contract-Enhancement Index (H/sec)†	Optimal Scanning Interval (sec)‡
3 ml/sec uniphasic	50 ± 8	385 ± 398	25 ± 13
2 ml/sec uniphasic	75 ± 7	397 ± 412	25 ± 16
3 ml/sec biphasic	119 ± 8	123 ± 194	16 ± 18

Note.—Values are mean ± 1 SD.
* Significant differences between all 3 protocols observed ($P < 0.0001$).
† 50-H threshold. Significant difference between biphasic and both uniphasic protocols observed ($P < 0.0001$).
‡ Significant differences between biphasic and both uniphasic protocols observed ($P < 0.01$).
(Courtesy of Birnbaum BA, Jacobs JE, Yin D: Hepatic enhancement during helical CT: A comparison of moderate rate uniphasic and biphasic contrast injection protocols. *AJR* 165:853–858, 1995.)

(50 mL) and 1 mL/sec (100 mL). The dynamic incremental CT data were used to create aortic and hepatic enhancement curves. The 3 protocols were compared for maximal hepatic enhancement. Also, contrast enhancement parameters were modeled for a 38-second helical acquisition.

Results.—Peak hepatic enhancement was 64 H for the 3 mL/sec uniphasic protocol and 62 H for the 2 mL/sec uniphasic protocol, compared with 52 H for the 3 mL/sec biphasic protocol (Table 3). Contrast enhancement indices were 385, 397, and 123 H/sec, respectively (Table 4). Optimal scan delay times were 50, 75, and 119 sec (Fig 1).

Conclusions.—In hepatic helical CT, a moderate-rate uniphasic injection protocol provides better hepatic enhancement without the long delay times required by a moderate-rate biphasic injection protocol. In contrast to previous reports, the new results suggest that the hepatic enhancement

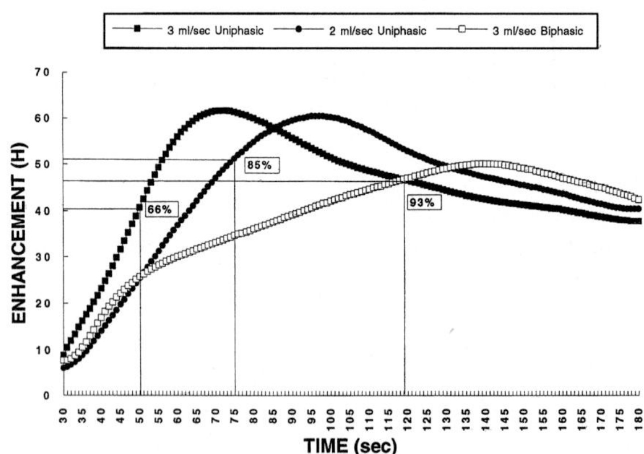

FIGURE 1.—Statistically fitted hepatic enhancement curves generated from pooled patient data: (**1**) 3 mL/sec uniphasic injection protocol: peak = 72 sec, equilibrium = 87 sec, 50-sec delay corresponds to 66% maximum enhancement; (**2**) 2 mL/sec uniphasic injection protocol: peak = 97 sec, equilibrium = 124 sec, 75-sec delay corresponds to 85% maximum enhancement; (**3**) 3 mL sec [50 mL], 1 mL/sec [100 mL] biphasic injection protocol: peak = 140 sec, equilibrium = 162 sec, 119-sec delay corresponds to 93% maximum hepatic enhancement. (Courtesy of Birnbaum BA, Jacobs JE, Yin D: Hepatic enhancement during helical CT: A comparison of moderate rate uniphasic and biphasic contrast injection protocols. *AJR* 165:853–858, 1995.)

provided by a uniphasic injection may be similar to that achieved with a high–flow-rate biphasic injection.

▶ Optimal hepatic CT imaging relies on maximum hepatic enhancement but must be completed before the onset of equilibrium, when the enhancement curves for aortic and hepatic parenchyma begin to decline in parallel fashion. For nonhelical CT scanners, the slower scanning repetition rates necessitated the use of biphasic contrast medium injections to allow hepatic imaging to be completed before equilibrium. However, for helical CT scanning of the liver, rapid uniphasic bolus infusion of contrast medium is clearly superior. Note that the more rapid rates of infusion cause the peak hepatic enhancement to occur earlier as well as higher, and so scanning should be initiated sooner than with slow (1–2 mL/sec) bolus infusions. The time to peak enhancement is actually somewhat variable, in large part due to variations in cardiac output and circulation time. Methods that allow on-line monitoring of vascular and liver enhancement (such as General Electric's "Smart Prep" program) offer optimal timing of CT scanning during bolus infusion.

M.P. Federle, M.D.

Effect of Rate of Contrast Medium Injection on Hepatic Enhancement at CT

Garcia PA, Bonaldi VM, Bret PM, et al (McGill Univ, Montreal)
Radiology 199:185–189, 1996 2–9

Purpose.—The best way to administer contrast material in the CT evaluation of hepatic tumors has been debated. The rate of injection is a key point, because conventional acquisitions require either monophasic low flow rates or biphasic injection with initial high flow rates, whereas helical acquisitions generally use high monophasic injection rates. The effects of contrast injection rates on CT liver enhancement were investigated.

Methods.—The analysis included 45 patients undergoing follow-up CT scans of the liver. Those with conditions that could affect portal venous flow were excluded. Fifty-three paired examinations were divided into 5 different groups, according to the rate of contrast material delivery, for comparison: group A, 2 vs. 3 mL/sec; group B, 2 vs. 4.5 mL/sec; group C, 3 vs. 4.5 mL/sec; group D, 3 vs. 6 mL/sec; and group E, 4.5 vs. 6 mL/sec.

Results.—Faster contrast injection rates were associated with shorter times to peak enhancement. This difference was significant only in groups B and D, which had extreme differences in contrast injection rates. Within each group of paired examinations, there was little difference in the maximum enhancement (Table 2). Also, no significant differences were detected on comparison of mean enhancement values measured at 3-second intervals (figure) or in the percentage of sections with enhancement of greater than 40 Hounsfield units (Table 4).

TABLE 2.—Live-Enhancement With Different Rates of Injection

Enhancement	Patient Group and Injection Rates (mL/sec)									
	A		B		C		D		E	
	2	3	2	4.5	3	4.5	3	6	4.5	6
Peak liver enhancement (HU)*	57	58	48	47	55	58	55	54	62	61
95% CI	(42, 72)	(49, 66)	(43, 53)	(39, 54)	(48, 63)	(49, 67)	(45, 64)	(44, 65)	(53, 71)	(52, 69)
Time to peak enhancement (sec)†	83	62	82	54	63	57	69	53	56	49
95% CI	(59, 106)	(50, 73)	(73, 91)	(46, 61)	(56, 69)	(51, 64)	(60, 77)	(46,61)	(49,63)	(42,57)

* *P* values for comparison of peak liver enhancement with the 2 injection rates within each group are as follows: group **A**, 0.88; group **B**, 0.69; group **C**, 0.62; group **D**, 0.97; group **E**, 0.58.
† *P* values for comparison of time to peak enhancement with the 2 injection rates within each group are as follows: group **A**, 0.08; group **B**, 0.001; group **C**, 0.07; group **D**, 0.02; group **E**, 0.18.
Abbreviations: HU, Hounsfield units; *CI*, confidence interval.
(Courtesy of Garcia PA, Bonaldi VM, Bret PM, et al: Effect of rate of contrast medium injection on hepatic enhancement at CT. *Radiology* 199:185–189, 1996. Radiological Society of North America.)

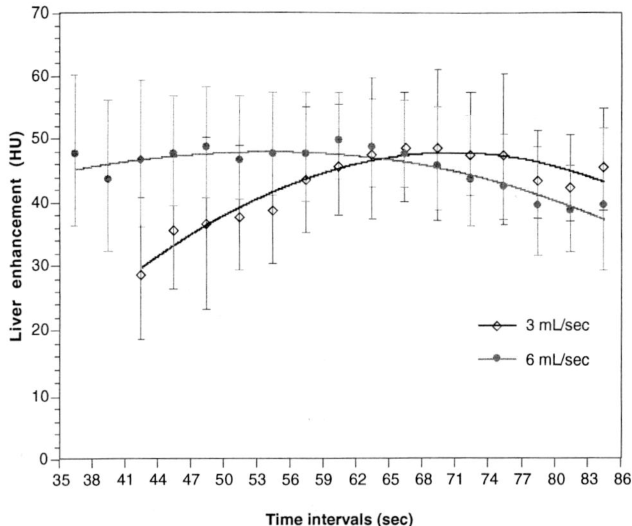

FIGURE.—Time-attenuation curves obtained at 3-second intervals at injection rates of 3 and 6 mL/sec (group D). *HU* denotes Hounsfield units. (Courtesy of Garcia PA, Bonaldi VM, Bret PM, et al: Effect of rate of contrast medium injecton on hepatic enhancement at CT. *Radiology* 199:185–189, 1996. Radiological Society of North America.)

Conclusion.—Increasing the rate of contrast injection on CT examination of the liver reduces the time to maximum liver enhancement. However, it has no effect on the maximum level of enhancement. Thus, high rates of contrast injection are of no practical value during routine CT scanning of the liver.

▶ This is an intriguing and well-performed study with important implications. Nevertheless, I urge caution and careful reading of the full manuscript before you rush out and change your CT protocols. Other authors have reported greater hepatic enhancement with rates of 5 vs. 2.5 mL/sec, and slower rates of infusion clearly produce suboptimal liver enhancement in our own studies.[1] Everyone agrees that keeping volume constant and increased rates of injection result in shorter time to peak liver enhancement and a faster fall to equilibrium phase. Therefore, when using a nonhelical scanner, you do not want to inject contrast medium at 4 or 5 mL/sec to evaluate the liver. Rates of 2.5 or 3 mL/sec, with a delay of about 45–50 seconds are preferable. However, when using a helical scanner, you should take advantage of more rapid infusion rates (4 or 5 mL/sec) and the faster scan time when examining the liver for possible hypervascular tumors, and you should scan the liver in both the arterial (20–45 seconds) and portal venous dominant (60–85) seconds phases.

M.P. Federle, M.D.

TABLE 4.—Ratios of Sections With Attenuation Value Greater than 40 Hounsfield Units

	Patient Group and Injection Rates (mL/sec)									
	A		B		C		D		E	
Sections	2	3	2	4.5	3	4.5	3	6	4.5	6
No. of sections >40 HU	71	105	73	59	104	114	65	65	154	121
Total no. of sections	111	129	117	117	137	145	101	107	163	154
Ratio	0.64	0.81	0.62	0.50	0.76	0.79	0.64	0.61	0.94	0.79

Note: In each group, $P > 0.05$ by means of the rank sum test.
Abbreviation: HU, Hounsfield units.
(Courtesy of Garcia PA, Bonaldi VM, Bret PM, et al: Effect of rate of contrast medium injection on hepatic enhancement at CT. *Radiology* 199:185–189, 1996. Radiological Society of North America.)

Reference

1. Chambers TP, Baron RL, Lush RM: Hepatic CT enhancement: II. Alterations in contrast medium volume and rate of injection within the same patients. *Radiology* 193:518–522, 1994.

Hepatic Helical CT: Effect of Reduction of Iodine Dose of Intravenous Contrast Material on Hepatic Contrast Enhancement

Freeny PC, Gardner JC, vonIngersleben G, et al (Univ of Washington, Seattle)

Radiology 197:89–93, 1995 2–10

Introduction.—Scan acquisition times are shorter with helical CT compared with incremental CT. Helical CT may therefore be able to reduce the volume of contrast material or the total iodine dose without compromising hepatic contrast enhancement (HCE). The effects of reducing the iodine dose during helical CT on HCE values were assessed.

Methods.—The randomized study included 111 patients who were suspected of having liver disease and were undergoing abdominal helical CT. The patients were assigned into 4 contrast protocol groups, based on the concentration (in milligrams of iodine per mL/volume [in mL] of iodine). Patients in group 1 received ioversol, 320/150/48; those in group 2 received ioversol, 320/100/32; those in group 3 received iohexol, 300/150/45; and those in group 2 received ioversol, 300/100/30. Otherwise, all 4 groups underwent the same helical CT scanning procedure. Time-attenuation curves were calculated for each group, as were the mean HCE, contrast enhancement index (CEI), and optimal liver scanning interval (OLSI).

Results.—Groups 1 and 3 had significantly better time-attenuation curves, mean HCE (Tables 1 and 2), CEI, and OLSI than groups 2 and 4 (Fig 1). When the volume of contrast agent was decreased from 150 to 100 mL, the mean HCE decreased by 27%, CEI decreased by 69%, and OLSI decreased from 80% to 100% to 0% to 43% at a threshold level of 40 to 60 HU (Fig 3).

TABLE 1.—Mean HCE: Individual Groups

				HCE (HU)				
Group	No. of Patients	Volume (mL)	Concentration (mg I/mL)	Mean	Minimum	Maximum	Standard Deviation	Standard Error
1	33	150	320	68	24	155	26.9	4.7
2	26	100	320	50	31	85	27.6	6.2
3	27	150	300	64	38	90	16.1	3.1
4	25	100	300	45	26	73	12.3	2.5

(Courtesy of Freeny PC, Gardner JC, vonIngersleben G, et al: Hepatic helical CT: Effect of reduction of iodine dose of intravenous contrast material on hepatic contrast enhancement. *Radiology* 197:89–93, 1995. Radiological Society of North America.)

TABLE 2.—Mean HCE: Group Comparisons

Groups	Volume (mL)	Concentration (mg I/mL)	Mean Difference in HCE	*P* Value*
1/3	150/150	320/300	4	NSS
2/4	100/100	320/300	5	NSS
1/2	150/100	320/320	18	<.01
1/4	150/100	320/300	23	<.01
3/2	150/100	300/320	11	<.05
3/4	150/100	300/300	19	<.01

* Scheffe and Tukey tests

Abbreviation: NSS, not statistically significant.

(Courtesy of Freeny PC, Gardner JC, vonIngersleben G, et al: Hepatic helical CT: Effect of reduction of iodine dose of intravenous contrast material on hepatic contrast enhancement. *Radiology* 197:89–93, 1995. Radiological Society of North America.)

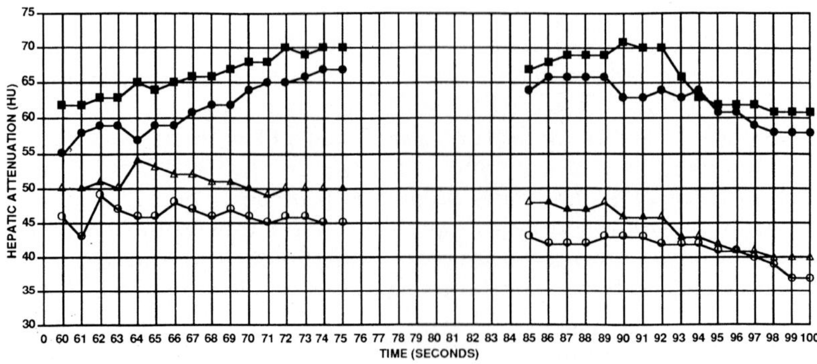

a.

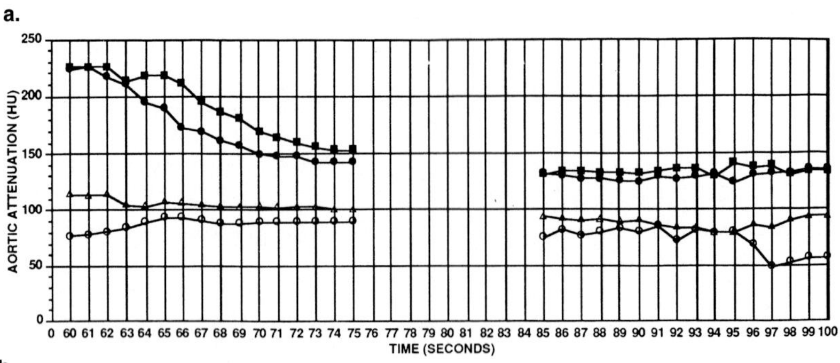

b.

FIGURE 1.—**A,** hepatic time-attenuation curves for helical CT groups 1–4. The gap between 75 and 85 seconds represents the 10-second interhelical delay. **B,** aortic time-attenuation curve for helical groups 1–4. *Solid square* = group 1, *open triangle* = group 2, *solid circle* = group 3, *open circle* = group 4. (Courtesy of Freeny PC, Gardner JC, vonIngersleben G, et al: Hepatic helical CT: Effect of reduction of iodine dose of intravenous contrast material on hepatic contrast enhancement. *Radiology* 197:89–93, 1995. Radiological Society of North America.)

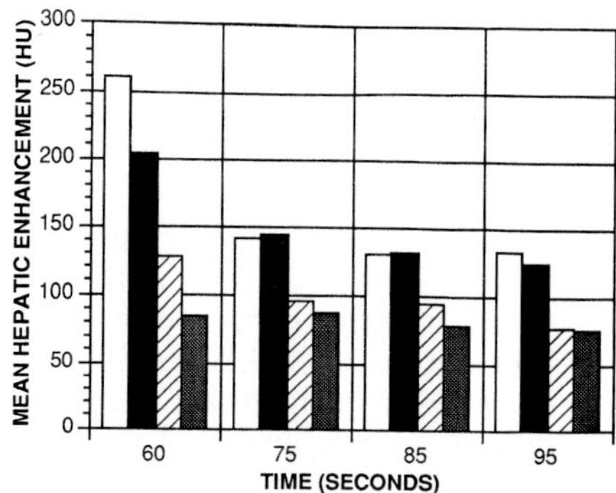

FIGURE 3.—Change in mean HCE for groups 1–4 at 4 times. Comparison of groups 1 (*white bar*) and 2 (*striped bar*) shows that HCE is greater for group 1 by 24%, 40%, 40%, and 53% at each of the 4 times. Comparison of groups 3 (*black bar*) and 4 (*cross-hatched bar*) shows that the HCE for group 3 is 20%, 49%, 49%, and 57% greater at each of the 4 times. (Courtesy of Freeny PC, Gardner JC, vonIngersleben G, et al: Hepatic helical CT: Effect of reduction of iodine dose of intravenous contrast material on hepatic contrast enhancement. *Radiology* 197:89–93, 1995. Radiological Society of North America.)

Conclusions.—Decreasing the iodine dose in contrast material for helical CT scanning can significantly decrease all HCE values, including CEI and OLSI. This could potentially decrease the detection of focal hypervascular hepatic lesions. The results suggest that diagnostic information may be lost when the contrast volume is reduced from 150 to 100 mL.

► One of the initial assumptions for helical CT was that it would allow a decrease in the concentration and/or volume of contrast material without compromising scan quality. In fact, if one is able to optimally time the arrival of the bolus on contrast material in the liver, "adequate" enhancement of the liver (50 H) can be achieved with 100 mL of 320 mg I/mL contrast agents, especially for smaller patients. However, as Freeny and his colleagues have shown in this article, the 2 most important measures of liver enhancement, the mean HCE and the CHI, are both consistently and significantly better with high volume (150 mL) vs. low volume (100 mL) injections. The larger volume also allows the entire liver helical scan sequence to be completed during optimal enhancement.

Let me put this into practical terms. If you are scanning an average-to-heavy patient and are using less than 150 mL of contrast medium, you are missing a *substantial* number of hepatic tumors.

M.P. Federle, M.D.

CT Evaluation of Hepatic Tumors: Comparison of CT With Arterial Portography CT with Infusion Hepatic Arteriography, and Simultaneous Use of Both Techniques

Irie T, Takeshita K, Wada Y, et al (Natl Defense Med College, Saitama, Japan)
AJR 164:1407–1412, 1995 2–11

Background.—Although CT with arterial portography (CTAP) is the most sensitive technique for detecting hepatic tumors, small tumors can go unnoticed. Also, the appearance of small nodules detected with CTAP alone can be nonspecific. Another sensitive method for detecting hepatic tumors is CT with infusion hepatic arteriography (CTIHA). It was hypothesized that CTAP and CTIHA may be able to detect tumors that are not detectable by one another.

Methods.—Fifty-four patients undergoing partial liver resection were assessed with CTAP and/or CTIHA preoperatively. Seventy-seven malignant and 15 benign nodules were confirmed histologically in these patients.

Findings.—Eighty-eight percent of the malignant nodules were identified by CTAP, 83% by CTIHA, and 90% by simultaneous interpretation of both images. The differences among these 3 modalities were nonsignificant. Sixteen malignant and 12 benign small nodules were identified by CTIHA. Rim enhancement was evident on 13 of these malignant tumors and on 2 benign ones. A diagnostic accuracy of 82% was associated with the use of rim enhancement as the criterion for malignancy of these small nodules (Fig 6).

Conclusions.—The ability of CTAP, CTIHA, and combined CTAP and CTIHA to identify malignant hepatic tumors is comparable. Computed tomography with arterial portography alone is the modality of choice for

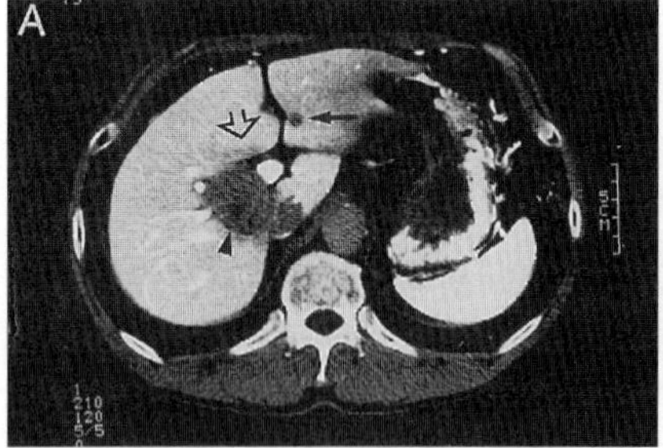

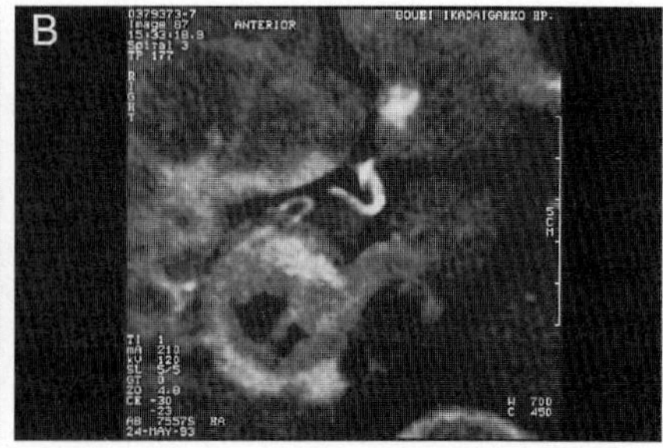

FIGURE 6.—Hemangioma of benign small nodule (8-mm diameter) without rim enhancement. Pathologic examination revealed small nodule to be a hemangioma and large one to be a hepatocellular carcinoma. **A,** CT scan obtained during arterial portography shows a small nodule (*solid arrow*) in lateral segment and a large one (*arrowhead*) in right lobe. *Open arrow* points to area of decreased portal perfusion anterior to porta hepatis. **B,** on CT scan obtained during infusion hepatic arteriography, the small nodule is hyperattenuating (*solid arrow*), but no rim enhancement is seen. Large nodule has rim enhancement (*arrowhead*). Area of decreased portal perfusion anterior to porta hepatis on **A** is homogeneously enhanced on **B** (*open arrow*); however, surgical findings revealed no abnormality there. (Courtesy of Irie T, Takeshita K, Wada Y, et al: CT evaluation of hepatic tumors: Comparison of CT with arterial portography, CT with infusion hepatic arteriography, and simultaneous use of both techniques. *AJR* 164:1407–1412, 1995.)

detecting malignant hepatic tumors. Distinguishing between malignant and benign small nodules can be facilitated by CTIHA.

► I agree that CTAP is the most sensitive and useful final test for potentially resectable hepatic tumors in most cases. However, in patients with cirrhosis with portal hypertension, CTAP is frequently nondiagnostic due to hepatofugal shunting of blood (and contrast medium). I would add that neither CTAP nor CT arteriography should ever be interpreted in isolation, as they are nonspecific and frequently show pseudotumors. We still find that a good IV bolus-enhanced CT scan is the best and most practical way to screen for and to characterize hepatic masses.

M.P. Federle, M.D.

Nontumorous Low-Attenuation Defects in the Liver on Helical CT During Arterial Portography: Frequency, Location, and Appearance

Bluemke DA, Soyer P, Fishman EK (Johns Hopkins Med Inst, Baltimore, Md; Centre Médico-Chirurgical Foch, Suresnes Cedex, France)

AJR 164:1141–1145, 1995 2–12

Background.—The use of helical CT during arterial portography (CTAP) can help detect low-attenuation defects in the liver that are the result of variations in the portal perfusion of the liver rather than intrahepatic tumor. The frequency, location, and appearance of these nontumorous low-attenuation defects as detected with helical CTAP were characterized.

Methods.—Three radiologists retrospectively reviewed the helical CTAP studies of 89 patients referred for the preoperative assessment of metastatic or primary liver tumors during 20 months. Findings on helical CTAP images were compared with findings at surgery in 53 patients, the results of the MR studies of 25 patients, and the findings of follow-up CT assessments in 11 patients.

TABLE 2.—Prevalence of Focal Nontumorous Perfusion Defects Detected on Helical CT During Arterial Portography

Location of Defect	No. (%) of Patients
Adjacent to gallbladder fossa	35 (39)
Porta hepatis	34 (38)
Subcapsular	13 (15)
Adjacent to falciform ligament	12 (13)
Hepatic surface, adjacent to rib	2 (2)
Posterior portion segment 2	1 (1)

Note: Total of 89 patients. Percentages do not add to 100% because some patients had more than 1 defect.

(Courtesy of Bluemke DA, Soyer P, Fishman EK: Nontumorous low-attenuation defects in the liver on helical CT during arterial portography: Frequency, location, and appearance. *AJR* 164:1141–1145, 1995.)

Findings.—A total of 97 nontumorous perfusion defects were detected in 68 patients. Thirty-five defects were found adjacent to the gallbladder fossa; 34, anterior to the porta hepatis; 13, in the subcapsular part of the liver; and 12, adjacent to the falciform ligament (Table 2). Nontumorous perfusion defects were typically wedge-shaped or flat and ranged from 8 to 20 mm.

Conclusions.—Nontumorous perfusion abnormalities have a characteristic appearance and location on helical CTAP images. These abnormalities are more common than reported previously with conventional CTAP. Clinicians must be familiar with the locations and typical appearances of nontumorous defects to avoid making false positive diagnoses (Figs 1 and 6).

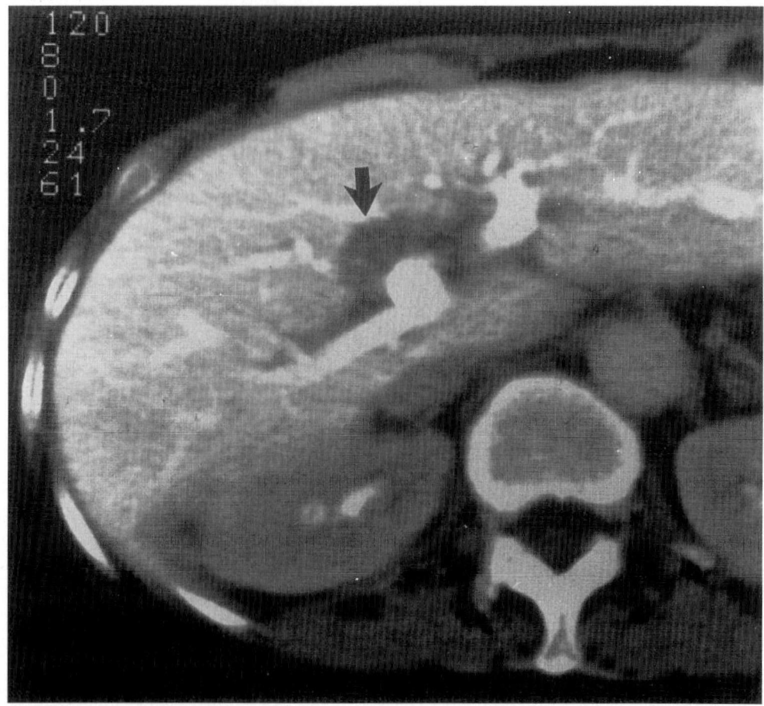

FIGURE 1.—Periportal perfusion defect. Helical CT scan obtained during arterial portography shows flat, nontumorous perfusion defect anterior to porta hepatis (*arrow*) in patient with hepatoma. Intraoperative sonography, surgical palpation, and inspection showed no evidence of tumor at that location. (Courtesy of Bluemke DA, Soyer P, Fishman EK: Nontumorous low-attenuation defects in the liver on helical CT during arterial portography: Frequency, location, and appearance. *AJR* 164:1141–1145, 1995.)

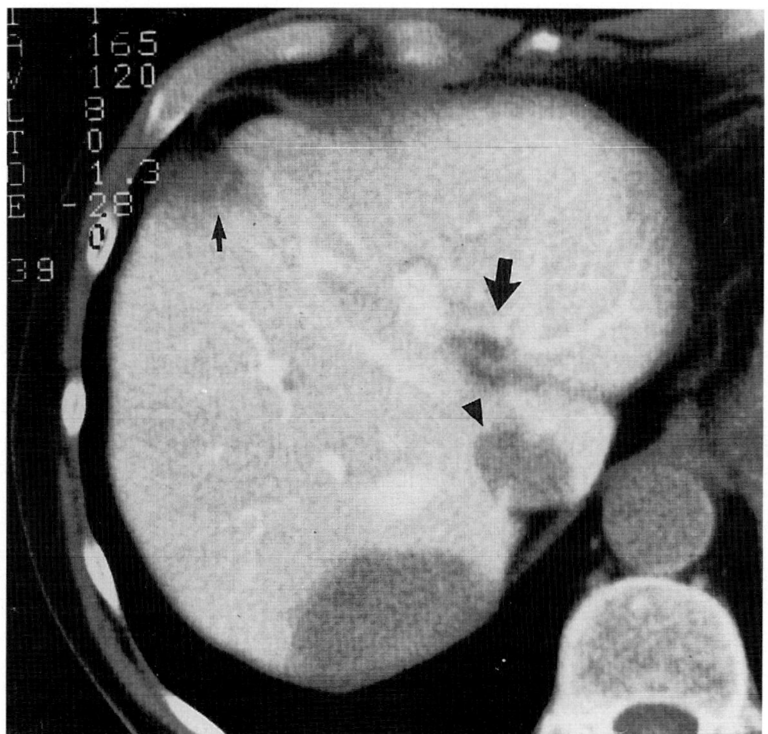

FIGURE 6.—Hepatic metastasis misinterpreted as perfusion defect. Helical CT scan obtained during arterial portography shows round, hypoattenuated perfusion defect (*large arrow*) extending along fissure of sinus venosum. A small vessel was retrospectively detected within lesion, which is not characteristic of nontumorous perfusion defects. At surgery, this defect was found to be due to metastatic colon cancer. A large metastasis is present posteriorly in right lobe (*large arrowhead*). Decreased attenuation anteriorly in right lobe is due to partial volume averaging with diaphragm (*small arrow*). *Small arrowhead* indicates the inferior vena cava. (Courtesy of Bluemke DA, Soyer P, Fishman EK: Nontumorous low-attenuation defects in the liver on helical CT during arterial portography: Frequency, location, and appearance. *AJR* 164:1141–1145, 1995.)

► We have also noted an increased incidence of perfusion defects on CTAP studies performed on helical CT scanners, compared with our earlier reported experience with conventional scanners. I believe that these can be minimized by delaying the CT scans beyond the 30–35 second postinjection that these authors used. We either delay scanning for 45–50 seconds or perform a second helical series through the liver after a 60-second delay. Although some arterial recirculation of contrast medium undoubtedly occurs, this does not seem to decrease detection of tumor defects, whereas benign perfusion defects definitively decrease. As these and other authors have noted, most perfusion defects have a characteristic subcapsular location, including the porta hepatis and gallbladder fossa, and are correlated with aberrant venous drainage.

M.P. Federle, M.D.

Focal Hypoechoic Regions in the Liver at the Porta Hepatis: Prevalence in Ambulatory Patients

Kester NL, Elmore SG (Smith-Glynn-Callaway Clinic, Springfield, Mo)

J Ultrasound Med 14:649–652, 1995 2–13

Purpose.—Previous reports have suggested that focal hypoechoic regions in the liver at the porta hepatis are an unusual finding. However, experience suggests that this finding may be more frequent than generally thought, especially in obese patients. The prevalence of focal hypoechoic regions in the liver at the porta hepatis was prospectively studied.

Methods.—The study included 534 consecutive ambulatory patients undergoing hepatic sonography. On review by a sonographer, scans with at least 1 focal hypoechoic region adjacent to the gallbladder or portal vein in 2 imaging planes were classified as positive.

Results.—Five percent of patients had at least 1 focal hypoechoic area (Fig 1). Eighty-two percent of the patients with positive scans had at least 1 hypoechoic area adjacent to the gallbladder. Sixty-five percent of the patients with positive scans were obese, compared with 43% of the remaining patients. Seventy-nine percent of the patients with positive scans also had sonographic evidence of diffuse fatty infiltration of the liver.

Conclusions.—Focal hypoechoic regions in the liver at the porta hepatis may be detected with hepatic sonography in about 5% of ambulatory patients. This finding is more frequent in obese patients than in nonobese

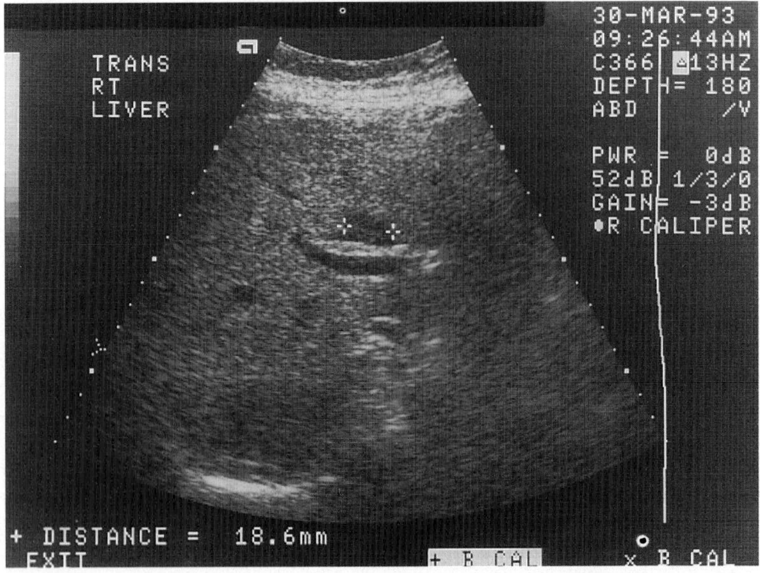

FIGURE 1.—Transverse ultrasonogram shows a small, well-defined hypoechoic focus anterior to the portal vein (*cursors*). (Courtesy of Kester NL, Elmore SG: Focal hypoechoic regions in the liver at the porta hepatis: Prevalence in ambulatory patients. *J Ultrasound Med* 14:649–652, 1995.)

patients. It is important not to mistake these hypoechoic areas for lesions of greater clinical significance.

► Focal sparing in an otherwise fatty liver has a characteristic appearance on ultrasound (focal hypoechoic region) as well as CT (focal area of increased density relative to the remainder of the liver, but isodense to spleen and muscle). The diffuse fatty liver (steatosis) may be less evident on US than the focal hypoechoic lesion, and the same may be true on CT. These authors have provided a valuable reminder of the frequency of this potential pitfall. The focal sparing appears usually to be due to local alterations in hepatic blood flow.

M.P. Federle, M.D.

Focal Sparing of Segment IV in Fatty Livers Shown by Sonography and CT: Correlation With Aberrant Gastric Venous Drainage

Matsui O, Kadoya M, Takahashi S, et al (Kanazawa Univ, Japan)

AJR 164:1137–1140, 1995 2–14

Background.—The posterior edge of segment IV is one of the most common sites of focal sparing in fatty livers demonstrated by CT or sonography. Differentiating focal spared area from tumor has been a diagnostic challenge. Whether the focal spared area at the posterior edge of segment IV in fatty liver is correlated with the decline in portal perfusion from the main portal vein caused by aberrant gastric venous drainage directed into segment IV was investigated.

Methods.—Seventeen patients with fatty liver diagnosed by sonography and CT scanning were included in the study. All had hepatic arteriography, CT, or both performed during arterial portography (CTAP). In 7 patients, there was a focal spared area of more than 2 cm in the longest diameter at the posterior edge of segment IV. Ten patients showed no evidence of a focal spared area. The frequencies of aberrant gastric venous drainage demonstrated by arteriography in 17 patients and by CTAP in 15 patients were compared.

Findings.—In all patients with a spared area, hepatic arteriography demonstrated aberrant gastric venous drainage. A portal perfusion defect at the posterior edge of segment IV was shown by CTAP in all 5 patients with a focal spared area undergoing this examination. However, none of the patients without a spared area had definite aberrant gastric venous drainage and portal perfusion defects. The between-group difference in the frequency of aberrant gastric venous drainage was significant (Fig 1).

Conclusions.—The focal spared area at the posterior edge of segment IV in fatty liver was strongly correlated with aberrant gastric venous drainage directed to segment IV. Focally reduced blood flow from the main portal vein related to aberrant gastric venous drainage is probably a cause of the focal spared region, which is important in the differential diagnosis of hepatic tumors.

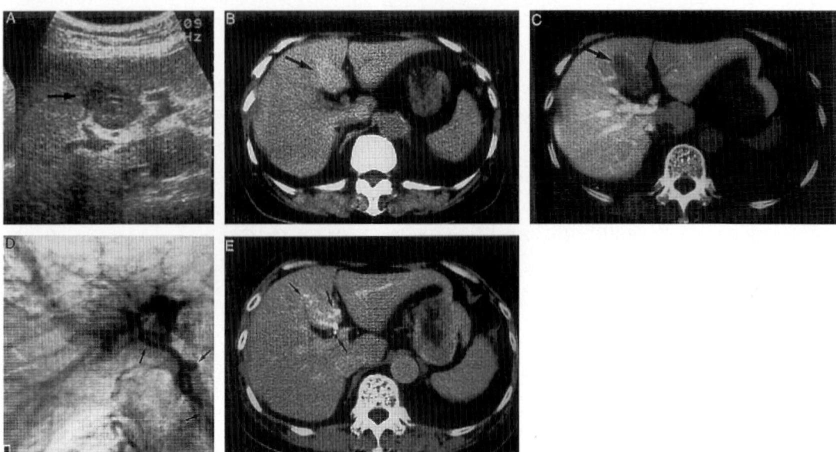

FIGURE 1.—Focal spared area at posterior edge of segment IV in fatty liver. **A**, sonogram shows hypoechoic area at posterior edge of segment IV (*arrow*) in diffusely hyperechoic liver with blurred intrahepatic portal veins. **B**, unenhanced CT scan shows relatively hyperdense area (*arrow*) in diffusely hypodense liver with unclear intrahepatic vessels. These findings are compatible with focal spared area in fatty liver. **C**, CT scan obtained during arterial portography shows portal perfusion defect (*arrow*) at posterior edge of segment IV, and its location and configuration are the same as those of focal spared area seen or unenhanced CT scan. **D**, venous phase of celiac angiogram shows aberrant right gastric venous drainage in direction of segment IV (*arrows*). **E**, CT scan obtained during injection of contrast medium into right gastric artery confirms direct drainage of right gastric vein selectively into area consistent with focal spared area. (*Arrows* indicate strongly enhanced aberrant right gastric vein and its ramification in segment IV). (Courtesy of Matsui O, Kadoya M, Takahashi S, et al: Focal sparing of segment IV in fatty livers shown by sonography and CT: Correlation with aberrant gastric venous drainage. *AJR* 164:1137–1140, 1995.)

► What an elegant and satisfying little paper! The authors have clearly defined the etiology of the commonly observed (but frequently confused) areas of focal sparing as a pseudotumor. Similar aberrant alterations in blood supply, such as cystic vein drainage into liver surrounding the gallbladder fossa, and peribiliary veins and capsular veins draining into other subcapsular sites, are surely the cause not only of focal fatty sparing but also of perfusion defects encountered on CT portography.

M.P. Federle, M.D.

Management of Focal Nodular Hyperplasia and Hepatocellular Adenoma in Young Women: A Series of 41 Patients With Clinical, Radiological, and Pathological Correlations

Cherqui D, Rahmouni A, Charlotte F, et al (Université Paris XII, Créteil)

Hepatology 22:1674–1681, 1995 2–15

Background.—Focal nodular hyperplasia (FNH) typically is managed conservatively, whereas hepatocellular adenoma (HA) usually requires surgical resection. Preoperative distinction between these 2 benign liver tumors therefore is important, but it is complicated by the fact that both tumors share certain characteristics. The frequency of FNH and HA was

TABLE 1.—Criteria Considered Typical for the Diagnosis of Focal Nodular Hyperplasia and Hepatocellular Adenoma

Imaging Technique	FNH	HA
CT	Arterial enhancement Presence of a central stellate hypodense element	Arterial enhancement Precontrast hyperdense areas (hemorrhage) Low-density areas (necrosis or fat)
MRI		
Unenhanced	Isointense or hypointense on T1 images Slightly hyperintense on T2 images Presence of a central stellate area hyperintense on T2 and hypointense on T1 images Homogeneous signal intensity	Hyperintense area(s) on T1 and T2 images (hemorrhage) Hypointense area(s) on T1 corresponding to hyperintense areas on T2 images (necrosis)
Enhanced (Gadolinium)	Arterial enhancement Accumulation of contrast agent within the central area on delayed T1 images	Arterial enhancement No accumulation of contrast agent within the tumor
Angiography	Hypervascular tumor Vascular supply arising centrally ("spoke wheel" appearance)	Hypervascular tumor Vascular supply arising peripherally
Color Doppler US	Arterial signals within the tumor	Venous signals within the tumor
Scintigraphy		
Colloids	Increased or normal uptake	Focal defect
TBIDA	Delayed hyperfixation in the tumor area (hot spot)	Unknown

Abbreviations: FNH, focal nodular hyperplasia; *HA* hepatocellular adenoma.

(Courtesy of Cherqui D, Rahmouni A, Charlotte F, et al: Management of focal nodular hyperplasia and hepatocellular adenoma in young women: A series of 41 patients with clinical, radiological, and pathological correlations. *Hepatology* 22:1674–1681, 1995.)

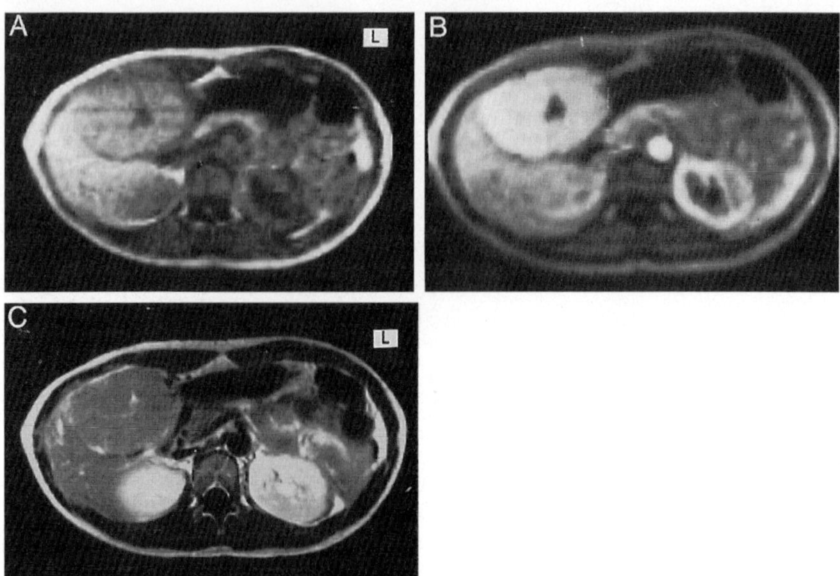

FIGURE 3—Contrast-enhanced dynamic MRI scans of a focal nodular hyperplasia (typical features). **A**, T1-weighted TurboFLASH (fast low-angle shot) before injection of paramagnetic contrast agent. The mass is slightly hypointense relative to the liver with marked hypointense central area. **B**, T1-weighted TurboFLASH obtained 20 seconds after injection of paramagnetic contrast agent. The tumor shows marked enhancement, whereas the central area remains hypointense. C, delayed contrast-enhanced T1-weighted spin echo image obtained 4 minutes after injection of paramagnetic contrast agent. A high-signal intensity is visible within the central element caused by the accumulation of the contrast agent. This shows that the central area is vascularized and consequently does not correspond to necrosis. (Courtesy of Cherqui D, Rahmouni A, Charlotte F, et al: Management of focal nodular hyperplasia and hepatocellular adenoma in young women: A series of 41 patients with clinical, radiological, and pathological correlations. *Hepatology* 22:1674–1681, 1995.)

evaluated in a series of patients with histologic diagnoses, as was the value of new imaging techniques in making preoperative diagnoses and of intraoperative frozen section studies.

Patients and Methods.—Thirty-five consecutive women with FNH and 6 with HA who had been treated between 1985 and 1992 were included in the study. New techniques, including enhanced MRI and color Doppler ultrasonography (US) were prospectively evaluated, along with CT, US, angiography, and scintigraphy. Findings were considered diagnostic when typical features were present and atypical when these features were not observed (Table 1). Histologic examination of all surgical specimens also was performed.

Results.—During the study, a six-fold increase in the number of patients with FNH was noted. In contrast, the number of patients with HA did not change. In 74% of the patients, FNHs were incidentally detected on US evaluation. Enhanced MRI was found to be the best imaging procedure for detection of FNH. Preoperative diagnoses of FNH were made with a sensitivity was 70% and specificity 98% with use of MRI. The presence of areas of hemorrhage or necrosis on MRI were, in contrast, indicative of

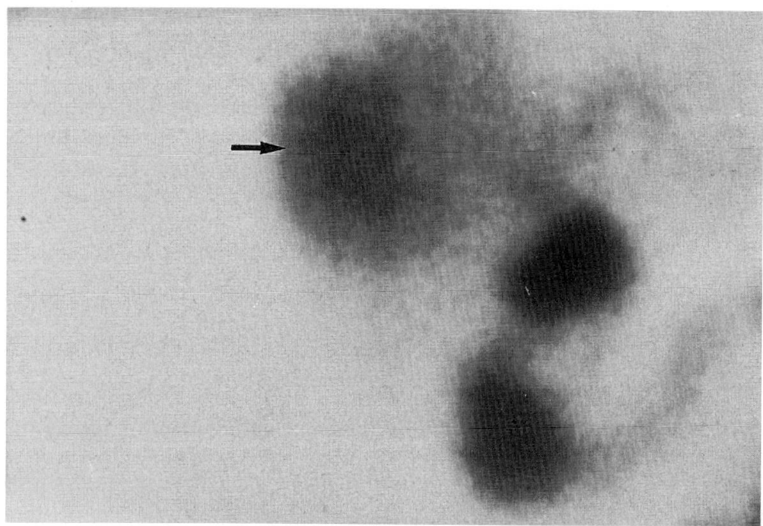

FIGURE 5.—Hepatobiliary scan of a focal nodular hyperplasia obtained 1 hour after injection of Tc-99m-labeled TBIDA. The tracer has been cleared by the liver parenchyma (tracer present in the bowel), but is retained by the tumor (*arrow*). Typical delayed hot spot. (Courtesy of Cherqui D, Rahmouni A, Charlotte F, et al: Management of focal nodular hyperplasia and hepatocellular adenoma in young women: A series of 41 patients with clinical, radiological, and pathological correlations. *Hepatology* 22:1674–1681, 1995.)

HA. These areas can imitate a central element, as shown by CT, but not on enhanced MRI (Fig 3). Color Doppler US may also differentiate FNH from HA by the detection of intratumoral arterial signals in FNHs and venous signals in HAs, although arterial signals may also be observed in malignant lesions. Because this technique cannot be used to rule out malignancy, it should be considered a useful adjunct. Hepatobiliary scans with injection of Tc-99m-labeled TBIDA revealed late hot spots in 24 of 27 FNHs, although specificity of this technique has not been adequately determined (Fig 5). Intraoperative frozen sections were done in 16 patients with 19 tumors. Sensitivity was 89% and specificity 100%.

Conclusions.—Focal nodular hyperplasia is currently detected more often than HA. Preoperative diagnoses of FNH can be achieved in 70% of patients using enhanced MRI, thus avoiding needless surgeries. When clinical, biochemical, or imaging data are atypical for FNH, histologic diagnosis is essential and can be obtained safely and dependably using large surgical biopsy specimens. Finally, frozen-section studies can assist the surgeon in determining when and whether to resect a lesion during operative procedures.

► The recent increase in the detection of FNH is surely due to the more common use of high resolution CT, US, and MR. The imaging characteristics of FNH are essentially identical on CT and MR, and I would alter the criteria and conclusions of these authors somewhat. Focal nodular hyperplasia shows rapid *uniform* enhancement during the arterial-early portal phase of enhancement after a rapid IV bolus of iodine (for CT) or gadolinium (for MR). The central scar is characteristic and shows delayed enhancement (CT and MR), due to its fibrotic nature. Malignant tumors almost never demonstrate such uniform enhancement, including fibrolamellar hepatoma. In this series, Tc-IDA was extremely useful, showing late "hot spots" in 24 of 27 FNHs, whereas earlier investigations found increased uptake of sulfur colloid in only about 50% of FNH. The incidence of hepatic adenomas appears to be decreasing, perhaps due to the use of low estrogen oral contraceptives for the past decade. I believe the diagnosis of FNH can be made confidently in the great majority of cases and that biopsy and surgery are rarely indicated for diagnosis or therapy.

M.P. Federle, M.D.

The Radiologic and Pathologic Spectrum of Biliary Hamartomas

Lev-Toaff AS, Bach AM, Wechsler RJ, et al (Thomas Jefferson Univ Hosp, Philadelphia; Jefferson Med College, Philadelphia)

AJR 165:309–313, 1995 2–16

Background.—Biliary hamartomas are benign liver malformations that typically appear as subcapsular or parenchymal whitish nodules measuring less than 0.5 cm in diameter. Multiple lesions are common, but few lesions and even solitary lesions have been reported. The range of radiologic and pathologic findings in a group of patients with biliary hamartomas was evaluated.

Patients and Methods.—Eighteen patients (mean age, 66 years), who had a primary malignant lesion and had undergone liver biopsy for possible metastatic disease were included. All patients received diagnoses of biliary hamartomas. Prebiopsy imaging studies had been performed, including CT in 16 and sonography in 11 patients. A retrospective review of the imaging studies was carried out. Findings were then correlated with those obtained at surgery and on pathologic assessment. Hamartomas were histologically classified based on the extent of cystic dilatation of bile ducts within the lesion.

Results.—Various radiologic findings were observed. Four patients had 1 or 2 circumscribed lesions measuring 5–10 mm in diameter, 1 patient had about 5 lesions measuring approximately 5 mm each, 2 patients had innumerable tiny, essentially uniform lesions measuring 2–5 mm, and 3 patients had innumerable, variably sized lesions measuring 2–15 mm (Fig 4). Throughout the livers of patients with innumerable lesions, nodules were either uniformly or nonuniformly dispersed. Contrast-enhanced CT showed hypodense lesions in all patients. On sonography, lesions were found to be hypoechoic. Imaging studies failed to identify lesions in 8 patients; however, biopsies were carried out at surgery when single or multiple tiny nodules were observed on the liver surface. Diagnoses were made by wedge or core-needle biopsy. Fine-needle aspirations were nondiagnostic. Single or multiple hamartomas of various sizes ranging from

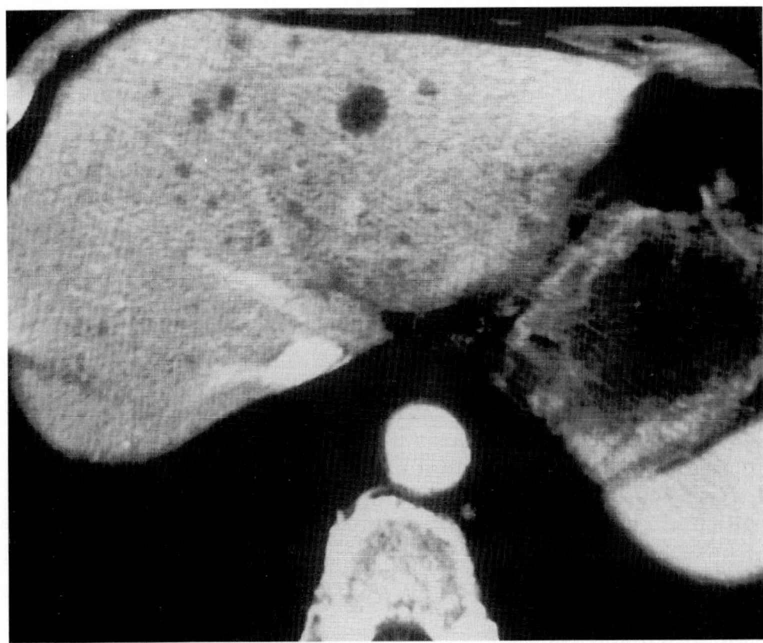

FIGURE 4.—Multiple biliary hamartomas in 75-year-old man with carcinoma of colon. Contrast-enhanced CT scan shows multiple hypodense nodules 2–15 mm in size scattered throughout liver. (Courtesy of Lev-Toaff AS, Bach AM, Wechsler RJ, et al: The radiologic and pathologic spectrum of biliary hamartomas. *AJR* 165:309–313, 1995.)

solid to largely cystic lesions were noted on pathologic review. No correlation between extent of cystic dilatation and imaging results was noted. There was a correlation between visibility on imaging and larger lesion size. Small surface lesions typically were occult.

Conclusions.—Single or multiple nonspecific lesions that can mimic metastatic disease may be caused by biliary hamartomas. In patients with primary malignant tumors and evidence of single or multiple hepatic lesions, biliary hamartomas should be considered as a possible diagnosis.

▶ The incidence of biliary hamartomas is about 1% in unselected autopsy series, at least for those macroscopic lesions likely to be detectable on modern imaging studies. Because most of these lesions are less than 1 cm in diameter, it is likely that we frequently miss them with lower resolution CT, ultrasound (US), and MR techniques. I believe it is useful to think of biliary hamartomas as part of the spectrum of hepatic cystic disease and congenital hepatic fibrosis. This is the largest series of cases reported of what had been regarded as a rare entity, but one that we are starting to encounter more frequently. Most importantly, lesions that are uniformly hypoechoic on US and nonenhancing on CT should be regarded as potentially benign, even in patients with cancer. Wedge or core-needle biopsy can confirm this diagnosis.

M.P. Federle, M.D.

Nodular Sarcoidosis of the Liver and Spleen: Analysis of 32 Cases
Warshauer DM, Molina PL, Hamman SM, et al (Univ of North Carolina, Chapel Hill; Univ of Alabama, Birmingham; Duke Univ, Durham, NC; et al)
Radiology 195:757–762, 1995 2–17

Introduction.—Most commonly affecting the pulmonary parenchyma and mediastinal lymph nodes, sarcoidosis is a generalized granulomatous disease. Hepatosplenic sarcoidosis usually is not seen on CT, or its appearance can be mistaken for lymphoma, metastatic disease or infection. Nodular hepatosplenic sarcoidosis was reviewed retrospectively to aid in differentiation of sarcoidosis from more threatening diseases.

Methods.—In the retrospective study, an evaluation was conducted of 32 patients (21 women, 1 man, aged 25–68 years) with nodular hepatosplenic sarcoidosis. The evaluation included chest radiographic stage, CT findings, level of angiotensin-converting enzyme, and clinical status. In 30 patients, biopsy findings revealed a diagnosis of sarcoidosis; in these 30 patients, there were 43 biopsy sites.

Results.—Nodules were of low attenuation, small, and multiple. Organomegaly was common. In 76% of patients, abdominal adenopathy was

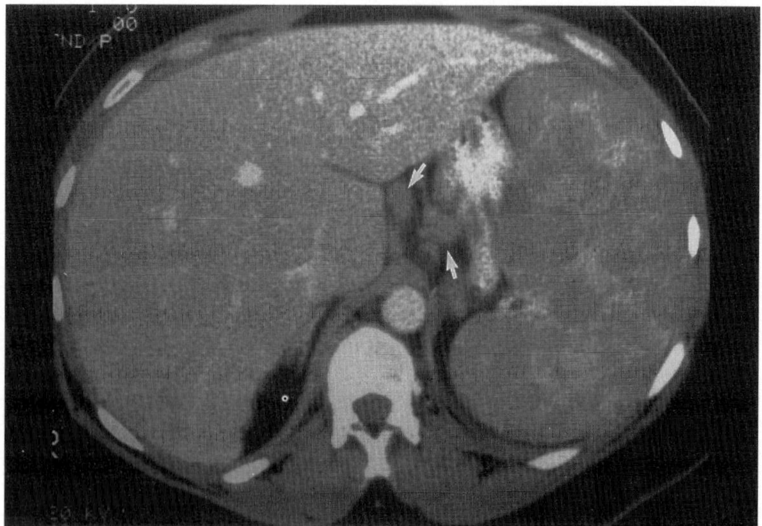

FIGURE 3B.—Confluent nodularity in sarcoidosis. Contrast-enhanced CT scan obtained in a 38-year-old woman demonstrates multiple, low-attenuation splenic nodules (conspicuity grade 3) that tend to become confluent. Note adenopathy of the celiac axis and gastrohepatic ligament (*arrows*). Liver is moderately enlarged (size grade 2). (Courtesy of Warshauer DM, Molina PL, Hamman SM, et al: Nodular sarcoidosis of the liver and spleen: Analysis of 32 cases. *Radiology* 195:757–762, 1995.)

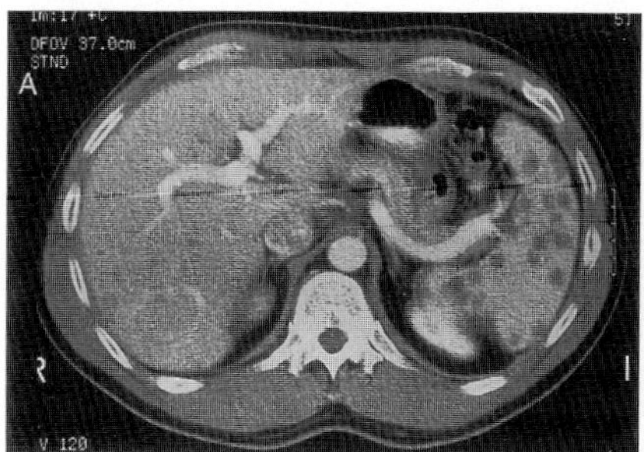

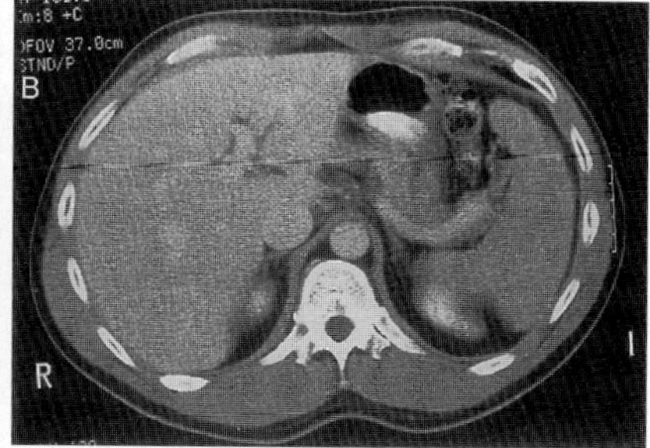

FIGURE 4.—Sarcoidosis in an asymptomatic 45-year-old man. **A**, contrast-enhanced spiral CT scan obtained during nonequilibrium hepatic parenchymal phase shows well-visualized nodules (conspicuity grade 3) in the spleen and smaller, faintly visualized nodules (conspicuity grade 1) in the liver (size grade 0). **B**, contrast-enhanced spiral CT scan obtained during the equilibrium phase 3.5 minutes after **A**. The splenic nodules are faintly visualized. Liver nodules are no longer seen. (Courtesy of Warshauer DM, Molina PL, Hamman SM, et al: Nodular sarcoidosis of the liver and spleen: Analysis of 32 cases. *Radiology* 195:757–762, 1995.)

present. In 25%, chest radiographs were normal; 61% of patients had stage 1 (hilar or mediastinal adenopathy only) or stage 2 (parenchymal infiltrate and adenopathy) radiographs. In 66% of patients, abdominal or systemic symptoms were present. In 10 (91%) of 11 patients tested, the level of angiotensin-converting enzyme was elevated. In 74% of patients with follow-up radiographs taken an average of 18 months after initial radiography, no change in chest radiographic stage was seen. With increasing size, the nodules became confluent on CT (Fig 3, B).

Conclusion.—Organomegaly, symptoms, and adenopathy are associated with nodular hepatosplenic sarcoidosis. Advanced lung disease was not associated with nodules. A change in radiographic stage was not heralded by nodules. An elevated level of angiotensin-converting enzyme may help with diagnosis. Differences in visibility of the nodule may be accounted for in part by variation in CT scanning techniques (Fig 4).

▶ The similarity of the abdominal CT findings between sarcoidosis and lymphoma is striking. One of my pet peeves is the initiation of an expensive imaging work-up for presumed lymphoma, based on the clinical or chest film finding of lymphadenopathy. Biopsy or other clinical markers (such as elevation of angiotensin-converting enzyme) should be obtained before CT, in my opinion.

M.P. Federle, M.D.

Detection of Liver Metastases: Comparison of Superparamagnetic Iron Oxide-Enhanced and Unenhanced MR Imaging at 1.5 T With Dynamic CT, Intraoperative US, and Percutaneous US

Hagspiel KD, Neidl KFW, Eichenberger AC, et al (Univ Hosp Zurich, Switzerland)

Radiology 196:471–478, 1995 2–18

Background.—The availability of more aggressive surgical procedures for the treatment of liver metastases has made the task of preoperative imaging more demanding. The role of superparamagnetic iron oxide (AMI)-25-enhanced MRI in the preoperative assessment of patients with liver metastases was evaluated.

Patients and Methods.—Eighteen patients with a limited number of lesions or with multiple lesions that spared some segments of the liver, and thus potentially curable with surgical treatment, were included in the study. Preoperative imaging with AMI-25-enhanced and unenhanced MRI at 1.5 T, percutaneous ultrasound (US), and CT were performed. Thirteen patients subsequently underwent surgery and intraoperative US (IOUS) after preoperative imaging. The sensitivity of AMI-25-enhanced and unenhanced MRI was evaluated and compared with US, CT, and IOUS.

Results.—The total number of lesions detected with any of the imaging techniques served as the standard of reference in the preoperative imaging group. Sixty-eight liver lesions were identified with all imaging techniques combined. The sensitivity of AMI-25-enhanced MRI was 99%. This was the most sensitive modality, followed by unenhanced MRI, dynamic CT, and US.

The total number of metastases identified at IOUS and pathologic examination served as the standard of reference in the surgical group. The sensitivity of IOUS was 80%. This was the most sensitive method, followed by AMI-25-enhanced MRI, with a sensitivity of 56%.

In 2 patients, the initially planned surgical approach was modified as a result of findings noted with AMI-25-enhanced MRI. In both patients, this technique detected the presence of lesions not identified through other modalities. These lesions were confirmed at surgery in both patients (Fig 3).

The majority of patients receiving AMI-25 did not experience any side effects, and clinically significant changes in blood pressure or pulse rate were not observed after administration. An increase in serum iron and ferritin levels was noted on laboratory tests; otherwise, no other changes in serum or urine occurred. There also were no late complications at 3 to 12 months post-AMI-25 administration. In 1 patient, lumbar pain was reported approximately 2 minutes after AMI-25 was given. The infusion was rapidly terminated, and the pain gradually improved during the next several hours. No treatment was required, and no late complications were noted. The cause of this back pain has not been determined.

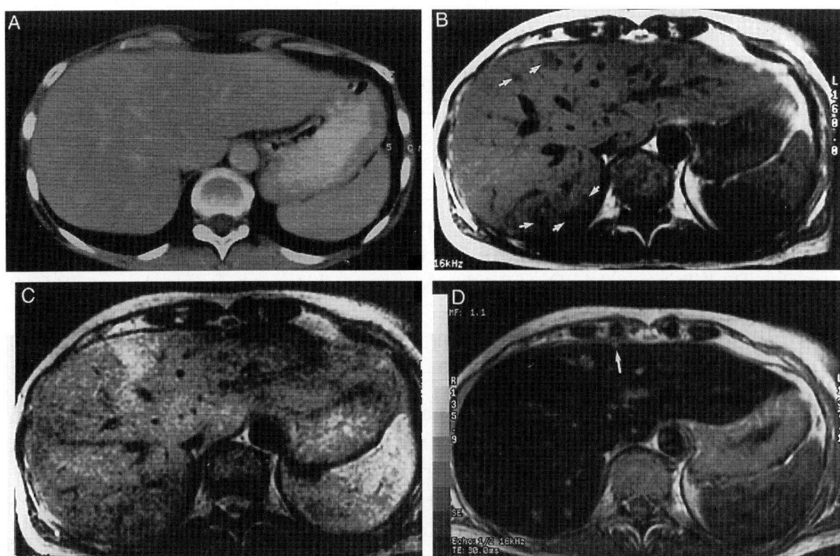

FIGURE 3.—Multiple liver metastases from a gallbladder carcinoma in a 46-year-old woman. Preoperative imaging studies showed no evidence of tumor in segments II and III. **A**, dynamic CT scan through the upper part of the liver shows no definite metastates. **B**, unenhanced T1-weighted MR image (500/11), however, shows 5 lesions (*arrows*). **C**, unenhanced T2-weighted MR image (2,500/80) shows diffuse edema to metastases but does not depict individual lesions. **D**, an AMI-25-enhanced long TR/short MR image (2,500/30) shows 6 lesions (the additional lesion is marked with an *arrow*) but still no lesion in segments II and III. At surgery, 3 previously undetected metastases were found in hepatic segments II and III (10, 3, and 3 mm in diameter, all on the liver surface). (Courtesy of Hagspiel KD, Neidl KFW, Eichenberger AC, et al: Detection of liver metastases: Comparison of superparamagnetic iron oxide-enhanced and unenhanced MR imaging at 1.5 T with dynamic CT, intraoperative US, and percutaneous US. *Radiology* 196:471–478, 1995. Radiological Society of North America.)

Conclusions.—Preoperative evaluation of patients with potentially curable metastatic liver disease is facilitated by the use of AMI-25-enhanced high-field-strength MRI.

► It is noteworthy that the contrast-enhanced MR scans would have been judged to be nearly 100% sensitive for detecting liver metastases, compared with other preoperative imaging studies. However, it is humbling to see how relatively poorly noninvasive imaging studies perform compared with IOUS (or CT portography, or pathologic findings at hepatic resection for that matter). The performance of CT can definitely be improved over that achieved in this study, which used thick (10 mm) sections, slow acquisition (2–3 minutes), and slow infusion of contrast material. In my opinion, a safe and effective, liver-specific contrast medium will have to be developed before MR can compete with good quality CT in detecting liver tumors. Other investigators have reported less encouraging results with AMI-25, the agent used in this study.

M.P. Federle, M.D.

Suggested Reading

Marchal G, Van Hecke P, Demaerel P, et al: Detection of liver metastases with superparamagnetic iron oxide in 15 patients: Results of MR imaging at 1.5 T. *AJR* 152:771–775, 1989.

Dynamic GD-Enhanced MR Imaging of Hepatic Hemangioma: Is High Temporal Resolution Requisite for Characterization?

Urhahn R, Kilbinger M, Drobnitzky M, et al (Univ of Technology (RWTH) Aachen, Germany)

Magn Reson Imaging 14:31–41, 1996 2–19

Background.—Patients with hemangiomas (the most common benign hepatic tumor) typically do not require therapeutic intervention; therefore, noninvasive diagnostic techniques are essential to avoid unnecessary laparotomy and/or biopsy. The magnetization-prepared gradient-echo (MP-GRE) MR imaging technique provides a noninvasive means of evaluating the perfusion kinetics of hepatic lesions, with a temporal resolution comparable to that of high-speed CT scanners. The utility of high temporal resolution in the dynamic characterization of hepatic hemangiomas was evaluated, using a contrast-optimized fast MP-GRE MR imaging method coupled with IV bolus injection of Gd-DTPA.

Patients and Methods.—Twenty-six patients with 34 hemangiomas previously verified by CT and ultrasound were included in the study. Single-level inversion recovery incremental flip angle MP-GRE images were obtained in all patients before and after injection of Gd-DTPA (30 images per minute postinjection) without breath-holding. Enhancement patterns and associated temporal changes were evaluated. Small hemangiomas were defined as those less than 2.0 cm, medium lesions as those measuring 2.0–5.0 cm, and large lesions as those greater than 5 cm.

Results.—Lesion size ranged from 1.4 to 12.5 cm, with a mean size of 3.1 cm. There were 10 small, 20 medium, and 4 large hemangiomas. One to 3 lesions were noted per patient (mean, 1.3 per patient). In 31 of the lesions (91%), classic early peripheral nodular enhancement (PNE; defined as sharp peripheral nodules of intense enhancement proximal to areas of nonenhancement during the arterial and portal perfusion phase), with subsequent progressive hyperintense fill-in was noted. Complete fill-in (defined as homogenous hyperintensity), was observed in 19 lesions (pattern A), and partial fill-in was noted in 12 of the 31 lesions (pattern B).

In 3 of the pattern A lesions (1 medium and 2 small), fill-in was complete within 10 seconds (Fig 5). In an additional 4 lesions (1 medium and 3 small), complete fill-in was observed within 45 seconds. The remaining 12 lesions (8 medium and 4 small) required more than 45 seconds to achieve homogeneous hyperintensity. Immediate homogeneous hyperintensity was not observed in any hemangioma without preceding PNE.

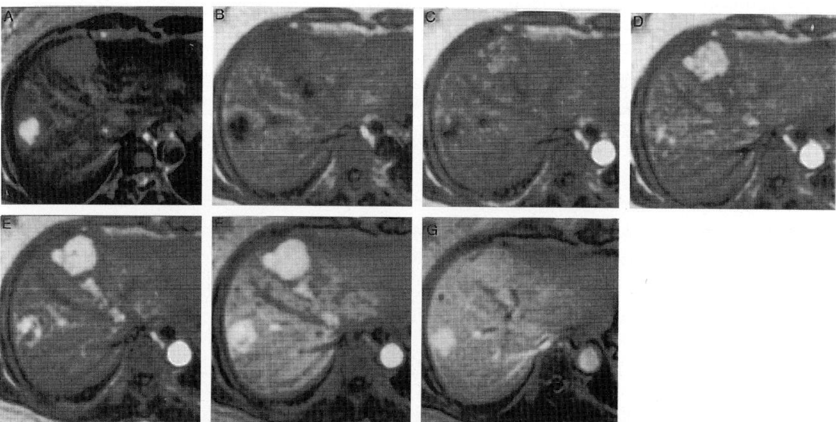

FIGURE 5.—Hemangioma (2.1 cm diameter) and focal nodular hyperplasia. **A** transaxial T_2-weighted spin-echo image. **B,** transaxial precontract magnetization-prepared gradient-echo (MP-GRE) images with inversion delay = 300 ms C: Postcontrast MP-GRE images obtained 4 seconds after appearance of the contrast bolus in the abdominal aorta. **D–F,** postcontrast images obtained 2, 4, and 6 seconds after **C. G,** delayed postcontrast image 100 seconds after **C.** Marked hyperintensity of hemangioma and slight hyperintensity of focal nodular hyperplasia in **A.** The FNH shows immediate homogenous hyperintensity in **C–D.** The hemangioma demonstrate early peripheral nodular enhancement (**c**) with subsequent fast centripetally oriented fill-in (**D–E**). Both lesions are nearly homogenous hyperintense in **F.** On delayed images, the hemangioma shows hyperintensity compared with isointense FNH. *Abbreviation*: FNH, focal nodular hyperplasia. (Courtesy of Urhahn R, Kilbinger M, Drobnitzky M, et al: Dynamic GD-enhanced MR imaging of hepatic hemangioma: Is high temporal resolution requisite for characterization? Reprinted from *Magn Reson Imaging* 14:31–41, 1996. With kind permission from Elsevier Science Ltd, The Boulevard, Lanford Lane, Kidlington OX5 1GB, UK.)

Conclusion.—High temporal resolution is important in the dynamic characterization of hepatic hemangioma. Regardless of enhancement speed, the dynamic Gd-enhanced MP-GRE MRI technique can reliably assess the hemokinetics of hepatic hemangiomas. The time resolution of routine breath-hold GRE methods may be sufficient for most hemangiomas when patients are able to hold their breath. In instances of primarily small high-flow hemangiomas, however, a temporal resolution of fewer than 10 seconds during the early perfusion phase does appear to be necessary.

▶ The ability to acquire MR images through cavernous hemangiomas every 2 seconds after bolus gadolinium administration provides important keys to understanding the pathology and optimal imaging of hemangiomas and other liver masses. *All* hemangiomas demonstrated nodular peripheral enhancement and, as beautifully illustrated by the accompanying figures, this allowed confident differentiation from other "hypervascular" masses. The liver handles Gd as it does iodinated contrast media, so these results can be extrapolated to the expected enhancement pattern of hemangiomas on CT after bolus contrast administration. If the timing of CT sections is ideal, nodular peripheral enhancement is seen in almost all cavernous hemangiomas. Lesions of less than 2 cm may fill in completely by 10 seconds, making it impractical to detect nodular enhancement in all cases, even with helical scanning during the arterial phase of liver enhancement. However, to determine the nature of a specific liver lesion suspected to be a hemangioma, rapid acquisition of scans through the lesion without table incrementation would allow detection of diagnostic CT or MR criteria in virtually all cases.

M.P. Federle, M.D.

Pyogenic Liver Abscesses: 13 Years of Experience in Percutaneous Needle Aspiration With US Guidance

Giorgio A, Tarantino L, Mariniello N, et al (Cotugno Hosp for Infectious Disease, Naples, Italy; Ospedale Civile di Gorizia, Italy)

Radiology 195:122–124, 1995 2–20

Background.—Percutaneous placement of a catheter, a widely used method for drainage of pyogenic liver abscesses (PLA), has a low cure rate and carries a risk of complications. At the study institution, liver abscesses are treated with ultrasound–guided needle aspiration and antibiotic therapy, a procedure that is simpler and less costly than catheter placement. The efficacy of percutaneous needle aspiration (PNA) and antibiotic therapy for PLA was assessed in a series of 115 patients.

Methods.—The patients, 59 men and 56 women, had a mean age of 45.3 years. All had fevers and 97 had leukocytosis. A total of 301 PNAs were performed in 147 PLAs. Fifty-seven patients had a single puncture; the rest had a mean of 2.2 aspirations per PLA. Coagulation status was assessed before the procedure to confirm prothrombin time in the normal range. Patients were placed in a supine position for an anterior abdominal wall approach or on the left side for access through the ribs. Local anesthesia was then administered, gentamicin sulfate or metronidazole was injected into the cavity, and broad-spectrum antibiotics were administered once the cause of the disease was determined (Table 3). Needle caliber (22 to 16 gauge) was selected according to PLA volume. A saline lavage solution was used after the cavity contents were aspirated as much as possible. When necessary, PLA was repeated every 3–7 days.

Results.—The cure rate for PNA in the series of patients was 98.3%. Cure was defined as normalization of clinical and laboratory parameters and resolution of hepatic lesions. Temperature returned to normal at an average of 1.2 days after PNA; PLAs were completely healed, as demonstrated at ultrasound, at a mean of 37 days. Two patients with a single large abscess (8.0 and 8.5 cm) required surgery. There were no complications or deaths; clinical and ultrasound follow-up at a mean of 18 months showed no recurrence.

Conclusion.—Percutaneous needle aspiration with ultrasound guidance and antibiotic treatment cured 113 of 117 patients with pyogenic liver abscesses. Compared with a drainage catheter set, a needle is 30–40 times cheaper, and less medical or nursing care is required with PNA. The outcome of the procedure was not affected by the size, number, or presence of multiloculated cavities, although high viscosity of the content of the

TABLE 3.—Causes of PLA in 115 Patients

Causes	Patients
Cryptogenic	32 (27.8)
Lithiasic cholangitis	27 (23.5)
Complication of surgery	16 (13.9)
Neoplastic stenosis of biliary ducts	15 (13.0)
Diverticulitis	7 (6.1)
Retrocecal abscess	4 (3.5)
Chronic pancreatitis	5 (4.3)
Duodenal ulcer	3 (2.6)
Appendicitis	3 (2.6)
Hematogenous sepsis	2 (1.7)
Ovarian abscess	1 (.9)

Note: Numbers in parentheses are percentages.
Abbreviation: PLA, pyogenic liver abscesses.
(Courtesy of Giorgio A, Tarantino L, Mariniello N, et al: Pyogenic liver abscesses: 13 years of experience in percutaneous needle aspiration with US guidance. *Radiology* 195:122–124, 1995. Radiological Society of North America.)

cavity caused 2 failures. Previous studies in which PNA was less successful had more immunocompromised patients and patients with postsurgical abscesses.

► There has been a striking evolution in the management of liver abscesses during the past 15 years, generally favoring less invasive therapy. There are obvious advantages in both cost and morbidity, to a nonsurgical and even a noncatheter approach, although success rates will decrease if the study population includes patients with infected necrotic neoplasms, biliary obstruction, or immunocompromise, the underlying cause of the abscesses in this series is probably similar to that encountered in many community hospitals. We have had similar success, and the key seems to be to aspirate most of the pus at the initial intervention and to administer a suitable parenteral antibiotic. Prior emphasis on complete drainage by surgery or multiple catheters does not seem warranted.

M.P. Federle, M.D.

Image-Guided Percutaneous Hepatic Biopsy: Effect of Ascites on the Complication Rate

Little AF, Ferris JV, Dodd GD III, et al (Univ of Pittsburgh, Pa)
Radiology 199:79–83, 1996 2–21

Introduction.—Image-guided percutaneous hepatic biopsy is widely used for diagnostic evaluation of local or diffuse hepatic conditions. Ascites are sometimes regarded as a contraindication to this technique because of concerns about bleeding. A large experience with image-guided percutaneous hepatic biopsy was reviewed to determine the complication rate in patients with ascites.

Methods.—The review included 476 patients undergoing percutaneous hepatic biopsy under ultrasound or CT guidance. One hundred seventy-three patients had ascites and 303 did not. All patients with coagulopathy received appropriate blood products before undergoing biopsy. Decreases in hematocrit or hemoglobin not requiring treatment were classified as minor complications, whereas hemorrhage requiring transfusion or surgery or resulting in death was classified as a major complication.

Results.—Six patients with and 10 without ascites experienced major complications. The numbers of patents with minor complications were 10 and 15, respectively. In the ascites group, the major complications required blood transfusion but not surgery. Five of the 6 ascitic patients with major complications had a moderate or severe amount of perihepatic ascites. One of the nonascitic patients with major complications required surgery; the rest required transfusion only. No patient in either group died of hemorrhagic complications.

Conclusions.—Patients with ascites can undergo image-guided percutaneous hepatic biopsy with no significant increase in the risk of major or minor complications. This is the case regardless of the type of needle used, the number of biopsy passes made, or the imaging technique used. Ascites should not be regarded as a contraindication to image-guided percutaneous hepatic biopsy.

▶ Neither major nor minor complications were significantly more frequent when image-guided liver biopsies were performed in patients with ascites vs. those without ascites. The markedly lower complication rate in this series when compared with the reported experience with bedside, blind percutaneous liver biopsy is likely the result of several factors. The authors stress the advantages of ultrasound rather than CT guidance (much faster, less time for needle laceration of the liver); automated gun use for core biopsies; and choosing a needle track that interposes normal parenchyma between the lesion and the hepatic capsule.

M.P. Federle, M.D.

Biliary

Is ERCP Necessary for Symptomatic Gallbladder Stone Patients Before Laparoscopic Cholecystectomy?

Changchien C-S, Chuah S-K, Chiu K-W (Chang Gung Mem Hosp, Taiwan, Republic of China)

Am J Gastroenterol 90:2124–2127, 1995 2–22

Background.—Laparoscopic cholecystectomy (LC), the procedure of choice for symptomatic cholethiasis, generally produces a good outcome in patients with simple gallbladder stones. The modality of choice for demonstrating the biliary tree in patients with gallbladder stones is endoscopic retrograde cholangiopancreaticography (ERCP), an invasive procedure. The necessity of ERCP in patients with symptomatic gallstones before LC

TABLE 2.—Predictability of Common Ductal Pathology by Both Sonography and Liver Biochemistry

	Sono (+) LB (+) (n = 37) No (%)	Sono (+) LB (−) (n = 9) No (%)	Sono (−) LB (+) (n = 27) No (%)	Sono (−) LB (−) (n = 42) No (%)
Positive ERCP findings	34 (91.9)	6 (66.7)	11 (40.7)	1 (2.4)*
Negative ERCP findings	3 (8.1)	3 (33.3)	16 (59.3)	41 (97.6)

*Normal common bile duct with a small stone on ERCP.

Abbreviations: Sono (+), a dilated common bile duct; *Sono (−),* a normal common bile duct on sonogram; *LB (+),* an abnormal liver biochemistry; *LB (−),* a normal liver biochemistry.

(Courtesy of Changchien C-S, Chuah S-K, Chiu K-W: Is ERCP necessary for symptomatic gallbladder stone patients before laparoscopic cholecystectomy? *Am J Gastroenterol* 90:2124–2127, 1995.)

was investigated using noninvasive methods such as sonography and liver function tests (LFTs).

Methods.—One hundred fifteen patients with symptomatic gallbladder stones underwent LFT and ERCP before LC. In all patients, diagnosis was confirmed sonographically. Patients who had tumors or intrahepatic biliary stones shown on sonography were excluded. Based on sonographic findings, patients were classified as having normal or dilated biliary trees. Patients were also divided into normal and abnormal LFT groups.

Findings.—Ninety-eight percent of the patients with both normal biliary sonograms and LFT results had negative ERCP findings. The positive predictability of biliary tree dilation on sonogram for ductal abnormalities on ERCP was 87%. The sonographic finding of a normal biliary tree was associated with a 17.4% incidence of positive ductal abnormality on ERCP. The finding of a single abnormal LFT was correlated with a 68.8% positive predictability for ductal abnormality on ERCP (Table 2).

Conclusions.—Patients with symptomatic gallbladder stones who have a normal biliary tree on sonography and a normal LFT do not need to undergo ERCP. Assessment with ERCP is necessary for patients with either a dilated bile duct on sonogram or an abnormal LFT.

▶ The excellent positive and negative predictive values for a combination of ultrasound and LFT studies achieved in this investigation are both compelling and consistent with those from other studies. The selective use of preoperative ERCP did not result in a higher surgical complication rate than that reported by groups who have recommended routine pre- or intraoperative cholangiography.

M.P. Federle, M.D.

Prospective Evaluation of Ultrasonography and Liver Function Tests for Preoperative Assessment of the Bile Duct

Welbourn CRB, Haworth JM, Leaper DJ, et al (Southmead Hosp, Bristol, England)

Br J Surg 82:1371–1373, 1995 2–23

Introduction.—An accurate, straightforward preoperative test to predict the presence of bile duct stones is currently unavailable. Such a test would allow patients to avoid unnecessary invasive investigation. Ultrasonography (US) and liver function tests (LFTs) have a poor positive predictive value for stones, and algorithms based on bile duct diameter and liver function are impractical to use. Researchers examined a large group of patients to assess the value of US and LFTs in combination with measurements taken as close as possible to the planned operation.

Methods.—The prospective study included a consecutive cohort of patients with symptomatic gallstones. All underwent US of the bile duct and measurement of LFTs on the day before surgery. A normal diameter of the internal bile duct as seen at US was 5 mm or less up to age 50, then increasing by 1 mm per decade. Abnormal findings were a dilated duct or a rise in 1 or more of serum bilirubin, alanine aminotransferase, or alkaline phosphatase levels above the reference range.

Results.—Laparascopic cholecystectomy alone was performed in 494 patients; 51 underwent treatment of confirmed bile duct stones. No bile duct injuries occurred. Depending on the number of abnormalities used, sensitivity of US and LFTs ranged from 46% to 96%. The positive predictive value was 35% when duct diameter or a single abnormality on LFTs was used, but this rose to 77% for duct diameter plus 2 or more LFTs (Table 1). At least 1 abnormality was recorded in 103 patients who did not have bile duct stones; 2 patients with no preoperative abnormality had stones. Two of 6 patients who had stones without having a dilated duct had incorrect US measurements of the bile duct. Although all groupings yielded at least a 96% negative predictive value for the absence of stones, none combined high sensitivity and high positive predictive value.

TABLE 1.—Values of Predictive Ability (Percent)

	Abnormal test			
	Duct diameter or any LFT	Duct diameter alone	Two or more LFTs alone	Duct diameter + two or more LFTs
Sensitivity	96	89	46	46
Specificity	78	89	98	99
Positive predictive value	35	47	63	77
Negative predictive value	99	99	96	96

Abbreviation: LFT, liver function test.

(Courtesy of Welbourn CRB, Haworth JM, Leaper DJ, et al: Prospective evaluation of ultrasonography and liver function tests for preoperative assessment of the bile duct. *Br J Surg*, Blackwell Science Ltd, 82:1371–1373, 1995.)

Conclusion.—A high degree of accuracy in predicting stones would be helpful in clinical practice. Because many patients spontaneously pass bile duct stones, assessments should be performed as close as possible to the planned surgery. The best predictive value of the state of the bile duct is given by a combination of US and LFTs. Predictive criteria still need to be refined.

▶ Both US and LFTs, alone or together, have high specificity and negative predictive value in the evaluation of bile duct calculi. If cholangiography is performed for any 1 abnormality on US or LFT, it would be normal in two thirds of patients. If the indication for cholangiography is taken as a dilated duct plus 2 abnormal LFTs, the positive predictive value would improve to 77%, but at the cost of missing more than half the bile duct stones. The authors point out that many ductal stones pass spontaneously, implying that US and LFT should be repeated shortly before any planned therapeutic intervention.

M.P. Federle, M.D.

Imaging of the Common Bile Duct During Laparoscopic Cholecystectomy: Sonography Versus Videofluoroscopic Cholangiography
Teefey SA, Soper NJ, Middleton WD, et al (Washington Univ, St Louis, Mo)
AJR 165:847–851, 1995 2–24

Introduction.—Intraoperative evaluation during open cholecystectomy has included laparoscopic sonography and cholangiography; however, videofluoroscopy can further enhance the detection of bile duct calculi and delineating ductal anatomy because of its ability to show real-time video images of the injection of contrast material. During laparoscopic cholecystectomy, the accuracies of laparoscopic sonography and laparoscopic videofluoroscopic cholangiography were compared in their ability to detect common bile duct stones and identify ductal anomalies.

Methods.—Laparoscopic sonography and laparoscopic videofluoroscopic cholangiography were performed on 95 patients who underwent laparoscopic videofluoroscopic cholecystectomy. The sonographs were obtained by a gastrointestinal surgeon using a linear-array transducer, in which the real-time video images of the studies were relayed to a remote viewing site for interpretation by an experienced radiologist. The laparoscopic cholangiograms were also performed by a gastrointestinal surgeon using a standard C-arm digital fluoroscopy unit, in which the real-time video images of the injection of contrast material were recorded using a standard videocassette recorder and relayed to a remote viewing site for interpretation by an experienced radiologist. The evaluation included the number of successful studies; the time required to complete the study; complications; and the ability to completely visualize the common bile duct, cystic duct, ductal anomalies, maximum diameter of the common bile duct, stones, or debris.

Results.—Laparoscopic videofluoroscopic cholangiography was successfully performed in 90 of 95 patients, and laparoscopic sonography was successfully performed in 93 of 95 patients. Laparoscopic cholangiography took a mean of 14 ± 6 minutes to perform, whereas laparoscopic sonography took a mean of 8 ± 3 minutes to perform. The common bile duct was completely visualized in 84 of 93 patients with sonography, whereas cholangiography depicted the common bile duct in 86 of 90 patients. The cystic duct was shown in 87 of 93 patients with sonography, whereas cholangiography revealed the cystic duct in 80 of 90 patients. No ductal anomalies were seen in any of the 93 patients using sonography, whereas cholangiography showed ductal variants in 13 of 90 patients. Common bile duct stones were seen in 12 of 93 patients using sonography, whereas 5 of 90 patients were found to have common bile duct stones with cholangiography. In 2 of 93 patients, sonography altered operative management.

Conclusion.—In visualizing the common bile duct and cystic duct and in detecting common bile duct stones, laparoscopic sonography is as accurate as laparoscopic videofluoroscopic cholangiography. However, regarding the detection of ductal anomalies, data are limited to determine whether laparoscopic sonography is as accurate as laparoscopic cholangiography.

► This study offers convincing evidence that an experienced operator (a surgeon in this case) can quickly and accurately assess the common bile duct for stones with laparoscopic sonography. Laparoscopic cholangiography took a bit longer to perform in this study and was judged to be more technically challenging. Cholangiography has the advantage of depicting ductal anomalies as well as stones, although these authors (and others) believe that meticulous surgical dissection obviates inadvertent damage to ducts regardless of the anatomy. As addressed in other abstracts in this section, preoperative screening for ductal calculi by transabdominal sonography and liver function tests will detect most common duct stones. It is important for laparoscopic surgeons, in my opinion, to become expert at either laparoscopic sonography or cholangiography to evaluate the minority of patients who require intraoperative evaluation.

M.P. Federle, M.D.

Postsurgical Bile Leaks: Endoscopic Obliteration of the Transpapillary Pressure Gradient is Enough

Bjorkman DJ, Carr-Locke DL, Lichtenstein DR, et al (Brigham and Women's Hosp, Boston; Univ of Utah, Salt Lake City)

Am J Gastroenterol 90:2128–2133, 1995 2–25

Background.—Biliary surgery is sometimes complicated by postoperative bile leaks. This uncommon but well-documented complication is seen more often after laparoscopic procedures. One effective treatment for bile leaks is endoscopic therapy with a long biliary endoprosthesis traversing

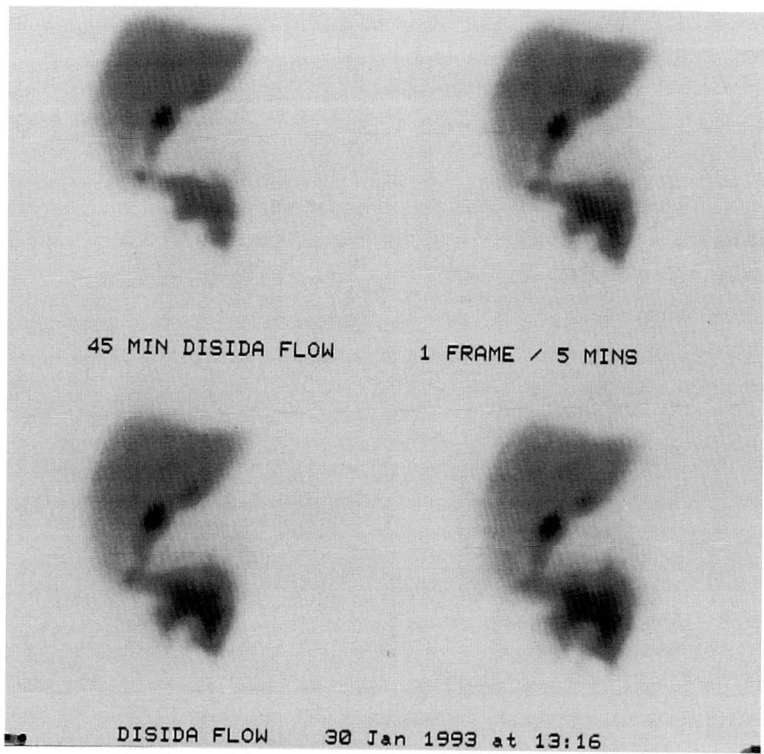

FIGURE 1.—Sequential 2-minute images of a DISIDA scan during 30 minutes from a patient with a bile leak showing liver uptake but no visualization of the bile duct or bowel. During the time of the scan, there is increasing activity outside the bowel. *Abbreviation: DISIDA*, diisopropyliminodiacetic acid. (Courtesy of Bjorkman DJ, Carr-Locke DL, Lichtenstein DR, et al: Postsurgical bile leaks: Endoscopic obliteration of the transpapillary pressure gradient is enough. *Am J Gastroenterol* 90(12): 2128–2133, 1995.)

the site of the leak. However, equalizing biliary and duodenal pressures with a short transpapillary stent may be equally effective.

Methods.—Thirty-one patients seen consecutively with postoperative bile leaks during a 52-month period were studied to determine the value of endoscopic obliteration of the transpapillary pressure gradient. Treatment consisted of long endoprostheses, sphincterotomy, or short transpapillary stents.

Findings.—All 25 patients in whom a bile leak was documented responded to endoscopic treatment. All treatment modalities were associated with comparable clinical success rates, the need for radiologic drainage, length of hospitalization, and the incidence of pancreatitis (Figs 1 and 4).

Conclusions.—Endoscopic treatment is very successful in the treatment of postoperative bile leaks. The mechanism of healing appears to be the equalization of bile duct and duodenal pressure, permitting bile flow into the duodenum. Endoscopically placing short transpapillary stents without

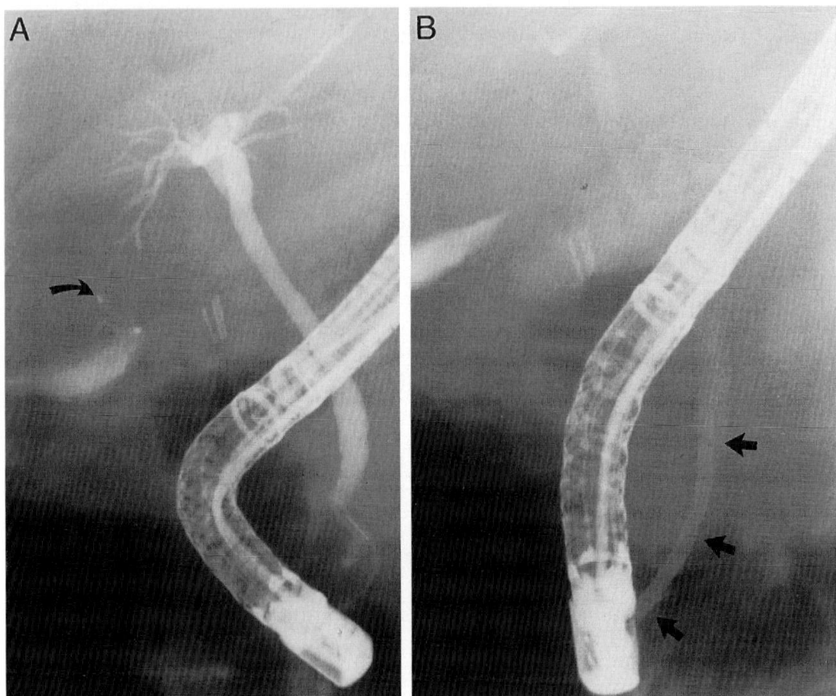

FIGURE 4.—Endoscopic retrograde cholangiography demonstrating (**A**) bile leak from a duct of Luschka (*arrow*) in the gallbladder bed and (**B**) its treatment by insertion of a 10 Fr 2 cm endoprosthesis (*arrow*). (Courtesy of Bjorkman DJ, Carr-Locke DL, Lichtenstein DR, et al: Postsurgical bile leaks: Endoscopic obliteration of the transpapillary pressure gradient is enough. *Am J Gastroenterol* 90(12): 2128–2133, 1995.)

sphincterotomy is a temporary, effective, and technically simple way to equalize pressure. It should be considered primary treatment for most postoperative bile leaks.

► The incidence of bile duct injury during laparascopic cholecystectomy (LC) is 1% to 3%. Given the huge number of patients who undergo laparoscopic cholecystectomy and the potential morbidity and mortality of bile duct leaks, this investigation is both timely and important. Biliary leaks may be detected and corrected at initial surgery, but delayed diagnosis (days to weeks) is more common. Because other groups have now reported similar excellent results, it seems clear that endoscopic sphincterotomy or stenting can obviate surgical intervention in most areas of iatrogenic bile leaks after LC.

M.P. Federle, M.D.

Does the Common Bile Duct Dilate After Cholecystectomy? Sonographic Evaluation in 234 Patients

Feng B, Song Q (Shanxi Provincial People's Hosp, Taiyuan, Shanxi, People's Republic of China)

AJR 165:859–861, 1995 2–26

Introduction.—Considerable controversy has been generated since the dilatation of the common bile duct after cholecystectomy was reported in 3 dogs in 1887. It is still uncertain whether postcholecystectomy bile-duct dilatation is a myth or a fact. An attempt was made to determine whether the common bile duct dilates after cholecystectomy.

Methods.—The luminal diameter of the proximal segment of the common bile duct was measured on 234 patients on anteroposterior transverse sonograms 4 to 15 days before their cholecystectomy. Seven to 2,160 days after surgery, the luminal diameter was measured again on sonograms for all of the patients. Normal was considered to be a diameter of 6 mm or less, which was found in 197 patients, whereas 37 patients had a dilated common bile duct of greater than 6 mm. Measurements were conducted on 1 machine by 1 physician who was blinded to the results of previous examinations.

Results.—Before cholecystectomy, the mean diameter of the common bile duct measured on sonograms was 5.9 mm; after surgery, it was 6.1 mm, which was statistically significant. In 110 patients, the common bile duct diameter increased. In 61 patients, the diameter decreased, and in 63 patients the diameter stayed the same. After surgery, 167 of the 234 patients (71%) had a normal diameter of the common bile duct. Twenty-nine percent of asymptomatic patients had dilatation, with the maximum diameter being 13 mm, but because they were asymptomatic, they did not undergo further workup.

Conclusion.—After cholecystectomy, the diameters of the common bile duct measured on sonograms increased slightly, less than 1 mm, in asymptompatic patients. After cholecystectomy, most patients do not have significant compensatory dilatation.

► This investigation has several advantages over others that have addressed the same clinical concern. A single physician performed all the ultrasound examinations; a very large number of patients were studied; and patients were excluded who had had bile duct manipulation. After cholecystectomy, the bile duct dilates slightly (from 5.0 mm to 5.5 mm) and then stays stable in most cases. In 167 of 234 patients, the increased diameter did not exceed the usually cited upper limit of normal (6 mm), and this is probably of no clinical significance. Unfortunately, we don't know the fate of the 29% of patients who had common bile duct diameters exceeding 6 mm, because asymptomatic patients were not investigated further. Even in this group, however, compensatory and progressive dilation did not seem to occur.

M.P. Federle, M.D.

Evaluation of a Non–Breath-Hold MR Cholangiography Technique

Macaulay SE, Schulte SJ, Sekijima JH, et al (VA Med Ctr, Seattle; Univ of Washington, Seattle; Philips Med Systems, Shelton, Conn)

Radiology 196:227–232, 1995 2–27

Background.—Various MR cholangiography techniques have been used that require patients to hold their breath for up to 30 seconds. A non–breath-hold technique was developed to allow imaging of patients who are unable to hold their breath for the required period of time with current techniques. The new sequence is a heavily T2-weighted, turbo spin-echo technique. Six signals are averaged to compensate for loss of signal from respiratory motion. The ability of this new MR technique to visualize the biliary system was assessed.

Methods.—In 28 patients with various biliary diseases, 29 non–breath-hold MR cholangiographic studies were performed. Results were compared to 28 direct cholangiographic studies in 24 patients.

Results.—Magnetic resonance cholangiography showed intrahepatic ducts in the peripheral third of the liver and in the 4 hepatic segments in 100% of dilated ducts (Fig 1). Magnetic resonance cholangiography showed intrahepatic ducts in the peripheral third of the liver in 82% of nondilated ducts and in the 4 hepatic segments in 91% of nondilated ducts (Table). Extrahepatic ducts were seen in 90% of studies. Filling defects were detected in the extrahepatic ducts in 71% of studies (Fig 4). Filling defects were detected in the gallbladder in 100% of the studies. The site and character of obstructions were accurately shown in the majority of cases. Intrahepatic duct dilatation was also accurately shown. Measure-

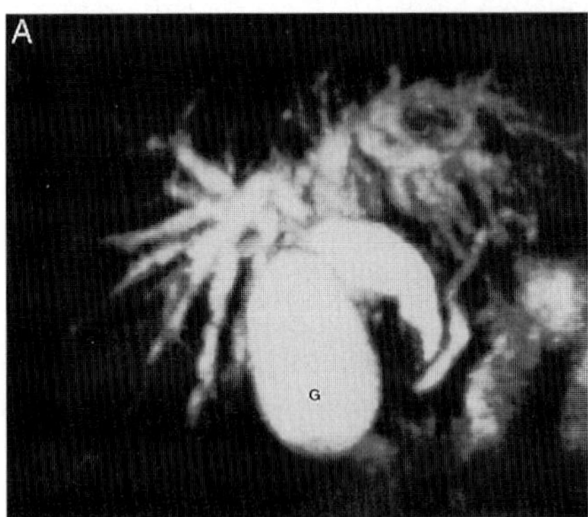

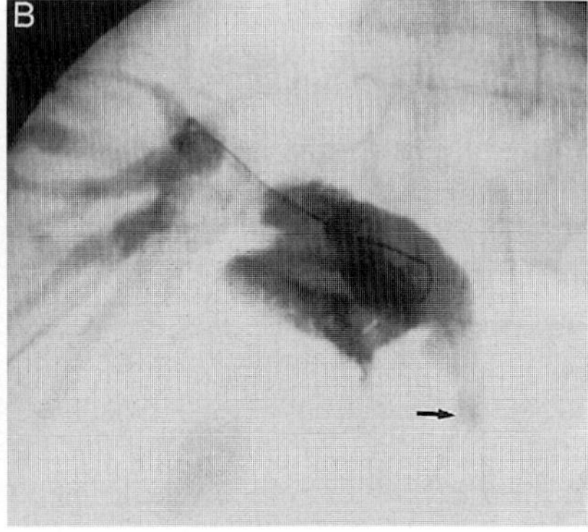

FIGURE 1.—Images of a 71-year-old man with weight loss and painless jaundice caused by adenocarcinoma of the pancreatic head. **A**, MR cholangiographic maximum intensity projection image shows markedly dilated intrahepatic ducts in all hepatic segments. The extrahepatic duct is also severely dilated to its intrapancreatic portion, where there is a tapered stenosis (*arrow*). The main pancreatic duct abruptly narrows in the same region (*arrowhead*) and is moderately dilated. **B**, percutaneous transhepatic cholangiographic image correlates with the MR cholangiogram, showing severe biliary dilatation and a tapered stenosis in the distal extrahepatic duct (*arrow*). Note wire extending through the stenosis. *Abbreviation*: *g*, gallbladder. (Courtesy of Macaulay SE, Schulte SJ, Sekijima JH, et al: Evaluation of a non–breath-hold MR cholangiography technique. *Radiology* 196:227–232, 1995. Radiological Society of North America.)

TABLE.—Intrahepatic Bile Duct Visualization

Modality	To Peripheral Third of Liver		All Four Hepatic Segments	
	Dilated	Non-dilated	Dilated	Non-dilated
MRC	18/18	9/11	18/18	10/11
ERC	12/14	7/7	10/14	5/7
PTC	5/5	1/1	2/5	0/1
IOC	NA	1/1	NA	1/1

Note: Numbers represent the number of cases in which duct is visualized/total number of cases.
Abbreviations: MRC, magnetic resonance cholangiography; *NA,* not applicable.
(Courtesy of Macaulay SE, Schulte SJ, Sekijima JH, et al: Evaluation of a non–breath-hold MR cholangiography technique. *Radiology* 196:227–232, 1995. Radiological Society of North America.)

ments of extrahepatic duct and main pancreatic duct caliber by MR and direct cholangiography were closely correlated.

Conclusions.—For depicting intrahepatic ducts in general, this non–breath-hold MR technique is comparable to endoscopic retrograde cholangiography and percutaneous transhepatic cholangiography. For depicting dilated intrahepatic ducts, this technique may be superior to either

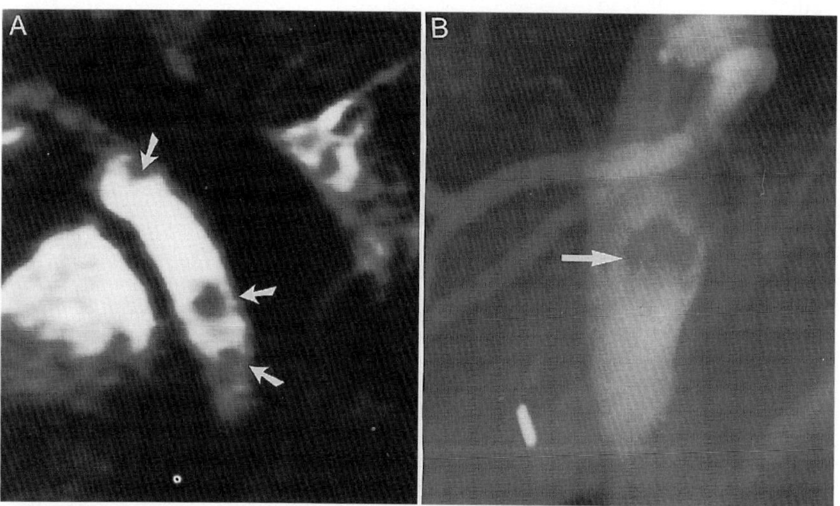

FIGURE 4.—Images of a 57-year-old man with abdominal pain, nausea, and vomiting. Stones and sludge were present in the extrahepatic duct at endoscopic retrograde cholangiography. **A,** MR cholangiographic source image shows filling defects in the extrahepatic duct. **B,** endoscopic retrograde cholangiographic image demonstrates 1 of the stones (*arrow*). (Courtesy of Macaulay SE, Schulte SJ, Sekijima JH, et al: Evaluation of a non-breath-hold MR cholangiography technique. *Radiology* 196:227–232, 1995. Radiological Society of North America.)

of the other techniques. Extrahepatic duct caliber can be visualized and measured in the majority of cases.

▶ The quality of MR cholangiograms has improved remarkably within a few years, but I am still uncertain as to the clinical role of this technique. Most patients with upper abdominal pain and/or jaundice will have CT or US and will receive an accurate diagnosis as to the presence, level, and nature of biliary obstruction. If 1 more (expensive) test needs to be performed for further evaluation and possible intervention, I believe direct cholangiography will be it. Endoscopic retrograde cholangiopancreaticography or transhepatic cholangiography are still the most precise diagnostic tools for evaluating biliary obstruction. They also serve to guide interventional techniques, such as endoluminal stenting. Magnetic resonance cholangiography is a promising and exciting tool to have available in certain problem cases.

M.P. Federle, M.D.

Pancreas

Quantitative Evaluation of Pancreatic Enhancement During Dual-Phase Helical CT

Hollett MD, Jorgensen MJ, Jeffrey RB Jr (Stanford Univ, Calif)
Radiology 195:359–361, 1995 2–28

Objective.—The quality of pancreatic enhancement in dual-phase helical CT was compared with an early and standard delay.

Background.—Pancreatic enhancement in CT is greatest when the contrast material is rapidly infused. Standard CT results in compromise between imaging during peak pancreatic or peak hepatic enhancement. Dual-phase scanning of the abdomen with a single bolus of contrast material during the arterial phase and portal venous phase is now possible with helical CT.

Methods.—A dual-phase helical CT examination of the abdomen was performed in 120 patients to evaluate or exclude various conditions. A rapidly infused 150-mL bolus of contrast material was administered, and early delayed scanning was performed beginning at 20 seconds. Standard delayed scanning began between 49 and 71 seconds. In 92 patients, the head, body, and tail of the pancreas were measured.

Results.—With an early delay of 20 seconds, the mean pancreatic enhancement was 82 Hounsfield units (HU) ± 3. With the standard delay, the mean pancreatic enhancement was 62 HU ± 2. In 66 of 92 patients, the improvement in enhancement was more than 10 HU.

Discussion.—Pancreatic enhancement is often significantly greater in helical CT with an early delay after administration of a rapidly infused contrast material than with standard delay. At this facility, arterial phase scanning in patients with suspected pancreatic abnormalities is limited to the pancreas region, except when hypervascular liver metastasis is also suspected.

▶ There are several reasons to strive for optimal pancreatic enhancement. Pancreatic ductal carcinoma and pancreatitis with necrosis are diagnosed primarily by relatively less enhancement than normal pancreatic parenchyma. Conversely, most islet cell tumors are hypervascular (and thus, hyperdense) to normal pancreas during the arterial-dominant phase of enhancement. Encasement or occlusion of peripancreatic blood vessels from malignant or benign causes is also more evident with optimal vascular enhancement. With a nonhelical scanner, you cannot achieve optimal evaluation of liver, pancreas, and blood vessels. Even with helical CT, the optimal phase for pancreatic parenchymal enhancement precedes the optimal timing for liver enhancement (due to the predominant influence of portal venous flow). Dual-phase helical CT for pancreatic evaluation is clearly superior to earlier methods.

M.P. Federle, M.D.

Potentially Resectable Pancreatic Adenocarcinoma: Spiral CT Assessment With Surgical and Pathologic Correlation

Bluemke DA, Cameron JL, Hruban RH, et al (Johns Hopkins Med Inst, Baltimore, Md)

Radiology 197:381–385, 1995 2–29

Introduction.—No more than 15% of patients with pancreatic adenocarcinoma will have resectable disease at the time of diagnosis. Significant advances in CT technology have occurred since the imaging features of these resectable tumors were described. Spiral CT was evaluated for its accuracy in assessing the resectability of small pancreatic ductal adenocarcinomas, including histopathologic and surgical correlation.

Methods.—The study included spiral CT scans from 64 patients undergoing surgery for potentially resectable pancreatic adenocarcinoma. The scans, made after injection of nonionic iodinated contrast material, were prospectively evaluated for tumor resectability. The CT findings were correlated with the surgical and pathologic findings.

Results.—Spiral CT depicted 89% of the tumors. Of these 64 carcinomas, 24 were found to be resectable at surgery (Figs 1 and 2). The resectable tumors averaged about 3 cm. Spiral CT was 70% accurate in assessing resectability. Fifty-eight percent of the resected tumors were hypoattenuating with regard to the rest of the pancreas, and the remainder were isoattenuating. At histologic examination, 11 carcinomas showed arteriolar neointimal proliferation (Table).

Conclusions.—Spiral CT can identify most small, potentially resectable pancreatic tumors. However, more than 40% of tumors that appear resectable on CT scans are actually unresectable at surgery, often because of small liver metastases. Future efforts to improve preoperative tumor staging for pancreatic ductal adenocarcinomas should focus on the detection of small pancreatic tumors and early metastases.

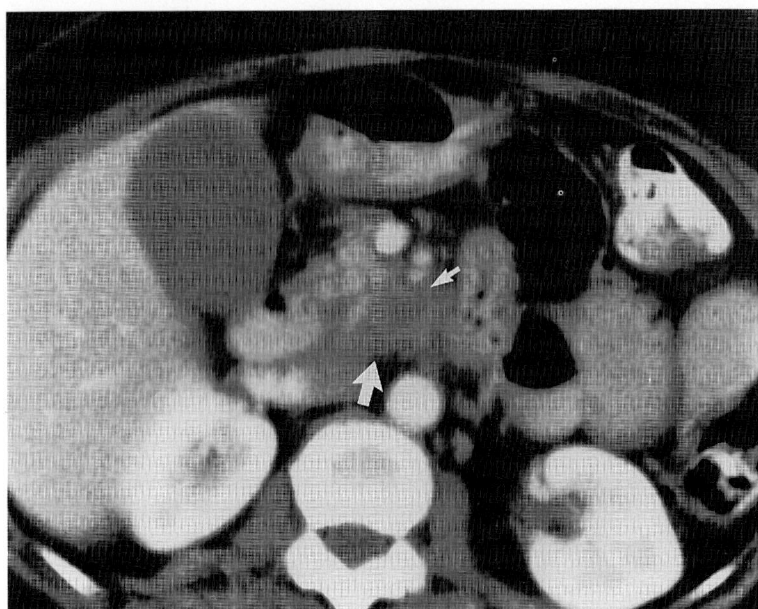

FIGURE 1.—Unresectable pancreatic adenocarcinoma. Spiral CT scan shows a hypoattenuating tumor (*large arrow*) arising from the head and uncinate process of the pancreas and extending posteriorly and caudally to surround the superior mesenteric artery as it branches (*small arrow*). The fat plane between the artery and tumor is obliterated. The tumor was predicated to be unresectable on the basis of the findings in the spiral CT examination. At surgery, the main bulk of the tumor was resected, but the gross tumor around the superior mesenteric artery was left behind. (Courtesy of Bluemke DA, Cameron JL, Hruban RH, et al: Potentially resectable pancreatic adenocarcinoma: Spiral CT assessment with surgical and pathologic correlation. *Radiology* 197:381–385, 1995. Radiological Society of North America.)

► The accuracy of CT in this group of patients with pancreatic cancer might seem unusually low, but these patients were highly selected on the basis of having small, presumably resectable tumors. Even though a helical scanner was used, I think the technique might have been improved, yielding even better results. The pancreatic parenchyma is optimally enhanced and distinguished from the typical nonenhancing carcinoma during the arterial phase of enhancement (roughly 30 to 45 seconds), rather than the somewhat delayed scanning used in the study (initiated after a 40- to 60-second delay). Other diagnostic pitfalls, including the coexistence of tumor and pancreatitis, as well as small liver or peritoneal metastases, remain challenging. Optimal CT scanning for suspected pancreatic cancer includes arterial phase imaging through the pancreas with thin collimation (3 to 5 mm) followed by portal vein dominant phase imaging through the liver and pancreas to optimize detection of metastases and venous involvement. The great majority of pancreatic adenocarcinomas are unresectable for cure, and CT signs of unresectability are highly specific. We can reduce the 40% error rate of cases thought to be resectable by CT criteria by improving our CT technique.

M.P. Federle, M.D.

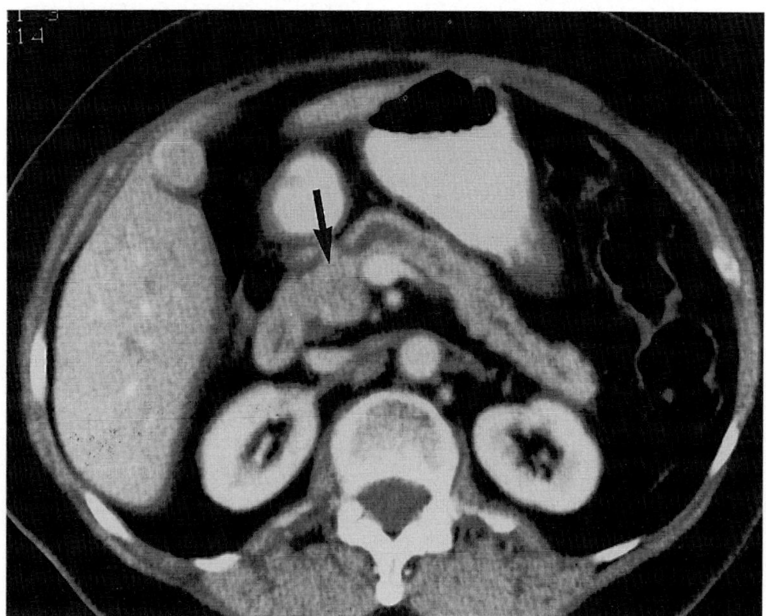

FIGURE 2.—Resectable pancreatic adenocarcinoma. Spiral CT scan shows the tumor in the pancreatic head (*arrow*) to have similar attenuation to the remainder of the pancreas. The pancreatic duct is dilated. At surgery, a 2.5-cm moderately differentiated adenocarcinoma was present, with invasion of the peripancreatic fat and tumor in 2 of 8 peripancreatic lymph nodes. (Courtesy of Bluemke DA, Cameron JL, Hruban RH, et al: Potentially resectable pancreatic adenocarcinoma: Spiral CT assessment with surgical and pathologic correlation. *Radiology* 197:381—385, 1995. Radiological Society of North America.)

TABLE.—Pathologic Findings in 24 Patients With Resected Pancreatic Adenocarcinoma

Pathologic Finding	No. of Patients
Peripancreatic lymph nodes	18 (75)
Perineural invasion	18 (75)
Duodenal invasion	17 (71)
Peripancreatic fat invasion	17 (71)
Bile duct invasion	16 (67)
Microvascular invasion	12 (50)
Neointimal proliferation	11 (46)

Note: Numbers in parentheses are percentages.

(Courtesy of Bluemke DA, Cameron JL, Hruban RH, et al: Potentially resectable pancreatic adenocarcinoma: Spiral CT assessment with surgical and pathologic correlation. *Radiology* 197:381–385, 1995. Radiological Society of North America.)

Pancreatic Adenocarcinoma: CT Versus MR Imaging in the Evaluation of Resectability: Report of the Radiology Diagnostic Oncology Group

Megibow AJ, Zhou XH, Rotterdam H, et al (New York Univ; Harvard Med School, Boston; Univ of Michigan Hosps, Ann Arbor; et al)

Radiology 195:327–332, 1995 2–30

Objective.—An attempt was made to compare findings from CT and MRI in patients with pancreatic adenocarcinoma and to determine the best imaging sequences for MRI.

Background.—Pancreatic cancer is unlikely to be confirmed to the organ of origin, which explains the poor outcome of surgical management. Imaging has allowed surgeons to select patients that may benefit from surgery. Computed tomography is most often used, but MRI is beginning to be used to assess pancreatic disease.

Methods.—There were 189 patients with adenocarcinoma of the pancreas chosen from 4 medical centers. Computed tomography was performed, but spiral CT was not used. The CT scans and MR studies were interpreted separately using a 5-point scale. Diagnostic features included the presence of peripancreatic vascular invasion, lymphadenopathy, and hepatic masses. For MR studies, 4 pulse sequences were ranked in order of usefulness. Then, CT scans and MR studies were reinterpreted together.

TABLE 1.—Correlation With Surgical or Pathologic Standard of Reference

Modality	No. of Lesions in Standard of Reference	No. of Positive (Unresectable) Lesions*	No. of Negative (Resectable) Lesions†
		Overall Resectability	
CT alone	143	121 (84.6)	22 (15.4)
MR imaging alone	138	117 (84.8)	21 (15.2)
CT plus MR imaging	126	18 (14)	108 (86)
		Vascular Invasion	
CT alone	118	42 (35.6)	76 (64.4)
MR imaging alone	115	41 (35.6)	74 (64.3)
CT plus MR imaging	103	37 (35.9)	66 (64.0)
		Lymph Node Involvement	
CT alone	108	59 (54.6)	49 (45.4)
MR imaging alone	105	55 (52.4)	50 (47.6)
CT plus MR imaging	95	50 (53)	45 (47)
		Liver Metastases	
CT alone	123	104 (84.6)	19 (15.4)
MR imaging alone	120	101 (84.2)	19 (15.8)
CT plus MR imaging	108	91 (84.2)	17 (15.7)

Note: Numbers in parentheses are percentages. Percentages do not total 100 because of rounding.
* Surgical specimens were from truly unresectable lesions.
† Surgical specimens were from truly resectable lesions.
(Courtesy of Megibow AJ, Zhou XH, Rotterdam H, et al: Pancreatic adenocarcinoma: CT versus MR imaging in the evaluation of resectability: Report of the Radiology Diagnostic Oncology Group. *Radiology* 195:327–332, 1995. Radiological Society of North America.)

Findings from imaging were correlated with surgical or pathologic evaluations (Table 1).

Results.—The accuracy was 0.73 for CT and 0.70 for MRI. The negative predictive value was 0.28 for CT and 0.23 for MRI. The positive predictive value was 0.89 for CT and 0.88 for MRI. For evaluation of vascular invasion, gradient-echo and T1-weighted spin-echo sequences were ranked equally. For evaluation of lymphadenopathy, T1-weighted spin-echo sequences were preferred. For evaluating hepatic metastases, T2-weighted spin-echo sequences were preferred.

Discussion.—There were no significant differences between CT and MRI in predicting resectability in these patients. Although the various participating institutions allowed for a large study population, the variety of readers naturally introduces error into the data. Note that the state-of-the-art pulse sequences that were assessed are no longer state-of-the-art.

▶ The Radiology Diagnostic Oncology Group (RDOP) studies were a noble attempt to respond to the criticism that radiology research is insufficiently scientific, not hypothesis-driven, or inconclusive in proving the merit of competing imaging studies. Of course, now that these multi-institutional, large-scale, expensive studies have been done, no one believes the results, including the investigators who participated! A major problem is the rapid evolution of imaging techniques, with the MR and CT techniques used in the study considered outmoded by the investigators before the manuscript was even published. This is not a criticism of this investigation, which does provide a useful snapshot of the results that can be expected using the CT and MR techniques that were stipulated. It is important to filter all clinical research through your own prism, taking into account your training, experience, and imaging equipment. All clinical research reflects these variables and other inevitable biases, no matter how honest the investigators are.

M.P. Federle, M.D.

Kidney

Renal Masses: Assessment of Corticomedullary-Phase and Nephrographic-Phase CT Scans

Cohan RH, Sherman LS, Korobkin M, et al (Univ of Michigan, Ann Arbor)
Radiology 196:445–451, 1995 2–31

Objective.—The renal CT scans of 33 patients were retrospectively reviewed to compare the value of thin-section helical CT performed during the corticomedullary phase (CMP) and during the nephrographic phase (NP) of contrast enhancement in the identification and characterization of renal masses.

Methods.—The same technique was used for all scans. For CMP scans, 5-mm thick, continuous helical mode scans were obtained before and 40 seconds after initiation of dynamic bolus injection of contrast material. For NP scans, 5-mm-thick, contiguous, axial-mode scans were obtained after

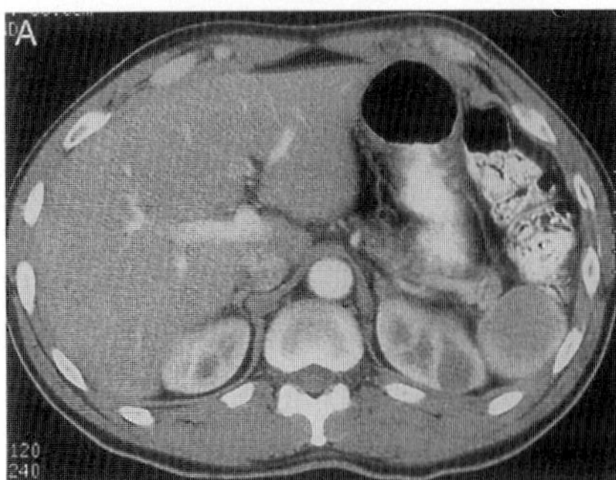

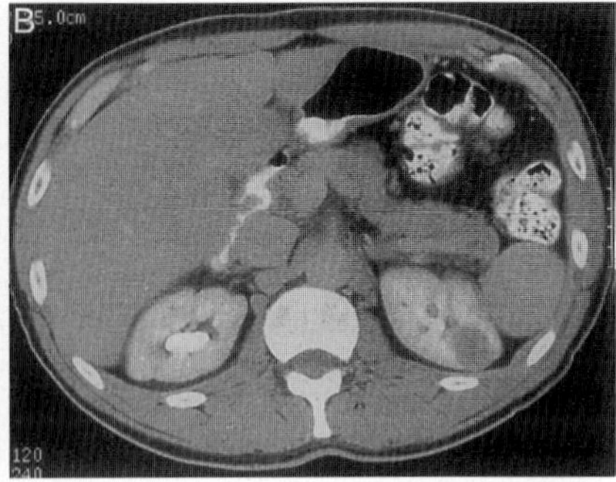

FIGURE 3.—Depiction of cortical lesions at CT in a patient who has not yet undergone surgery. **A**, no renal masses were prospectively identified on this CMP image. A low-attenuation splenic mass *(M)* was noted. **B**, a solid renal mass can be easily detected in the posterolateral aspect of the middle of the left kidney on an NP image obtained at a similar level. *Abbreviations: CMP,* corticomedullary phase; *NP,* nephrographic phase. (Courtesy of Cohan RH, Sherman LS, Korobkin M, et al: Renal masses: Assessment of corticomedullary-phase and nephrographic-phase CT scans. *Radiology* 196:445–451, 1995. Radiological Society of North America.

completion of CMP scanning. The scans were reviewed in a blinded manner during 3 separate sessions. The size and location of the lesion and its classification as a simple cyst, complex cyst, solid mass, or indeterminate mass were recorded.

Results.—A review of the scans, separately and in combination, led to the identification of 259 lesions with CMP, 389 with NP, and 417 with CMP and NP together. The higher sensitivity noted when CMP and NP scans were reviewed together was attributed to the improved detection of small lesions with NP. One large mass was not seen on CMP (Fig 3). The greatest difference between the methods occurred in the detection of renal medulla; 111 lesions were identified on NP scans vs. 25 on CMP scans.

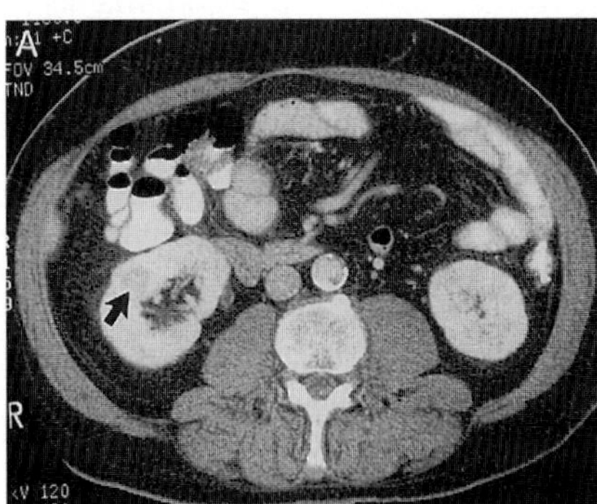

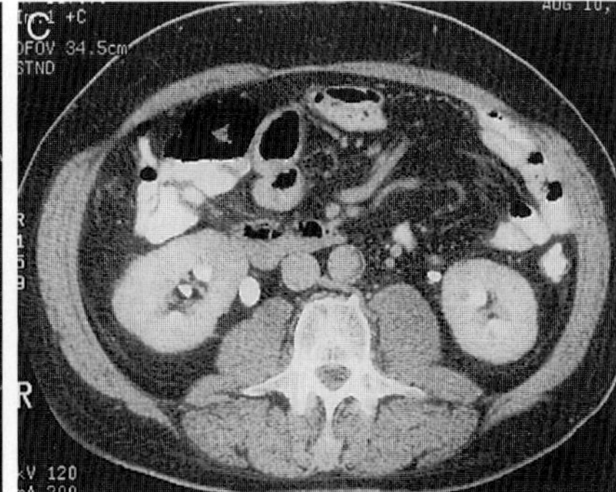

FIGURE 5.—False positive identification of a mass at NP imaging. **A**, NP image shows a rounded area of decreased attenuation in the anterior aspect of the middle of the right kidney *(arrow)*. This was suspected to be a solid heterogeneously enhancing mass. **C**, delayed images fail to demonstrate any abnormality in this region. In retrospect, the low-attenuation area was believed to represent normal renal medulla that had not yet enhanced homogeneously and to the same extent as the renal cortex. *Abbreviations: CMP,* corticomedullary phase; *NP,* nephrographic phase. (Courtesy of Cohan RH, Sherman LS, Korobkin M, et al: Renal masses: Assessment of corticomedullary-phase and nephrographic-phase CT scans. *Radiology* 196:445–451, 1995. Radiological Society of North America.)

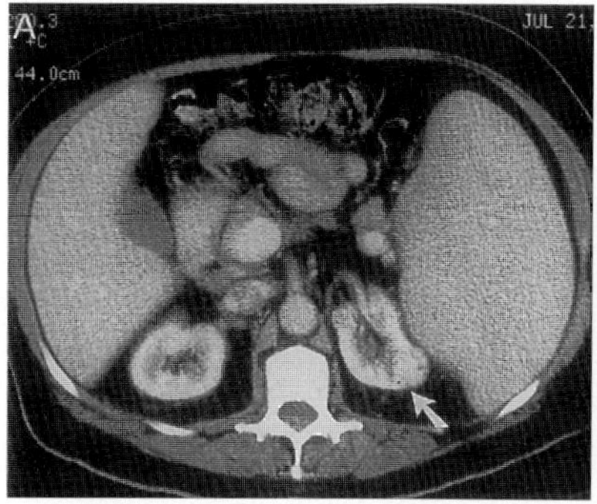

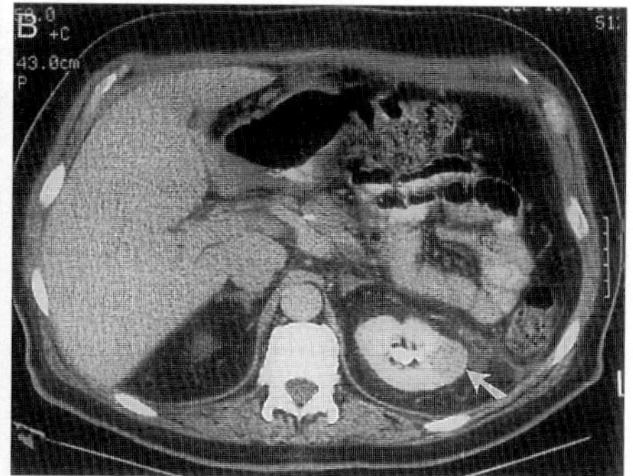

FIGURE 7.—Limitation of scanning in the CMP in the detection of hypervascular renal masses. **A**, a small, hypervascular renal mass *(arrow)* is barely visible on this scan obtained during the CMP of contrast enhancement in a patient with splenomegaly due to chronic lymphocytic leukemia. The patient subsequently underwent splenectomy. **B**, on a postoperative CT scan obtained 2 months later during the EP of renal enhancement, the mass *(arrow)* can be easily visualized. The mass was subsequently removed and was found to be a renal carcinoma. *Abbreviations: CMP*, corticomedullary phase; *EP*, excretary phase. (Courtesy of Cohan RH, Sherman LS, Korobkin M, et al: Renal masses: Assessment of corticomedullary-phase and nephrographic-phase CT scans. *Radiology* 196:445–451, 1995.)

False positive findings occurred when CMP scans alone were reviewed and when NP scans were obtained immediately after CMP scans (Fig 5). Some small renal neoplasms were not easily distinguished from normal parenchyma with CMP helical CT (Fig 7).

Conclusion.—In this group of patients with a variety of renal masses, more of the masses were detected with NP helical CT than with CMP helical CT. The difference in detection rate was greatest for medullary lesions < 11 mm, but even large masses can be obscured when CMP contrast–enhanced CT scans are obtained.

▶ As helical CT scanning becomes routine, careful attention must be paid to the timing of images relative to the contrast administration. We need to learn a new vocabulary of CT terms that relates to renal imaging CMP vs. NP or liver imaging (arterial dominant or portal venous dominant phases) that have a striking impact on the appearance and detectability of lesions. This is a timely and informative study of helical CT of the kidney.

M.P. Federle, M.D.

Renal Artery Stenosis: Evaluation of Doppler US After Inhibition of Angiotensin-Converting Enzyme With Captopril

René PC, Oliva VL, Bui BT, et al (Hôpital Notre-Dame, Montreal)
Radiology 196:675–679, 1995 2–32

Background.—Several researchers have recently studied the Doppler waveform recorded distal to an arterial stenosis rather than at the stenosis itself in patients with renal artery stenosis (RAS). The presence of a pulsus tardus—a delayed or prolonged early acceleration—was described originally in the carotid arteries. By using an "acceleration index," some of these studies have shown a marked reduction in systolic acceleration distal to a severe RAS. Renal vascular resistance is reduced by angiotensin-converting enzyme (ACE) inhibitors, which interrupt the integrity of the intrarenal renin-angiotensin system.

Methods.—Sixty-two renal arteries in 31 patients with hypertension were studied. The patients had undergone Doppler scanning before and 1 hour after the administration of captopril before angiography was performed. Doppler waveforms were classified as having a normal or pulsus tardus configuration using pattern recognition criteria.

Findings.—Based on recognition of the pulsus tardus, precaptopril Doppler scanning demonstrated 68% of 19 significant renal artery stenoses subsequently detected on angiography. By contrast, all 19 stenoses were identified with postcaptopril Doppler scanning.

Conclusions.—Captopril administration significantly enhances the sensitivity of Doppler ultrasound in detecting RAS when waveforms are analyzed using pattern recognition criteria. In severe cases, standard renal Doppler ultrasound without captopril intake is adequate for detection. The diagnosis of more moderate cases apparently requires the addition of captopril.

▶ Renal artery stenosis accounts for about 5% of hypertension cases, but it is important to diagnose because medical antihypertensive treatment is likely to be ineffective, whereas angioplasty (or surgery) can be curative. We definitely need an effective noninvasive screening test for renovascular hypertension because clinicians are understandably reluctant to obtain angiography without a high degree of suspicion. The net result in our practice is that we rarely get a chance to diagnose or treat renovascular hypertension. The use of captopril seems to improve substantially the capability of ultrasound to depict flow alterations caused by moderate degrees of RAS. I hope these promising results can be confirmed in large-scale studies.

M.P. Federle, M.D.

High Diagnostic Performance of CT Scan for Analgesic Nephropathy in Patients With Incipient to Severe Renal Failure

Elseviers MM, de Schepper A, Corthouts R, et al (Universitair Ziekenhuis Antwerpen, Belgium; St Augustinusziekenhuis, Antwerpen, Belgium; Algemeen Ziekenhuis Stuivenberg, Antwerpen, Belgium; et al)

Kidney Int 48:1316–1323, 1995 2–33

Introduction.—Analgesic nephropathy in end-stage renal failure (ESRF) can be diagnosed by demonstrating a bilateral decrease in renal volume together with either bumpy contours or papillary calcifications, but the diagnostic value of CT in this setting has not been compared with sonog-

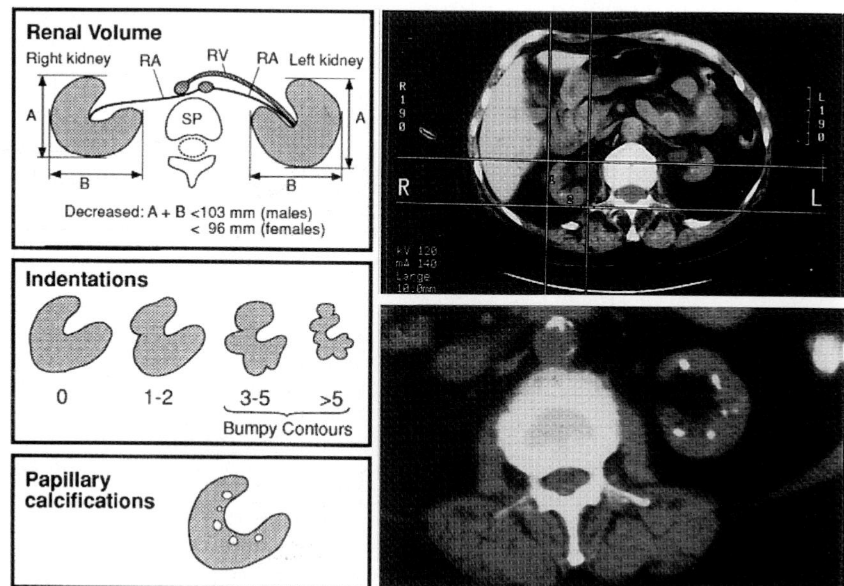

FIGURE 1.—Description of the renal imaging criteria of analgesic nephropathy as observed on CT scan including a decreased renal volume, bumpy contours, and papillary calcifications. Renal size was measured by the sum of both sides of the rectangle enclosing the kidney at the level of the renal vessels. Indentations were counted at the level where most indentations were present. Triangular, ringlike, or polygonic calcifications on the papillary line were considered as signs of renal papillar necrosis. (Courtesy of Elseviers MM, de Schepper A, Corthouts R, et al: High diagnostic performance of CT scan for analgesic nephropathy in patients with incipient to severe renal failure. *Kidney Int* 48:1316–1323, 1995. Reprinted by permission of Blackwell Science, Inc.

raphy and conventional tomography. A study of analgesic abusers and control subjects with ESRF and no clear renal diagnosis evaluated the diagnostic performance of CT.

Methods.—Eligible patients had a measured creatinine clearance below 20 mL/min. Analgesic abuse was defined as the long-term (5 years or more) daily use of analgesic mixtures—products containing 2 analgesic components combined with potentially addictive substances. All patients were examined with sonography, tomography, and CT (without iodinated contrast material) for signs of analgesic nephropathy. Renal contours were considered bumpy if at least 3 indentations were seen. Renal papillary necrosis, considered the hallmark of analgesic nephropathy, was signaled by triangular, ringlike, or polygonic calcifications on the papillary line (Fig 1).

Results.—The 3 imaging methods were comparable in their ability to evaluate renal size. Detection of papillary calcifications was superior with CT (87% sensitivity, 97% specificity). In a second study of 53 known analgesic abusers with incipient to moderate renal failure, the CT renal image of analgesic nephropathy was comparable to observations made in patients with ESRF. It was possible to demonstrate decreasing renal volume, irregular contours, and signs of papillary necrosis even in abusers

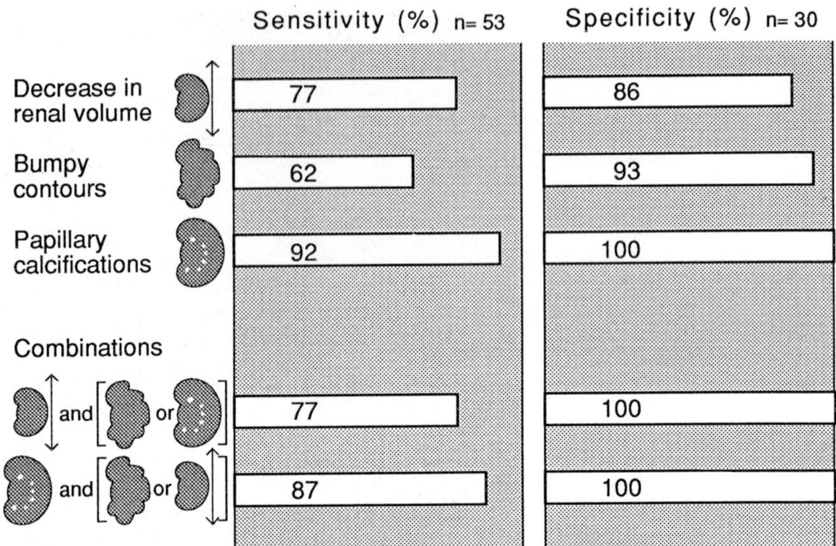

FIGURE 8.—Performance of the renal imaging criteria using CT in patients with incipient to moderate renal failure (S_{Cr}) = 1.5 to 4 mg/dL or 170 to 450 mmol/L). Combination 1 can be defined as a decreased renal volume combined with either bumpy contours or papillary calcifications. Combination 2 can be defined as papillary calcifications combined with either bumpy contours or decreased renal volume. (Courtesy of Elseviers MM, de Schepper A, Corthouts R, et al: High diagnostic performance of CT scan for analgesic nephropathy in patients with incipient to severe renal failure. *Kidney Int* 48:1316–1323, 1995. Reprinted by permission of Blackwell Science, Inc.)

with a serum creatinine level less than 2 mg/dL. These signs could be observed with scanners of varied technical specifications (Fig 8).

Conclusion.—Until recently, a diagnosis of analgesic nephropathy was based on history and exclusion of other causes of renal failure. Evaluation with CT and the criteria described here can provide an early diagnosis of this condition.

▶ Chronic renal injury caused by analgesic use is a major health problem that is thought to be both underrecognized and underreported. Clinical signs and symptoms are nonspecific; patients frequently hide their true analgesic consumption; and prior imaging criteria have been inadequate. This fascinating study reveals an important role for CT in all patients with renal failure of uncertain etiology. The CT criteria seem remarkably simple, accurate, and clinically useful.

M.P. Federle, M.D.

Bilateral Solid Multifocal Intrarenal and Perirenal Lesions: Differentiation With Ultrasonography, Computed Tomography and Magnetic Resonance Imaging

Hauser M, Krestin GP, Hagspiel KD (Zurich Univ Hosp, Switzerland)

Clin Radiol 50:288–294, 1995 2–34

Background.—Increasingly, focal masses of the kidney and perirenal region are being detected as incidental findings by cross-sectional imaging methods. Frequently, multiple lesions are present on both sides. Whereas cystic masses are usually not a diagnostic problem, more solid-appearing masses may represent a wide range of conditions, both benign and malignant.

Objective.—The findings on ultrasonography (US), CT scanning, and MR imaging were reviewed in 24 patients seen in the years 1988–1991, who had bilateral and multifocal solid intrarenal and/or perirenal lesions. Each patient had at least 2 lesions containing internal echoes or having a CT attenuation value of at least 18 Hounsfield units (HU). A total of 560 solid lesions were analyzed. The most frequent diagnoses were non-Hodgkin's lymphoma and metastasizing primary neoplasm, but some patients had inflammatory renal disorders or other benign conditions.

Methods.—Six patients had US, 17 had CT, and 10 underwent MR imaging. The US studies used a 3.5- or 5-MHz curvilinear or sector array device. When necessary, both linear and sector methods were used. Patients were scanned in both the sagittal and coronal planes. The CT studies were done using third-generation equipment, both before and after contrast administration. Spin-echo MR studies were done in all patients, and T1-weighted images were acquired after IV contrast.

Findings.—Four patients had both intrarenal and perirenal masses, but 80% of all lesions were within the kidney. The angiomyolipomas and renal-cell adenomas nearly always had clearly defined margins, but most focal inflammatory lesions and some lymphomatous lesions had poorly

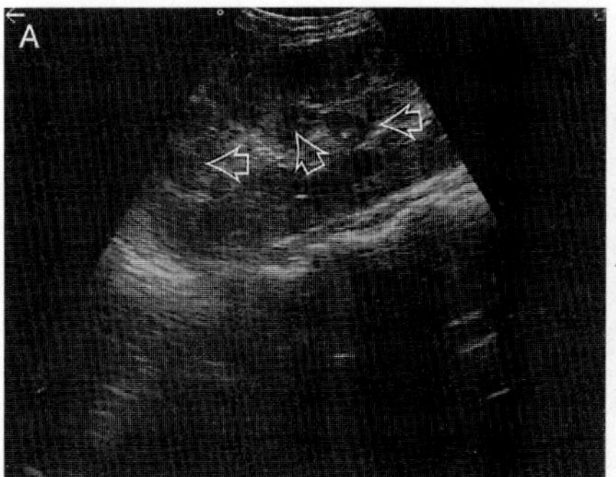

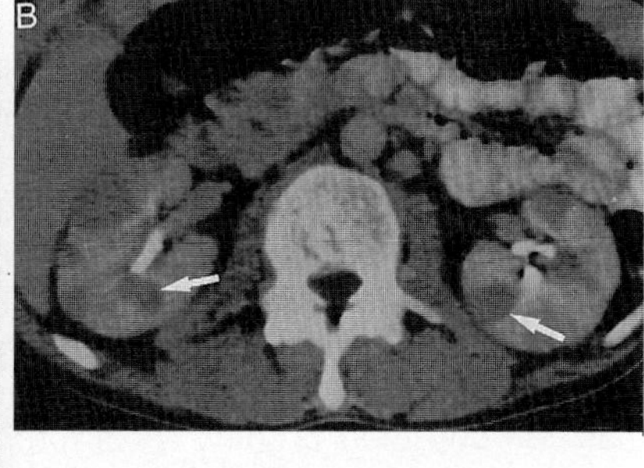

FIGURE 2.—Longitudinal US (**A**) of a right kidney and axial contrast-enhanced CT (**B**) of multiple intrarenal lymphomas (*open arrows*) in a patient with non-Hodgkin's lymphoma. (Courtesy of Hauser M, Krestin GP, Hagspiel KD: Bilateral solid multifocal intrarenal and perirenal: Differentiation with ultrasonography, computed tomography and magnetic resonance imaging. *Clin Radiol* 50:288–294, 1995.)

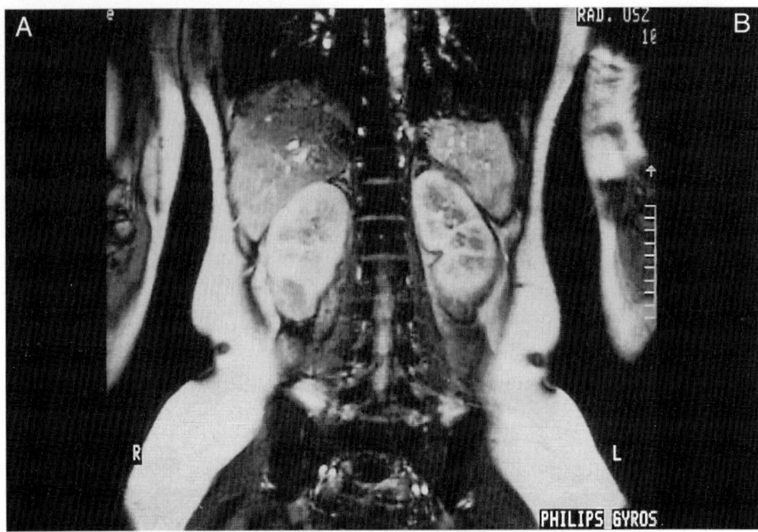

FIGURE 4.—Axial contrast-enhanced CT (**A**) and coronal contrast-enhanced T1-weighted SE MRI (**B**) in a patient with multifocal bacterial nephritis and multifocal renal abscesses (*arrows*). (Courtesy of Hauser M, Krestin GP, Hagspiel KD: Bilateral solid multifocal intrarenal and perirenal: Differentiation with ultrasonography, computed tomography and magnetic resonance imaging. *Clin Radiol* 50:288–294, 1995.)

defined contours. Postcontrast CT and MR images were most revealing. US failed to detect 14% of the lesions documented by the other modalities. In MR studies, lymphomatous and metastatic lesions tended to enhance markedly after contrast administration. Both CT scanning and MR imaging were clearly better than US in detecting nodular renal lesions (Fig 2). Inflammatory lesions tended to enhance poorly on MR imaging (Fig 4). Most angiomyolipomas had a homogeneous hyperechoic appearance with an average attenuation of −82 HU. Multiple renal adenomas or renal-cell carcinomas could not be reliably distinguished from other conditions.

► Imaging findings are unreliable in distinguishing neoplastic and inflammatory renal masses. Aside from angiomyolipomas, imaging also fails to distinguish among the various neoplastic masses. Our policy is to recommend guided biopsy of a solid renal mass when there is a known primary malignancy elsewhere or a high likelihood of lymphoma (e.g., in a patient with AIDS or one with a solid organ transplant). Patients at risk for pyelonephritis are followed up clinically and with imaging until resolution. I disagree with these authors who diagnosed 27 "adenomas" and only 7 "renal carcinomas" among their primary renal tumors. Most pathologists doubt the existence of "adenomas" and regard these as relatively small, well-differentiated carcinomas. Overall, though, this is an impressive compilation of renal masses with some useful observations.

M.P. Federle, M.D.

A Three Centre Audit of IVU Referrals in Patients With Asymptomatic Microscopic Haematuria

Rockall AG, Wetton CWN, Thomas KE, et al (St Mary's Hosp, London; Middlesex Hosp, London)

Clin Radiol 51:282–284, 1996 2–35

Background.—Several different chemical reagent dipstick tests are used to screen for microscopic hematuria. These tests are sensitive, but false positive rates as high as 15% have been reported. It is generally agreed that

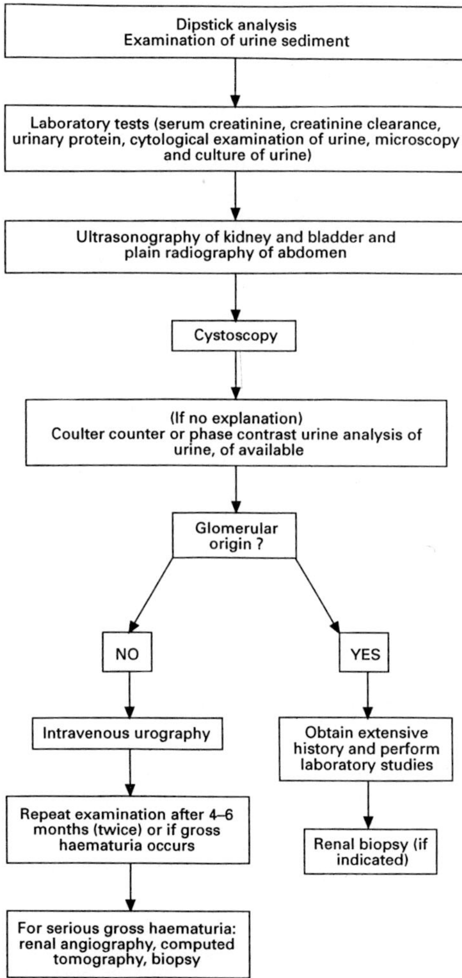

FIGURE 1.—Algorithm of diagnostic tests recommended for microscopic hematuria. (From Rockall AG, Wetton CWN, Thomas KE, et al: A three centre audit of IVU referrals in patients with asymptomatic microscopic haematuria. *Clin Radiol* 51:282–284, 1996. Courtesy of Schröder FH: Microscopic heamaturia. *BMJ* 309:70–72, 1994.)

the finding of hematuria should be confirmed by urine microscopy. An attempt was made to determine whether positive dipstick results were routinely confirmed by microscopy before IV urography (IVU) was performed.

Methods.—The study evaluated IVU request forms from 3 British hospitals during a 9-month period: a district general hospital, a teaching hospital, and a uroradiologic referral center. For all patients with asymptomatic microscopic hematuria, the case notes and urine microscopy results were evaluated. The date and results of dipstick testing and urine microscopy were recorded, as was the interval between urine microscopy and IVU.

Results.—The audit included 102 patients (mean age, 53 years; 17% younger than 40 years of age). Microscopy revealed significant hematuria in 37 patients, and the microscopy results were available before IVU was requested in 32 cases. These cases represented 31% of the total. The performance of urine microscopy was not recorded for 8 patients. Urinary tract infection was present in 14 patients. Microscopic confirmation was most likely to be obtained at the district general hospital.

Conclusion.—Radiology departments commonly receive requests for IVU in patients who have undergone dipstick testing only. The presence of significant hematuria is frequently unconfirmed when IVU is ordered; in some cases, infection is not yet excluded. The diagnosis of microscopic hematuria must be confirmed before IVU is ordered (Fig 1).

► In the new medical socioeconomic environment, radiologists may be more attuned to reducing unnecessary imaging tests. This is a nice review of a common clinical problem, and it presents a well-reasoned plan of assessment (first proposed by Schröder FH[1]). Dipstick testing of urine is known to have a false positive rate and may detect myoglobin and hemoglobin as well as red cells. Microscopy is necessary to confirm the dipstick results. Up to 10 red blood cells per high power field is usually considered normal, although not always recognized as such by referring physicians. Young women commonly have urinary tract infections, a known cause of microscopic hematuria. Conversely, individuals younger than 40 years of age are unlikely to have a malignancy, and even less likely to have 1 detected by excretory urography.

M.P. Federle, M.D.

Reference

1. Schröder FH: Microscopic haematuria. *BMJ* 309:70-72, 1994.

Acute Gas-producing Bacterial Renal Infection: Correlation Between Imaging Findings and Clinical Outcome

Wan Y-L, Lee T-Y, Bullard MJ, et al (Chang Gung College of Medicine and Technology, Tao-Yuan, Taiwan)

Radiology 198:433–438, 1996 2–36

Introduction.—Patients with severe, acute, gas-producing infections of the renal parenchyma and surrounding tissues are said to have emphysematous pyelonephritis (EPN). In the authors' experience, some patients with EPN have a fulminant clinical course and a poor prognosis, whereas others have a slower course with a better outcome. The imaging findings and clinical outcomes of patients with EPN were correlated.

Methods.—The retrospective study included 38 patients with EPN. The imaging studies included radiography in 33 patients, CT in 31, and ultrasonography in 35. Two radiologically identifiable subytpes of EPN were proposed: type I, which featured parenchymal destruction with either no fluid collection or the presence of streaky or mottled gas, and type II, characterized by renal or perirenal fluid collections with bubbly or loculated gas in the collecting system.

Results.—The imaging findings were consistent with type I EPN in 16 patients (Fig 4) and type II EPN in 22 (Fig 7). Almost all patients in both groups had diabetes. The clinical course was much more fulminant for patients with type I EPN, with a significantly shorter interval from symptom onset to death. Sixty-nine percent of patients with type I EPN died,

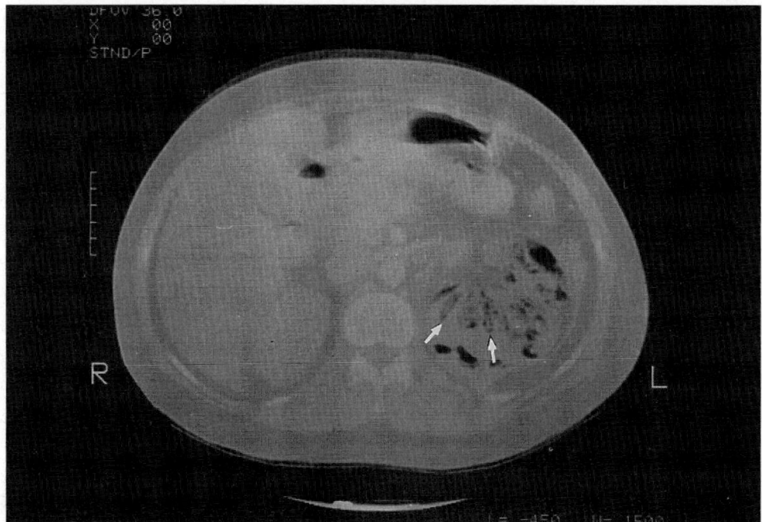

FIGURE 4.—Type I emphysematous pyelonephritis with extensive parenchymal destruction in a 43-year-old woman. Computed tomography scan with a modified lung window display shows an area of streaky gas (*arrows*) that was not seen on the radiograph (not shown). (Courtesy of Wan Y-L, Lee T-Y Bullard MJ, et al: Acute gas-producing bacterial renal infection. Correlation between imaging findings and clinical outcome. *Radiology* 198:433–438, 1996, Radiological Society of North America.)

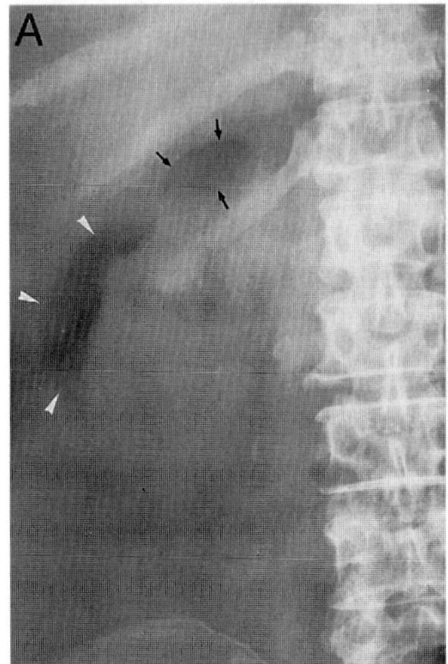

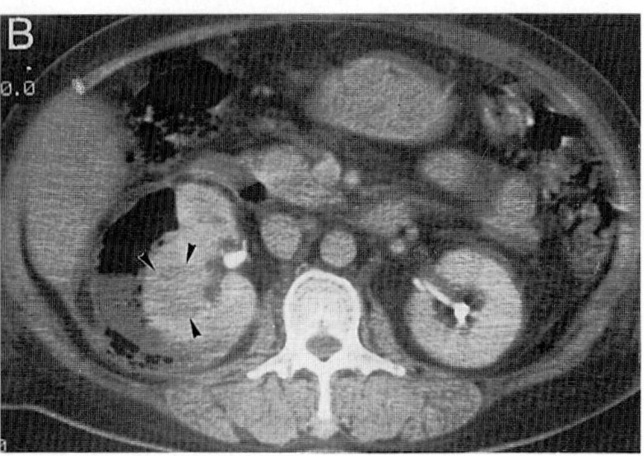

FIGURE 7.—Type II emphysematous pyelonephritis in a 57-year-old woman. **A:** Radiograph shows crescent-shaped (*arrowheads*) and loculated (*arrows*) gas in the right renal area. **B:** Computed tomography image obtained after administration of contrast material shows a low-attenuation area (*arrowheads*) in the right kidney caused by acute pyelonephritis as well as a subcapsular abscess with fluid and bubbly and loculated gas. (Courtesy of Wan Y-L, Lee T-Y, Bullard MJ, et al: Acute gas-producing bacterial renal infection: Correlation between imaging findings and clinical outcome. *Radiology* 198:433–438, 1996. Radiological Society of North America.)

compared with 18% of those with type II EPN. The imaging studies of patients with type I EPN were characterized by the absence of fluid or pus.

Conclusion.—Types I and II EPN can be distinguished on the basis of imaging studies, and this distinction is of great prognostic importance. Type I EPN, characterized by parenchymal destruction with lack of fluid content and the presence of a parenchymal streaky or mottled gas pattern on imaging studies, has a higher mortality rate and a fulminant course.

► What these authors have termed type I EPN, renal parenchymal destruction with little or no fluid component, is a deadly renal infection almost always demanding urgent nephrectomy for cure. Other authors, unfortunately, have included any form of gas-containing renal or perirenal abscess (or simple pyelitis) within their definition of EPN. These are fundamentally different processes with significantly different prognoses and recommended therapy. The treatment of choice for pyogenic renal and perirenal abscesses is percutaneous drainage of collections of pus, coupled with parenteral antibiotics. The absence of liquid pus in true EPN ("type I EPN") serves as an important diagnostic and prognostic feature.

M.P. Federle, M.D.

Adrenal

Differentiation of Adrenal Adenomas From Nonadenomas Using CT Attenuation Values

Korobkin M, Brodeur FJ, Yutzy GG, et al (Univ of Michigan, Ann Arbor; Associated Radiologists of Oakland County PC, Bloomfield Hills, Mich)
AJR 166:531–536, 1996 2–37

Background.—Characterization of adrenal masses is an important, ongoing clinical problem. Several recent studies have reported that the attenuation values of an adrenal mass on unenhanced CT scans may be used to distinguish adenomas from other anomalies. The efficacy of unenhanced CT attenuation values, enhanced CT attenuation values, and lesion size in differentiating adrenal adenomas from nonadenomatous adrenal masses was evaluated.

Patients and Methods.—The CT scans of 124 patients with 135 adrenal masses were reviewed retrospectively. There were 93 cortical adenomas—including 85 hyperfunctioning, 4 Cushing's, and 4 primary aldosteronism adenomas—and 42 nonadenomas—including 34 metastases, 4 cortical carcinomas, and 4 pheochromocytomas. Scattergrams and mean size and attenuation values on enhanced and unenhanced scans were correlated with final diagnoses. Receiver operating characteristic analysis was also carried out.

Results.—Unenhanced CT scans were available for 41 adenomas and 20 nonadenomas. A significantly lower mean attenuation value was noted in the adenomas, at 2.5 H compared with 32 H in the nonadenomas. Thirty-five of the 41 adenomas had attenuation values of less than 18 H, com-

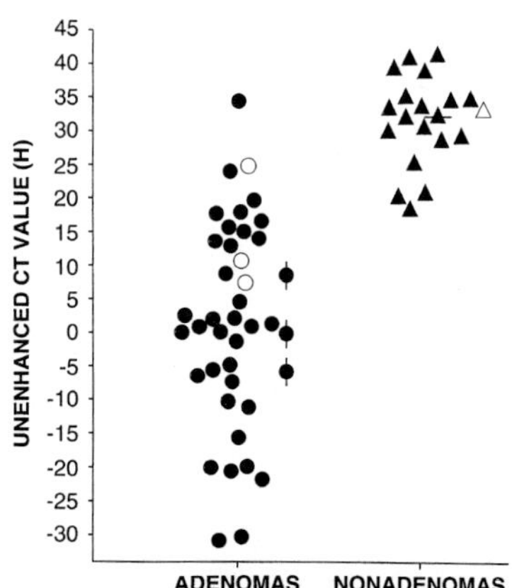

FIGURE 1.—Scattergram of attenuation values on unenhanced CT of adrenal adenomas and nonadenomas. All masses with H values of less than 18 were adenomas. *Solid circles* indicate nonhyperfunctioning adenomas; *open circles*, Cushing's adenomas; *solid circles with vertical lines*, primary aldosteronism adenomas; *solid triangles*, metastases; *open triangles*, pheochromocytomas; *solid triangle with horizontal lines*, cortical carcinomas. (Courtesy of Korobkin M, Brodeur FJ, Yutzy GG, et al: Differentiation of adrenal adenomas from nonadenomas using CT attenuation values. *AJR* 166:531–536, 1996.)

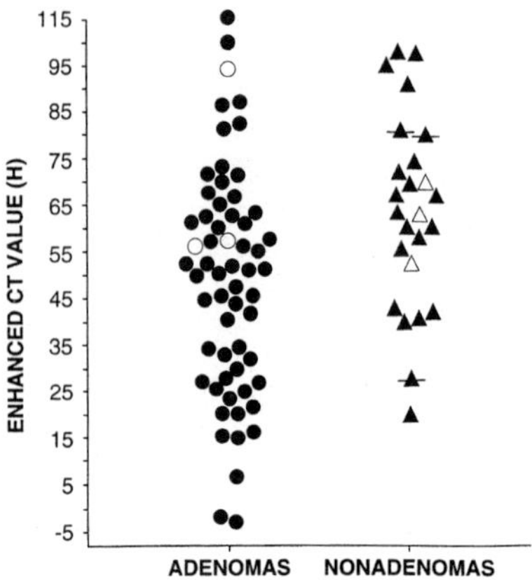

FIGURE 2.—Scattergram of attenuation values on enhanced CT of adrenal adenomas and nonadenomas. All masses with H values of less than 18 were adenomas, but only 10% of adenomas fit that criterion. *Solid circles* indicate nonhyperfunctioning adenomas; *open circles*, Cushing's adenomas; *solid triangles*, metastases; *open triangles*, pheochromocytomas; *solid triangle with horizontal lines*, cortical carcinomas. (Courtesy of Korobkin M, Brodeur FJ, Yutzy GG, et al: Differentiation of adrenal adenomas from nonadenomas using CT attenuation values. *AJR* 166:531–536, 1996.)

pared with none of the nonadenomas. The sensitivity:specificity ratio for the diagnosis of adrenal adenomas was, thus, 85%:100% at a threshold of 18 H, and positive and negative predictive values were 100% and 77%, respectively (Fig 1). Enhanced CT images were available for 60 adenomas and 25 nonadenomas, with the mean attenuation values also found to be significantly lower for adenomas, at 47 H vs. 62 H for nonadenomas. As with the unenhanced CT values, the lowest enhanced CT attenuation values of the nonadenoma was 18 H; however, the sensitivity:specificity ratio was just 10%:100% for this threshold value (Fig 2). The mean

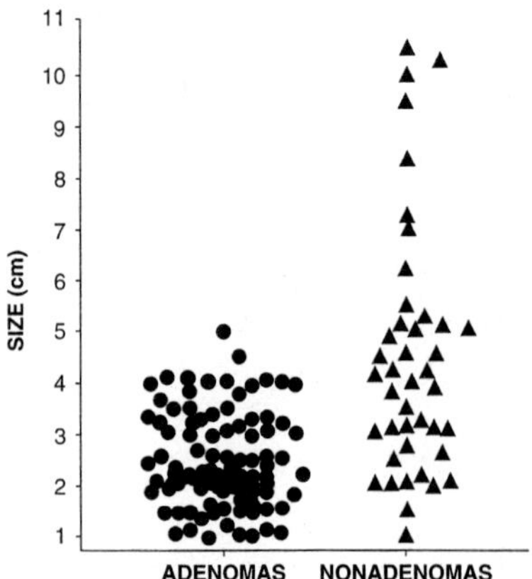

FIGURE 3.—Scattergram of size of adrenal adenomas. There was no size threshold below which all masses were adenomas. *Solid circles* indicate all adenomas; *solid triangles*, all nonadenomas. (Courtesy of Korobkin M, Brodeur FJ, Yutzy GG, et al: Differentiation of adrenal adenomas from nonadenomas using CT attenuation values. *AJR* 166:531–536, 1996.)

diameter of the adenomas was significantly lower compared with nonadenomas, at 2.4 cm vs. 4.5 cm. There was, however, considerable overlap between the 2 groups at the smallest size, meaning that there was no size threshold below which all masses were adenomas (Fig 3). A significantly greater area under the receiver operating characteristic curve was noted for unenhanced CT attenuation values, at 0.98 vs. 0.68 for the enhanced CT values and 0.79 for the area for size.

Conclusion.—Benign adrenal masses can be differentiated from other abnormalities with high specificity and sensitivity with the use of unenhanced CT attenuation values. In contrast, enhanced CT attenuation values and lesion size are not able to effectively characterize adrenal masses.

▶ This investigation offers further proof that non–contrast-enhanced CT can distinguish adenomas and metastases reliably, with 100% specificity if the attenuation value of the mass is water density or less. But what happens when you discover the adrenal mass on your routine enhanced CT of the abdomen for "rule-out mets?" During the period of contrast administration, the overlap in densities between adenomas and nonadenomas makes distinction impossible. However, the same group of investigators has subsequently reported that delayed CT scans result in a return to diagnostic low attenuation for adrenal adenomas. So the answer to the question posed above is, "Put the patient aside for 45 minutes and repeat thin sections (3–5 mm) through the adrenal mass." If the region of interest is near water density (10 H or less), it is an adenoma.

M.P. Federle, M.D.

Adrenal Nonhyperfunctioning Adenoma and Nonadenoma: CT Attenuation Value as Discriminative Index

Miyake H, Takaki H, Matsumoto S, et al (Oita Med Univ, Japan)
Abdominal Imaging 20:559–562, 1995 2–38

Background.—Most adrenal masses found incidentally on abdominal CT are nonhyperfunctioning adenomas. It is important to differentiate these masses from metastasis in patients with primary extra-adrenal malignancy. Thirty-six adrenal masses in 34 patients were retrospectively studied to determine the sensitivity of CT attenuation values in distinguishing between adrenal nonhyperfunctioning adenomas and nonadenomas.

Patients and Methods.—No patient had evidence of hormonal hypersecretion. Fourteen masses proved to be nonhyperfunctioning adenomas and 22 were nonadenomas. In the latter group, there were 17 metastases; 2 periadrenal tumors, and 1 case each of adrenocortical carcinoma, nonfunctioning pheochromocytoma, and adrenal cyst. Diagnosis was pathologically confirmed in 10 masses and clinically determined in the remaining 26 masses with follow-up CT, US, or adrenal cortical scintigraphy. Computed tomography scans were obtained in all patients; 7 had noncontrast

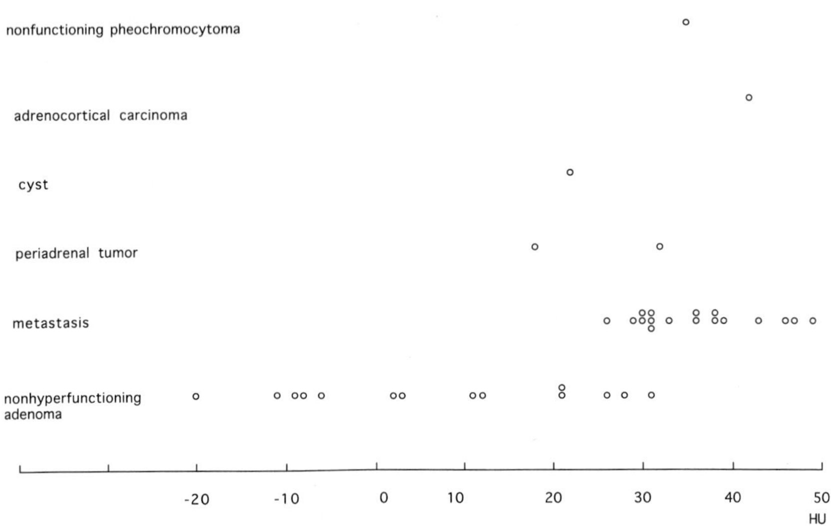

FIGURE 2.—Scattergram of noncontrast CT attenuation values in adrenal tumors. (Courtesy of Miyake H, Takaki H, Matsumoto S, et al: Adrenal nonhyperfunctioning adenoma and nonadenoma: CT attenuation value as discriminative index. *Abdom Imaging* 20:559–562, 1995.)

scans and 27 were examined before and after IV infusion of contrast medium. Attenuation values were calculated by setting a circular region of interest as large as possible in the center of each mass.

Results.—The mean diameter of nonadenomas (3.5 cm) was greater than that of nonhyperfunctioning adenomas (2.2 cm). Although no nonhyperfunctioning adenomas were larger than 4.0 cm in diameter, 15 of 17 metastases were equal to or smaller than 4 cm. Thus size alone could not definitively rule out metastasis. Except for 1 case of ganglioneuroma with myxomatous change, all adrenal masses below 20 Hounsfield units (HU) were nonhyperfunctioning adenomas (Fig 2). Using a threshold of 20 HU, CT attenuation values distinguished nonhyperfunctioning adenomas with a sensitivity of 64%, a specificity of 95%, and an accuracy of 83%. Specificity increased to 100% when the threshold was decreased to 15 HU.

Conclusion.—Nonhyperfunctioning adenomas are generally smaller than 4 cm and are less likely than nonadenomas to have a heterogeneous interior after contrast enhancement with CT. The use of CT attenuation values yields a more specific diagnosis. No further examinations are required for small (4 cm or smaller) asymptomatic adrenal masses with homogeneous low attenuation (15 HU or less).

▶ The findings in this study are important and consistent with other recent investigations. A small adrenal mass that has homogeneous low attenuation on *noncontrast* CT scans is an adrenal adenoma and requires no further evaluation. With this 1 simple criterion, you can provide a definite diagnosis in two thirds of cases, reserving biopsy or MR evaluation for equivocal cases or ones likely to represent a malignant mass.

M.P. Federle, M.D.

Distinction Between Benign and Malignant Adrenal Masses: Value of T1-Weighted Chemical-Shift MR Imaging

Outwater EK, Siegelman ES, Radecki PD, et al (Thomas Jefferson Univ, Philadelphia; Univ of Pennsylvania, Philadelphia; Suburban Hosp, Bethesda, Md)

AJR 165:579–583, 1995 2–39

Introduction.—The presence of lipid accumulation can help differentiate benign from malignant adrenal masses. Because T1-weighted opposed-phase imaging techniques can depict small proportions of lipid in tissues, these techniques may be useful with quantitative measurements. Patients with adrenal masses were examined to assess the accuracy of T1-weighted chemical-shift MR imaging in identifying benign and malignant lesions.

Methods.—The nature of the 58 masses had proved benign in 38 cases, based on stable size for at least 1 year, and malignant in 20, based on surgery or growth. Detection of lipid in the masses was compared for in-phase spin-echo sequences or in-phase breath-hold fast multiplanar spoiled gradient-recalled echo (FMPSPGR) sequences with a TE of 4.2 msec and opposed-phase breath-hold FMPSPGR sequences with a TR/TE of 35–155/2.2–2.9 and a 90-degree flip angle. Using a 5-point scale of

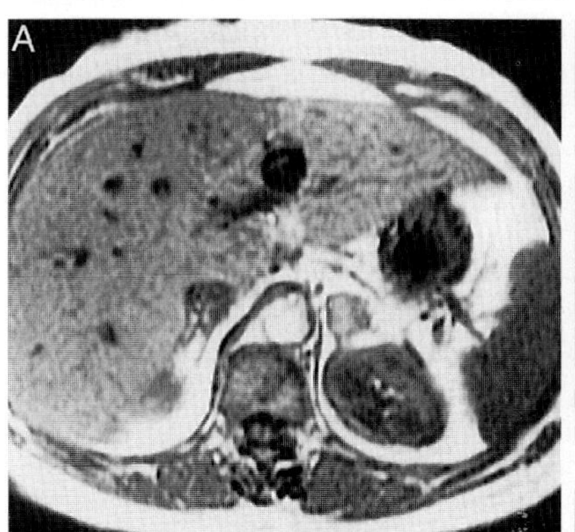

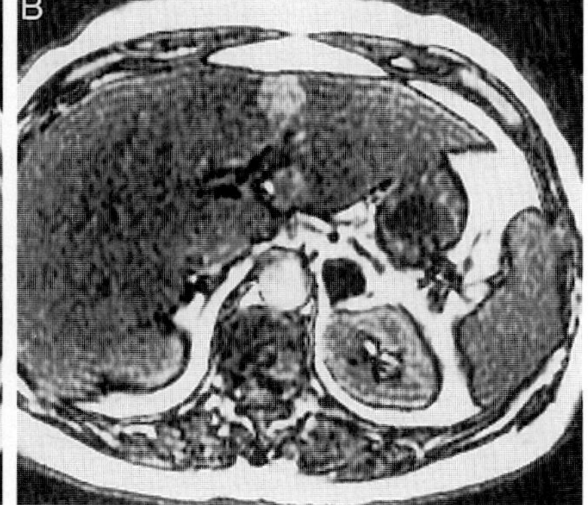

FIGURE 1.—Chemical-shift MR imaging of adrenal adenoma, 67-year-old woman with lung carcinoma. **A** and **B**, in-phase gradient-echo MR image (TE = 4.2 msec) **A** and opposed-phase fast multiplanar spoiled gradient-recalled echo sequence (TE = 2.4 msec) **B** show a left adrenal mass that is slightly hyperintense compared with spleen on in-phase image and markedly hypointense compared with spleen on opposed-phase image, indicating presence of lipid. Note loss of signal in fatty-infiltrated liver, making this an unreliable standard for comparison of signal intensity. Lesion was unchanged in size on serial CT scans obtained more than 1 year apart. (Courtesy of Outwater EK, Siegelman ES, Radecki PD, et al: Distinction between benign and malignant adrenal masses: Value of T1-weighted chemical-shift MR imaging. *AJR* 165:579–583, 1995.)

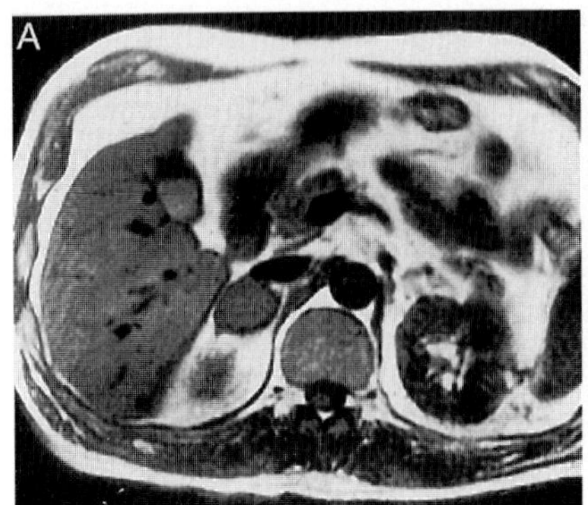

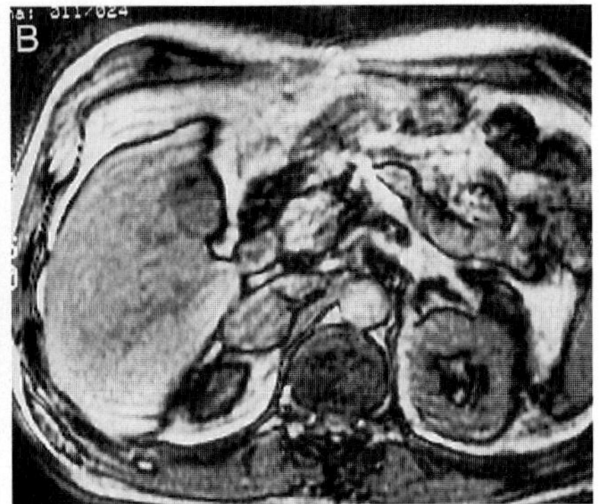

FIGURE 2.—Opposed-phase MR imaging diagnosis of metastasis in 57-year-old man with renal clear-cell carcinoma metastatic to the right adrenal gland. **A** and **B**, spin-echo in-phase image **A** and opposed-phase breath-hold fast multiplanar spoiled gradient-recalled echo image **B** show right adrenal mass that is isointense with spleen on T1-weighted images and isointense or slightly hyperintense on opposed-phase gradient-echo image. Thus, no evidence of loss of signal is apparent on opposed-phase image, consistent with metastasis. Lesion showed growth in parallel with a bone metastasis on serial studies obtained 4 months apart. (Courtesy of Outwater EK, Siegelman ES, Radecki PD, et al: Distinction between benign and malignant adrenal masses: Value of T1-weighted chemical-shift MR imaging. *AJR* 165:579–583, 1995.)

confidence, 3 radiologists blinded to clinical data and diagnosis classified the images as benign or malignant.

Results.—Benign lesions did not consistently have a higher signal intensity (relative to spleen) than malignant lesions, and detection of lipid within the lesion was a better indication of its benign nature than signal intensity. Nevertheless, the overall impression of the benignity of the lesion had better diagnostic performance than the presence of lipid alone. Comparison of the in-phase and opposed-phase images was important for diagnosis of lipid within adenomas (Fig 1) and for exclusion of lipid in metastases (Fig 2). The mean sensitivity for a definite or probable diagnosis of a benign lesion by the three observers was 87%, specificity was 92%, and the positive predictive value was 95%. At the highest confidence level of a benign mass, the mean positive predictive value increased to 99%, but sensitivity fell to 54%. There was good interobserver agreement.

Conclusion.—Most benign adrenal masses can be diagnosed at the highest threshold of confidence using chemical-shift imaging with breath-hold opposed-phase T1-weighted MR images. With such a level of accuracy, only a small number of indeterminate lesions should require follow-up examination or biopsy.

▶ Chemical-shift MR imaging is a substantial improvement over standard MR techniques in distinguishing adrenal adenomas from metastases. One contribution of this study was to note that the subjective evaluation of signal suppression on opposed-phase images was as accurate as any quantitative measure of signal intensity (which appeals to my laziness and aversion to measuring and memorizing numbers). Note that MR imaging is not necessary if a nonenhanced CT scan has already confirmed that the adrenal mass is an adenoma by virtue of having a homogeneous low attenuation (15 HU or less). (See Abstract 2–38.)

M.P. Federle, M.D.

Spontaneous Unilateral Adrenal Hemorrhage: Computerized Tomography and Magnetic Resonance Imaging Findings in 8 Cases

Hoeffel C, Legmann P, Luton JP, et al (Hôpital Cochin, Paris)
J Urol 154:1647–1651, 1995 2–40

Background.—Spontaneous unilateral adrenal hematomas are rare. Confidentally diagnosing adrenal hematoma and determining whether there is an underlying cause indicating surgery are difficult. The imaging features of spontaneous unilateral adrenal hematomas in 8 patients were reported.

Methods.—The CT and MRI findings and clinical histories of 8 patients with unilateral spontaneous adrenal hemorrhage seen during a 6-year period were reviewed. Eight patients underwent CT; 5, MRI; and 5, both. The imaging findings were correlated with histologic results.

Findings.—Magnetic resonance imaging was the most accurate imaging method, demonstrating variable appearances. On T1-weighted images, a heterogeneous mass was evident in all patients. Three had primarily low signal intensities. In 2 patients, the signal intensity was the same as the liver. Small foci of high signal intensity were noted in 4 patients. On T2-weighted images, masses in all but 1 patient had a heterogeneous high signal intensity with some lower signal areas. In 1 patient, this was serpiginous (Fig 6). Another patient had a peripheral rim of markedly high signal intensity. In another patient, the center of the mass had a lower signal. Computed tomographic findings included a mass in the adrenal bed

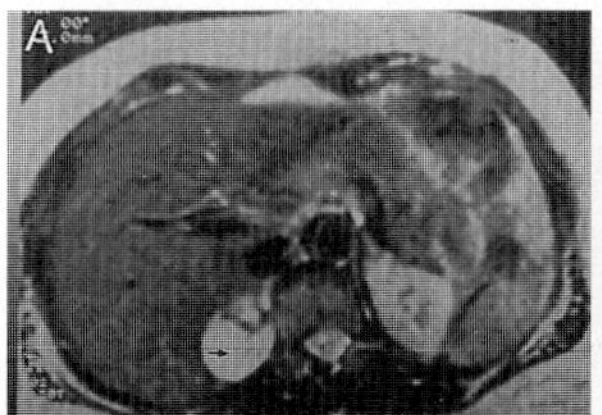

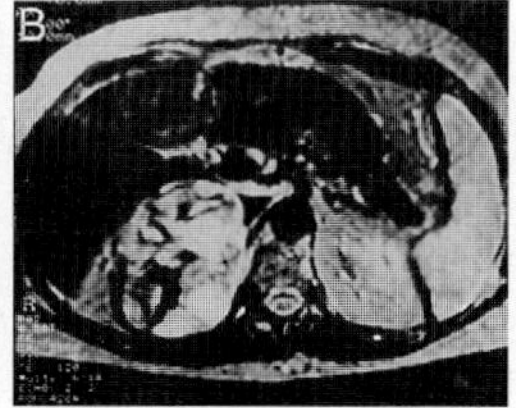

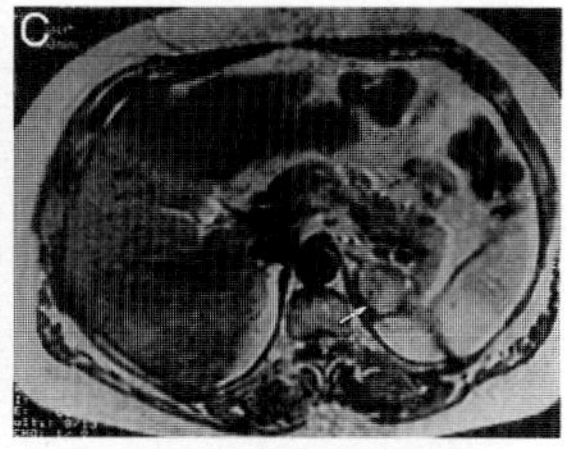

FIGURE 6.—Magnetic resonance imaging. **A,** axial spin echo (TR/2020, TE/120) T2-weighted image shows extremely high signal intensity with some serpiginous areas of lower signal (*arrow*) of right adrenal mass. **B,** T2-weighted image (TR/2100, TE/120) reveals heterogeneous right adrenal mass with numerous areas of low signal intensity, many of which have higher signal intensity centrally. Pathologic examination demonstrated old hematoma as assessed by presence of calcifications, capsule, and small benign tumor associated with hematoma. **C,** axial spin echo image (TR/2020, TE/60) demonstrates heterogeneous signal intensity with serpiginous pattern of low signal intensity and predominant areas of high signal intensity (*arrow*). Histopathology revealed idiopathic left adrenal hematoma composed of hemorrhagic necrosis and incompletely surrounded by fibrous capsule. (Courtesy of Hoeffel C, Legmann P, Luton JP, et al: Spontaneous unilateral adrenal hemorrhage: Computerized tomography and magnetic resonance imaging findings in 8 cases. *J Urol* 154:1647–1651, 1995.)

that obscured the tails and limbs. The lesions were round to oval, and the margins were well defined. In 6 patients, delineation was clearly marked from surrounding tissues. In 5 patients, the right adrenal gland was involved. There was no contrast enhancement on CT or MRI. Pathologic assessment demonstrated hematomas that were old and organized.

Conclusions.—An incidentally discovered large adrenal mass with no abnormal biochemical studies may be interpreted as a malignant tumor or intermittently functioning pheochromocytoma. The diagnosis of idiopathic adrenal hematoma is strongly suggested by MR signs of adrenal hemorrhage and the absence of significant MR enhancement of the mass. In such patients, surgery can be delayed until further imaging is done.

► Adrenal hemorrhage in adults is said to be rare, but we have seen many cases after trauma, liver transplantation, anticoagulant therapy, severe physical stress, and septicemia. The possibility of an underlying adrenal tumor must always be considered. This article reports on an interesting group of patients with "spontaneous" adrenal hemorrhage, but I question how diligent the authors were in screening for a history of likely cause of adrenal hemorrhage, as this was not addressed in the article. In the absense of such a history, any large adrenal mass will probably require surgical removal because an adrenal tumor cannot be reliably distinguished from subacute hemorrhage.

M.P. Federle, M.D.

Male Reproductive Tract

Ultrasonographic Evaluation and Clinical Correlation of Intratesticular Lesions: A Series of 39 Cases

Coret A, Leibovitch I, Heyman Z, et al (Tel Aviv Univ, Israel)
Br J Urol 76:216–219, 1995 2–41

Background.—Most patients with testicular neoplasms initially have a painless testicular mass or diffuse testicular enlargement clinically. However, swelling and hydrocele, tenderness after minor trauma, or a painful and tender scrotum with epididymo-orchitis have also been noted. Because the clinical presentation and assessment of patients with testicular tumors can be nonspecific and nondiagnostic, the accuracy of ultrasound (US) in the diagnosis of testicular tumors was investigated.

Methods and Findings.—Thirty-nine patients referred because of pain, tenderness, and the appearance of a mass in the scrotum or scrotal swelling after trauma underwent US. Patients ranged in age from 3 to 61 years, with a mean age of 20.3 years. In 35 patients, intratesticular lesions were found on US. The remaining 4 had no suspicious findings after surgical exploration of the scrotum based on clinical findings only. Findings on US were consistent with neoplasm in 5 patients, but no tumor was discovered at surgery or on follow-up. In 1 patient, in whom the US findings suggested inflammation, an embryonal cell carcinoma was found on exploration 3 weeks later.

Conclusions.—Although US is very sensitive in helping to differentiate an intratesticular lesion from an extratesticular 1 and in excluding a testicular tumor, the pattern of different benign processes on US may be similar to those of tumors. Ultrasonography had a sensitivity of 96.6% and a specificity of 44.4% in the diagnosis of testicular lesions. Its positive predictive value and accuracy were 85.3% and 84.6%, respectively, indicating that scrotal exploration is needed when an intratesticular lesion is found on US, even when there is no clinical suspicion of such a neoplasm.

▶ Ultrasound is very sensitive in depicting testicular pathology and distinguishing testicular from extratesticular processes. However, morphologic (and in other investigations, color Doppler) features do not distinguish neoplastic from inflammatory or traumatic testicular masses reliably. The clinical setting usually indicates the likely cause. It should be noted that in an asymptomatic patient or in a young man with metastatic disease, any US-detected intratesticular mass is likely to be neoplastic, and surgical exploration of the scrotum is indicated.

M.P. Federle, M.D.

Nonpalpable Intratesticular Masses Detected Sonographically
Comiter CV, Benson CJ, Capelouto CC, et al (Harvard Med School, Boston)
J Urol 154:1367–1369, 1995 2–42

Background.—Most testicular cancers are palpable. However, sometimes an impalpable testicular cancer will be detected with scrotal ultrasound in a patient with scrotal trauma, scrotal pain, infertility, hydrocele, epididymal disease, or a contralateral scrotal mass. The implications of impalpable testicular masses are debated. The sonographic and pathologic findings of 15 impalpable testicular masses are reported.

Patients and Findings.—The patients were identified from a series of 3,019 scrotal ultrasound studies performed during a 9-year period. The patients' mean age was 34 years. All had an intratesticular lesion identified on sonography that did not meet the criteria for a simple cyst. The mean mass size was 12 mm, and 12 of 15 masses were predominantly hypoechoic. Eighty-seven percent of the masses proved to be malignant—there were 5 seminomas, 6 nonseminomas, 2 burned-out tumors, 1 lipoma, and 1 granuloma. Five of 6 patients with persistent scrotal pain were found to have a viable testicular cancer.

Conclusions.—Most intratesticular masses that are impalpable and detected only with sonography will prove to be malignant. Scrotal ultrasound should be performed in any young man with a retroperitoneal or visceral mass. The testicular mass will most often represent a primary cancer, but regression is possible. Ultrasound is also indicated for patients with persistent scrotal pain.

▶ Testicular cancer is the most common malignancy in young men, usually presenting as a palpable mass. Ninety-five percent of all palpable intratesticular masses are malignant germ cell tumors. In a young man with retroperitoneal nodal or abdominal visceral masses, an impalpable but sonograpically visible testicular tumor is the likely cause. In the setting of testicular pain, a contralateral mass or a history of other scrotal pathology, these authors found testicular tumors in many cases. However, other investigators have found benign conditions (including Sertoli or Leydig cell tumors) to be more frequent.[1] Regardless, histologic diagnosis is mandatory. The true incidentally discovered mass might be approached with a conservative surgical approach (inguinal approach, ultrasound-guided excision of the lesion, and frozen section analysis) before committing to orchiectomy.

M.P. Federle, M.D.

Reference

1. Horstman WG, Haluszka MM, Burkhard TK: Management of testicular masses incidentally discovered by ultrasound. *J Urol* 151:1263, 1994.

Improved Accuracy of Computerized Tomography Based Clinical Staging in Low Stage Nonseminomatous Germ Cell Cancer Using Size Criteria of Retroperitoneal Lymph Nodes

Leibovitch I, Foster RS, Kopecky KK, et al (Indiana Univ, Indianapolis)
J Urol 154:1759–1763, 1995 2–43

Background.—The accuracy of radiologic diagnosis of low-stage nonseminomatous germ cell tumor is relatively low, on the order of 67% to 82%. In the absence of definite criteria for CT categorization, some equivocal CT scans may be classified as questionable. The size of retroperitoneal lymph nodes was evaluated as a possible criterion for use in CT staging in patients with low-stage nonseminomatous germ-cell cancer.

Methods.—The retrospective study included 143 CT scans of selected patients with stage A to B1 nonseminomatous germ cell tumors who underwent primary retroperitoneal lymph node dissection (Fig 1). Pathologic examination revealed stage A disease in 62% of patients and stage B1 disease in 38%. The diameter of the retroperitoneal nodes demonstrated on CT scan was determined, and the relationship of lymph node size with disease stage was analyzed by multivariate logistic regression.

Results.—Eighty-one percent of the scans demonstrated retroperitoneal lymph nodes, the short transaxial diameter of which ranged from 0–25 mm. The mean diameter was 4 mm in patients with stage A disease (Fig 2) and 11 mm in those with stage B disease. On the multivariate logistic

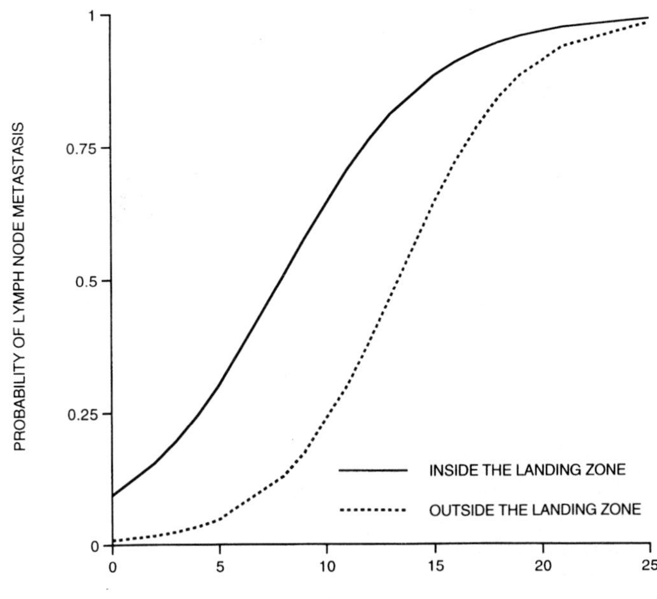

FIGURE 5.—Multivariate logistic regression model demonstrates relation between measured short transaxial diameter of detected retroperitoneal lymph nodes and histopathologic status of these nodes. Probability of metastatic tumor in retroperitoneal lymph nodes at given lymph node diameter is significantly affected by correlation between reported site of lymph nodes and expected primary landing zone (Wald chi-square test, $P = 0.0007$). (Courtesy of Leibovitch I, Foster RS, Kopecky KK, et al: Improved accuracy of computerized tomography based clinical staging in low stage nonseminomatous germ cell cancer using size criteria of retroperitoneal lymph nodes. *J Urol* 154:1759–1763, 1995.)

Female Reproductive Tract

MR Imaging of Tubo-Ovarian Abscess

Ha HK, Lim GY, Cha ES, et al (Catholic Univ, Seoul, Korea)
Acta Radiol 36:510–514, 1995 2–44

Introduction.—As a result of inadequate or delayed treatment of pelvic inflammatory disease, a tubo-ovarian abscess can develop. An inflammatory adnexal mass must be demonstrated to differentiate between uncomplicated salpingitis and a tubo-ovarian abscess. Magnetic resonance imaging has been shown recently to demonstrate adnexal mass. An analysis of MR findings of tubo-ovarian abscesses was conducted in 8 women.

Methods.—The MR images of 9 surgically proven tubo-ovarian abscesses of 8 women (35–72 years of age) were analyzed. Clinical symptoms included lower abdominal mass in 4 women, abdominal pain in all women, and generalized weakness in 2 women. Reasons for surgery were a large abscess larger than 10 cm in 3 women, clinical signs of sepsis or abscess rupture in 3 women, and failed medical therapy in 2. Signal intensity characteristics and the morphologic appearance of the mass were

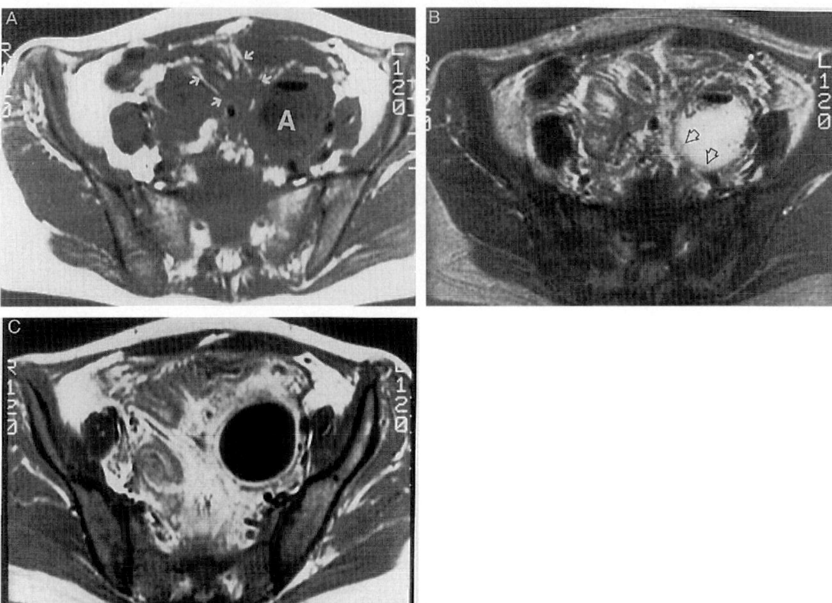

FIGURE 2.—Tubo-ovarian abscess in a 39-year-old woman. **A,** axial T1-weighted MR image (417/17) shows a hypointense mass (*A*) with ill-defined margins and an air-fluid level in the left adnexal region. "Mesh-like" linear strand (*arrows*) in the fat planes surrounding the abscess. **B,** axial T2-weighted image (1 800/80) shows shading (*arrows*) in the periphery of the hyperintense, pus-filled abscess cavity, as well as the air-fluid level. **C,** contrast-enhanced image (750/11) shows dense enhancement of a thin rim of the abscess wall. (Courtesy of Ha HK, Lim GY, Cha ES, et al: MR imaging of tubo-ovarian abscess. *Acta Radiol* 36:510–514, 1995.)

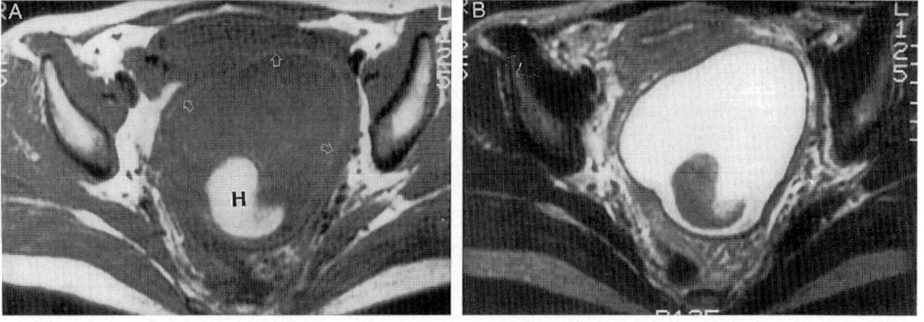

FIGURE 1.—Tubo-ovarian abscess in a 35-year-old woman. **A,** axial T1-weighted MR image (650/11) shows a large, thick-walled mass in the cul-de-sac, filled with pus. The content is isointense to the surrounding muscle and myometrium except for the focal hemorrhage (*H*) of hyperintensity. A thin, hyperintense rim (*arrows*) is seen in the innermost portion of the abscess wall. There are "mesh-like" linear strands in the para- and perirectal spaces. **B,** axial T2-weighted MR image (1 800/80) shows the thin rim of the abscess wall and the focal hemorrhage within the abscess to be hypointense. (Courtesy of Ha HK, Lim GY, Cha ES, et al: MR imaging of tubo-ovarian abscess. *Acta Radiol* 36:510-514, 1995.)

TABLE 1.—Magnetic Resonance Characteristics of Masses in 9 Tubo-Ovarian Abscesses in 8 Patients

Findings	In Case 1	2	3	4	5	6	7	8	9
Hyperintense rim, 1–3 mm (T1WI)	+	−	+	+	+	+	+	+	+
Thickened wall	+	−	+	+	+	+	+	+	+
Ill-defined margins	+	−	+	+	+	+	+	+	+
Multiple internal septations	+	−	+	+	+	−	+	+	+
Shading (T2WI)	−	+	−	+	+	+	+	+	+
Gas collection	−	−	−	+	+	−	−	−	−

Note: Unilateral abscess in 7 and bilateral in 1.
(Courtesy of Ha HK, Lim GY, Cha ES, et al: MR imaging of tubo-ovarian abscess. *Acta Radiol* 36:510–514, 1995.)

evaluated on the MR images, as was the presence of secondary changes in adjacent pelvic organs and structures.

Results.—In 5 women, the signal intensity of the lesions on T1-weighted images was hypointense to the surrounding muscle and myometrium (Fig 2); in 3 abscesses, the signal intensity was isointense, and in 1 abscess, it was hyperintense. On T2-weighted images, the signal intensity was heterogeneous in 3 abscesses and hyperintense in 6 abscesses. In the innermost aspect of the masses, a thin rim of 1–3 mm with hyperintensity on T1-weighted images was noted (Fig 1). Gas collection, shading, multiple internal septa, thickened wall, and an ill-defined margin were other findings (Table 1). In all women, "mesh-like" linear strands were seen in the pelvis with involvement of adjacent pelvic organs in 7 abscesses and lymphadenopathy in 3 abscesses.

Conclusion.—Magnetic resonance imaging was successful in demonstrating the extent of the disease, making a specific diagnosis, and characterizing the lesions. However, in terms of cost-effectiveness, MR imaging may be questionable, because ultrasound and CT have a high accuracy for specific diagnosis of this kind of lesion. Magnetic resonance imaging is useful when ultrasound or CT findings are equivocal.

► Because ultrasound and CT can confirm the presence of a tubo-ovarian abscess (TOA) that is suspected on clinical grounds, I am unsure of the exact role of MR in this context. The extensive mesh-like adhesions and the focal hemorrhage were all shown by MR and correspond well to the known pathophysiology of TOA. In cases of pelvic masses of unknown origin, MR is surely valuable, and some of these signs may prove to be relatively specific in distinguishing TOA from tumor.

M.P. Federle, M.D.

Fetal/Obstetric

Community-Based Obstetrical Ultrasound Reports: Documentation of Compliance With Suggested Minimum Standards

Smulian JC, Vintzileos AM, Rodis JF, et al (Univ of Connecticut, Farmington; Univ of Medicine and Dentistry of New Jersey, New Brunswick)

J Clin Ultrasound 24:123–127, 1996 2–45

Objective.—Few studies have examined the obstetric sonography performed by various community-based physicians, including obstetricians, radiologists, and family practitioners. Standards and guidelines for obstetric ultrasound (US) have been put forth by both the American College of Obstetrics and Gynecology (ACOG) and the American Institute of Ultrasound in Medicine (AIUM). The degree of compliance with these guidelines by community-based practitioners performing obstetric US was assessed.

Methods.—One hundred seventy-five obstetric US reports were obtained from various nontertiary referral facilities. Fifty-five reports came from obstetricians' offices and 120 came from radiologic facilities. Thirty-five percent and 22%, respectively, of the examinations were first-trimester examinations. The reports were reviewed for documentation of individual components of the ACOG and AIUM standards for obstetric US. General statements such as "normal fetal anatomy" were considered inadequate.

Results.—Of the first-trimester reports from obstetric offices, 35% demonstrated complete compliance with ACOG guidelines and 15% with AIUM standards. Compliance rates were lower for first-trimester reports from radiologic facilities: 12% and 4%, respectively (Table 2). None of the second- or third-trimester reports from either type of facility complied completely with either set of standards (Table 3). Obstetric reports tended

TABLE 2.—Documentation of First Trimester Components Suggested by ACOG and AIUM

	Obstetrical (n = 20)	Radiological (n = 26)	P
	(%)	(%)	
Fetal number	20 (100)	24 (92.3)	NS
Fetal viability	20 (100)	26 (100)	NS
Gestational sac location	16 (80)	25 (96.2)	NS
Fetal pole	20 (100)	25 (96.2)	NS
Crown-rump length	20 (100)	24 (92.3)	NS
Yolk sac	9 (45)	7 (26.9)	NS
Uterus	12 (60)	6 (23.1)	.025
Adnexa	14 (70)	14 (53.8)	NS
Cervix*	3 (15)	3 (11.5)	NS

* Applies only to AIUM standards.

Abbreviations: ACOG, American College of Obstetrics and Gynecology; *AIUM*, American Institute of Ultrasound in Medicine.

(Courtesy of Smulian JC, Vintzileos AM, Rodis JF, et al: Community-based obstetrical ultrasound reports: Documentation of compliance with suggested minimum standards. *J Clin Ultrasound* 24:123–127, 1996. Reprinted by permission of John Wiley & Sons, Inc.)

TABLE 3.—Documentation of Second/Third Trimester Components Suggested by ACOG and AIUM: General Information

	Obstetrical (n = 35)	Radiological (n = 94)	P
	(%)	(%)	
Fetal number	30 (85.7)	92 (97.9)	0.023
Fetal viability	31 (88.6)	93 (98.9)	0.028
Presentation	34 (97.1)	90 (95.7)	NS
Amniotic fluid volume	34 (97.1)	83 (88.3)	NS
Placental location	34 (97.1)	92 (97.9)	NS
Placental appearance*	25 (71.4)	52 (55.3)	NS
Relation of placenta to cervical os*	18 (51.4)	41 (43.6)	NS
Uterus	8 (22.9)	8 (8.5)	NS
Adnexa	8 (22.9)	3 (3.2)	0.001

* Applies only to AIUM standards.
Abbreviations: ACOG, American College of Obstetrics and Gynecology; *AIUM*, American Institute of Ultrasound in Medicine.
(Courtesy of Smulian JC, Vintzileos AM, Rodis JF, et al: Community-based obstetrical ultrasound reports: Documentation of compliance with suggested minimum standards. *J Clin Ultrasound* 24:123–127, 1996. Reprinted by permission of John Wiley & Sons, Inc.)

to include more components, perhaps because they were more likely to use US software or preprinted forms, rather than relying on dictated reports as the radiologists did.

Conclusion.—Obstetric US reports by community-based practitioners show poor compliance with published guidelines. This is especially true for examinations performed by radiologists. Using specific examination checklists would reduce the chances that some component of the US examination is omitted, thus reducing the risk of liability because of poor documentation.

▶ To my knowledge, this is the first attempt to document compliance with ACOG and AIUM guidelines for obstetrical US practice, and the results are not encouraging. Reports generated from obstetricians' offices tended to be more complete than those from radiologic facilities. The authors speculate that this may be, in part, the result of a greater use of US software and preprinted forms in obstetricians' offices rather than just dictation, as favored by radiologists. Although various components of the ultrasound report are surely of varying degrees of importance, it is hard to dismiss many of the omissions. Adherence to the guidelines would improve the assessment of adequacy of fetal growth and the screen for fetal abnormalities. Presumably it would also lead to reduced liability caused by poor documentation. Others have documented that nontertiary care centers were able to detect only 13% of malformed fetuses.[1]

M.P. Federle, M.D.

Reference

1. Goncalves LF, Romero R: A critical appraisal of the RADIUS study. *Fetus* 3:7–11, 1993.

End-Result of Routine Ultrasound Screening for Congenital Anomalies: The Belgian Multicentric Study 1984-92

Levi S, Schaaps JP, de Havay P, et al (Université Libre de Bruxelles, Brussels; Université de Liège, Belgium; Hopital Civil de Charleroi, Belgium; et al)

Ultrasound Obstet Gynecol 5:366–371, 1995 2–46

Introduction.—The value of routine ultrasound during pregnancy has been questioned. In an attempt to determine the ability of scanning to detect congenital anomalies in populations at normal risk for such anomalies, a prospective study was carried out in 5 US laboratories in Belgium.

Methods.—The study was conducted from 1984 to 1992 among patients attending a regular antenatal clinic. During the entire period, a total of 26,147 women attended the clinics; 96% (25,046 women and 25,469 fetuses) underwent at least 1 US scan. The results of prenatal US examinations were compared with pediatricians' reports on the neonates.

Results.—Abnormalities were present in 616 fetuses at birth or at pregnancy termination (Table 1), for a prevalence of anomalies of 2.42%. Abnormal fetuses detected with US numbered 274, yielding an overall sensitivity of 44.5% for routine scanning. The sensitivity of US was significantly higher in the later years of the study (51.1% for 1990 to 1992)

TABLE 1.—Patients and Principal Results

	1984–89	1990–92	1984–92
Pregnant women	16370	9777	26147
Pregnant women scanned	15654	9392	25046
Fetuses scanned	15868	9601	25469
Abnormal fetuses	381	235	616
Anomalies	415	270	685
Fetuses with one anomaly	324	202	526
Fetuses with ≥2 anomalies	57	33	90
total anomalies in this group	124	71	195
Abnormal fetuses detected (true positive)	154	120	274
Normal fetuses correctly described as normal (true negative)	15479	9357	24836
Normal fetuses erroneously considered as abnormal (false positive)	8	9	17
Abnormal fetuses not detected (false negative)	227	115	342
Pregnant women scanned (%)	96	96	96
Prevalence of abnormal fetuses (%)	2.40	2.45	2.42
Sensitivity (%)	40.4	51.1	44.5
Specificity (%)	99.95	99.90	99.93
False-positive rate (%)	0.05	0.10	0.07
False-negative rate (%)	59.6	48.9	55.5
Positive predictive value (%)	95.1	93.0	94.2
Negative predictive value (%)	98.6	98.8	98.6

(Courtesy of Levi S, Schaaps JP, de Havay P, et al: End-result of routine ultrasound screening for congenital anomalies: The Belgian multicentric study 1984–1992. *Ultrasound Obstet Gynecol* 5:366–371, 1995.)

than in the earlier period (40.4% for 1984 to 1989). The specificity of the test was high (99.9%). Overall, the positive predictive value was 94.2% and the negative predictive value was 98%. Taking into account the number of anomalies (685 defects), overall sensitivity was 52%; results from later years had a significantly greater sensitivity than those from the earlier years of the study (64% vs. 45%). The detection of anomalies before 23 weeks of gestation improved over the course of the study period. By the end of the study, US yielded the highest sensitivities in the detection of abnormalities of the nervous system (77%) and of the urogenital tract (72%); the lowest sensitivities were for cardiovascular (35%) and skeletal (34%) abnormalities.

Conclusion.—The routine US screening reported here was carried out by a team with mixed expertise. Detection of anomalies was generally better during 1990 to 1992 than during 1984 to 1989. A number of factors affect the detection rate, including gestational age, experience of the observer, image quality, and the types of anomalies encountered. The accuracy of routine screening is improving and its benefits are considerable.

► The authors of this important study point out several caveats in their discussion. The study was done in teaching hospitals, where scanning is performed by physicians with variable training and expertise. Their goal was to maximize the detection of serious anomalies during the first trimester of pregnancy, keeping false positive rates extremely low. Based on their earlier published research, the authors estimated that 55% of serious abnormalities might be detected, and they achieved a sensitivity of 51% in the second period of review. Perfect sensitivity is not achievable during the first trimester, because some abnormalities develop or progress only during later pregnancy (e.g., obstructive hydrocephalus and obstructive uropathy). High sensitivity achieved later in pregnancy has less potential impact on the decision for elective termination of pregnancy. The 2.4% prevalence of abnormal fetuses was a constant finding and represents the expected rate for a screening program in an unselected population.

M.P. Federle, M.D.

Imaging the Fetal Abdomen: How Efficacious Are the AIUM/ACR Guidelines?

Levine D, Callen PW, Goldstein RB, et al (Univ of California, San Francisco)
J Ultrasound Med 14:335–341, 1995 2–47

Objective.—The effectiveness of the guidelines of the American Institute of Ultrasound in Medicine/American College of Radiology in detecting fetal abdominal abnormalities was assessed.

Background.—The guidelines for routine obstetrical sonography recommend documentation of 5 regions of the fetal abdomen. These guidelines are designed to allow the majority of serious anomalies in the fetal abdomen to be detected, but there is little proof either that they are effective, or

TABLE 2.—Percentage of Abnormal Views According to Abdominal Location

Anomaly (No. of Cases)	Percentage of Views Abnormal				
	AC	CI	BL	ST	RA
Genitourinary (39)					
Duplication (4)	25	33	50	25	100
Renal dysplasia, Unilateral (6)	33	0	0	17	100
Renal dysplasia/agenesis, bilateral with oligohydramnios (10)	40	55	80	80	100
Hydronephrosis*/UPJ (10)	17	25	17	25†	100
Renal agenesis/ectopia, unilateral (3)	33	33‡	33‡	33‡	33
Posterior urethral valves (4)	25	67	100	25	100
Cloacal malformation (2)	100	0*	100	50	50
Abdominal wall (26)					
Omphalocele (10)	30	100	10	30	20
Gastroschisis (8)	12	75	12	36	12
Umbilical vein varix (2)	50	100	0	0	50
Abdominal wall defect (4)	100	75	50	75	75
Gastrointestinal (16)					
CDH (10)	30	0	0	100	20†
Duodenal/jejunal atresia (6)	33	40	0	83	50
Miscellaneous (26)					
Abdominopelvic cyst (9)	22	55	77	33	22
Hydrops/Lymphangiectasia/ meconium peritonitis (17)	94	100	57	94	82
Total	40	52*	37	52	61

* CI not seen in 10 studies; percentages do not include these studies. The CI site not seen in either case of cloacal malformation.

† CDH seen on ST view; hydronephrosis seen on RA view.

‡ One of 3 cases of unilateral renal agenesis identified on RA view. The AC, CI, ST, and BL views were abnormal in 1 case of a pelvic cyst with unilateral renal agenesis.

Abbreviations: AC, abdominal circumference; *CI*, cord insertion; *BL*, bladder; *ST*, stomach; *RA*, renal area; *UPJ*, ureteropelvic junction.

(Courtesy of Levine D, Callen PW, Goldstein RB, et al: Imaging the fetal abdomen: How efficacious are the AIUM/ACR guidelines? *J Ultrasound Med* 14:335–341, 1995.)

that the 5 views are equally effective. In part 1 of the study, the incidence of abnormal findings for each of the recommended views was established. In the second part, the ability of an individual without training in fetal sonography to identify image abnormalities was assessed.

Methods.—In part 1, 100 images from fetuses with abdominal abnormalities diagnosed sonographically were reviewed retrospectively. Images were masked, except for 1 view of the abdominal circumference, stomach, renal area, bladder, and cord insertion. In part 2, 70 normal images and 30 abnormal images were masked and shown to a fourth-year radiology resident and a sonographer.

Results.—In part 1, 2 sonologists recognized 96 of the 100 images as abnormal. The percentage of abnormal views according to abdominal region was calculated (Table 2). Four images had no abnormal views. In part 2, both the radiology resident and the sonographer indentified 29 of the 30 abnormalities. Both reviewers missed 1 case of gastroschisis. One reviewer had no false positive cases and the other had 7 false positive cases.

Discussion.—The majority of these abnormal fetuses were identified by examination of the 5 views recommended by the American Institute of Ultrasound in Medicine/American College of Radiology. These guidelines are effective for imaging the fetal abdomen. The sensitivity of sonography for detecting anomalies was not evaluated.

► The authors of this excellent and important paper point out several possible limitations that may decrease the applicability of the study to the general population. The University of California at San Francisco is a high obstetric referral center with superb ultrasonography (sonologists, in their parlance). Undoubtedly, the quality of the images obtained by these specialists would be hard to achieve in a general radiology practice. Nevertheless, senior radiology residents and sonographers, without the advantage of real-time evaluation, were able to recognize almost all significant abdominal abnormalities using only static images of the 5 standard regions of the fetal abdomen. This is a strong endorsement of the American Institute of Ultrasound in Medicine/American College of Radiology guidelines.

M.P. Federle, M.D.

Transvaginal Sonography and Serum hCG in Monitoring of Presumed Ectopic Pregnancies Selected for Expectant Management

Cacciatore B, Korhonen J, Stenman U-H, et al (Helsinki Univ)

Ultrasound Obstet Gynecol 5:297–300, 1995 2–48

Background.—The early treatment of ectopic pregnancy has been made possible with the advent of diagnostic techniques such as transvaginal ultrasonography and measures of human chorionic gonadotropin (hCG). Because a percentage of tubal pregnancies will resolve spontaneously, these 2 techniques were evaluated to determine their prognostic value.

Methods.—Patients with decreasing hCG levels, minimal clinical symptoms, an adnexal mass smaller than 5 cm, and hemoperitoneum of less than 50 mL were included in this study. Transvaginal sonography and serum hCG levels were performed initially, then every 2–3 days, then at 1–2-week intervals as the hCG decreased. Laparoscopy was performed if the patient worsened clinically or if the hCG level remained the same or increased on consecutive evaluations.

Results.—In 69% of patients, the hCG levels returned to normal within an average of 25 days; the ectopic mass took an average of 35 days to resolve (Fig 1). In this group of patients, the ectopic pregnancy was considered to have resolved spontaneously. Because their symptoms worsened or hCG level increased, the remaining 31% required laparoscopy. Free fluid was discovered in the cul-de-sac in 45% of patients and was found at the same rate in both groups. The mass decreased within 3 days in 55% of those who resolved and within 7 days in 84%. In patients who required surgery, the mass stayed the same size or increased in all patients. In those who recovered spontaneously, the hCG level decreased more

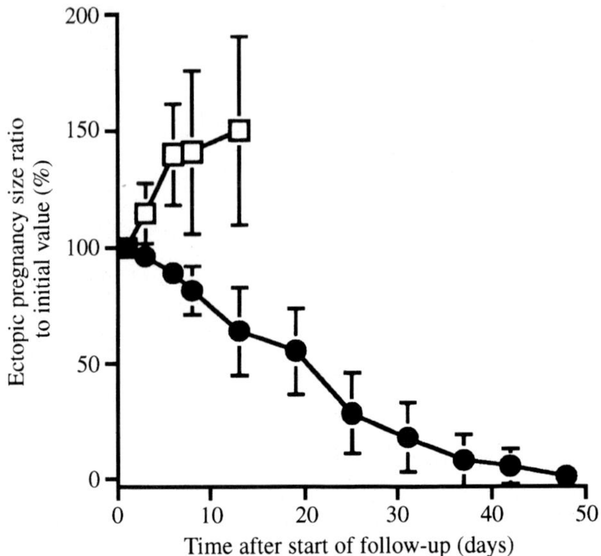

FIGURE 1.—Evolution (mean ± 95% confidence interval) of the ectopic pregnancy size ratio in patients with spontaneous resolution (*closed circles*) and in patients later treated by laparoscopy (*open squares*). Courtesy of Cacciatore B, Korhonen J, Stenman U-H, et al: Transvaginal sonography and serum hCG in monitoring of presumed ectopic pregnancies selected for expectant management. *Ultrasound Obstet Gynecol* 5:297–300, 1995.)

rapidly than in those who had surgery. Detection of a decreasing mass had a sensitivity of 84% and a specificity of 100%. The negative predictive value was 70% and the positive predictive value was 100%.

Discussion.—Patients with a declining serum hCG level that was below 2,000 IU/L initially have the best prognosis. Neither transvaginal sonography findings nor color Doppler measurement of blood flow had predictive value. The results reported here indicate that a repeat transvaginal ultrasound performed on day 7 will provide the most information on the status of the pregnancy. An increase in the size of the mass and the amount of fluid after 1 week is associated with a worsening clinical picture, whereas a decrease in mass is a good sign that an ectopic pregnancy is resolving on its own.

► This is a very practical and useful communication. The authors note several important caveats in their recommendation for expectant management. Excellent quality sonography is necessary to yield comparable results on the initial and follow-up scans. The patient must be reliable and return for re-evaluation, including accurate measurement of the serum hCG. Rapid access to surgery is essential and can usually be performed laparoscopically. Note that many patients were excluded from expectant management due to acute symptoms at the time of presentation.

M.P. Federle, M.D.

3 Musculoskeletal System

Introduction

The section on musculoskeletal imaging is replete with a considerable number of interesting articles encompassing multiple imaging modalities utilized in the evaluation of the musculoskeletal system.

The use of digitized radiography in comparing a work station to original film images was discussed in a single article, and I believe this will become more important in the future. Interobserver and intraobserver variability and clinical reproducibility were also covered in a number of important publications. The use of various imaging procedures and their diagnostic efficiency in specific cases was discussed.

The emphasis of the diagnostic articles was on newly described abnormalities, summary articles of high quality, and miscellaneous subjects of interests.

Murray K. Dalinka, M.D.

Spine

Digitized Radiographs in Skeletal Trauma: A Performance Comparison Between a Digital Workstation and the Original Film Images
Wilson AJ, Hodge JC (Washington Univ, St Louis)
Radiology 196:565–568, 1995 3–1

Background.—Teleradiology systems offer radiologists the opportunity to access images from multiple remote sites and read them in a single location. Before the concept of teleradiology can be fully accepted, the systems must be tested for accuracy against the standard of comparison: the conventional radiographic film. The diagnostic performance of a recently installed teleradiology system in routine skeletal trauma was evaluated.

Methods.—The study included radiographs of 180 patients with skeletal trauma. All of the films were digitized with a Kodak FD-1S laser digitizer, with a digital matrix of 2,000 × 2,500 × 12 bits/pixel and a spot size of

175 Ìm. Clinical and radiologic follow-up data from various sources were gathered for all patients. Four independent radiologist-readers interpreted both the digitized images on a work station and the original films. They identified fractures and dislocations on a 6-point scale ranging from definitely normal to definitely abnormal structure, then interpreted the images a second time at least 4 weeks later. For each reader and reading method, receiver operating characteristic curves were generated.

Results.—For all 4 readers, diagnostic performance in identifying fractures was significantly better with the original films than on the work station, though the patterns varied between readers. For subtle fractures, just 1 of the 4 readers showed significantly better performance with film. There were no significant differences in the identification of dislocations.

Conclusion.—For fractures but not dislocations the diagnostic performance of a digital teleradiology system appears to be inferior to that of the original films. The reason for the difference in fracture diagnosis is unknown; it does not appear to result from problems with spatial resolution or data loss during transmission. The limited dynamic range of the image resulting from displaying the data at 8 rather than 12 bits may play a role, but limited familiarity with the system is probably the most important factor. Though the system used in this study appears inadequate for routine reading of fracture films, clinically functional digitizing systems are probably achievable with existing technology.

► The results of digitalized studies are dependent on the digitilizer and digital viewing console. A more optimistic paper using equipment with higher resolution was published by DeCorato et al.[1]

M.K. Dalinka, M.D.

Reference

1. DeCorato DR, Kagetsu NJ, Ablow RC: Off-hours interpretation of radiologic images of patients admitted to the emergency department: Efficacy of teleradiology. *AJR* 165:1293, 1995.

Frequency and Significance of Fractures of the Upper Cervical Spine Detected by CT in Patients With Severe Neck Trauma

Blacksin MF, Lee HJ (Univ of Medicine and Dentistry of New Jersey, Newark)

AJR 165:1201–1204, 1995 3–2

Background.—For patients with severe trauma, it can be very difficult to perform a radiographic evaluation of the upper cervical spine. In particular, it can be difficult to obtain an adequate open-mouth view of the odontoid in these critically injured patients. Advanced imaging techniques such as CT and MRI have aided in identifying more subtle injuries of the cervical spine, particularly when plain radiographs are inadequate. The value of CT in detecting upper cervical spine fracture in patients with severe neck trauma was investigated.

Methods.—In 100 consecutive patients with severe trauma, CT of the cervicocranial junction was performed instead of the standard open-mouth radiograph. This policy was followed in all trauma patients with intubated airways and in patients in whom open-mouth positioning would be difficult. Plain radiographs obtained included a cross-table lateral view, an anteroposterior view, and a swimmer's view, if needed. All imaging studies were double-read by a musculoskeletal radiologist and a neuroradiologist who were unaware of the clinical findings. Clinical records were reviewed to see how the identification of fractures of the upper cervical spine altered patient treatment.

Results.—The CT scans identified 8 fractures in 7 patients: 3 fractures of the occipital condyle and 5 at the C1–C2 level. None of the 8 fractures was directly demonstrated by plain radiographs, though 2 of 7 patients were noted to have paravertebral soft-tissue swelling or other secondary signs of injury. The number of fractures detected was higher than expected. All surviving patients with fractures were managed with halo stabilization.

Conclusion.—Computed tomography can detect fractures of the occipital condyle and C1–C2 vertebrae that are not visible on cross-table lateral cervical spine radiographs. For victims of severe trauma in whom the standard open-mouth radiograph of the odontoid is impossible, CT is an efficient and accurate method of evaluation. There are currently no specific predictors to identify patients with potential fractures of the upper cervical spine.

► This paper seems to suggest that C1–C2 vertebrae should be studied by CT rather than an open-mouth view in trauma patients with intubated airways. The study did not obtain open-mouth views of patients whose airways were intubated, and hence there were no controls.

The high incidence (8%) of lesions in this area suggests that the study population is weighted toward patients with severe trauma. In addition, the possible complications inherent in missing these injuries were not addressed.

M.K. Dalinka, M.D.

Traumatic Isolation of the Cervical Articular Pillar: Imaging Observations in 21 Patients

Shanmuganathan K, Mirvis SE, Dowe M, et al (Univ of Maryland, Baltimore)

AJR 166:897–902, 1996 3–3

Background.—Traumatic isolation of a cervical spine articular pillar occurs with a simultaneous fracture through the lamina and ipsilateral pedicle. There is little understanding of the mechanisms involved in this rare injury, which is difficult to diagnose radiographically. The radiographs, CT scans, and medical records of patients with this injury were reviewed to characterize the mechanism of injury, associated injuries, and management.

Methods.—Twenty-one patients with a diagnosis of traumatic isolation of a cervical spine articular pillar were identified through a computer search. All patients underwent at least lateral cervical radiography and cervical CT scanning. These images and the clinical records were reviewed to determine the predominant mechanism of injury and other associated injuries.

Results.—The diagnosis of cervical spine injury that produced an isolated articular pillar accounted for 3% of the 703 cervical spine injuries seen during the 8-year study period. The fracture patterns indicated that the mechanism of injury was hyperflexion-rotation in 17 patients, hyperflexion-distraction in 3 patients, and hyperextension- rotation in 1 patient. In 19 patients, the isolated articular pillar was ipsilateral to the fracture through the transverse foramen. Fourteen patients had contralateral injuries at the level of the isolated articular pillar, and 13 patients had neurologic deficits. Management included surgical reduction and internal stabilization in 18 patients; 3 patients were managed nonsurgically with immobilization.

Conclusion.—Computed tomography provides useful information to detect articular process fractures, free fragments of bone, and articular pillar isolation. The mechanisms of injury typically involve hyperflexion. These findings have important clinical implications for management because of the presence of 2 levels of mechanical instability, which may require internal fixation of 3 contiguous vertebrae.

▶ This nice paper reviews a large number of patients with an uncommon injury. The authors have shown that these fractures are more often sustained in flexion rather than hyperextension, which the literature attributed to. I do have a problem with their definition, which I find confusing. In many of these cases multiple fractures are present, and although the articular pillar is isolated, the fracture is not isolated to the articular pillar.

M.K. Dalinka, M.D.

Radiographic Appearance of the Odontoid Lateral Mass Interspace in the Occipitoatlantoaxial Complex

Sutherland JP Jr, Yaszemski MJ, White AA III (Wilford Hall Med Ctr, Lackland AFB, Tex; Harvard Med School, Boston)

Spine 20:2221–2225, 1995 3–4

Objective.—There is ongoing debate about what happens to the odontoid lateral mass interspace (OLMI) during atlantoaxial rotation. Definitions of interspace asymmetry vary significantly. Because atlas fractures are a common feature of cervical spine fractures, it is essential to understand the radiographic anatomy of this area. The radiographic appearance of the OLMI was evaluated in various degrees of upper cervical spine rotation.

Methods.—Radiographic studies were performed in 10 cadaver cervical spines, which had been dissected of all but ligamentous soft tissue. The radiographs were analyzed to determine OLMI asymmetry in neutral position and in various positions of right and left rotation.

Results.—There was notable asymmetry on comparison of neutral positions and of rotated vs. neutral position. Although the asymmetry appeared clinically significant, it was not statistically significant. The 95% confidence interval for the measured difference between right and left OLMI in a cervical spine with no atlantoaxial rotation was 0.0–2.1 mm.

Conclusion.—Asymmetry measured in the atlantoaxial complex in neutral position does not necessarily reflect instability. The findings support the previous proposed concept of the "neutral zone." The OLMI tends to increase on the side to which the head is rotated, which makes it measurably larger than the contralateral OLMI. Therefore, OLMI asymmetry is not a useful marker of cervical instability in asymptomatic individuals.

► This paper is very helpful in clearing up much of the confusion with regard to asymmetry of the atlantoaxial complex and its overdiagnosis as rotary subluxation.

M.K. Dalinka, M.D

Magnetic Resonance Imaging of the Thoracic Spine: Evaluation of Asymptomatic Individuals

Wood KB, Garvey TA, Gundry C, et al (Univ of Minnesota, Minneapolis)

J Bone Joint Surg (Am) 77A:1631–1638, 1995 3–5

Introduction.—The rate of herniation of thoracic intervertebral disks is 0.15% to 4% of all patients with symptomatic protrusions of intervertebral disks. The rate of thoracic disk herniations reported by Love and Kiefer was 2 to 3 per 1,000 disk herniation. The low rate of symptoms may be attributed to the limited motion of the thoracic spine, secondary to the natural restraint provided by the ribs, sternum, and apophyseal joints. The MRI studies of the thoracic spines of 90 asymptomatic individuals were reviewed to determine prevalence of abnormal anatomical findings.

Methods.—Sixty individuals with no history of thoracic or lumbar pain, 30 research subjects with a history of low back pain only, 18 patients with surgically confirmed thoracic disk herniation, and 31 patients with thoracic pain underwent MRI of the thoracic spine. All disk levels were evaluated for herniation and compression of the spinal cord, height and disk space, signal intensity, annular integrity, and changes in the osseous end plate. Specific abnormalities of each disk had to be completely agreed on by 3 to 4 blinded observers to confirm diagnosis. Interobserver reliability was calculated.

Results.—There were no significant thoracic spine differences between the 30 patients with a history of low back pain only and the completely asymptomatic group. Of the 90 asymptomatic research subjects, 66 (73%) had evidence of intervertebral degenerative changes, annular disruption, or both. In 33 (55%) of 60 asymptomatic research subjects and 17 (57%)

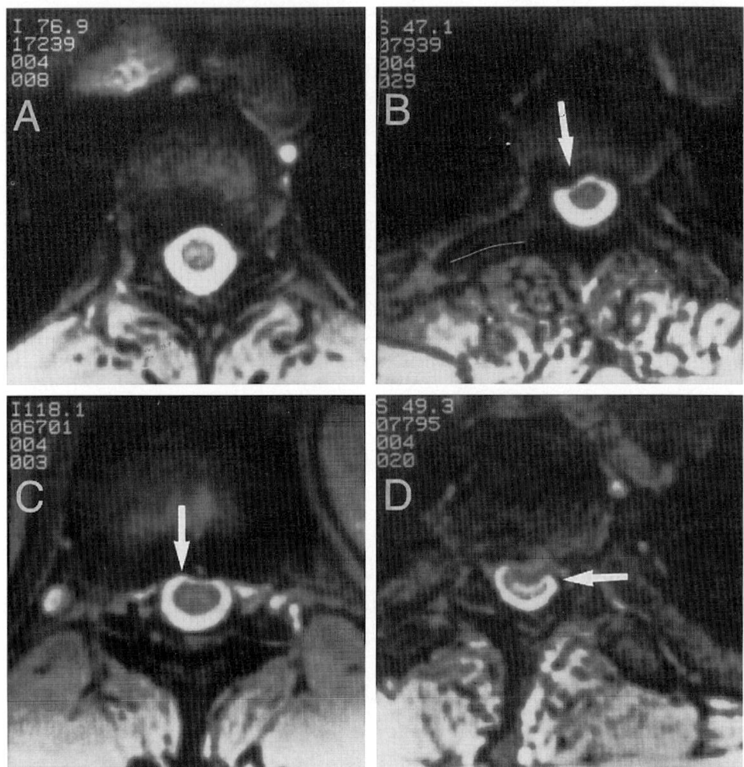

FIGURE 2.—Axial multiplanar gradient refocused MR images showing the spectrum of abnormalities of thoracic disks in asymptomatic individuals. **A,** the normal anatomy of a thoracic disk in a 38-year-old woman. **B,** images showing a right-sided bulge (*arrow*) of a disk in an asymptomatic 59-year-old man. **C,** a complete annular tear (*arrow*) in a 40-year-old woman. **D,** a 5-mm midline herniated nucleus pulposus (*arrow*), with deformation of the spinal cord in a 32-year-old man. (Courtesy of Wood KB, Garvey TA, Gundry C, et al: Magnetic resonance imaging of the thoracic spine: Evaluation of asymptomatic individuals. *J Bone Joint Surg [Am]* 77A:1631–1638, 1995.)

of 30 research subjects with a history of low back pain but no thoracic spine symptoms, multiple levels of disk degeneration were detected, as evidenced by loss of disk height and signal on T2-weighted multiplanar gradient refocused sequences (Fig 2). At least 1 bulging disk was detected in 48 (53%) of the 90 asymptomatic research subjects. At least 2 herniated disks were detected in 33 (37%) of 90 asymptomatic research subjects. Other findings included 52 (58%) annular tears, 26 (29%) deformations of the spinal cord, and 34 (38%) Scheuermann end-plate irregularities or kyphosis. No relationship was determined between age and the prevalence of herniation or the number of herniations. Of interest, 81% of deformations of the cord were detected in men. There were no significant differences between the asymptomatic group and the group with herniated thoracic disks in abnormal findings on MRI, sex, or age.

Conclusion.—It is estimated that the prevalence of herniated thoracic disks with an associated neurologic deficit is about 1 per 1 million population. Asymptomatic individuals had a greater incidence of abnormal thoracic disks than was previously supposed. There was no correlation between age and the prevalence of disk herniation. Most herniations (42 of 57) were detected caudal to the fifth thoracic level. Other reports have already established a relationship between symptomatic herniated disks in the thoracic spine with Scheuermann vertebral disease and its subsequent kyphosis. Specific diagnosis of herniated thoracic disks is difficult to determine because of the high rate of asymptomatic abnormalities and the diversity of symptoms that are manifested clinically. A high index of suspicion, strict clinical correlation, and proper additional studies are needed before patients should be recommended to undergo thoracic spine surgery with its high risk for complications and often disappointing results.

▶ This valuable paper should hopefully cut down on the overdiagnosis of abnormalities of the thoracic spine by MRI.

M.K. Dalinka, M.D.

Interobserver and Intraobserver Variability in Interpretation of Lumbar Disc Abnormalities: A Comparison of Two Nomenclatures

Brant-Zawadzki MN, Jensen MC, Obuchowski N, et al (Hoag Mem Hosp, Newport Beach, Calif; Cleveland Clinic, Ohio)

Spine 20:1257–1264, 1995 3–6

Introduction.—The lack of standardized terminology to describe degenerative disk disease has impeded attempts to develop practice guidelines. The use of disparate terms precludes a uniform system correlating the radiologic and operative findings. A wide range of imprecise terms have been used by radiologists to describe disk disease.

Objective.—Observer variability was quantified by asking 2 experienced neuroradiologists using separate nomenclature systems to prospectively assess the MR images of 98 asymptomatic individuals and 27 selected studies from patients with lumbar disk disease. The MR studies were done at a single institution. A total of 625 interspaces were evaluated.

Nomenclatures.—Initially the readers were asked to score each disk as normal, bulging, or herniated (nomenclature I). After 2 weeks they again read the studies using the terms normal, bulging, protruded, and extruded (nomenclature II). Finally, after 4 weeks, 70% of subjects had their scans read another time by both readers using nomenclature II. Precise definitions of each term were provided to the readers.

Results.—Interobserver agreement was 80% for both nomenclatures (Table 3). Intraobserver agreement was 86% for each of the readers. The most trouble was encountered for distinguishing between normal status and a bulge. Herniation was specified for 23% of asymptomatic individuals. When nomenclature II was used, 27% were said to have protrusion. Only 2 asymptomatic persons were thought to have a disk extrusion.

TABLE 3.—Interobserver Comparisons

Nomenclature I

Reader 1	Reader 2 Normal	Bulge	Herniation
Normal	368 (59%)	31 (5%)	1 (<1%)
Bulge	59 (9%)	89 (14%)	14 (2%)
Herniation	1 (<1%)	25 (4%)	37 (6%)

Nomenclature II

Reader 1	Reader 2 Normal	Bulge	Protrusion	Extrusion
Normal	374 (60%)	33 (5%)	1 (<1%)	
Bulge	48 (8%)	85 (14%)	12 (2%)	
Protrusion	4 (1%)	19 (3%)	36 (6%)	2 (<1%)
Extrusion		1 (<1%)	6 (1%)	4 (1%)

(Courtesy of Brant-Zawadzki MN, Jensen MC, Obuchowski N, et al: Interobserver and intraobserver variability in interpretation of lumbar disc abnormalities: A comparison of two nomenclatures. *Spine* 20:1257–1264, 1995.)

Discussion.—Experienced readers exhibit, at a minimum, moderate agreement when using standardized terms to interpret MR images of the lumbar spine. In asymptomatic subjects the term "herniation" is descriptively less precise than "extrusion," and it may mistakenly be given too much clinical significance by those who are less sophisticated. Spinal surgeons exhibit substantially more between- and within-observer variability. Standardized nomenclature will be necessary to develop appropriate diagnostic and therapeutic guidelines.

The Prevalence and Clinical Features of Internal Disc Disruption in Patients With Chronic Low Back Pain

Schwarzer AC, Aprill CN, Derby R, et al (Univ of Newcastle, Australia; Magnolia Diagnostics Inc, New Orleans, La; Spinecare, Daly City, Calif; et al)
Spine 20:1878–1883, 1995 3–7

Introduction.—The term "diskogenic pain" refers expressly to pain resulting from the intervertebral disk itself as opposed to nerve root pain caused by disk prolapse. Diskography is a physiologic test performed to determine whether a disk is painful, the important finding being whether stimulation of the disk reproduces the patient's pain. Internal disk disruption (IDD) is a condition in which disk pain results from changes in the internal structure of the disk while its external appearance remains normal. The definitive diagnosis of IDD requires reproduction of the patient's pain on disk stimulation and demonstration of internal disruption on CT diskography. False positive results were eliminated by requiring that stimulation of 1 or 2 other disks had to fail to reproduce pain. This study sought to determine whether these criteria for IDD could be met in patients with chronic low back pain and whether cases of IDD could be identified by conventional clinical findings.

Methods.—Ninety-two consecutive patients with low back pain who were referred for diskography were studied. A standard physical examination and CT diskography at at least 2 levels were performed in each patient. The diagnostic criteria for IDD of the International Association for the Study of Pain, as described earlier, were adopted. Disks with a CT finding of grade 3 or 4 radial fissure, according to the classification of Aprill and Bogduk, were regarded as abnormal. According to this classification, a grade 3 fissure reaches the outer third of the annulus fibrosis, and a grade 4 fissure also spreads circumferentially within the annulus with an arc of at least 30 degrees.

Results.—Thirty-nine percent of patients met all of the diagnosis criteria for IDD, most commonly at the L5–S1 and L4–L5 levels. All clinical tests showed significantly better agreement than expected by chance. The history and physical examination findings were unrelated to the finding of a positive diskogram. Pain referral patterns were also unable to distinguish between patients with and without diskogenic disease.

Conclusion.—The diagnostic criteria for IDD are met by a substantial proportion of patients with chronic low back pain. No clinical test or combination of tests can reliably differentiate between patients with and without diskogenic pain, though patients with central lumbar pain are unlikely to have IDD. The findings show that IDD is a demonstrable condition for many patients, but they offer no conclusions about how or whether these patients should be treated.

▶ This is an interesting study about a very controversial subject. Other interesting articles on this subject have been reported by Parfenchuck and Janssen[1] in *Spine* and by Kauppila and Videman[2] in the *Journal of Orthopaedic Rheumatology* and by Moneta et al.[3]

M.K. Dalinka, M.D.

References

1. Parfenchuck TA, Janssen ME: A correlation of cervical magnetic resonance imaging discography/computed tomographic discograms. *Spine* 19:2819–2825, 1994.
2. Kauppila LI, Videman T: Discographic findings and back pain history: An epidemiologic study of 58 cadavers. *J Orthop Rheumatol* 7:94–99, 1994.
3. Moneta GB, Videman T, Kaivanto K, et al: Reported pain during lumbar discography as a function of anular ruptures and disc degeneration: A re-analysis of 833 discograms. *Spine* 19:1968–1974, 1994.

Clinical Efficacy of SPECT Bone Imaging for Low Back Pain

Littenberg B, Siegel A, Tosteson ANA, et al (Dartmouth-Hitchcock Med Ctr, Lebanon, NH)

J Nucl Med 36:1707–1713, 1995 3–8

Objective.—The use of single-photon emission CT (SPECT) has been proposed as an accurate method of diagnosing low back pain. A careful literature search was performed to find evidence documenting the diagnostic accuracy, clinical usefulness, and cost effectiveness of SPECT in patients with low back pain.

Methods.—The review sought to summarize any valid clinical trials estimating the accuracy of SPECT in patients with low back pain, to identify any literature demonstrating the clinical usefulness of SPECT in this situation (i.e., its effect on patient management), and to locate any studies of the cost effectiveness or other societal benefits of SPECT. The study protocol was carefully designed to avoid bias and error.

Findings.—Of 13 reports that met the inclusion criteria, none included any information on the clinical usefulness or cost effectiveness of SPECT in low back pain. The most recent study provided data on 233 patients undergoing SPECT of the lumbar spine, including 75 patients with known malignancy but no known spinal metastases. Some SPECT abnormality was found in almost all patients, including the 28 with metastases and the 43 with benign conditions. There was a 1.01 likelihood ratio for a positive test result. The results suggested that lesions in the pedicle were more likely to be positive and those in the vertebral body to be benign; however, data were insufficient to determine the value of SPECT in differentiating between patients with and without metastatic spread.

In a study of athletes with back pain, SPECT abnormalities were common, but only 45% of them were also detected by planar bone scan. No external validation of the scintigraphic diagnoses and no clinical outcome data were provided. Another report suggested that SPECT is positive in patients with painful pars fractures and negative in those with asymptomatic fractures; again, no clinical outcome data were provided.

There were very few data on the accuracy of SPECT in low back pain. One small study concluded that SPECT is highly accurate in detecting pseudarthroses in patients with failed back surgery. A study of cancer patients found that SPECT was of little help in detecting spinal metastases because it was almost always positive. A small, retrospective study suggested that SPECT correctly classified 14 of 15 young patients with low back pain.

Discussion.—Few research data support the accuracy, clinical effect, or cost effectiveness of SPECT imaging for patients with low back pain. Truly useful studies of SPECT would require a large cohort, perhaps up to thousands of subjects; systematic enrolling of all subjects with back pain for whom SPECT might reasonably be helpful; and blinded use of SPECT as the index test and some reference test. Though SPECT could be useful in certain specific situations, no data justify its use in most patients with low back pain.

► The editors fully agree with this paper entitled "Clinical Efficacy of SPECT Bone Imaging for Low Back Pain." In our institution the cost of a bone scan with SPECT is more than the cost of an MRI, which we believe is the most efficacious imaging study in these patients.

M.K. Dalinka, M.D.

Spinal Dural Arteriovenous Fistulas: MR and Myelographic Findings

Gilbertson JR, Miller GM, Goldman MS, et al (Mayo Clinic and Mayo Found, Rochester, Minn)

Am J Neuroradiol 16:2049–2057, 1995 3–9

Introduction.—Spinal dural arteriovenous fistulas (AVFs) are cryptic acquired lesions typically occurring in older men. This is a rare but treatable myelopathy. The fistula, usually located within the dural sleeve of an existing thoracic or lumbar nerve, drains retrograde into the spinal coronal venous plexus. Symptoms can be traced to chronic venous ischemia from venous hypertension. The clinical and MRI findings from 132 patients with angiographically and surgically proven dural fistulas were compared with prone-supine myelography to determine the ability of MRI to screen patients adequately before spinal angiography.

Methods.—A review of 240 spinal angiograms in 132 patients indicated 97 vascular malformations, including 66 dural AVFs and 31 other spinal malformations. Sixteen patients with angiograms that were interpreted as normal had suspected spinal dural AVFs on myelogram or MRI. Imaging and clinical findings were reviewed retrospectively and compared.

Results.—Male patients outnumbered female patients 3.4:1. Average patient age was 62. The average length of time between symptom onset and diagnosis was 27 years. Fifteen patients had symptoms of 1 year or less, and 21 had symptoms of less than 2 years. Twenty-one of 31 patients experienced a chronic progressive clinical course. Remaining patients had a stepwise fluctuating clinical course. On initial clinical examination, 45% of patients had myelopathy, 39% had both myelopathy and lower motor neuron signs, and 16% had lower motor neuron signs only. By the time of diagnosis, most patients had developed some degree of sphincter dysfunction (Fig 8).

The MRI showed increased T2-weighted signal in the spinal cord in all 30 patients so examined. The T2-weighted signal was homogeneous in appearance. It was central in location, sparing a thin rim of the cord peripherally. The abnormal signal extended over an average of 7 levels and involved the tip of the conus in 26 of 30 studies. Flow voids were identified in 11 of 31 examinations on T1-weighted images and 14 of 31 T2-weighted images. A mass effect was present in 14 of 31 examinations. In

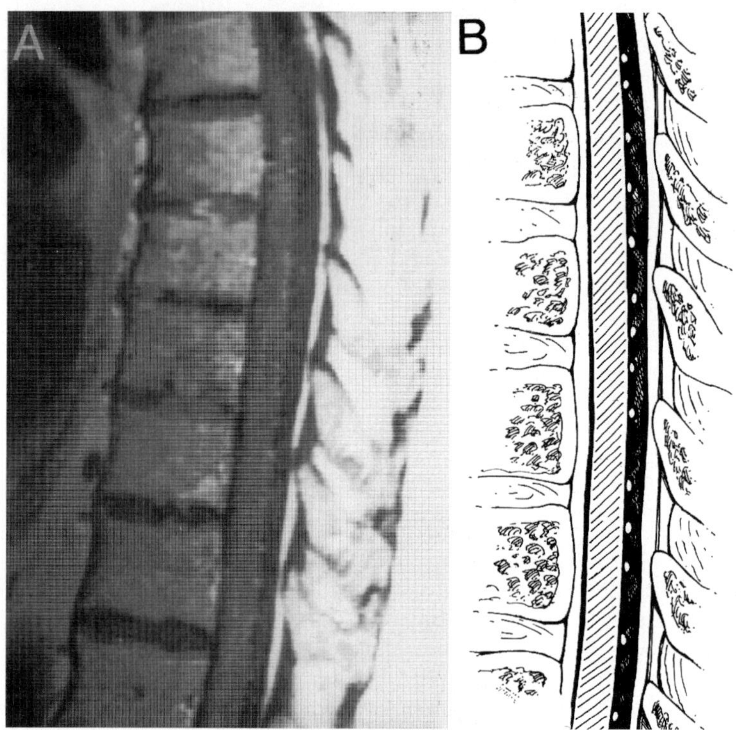

FIGURE 8.—**A,** circular dots of coronal venous plexus enhancement can be identified in this patient with a spinal dural atriovenous fistula at L1, as the dilated veins course in and out of the plane of section (pial veins in cross section) (recovery time 500 msec/echo time 19 msec/inversion time 2 msec). **B,** drawing depicts the same finding. (JR Gilbertson, GM Miller, MS Goldman, et al: Spinal dural arteriovenous fistulas: MR and myelographic findings. *Am J Neuroradiol* 16:2049–2057, 1995, Copyright by American Society of Neuroradiology.)

patients receiving contrast, abnormal enhancement was present in 22 of 25 examinations. Location of the enhancement was within the dilated coronal venous plexus in 13 patients, within the cord parenchyma in 5, and both in 4 patients.

Discussion and Conclusion.—Because the condition is potentially treatable, diagnosis of AVFs is important. The first suggestion of this diagnosis may be made by the radiologist. The most common spinal vascular malformation in this cohort was spinal dural AVF. Regardless of the location of the nidus, the symptom complex in these patients was progressive lower thoracic myelopathy. In all patients with a spinal dural AVF and in patients with a negative angiogram, vessels were identified on the spinal myelogram. The appearance of the vessels in the negative angiogram group were not as dilated or tortuous as those seen in the spinal dural group. Sensitivity and specificity of the MR examination was increased with gadolinium administration. Enhancement was present in 88% of patients with spinal dural AVFs. Flow voids were uncommon 35% on T1-weighted and 45% on T2-weighted sequences. Flow voids may be helpful but are not reliable and are often difficult to assess. The mass effect was seen in 45%

of patients with spinal dural AVFs. It should be emphasized that this finding corroborates the venous hypertension theory with resultant edema of the cord. The T2-weighted signal abnormality was never a single finding in any patients with a dural fistula. All patients with spinal dural AVF had additional findings, most frequently enhancement of the coronal venous plexus. Findings support the conclusion that MRI is the initial screening procedure of choice.

► This large series establishes criteria that may help exclude the diagnosis of spinal dural AVFs and should be helpful in eliminating unnecessary spinal angiograms in patients without abnormal signal on T2-weighted images.

M.K. Dalinka, M.D.

Hip and Pelvis

Traumatic Anterior Dislocation of the Hip: Spectrum of Plain Film and CT Findings

Erb RE, Steele JR, Nance EP Jr, et al (Vanderbilt Univ, Nashville, Tenn; Univ of Texas, Dallas)

AJR 165:1215–1219, 1995 3–10

Introduction.—Traumatic anterior dislocation of the hip represents 11% of all hip dislocations. The identification of traumatic anterior dislocation of the hip into superior and inferior types in plain radiographs was reviewed in 20 patients.

Discussion.—Inferior anterior hip dislocation is caused by forced abduction, external rotation, and flexion of the hip. The femoral head extrudes through the anterior capsule beneath the pubofemoral ligament and comes to rest anterior to the obturator ring. On plain radiographs, inferior hip dislocation is easily recognized, with the femoral head overlying the obturator foramen and with abduction and external rotation of the femur. Superior anterior hip dislocation is uncommon, accounting for less than 10% of anterior hip dislocations. With forced abduction, external rotation, and extension of the femur, the femoral head extrudes through the capsule between the iliofemoral and pubofemoral ligaments or avulses the anterior inferior iliac spine. Its radiographic appearance is less straightforward than inferior anterior hip dislocation and can be confused with posterior dislocation. However, whereas the hip is predictably held in external rotation and the lesser trochanter is prominent in superior anterior hip dislocation, the femur is typically rotated internally and the lesser trochanter is prominent in posterior dislocation (Fig 5).

Impaction fractures of the femoral head is a common complication of anterior hip dislocation, occurring in 12% to 87% of patients. These injuries are located in the superolateral aspect of the femoral head, appearing as a depressed fracture (similar to a Hill-Sachs deformity of the femoral head) or as mild flattening of the femoral head. Other skeletal injuries associated with anterior hip dislocation include ipsilateral frac-

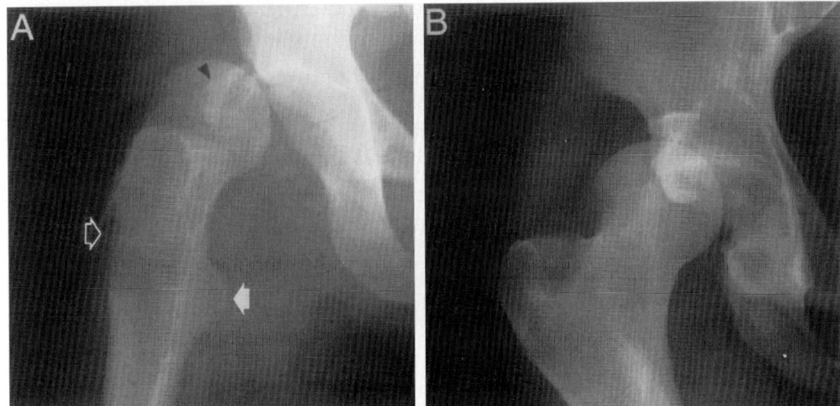

FIGURE 5.—Superior anterior hip dislocation vs. posterior hip dislocation. **A**, 27-year-old man with an anterior hip dislocation after motor vehicle accident. Anteroposterior view of the right hip demonstrates superolateral displacement of the femoral head with associated fractures of the anterior inferior iliac spine (*arrowhead*) and greater trochanter (*open arrow*). Note the prominent lesser trochanter (*solid arrow*), indicating external rotation of the femur. **B**, 20-year-old man with a posterior dislocation of the right hip after a motor vehicle accident. Anteroposterior view of the right hip demonstrates superolateral displacement of the femoral head and comminuted fracture of the posterior wall of the acetabulum. Note that the lesser trochanter is obscured, indicating internal rotation of the femur. (Courtesy of Erb RE, Steele JR, Nance EP Jr, et al: Traumatic anterior dislocation of the hip: Spectrum of plain film and CT findings. *AJR* 165:1215–1219, 1995.)

tures of the acetabulum, femoral neck, greater trochanter, and femoral shaft. Avulsion of the inferior iliac spine may occur, particularly in association with superior anterior hip dislocation. Arterial or venous injury also occurs in 1% of patients with anterior hip dislocation.

► This is a nice review article, and the original contains many excellent illustrations.

M.K. Dalinka, M.D.

MR Imaging in Evaluation of Suspected Hip Fracture: Frequency of Unsuspected Bone and Soft-Tissue Injury

Bogost GA, Lizerbram EK, Crues JV III (Cedars Sinai Med Ctr, Los Angeles)
Radiology 197:263–267, 1995 3–11

Background.—In patients with minimally impacted, nondisplaced hip fractures, radiographic findings may return as negative or equivocal, particularly when osteoporosis or advanced degenerative changes are noted. Multiple studies have demonstrated the accuracy of MRI in identifying occult hip fracture. In patients with pelvic fractures, the clinical manifestation may imitate that of hip fracture. Considerable soft-tissue or muscle injury also can occur with trauma. The prevalence of radiographically occult pelvic fractures and soft-tissue injuries in patients undergoing MRI for suspected hip fracture therefore was evaluated.

Patients and Methods.—Seventy consecutive patients with suspected hip fracture and negative radiographs who were referred for MRI over a 12-month period were studied. All patients underwent large field of view T1-weighted coronal MRI. Additional T2-weighted or short inversion time inversion recovery sequences also were performed. The numbers of MRI-detected soft-tissue and bone injuries were determined.

Results.—Bone or soft-tissue injuries were identified at MRI in 56 of the 70 patients. Occult femoral fractures were noted in 37% and occult pelvic fractures in 23% of the patients. Intertrochanteric fractures and femoral neck fractures occurred with essentially equal frequency (14 of the former and 11 of the latter). Soft-tissue abnormalities were noted in 74% of the patients, and muscle injuries also were commonly observed, with or without fracture. Pelvic fracture, muscle injury, and hematoma or seroma (or both), avascular necrosis, effusion, or bursitis were detected in 22 of 44 patients without hip fractures.

Conclusion.—The use of MRI facilitates detection of traumatic injuries on patients with suspected hip fracture but negative plain radiographs. In this study, 80% of patients with suspected hip fracture had some bone or soft-tissue injury noted on MRI. Twenty-three percent of patients also had occult pelvic fracture, emphasizing the need for large field of view MR images to include the entire pelvic region.

▶ This excellent paper points out both the cost effectiveness of evaluating patients with suspected hip fracture by MRI and the high prevalence of other abnormalities in the symptomatic patients.

M.K. Dalinka, M.D.

Quantifying the Extent of Osteonecrosis of the Femoral Head: A New Method Using MRI

Koo K-H, Kim R (Gyeong-Sang Natl Univ, Chinju, Republic of Korea; Harvard Med School, Boston)

J Bone Joint Surg (Br) 77B:875–880, 1995 3–12

Objective.—Thirty-three patients were studied to determine whether the extent of necrosis at initial scan MRI can predict the risk of collapse of the femoral head.

Background.—It has been suggested that the site and extent of the necrotic lesion affect the outcome of femoral head osteonecrosis, but the most reliable method of assessing this osteonecrosis has not been determined. Magnetic resonance imaging was used to assess the extent of the necrotic lesion in a randomized trial (Fig 1).

Methods.—In 33 patients, core-decompression with cancellous bone graft or conservative management was used to treat 37 hips with early-stage osteonecrosis. Evaluations were performed every 3 months. The extent of osteonecrosis in the MRI studies was based on abnormal signal intensity in the weight-bearing portion.

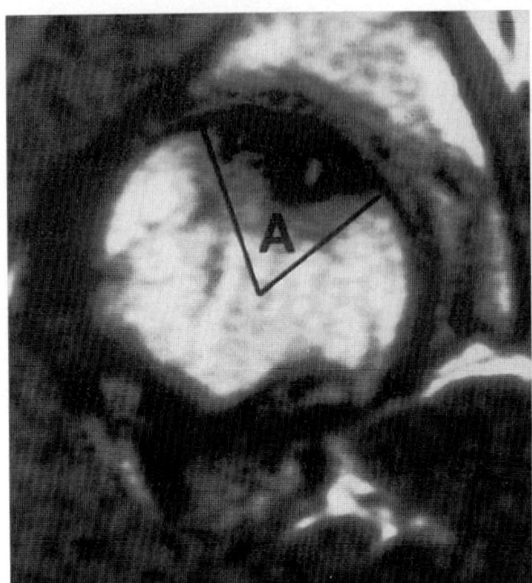

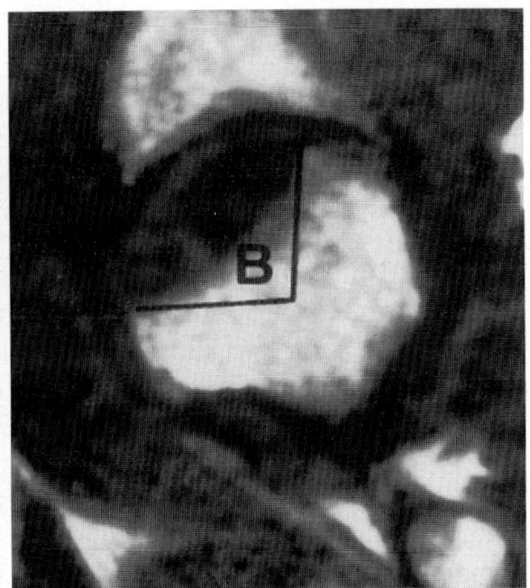

FIGURE 1.—Calculation of the index of necrotic extent using MRI. **A** is the angle of necrotic area in the midcoronal image, and **B** is the angle of necrotic area in the midsagittal image. The index for necrotic extent = (**A**/180) × (**B**/180) × 100. (Courtesy of Koo K-H, Kim R: Quantifying the extent of ostonecrosis of the femoral head: A new method using MRI. *J Bone Joint Surg [BR]* 77B:875–880, 1995.)

Results.—The arc of the necrotic portion in the midcoronal and midsagittal image was measured. These measurements were used in a formula to estimate the extent, or index, of necrosis. There was a strong correlation between this index and risk of collapse both before and after adjusting for age, gender, stage, and type of treatment.

Conclusion.—The extent of necrosis as measured by a new method based on MRI is a major predictor of adverse outcome in osteonecrosis of the femoral head. This method is relatively simple and is reproducible. This method may improve management of early stage osteonecrosis of the femoral head.

Preventing Collapse in Early Osteonecrosis of the Femoral Head: A Randomised Clinical Trial of Core Decompression

Koo K-H, Kim R, Ko G-H, et al (Gyeong-Sang Natl Univ, Chinju, Republic of Korea; Harvard Med School, Boston)

J Bone Joint Surg (Br) 77B:870–874, 1995 3–13

Objective.—Core decompression has been performed in attempts at joint preservation in patients with osteonecrosis of the femoral head. One study suggested that this procedure yielded more predictable pain relief and more consistent alteration of the indications for total hip arthroplasty compared with conservative therapy. Core decompression and conservative management were compared for their ability to prevent radiologic collapse of the femoral head in early-stage osteonecrosis.

Methods.—The randomized controlled trial included 37 hips of 33 patients with early-stage osteonecrosis as diagnosed by plain radiographs,

MRI, or both. They were assigned to undergo core decompression with cancellous bone grafting or conservative management. The primary end point of femoral head collapse was defined as a surface sinking of 2 mm or more seen on plain radiography compared with the normal contour of the initial radiograph. All patients but 2 had risk factors for osteonecrosis: alcohol abuse in 28 and a history of high-dose corticosteroids in 3. Most patients also had advanced osteonecrosis of the contralateral hip, for which they underwent total hip replacement before or after enrollment in the study.

Results.—In the core decompression group, pain was relieved in 9 of 10 initially symptomatic hips. In the conservative treatment group, by comparison, pain continued in 3 of 4 symptomatic hips. Collapse occurred in 14 hips in the core decompression group and 15 hips in the conservative management group. Collapse occurred in a median of 9 months, with no significant difference between groups. Two years after the initial diagnosis, total hip arthroplasty had been performed in 72% of hips in the core decompression group and 68% of hips in the conservative treatment group.

Conclusion.—In patients with osteonecrosis of the femoral head, core decompression can provide temporary relief of pain. However, it neither prevents nor delays collapse of the femoral head.

► These 2 papers show that the size and location of the lesion in avascular necrosis of the hip is the major determinant of the outcome. Their work casts doubt on the use of core decompression for other than symptomatic relief.

M.K. Dalinka, M.D.

Increasing Prevalence of Femoral Lysis in Cementless Total Hip Arthroplasty

Smith E, Harris WH (Massachusetts Gen Hosp, Boston; Harvard Med School, Boston)

J Arthroplasty 10:407–412, 1996 3–14

Introduction.—Femoral osteolysis around loose cemented femoral implants was first described as a destructive, macrophage-associated process in 1976. Since then, endosteal cortical erosions have been associated with loose cemented femoral components and stable cemented components, and bone lysis has been associated with both unstable and stable cementless femoral components. Wear debris consisting of particular polyethylene, bone cement, and metal has been shown to cause a foreign body granulomatous reaction and periprosthetic osteolysis. Cementless total hip arthroplasties have been recommended for younger, more active patients partly in the hope that avoiding cement would avoid femoral osteolysis. Unfortunately, this has not been the result. "Clinically silent" osteolysis occurring around cementless femoral components was described.

Methods.—The study included 94 hips in 86 patients who had undergone cementless primary total hip replacement. Sixty-one patients were men and 25 women, with a mean age of 54, mean weight of 78 kg, and mean height of 176 cm. The patients were followed for a mean of 53 months, though several were found to have osteolysis before 24 months. All radiographs were reviewed, and femoral osteolysis was recorded in terms of 7 zones on the anteroposterior and lateral radiographs. Sequential radiographs were used to assess progression of lysis. Uneven or scalloped areas of endosteal erosion were classified as erosive lysis, whereas generalized canal enlargement with endosteal resorption was classified as linear lysis. Stability of the femoral component was assessed in terms of radiographic evidence of migration and the demonstration of nonelastic motion between the prosthetic stem and femur at reoperation.

Findings.—Femoral lysis was found in 29 femurs, for a prevalence of 31%. The lysis was graded as extensive in 11 of the 29 hips. The femoral component was considered loose in 14 hips, 12 of which had femoral osteolysis. However, the Harris hip score for the hips with osteolysis was 88 points, and 25 of 29 were classified in the good or excellent category. The patients were included in a previous report of femoral lysis in Harris-Galante porous and Porous-Coated Anatomic femoral components, at which time the incidence of femoral lysis was 3%. All patients had progression of their lesions since then.

Conclusion.—Femoral osteolysis is an increasingly common problem in hips with a cementless femoral component. Over time, the endosteal lesions enlarge, and the prevalence of osteolysis increases. Compared with cemented femoral stems placed with second-generation cementing techniques, the results with uncemented femoral components have generally been less successful. Proactive follow-up is needed to document the progression of the lytic process in patients with cementless arthroplasties.

▶ This nice paper shows that "cement disease" can occur in the absence of cement. The authors also make the point that uncemented femoral components are not as successful as cemented stems with second-generation cementing techniques.

The authors believe that patients should have periodic radiographs after total hip replacement surgery; treatment, however, is purely dependent on symptoms. The periodic filming is therefore difficult to justify, particularly in the area of cost containment.

M.K. Dalinka, M.D.

Knee and Lower Extremity

Computerized Tomography for the Evaluation of Posttraumatic Multiplane Deformities of the Tibia

Westrich GH, Borrelli J Jr, Ghelman B, et al (Hosp for Special Surgery, New York; Cornell Univ, New York)
Am J Orthop May:7–10, 1995 3–15

Introduction.—Tibial malunion is common after high-energy trauma, with deformity occurring in the coronal and sagittal planes and often additional rotational deformity. This deformity can affect the mechanics of gait and hasten the development of degenerative arthritis. Surgical planning for the correction of such deformities depend on thorough radiographic evaluation, usually including anteroposterior, lateral, and oblique radiographs, to assess coronal and sagittal deformity, and scanograms, teleroentgenograms, or orthoroentgenograms, to determine limb length. However, the accuracy and cost effectiveness of CT scans were investigated in the evaluation of multiplane deformities of the tibia.

Methods.—Ten patients with posttraumatic multiplane deformities of the tibia were evaluated with a CT examination with anteroposterior (to evaluate varus-valgus angulation, displacement, and length discrepancy), lateral (to determine anteroposterior bowing and displacement), and selected axial (to evaluate rotational malalignment) images. The varus-valgus angulation in the coronal plane seen with the anteroposterior view and anterior bowing in the sagittal plane seen with the lateral view were determined by drawing a computer-generated line from either end through the long axis of the tibia to the deformity site, whereas leg length discrepancy could be determined by drawing a vertical line perpendicular to a horizontal line at the level of the ankle joint and extending to the knee (Fig 1). Angular deformity was assessed by determination of the angle of a tangential line drawn across the posterior femoral condyles on an axial view of the distal femur and of a tangential line drawn across the posterior aspect of the medial and lateral malleoli on an axial view of the ankle mortise to the horizontal axis (Fig 2).

Results.—This CT examination protocol enabled the determination of varus-valgus angulation, anteroposterior bowing, displacement, leg length discrepancy, and rotational malalignment in all 10 patients. The findings were accurate and reproducible. The examination took only 15 minutes and reduced the patient's radiation exposure by 80% compared with a standard radiographic examination. The cost of the CT examination was significantly less than that of a standard radiographic examination ($415 vs. $564).

Conclusion.—The selected CT examination is accurate and safe, exposing the patients to less radiation than typical evaluation techniques. Computed tomography is also cost effective in the evaluation of multiplane

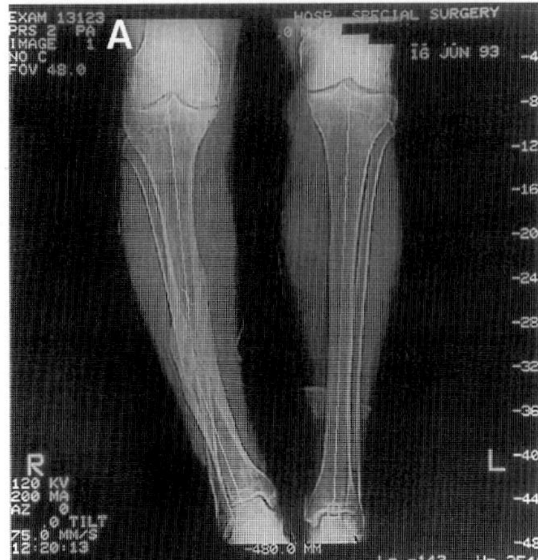

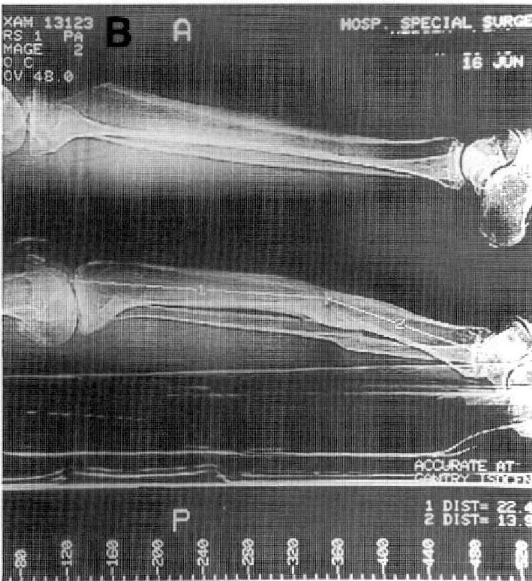

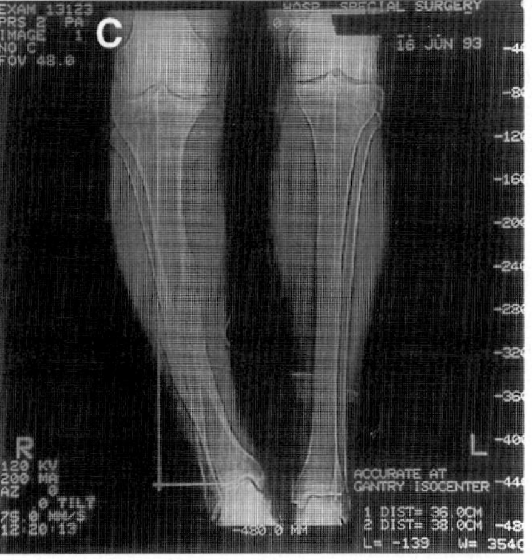

FIGURE 1.—Evaluation of posttraumatic multiplane deformity of the tibia. Varus-valgus angulation in the coronal plane and anterior bowing in the sagittal plane were determined by the angle of intersection between 2 lines drawn through the long axis of the tibia from each end to the site of the deformaity. Anteroposterior scout view (**A**) shows varus angulation of 15 degrees without medial displacement; lateral scout view (**B**) shows anterior tibial bowing of 15 degrees without lateral displacement. Leg-length discrepancy was determined from the anteroposterior scout view (**C**) by using the computer to erect a horizontal line at the level of the ankle joint and then measure the perpendicular vertical distance to the knee joint. The discrepancy, which is 2 cm in this example, is found by subtracting the value for the injured tibia from that of the normal tibia. (Reprinted by permission of the publisher from Westrich GH, Borrelli J Jr, Ghelman B, et al: Computerized tomography for the evaluation of posttraumatic multiplane deformities of the tibia. *Am J Orthop* May:7–10, Copyright 1995 by Quadrant Healthcom Inc.)

deformities of the tibia. It is likely that the technique could also be used in the evaluation of deformities of other long bones.

► The authors describe another use of CT, this 1 being simple to perform and cost effective.

M.K. Dalinka, M.D.

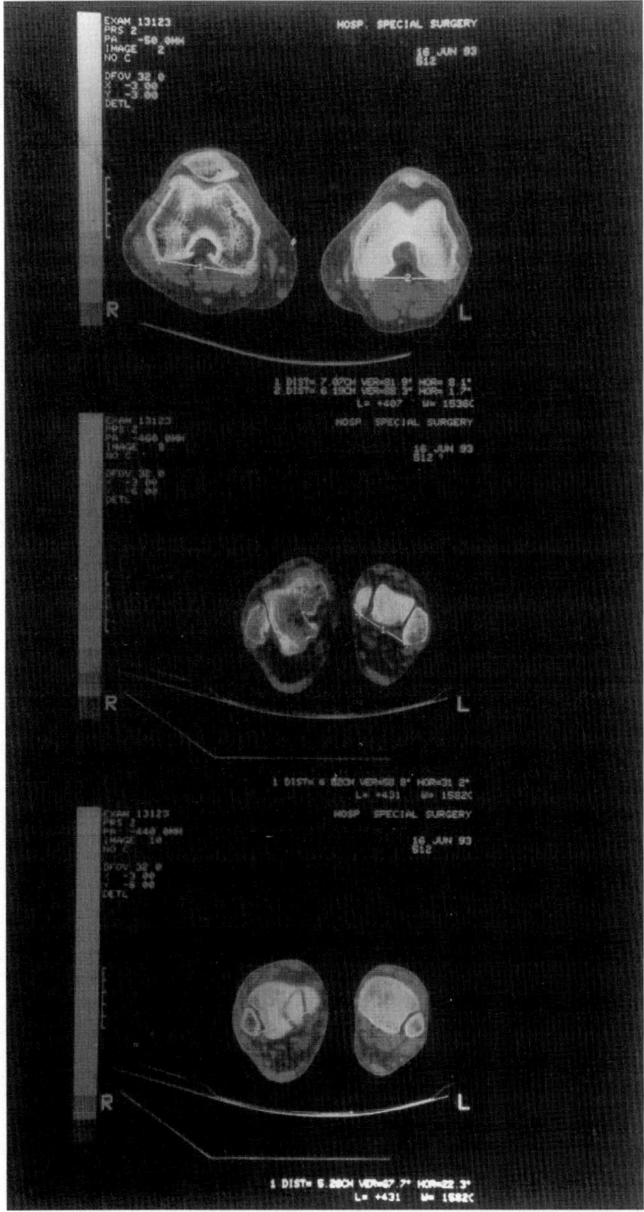

FIGURE 2.—An axial view at the level of the distal femur can be used to determine the angular deformity of the tibia of the patient shown in Figure 1. Computer-generated lines are placed tangentially across both posterior femoral condyles, and, with a second axial view at the level of the ankle mortise, the posterior aspect of the medial and lateral malleoli. Computerized measurement of the angles can determine the degree of deformity, and comparison with normal tibia can determine rotational malalignment. In this case, there was an insignificant malrotation (1 degree) of the extremity. (Reprinted by permission of the publisher from Westrich GH, Borrelli J Jr, Ghelman B, et al: Computerized tomography for the evaluation of posttraumatic multiplane deformities of the tibia. *Am J Orthop* May: 7–10, Copyright 1995 by Quadrant Healthcom Inc.)

MRI in the Management of Tibial Plateau Fractures

Holt MD, Williams LA, Dent CM (Cardiff Royal Infirmary, Wales, England)

Injury 26:595–599, 1995 3–16

Background.—Accurate reduction must be achieved and maintained to optimize the results of treatment for tibial plateau fractures, so a complete assessment of the fracture anatomy is an essential part of surgical planning. Plain radiographs may fail to demonstrate the fracture adequately. Even with oblique views, it can be difficult to evaluate the extent of the fracture and the degree of comminution. The use of MRI in investigating tibial plateau fractures was evaluated.

Methods and Findings.—The study included 21 patients with known tibial plateau fractures who underwent standard radiography and MRI scanning before receiving treatment. Magnetic resonance imaging led to reclassification to a worse prognostic group for 48% of fractures. In addition, the information provided by MRI led to a change in management for 19% of patients. The main problem with plain radiographs was that they failed to recognize the "split" part of "split-depression" type of fractures. In fractures with fragment displacement, plain radiographs underestimated the extent of displacement by an average of 35% (Fig 5). Intra-articular or extra-articular soft-tissue injuries (i.e., of the cruciate and collateral ligaments or menisci) were detected by MRI in 48% of patients.

Conclusion.—Magnetic resonance imaging overcomes many of the limitations of plain radiographs in the evaluation of tibial plateau fractures. Because the use of MRI has a significant impact on fracture classification and patient management, MRI is the imaging technique of choice in patients with tibial plateau fractures.

► We all should be aware of the value of MRI in patients with tibial plateau fractures. Although CT is still done in many institutions, it provides much less information.

M.K. Dalinka, M.D.

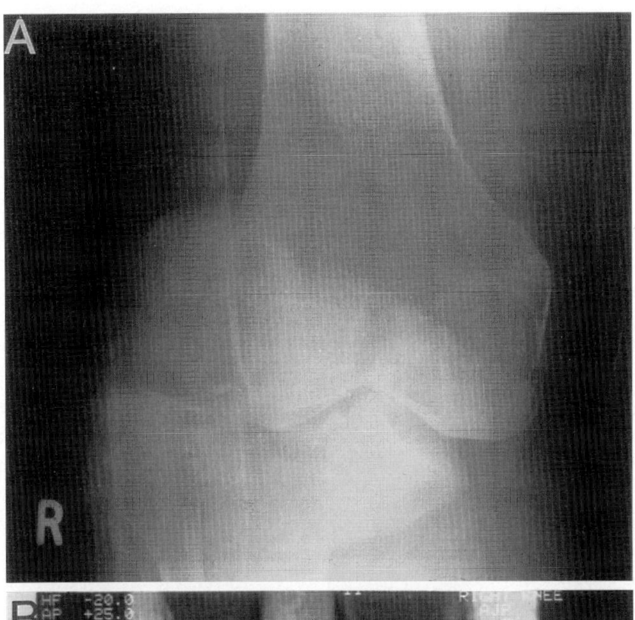

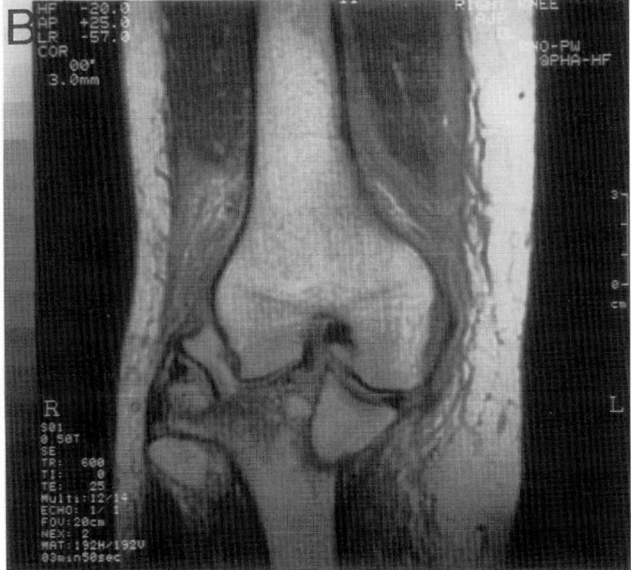

FIGURE 5.—Plain film (**A**) and MR image (**B**) of fracture-dislocation of the knee, irreducible because of a fragment of the lateral articular surface seen only on the MRI scan. (Reprinted from *Injury*; vol 26; Holt MD, Williams LA, Dent CM: MRI in the management of tibial plateau fractures; pp 595–599; Copyright 1995; with permission from Elsevier Science Ltd, The Boulevard, Langford Lane, Kidlington OX5 1GB, UK.)

Error Patterns in the MR Imaging Evaluation of Menisci of the Knee

Justice WW, Quinn SF (Oregon Health Sciences Univ, Portland; Good Samaritan Hosp and Med Ctr, Portland, Ore)

Radiology 196:617–621, 1995 3–17

Background.—Magnetic resonance imaging has been shown to be highly accurate in the diagnosis of meniscal tears. Though sensitivity and specificity figures are very encouraging, the reasons for the errors that do occur are unclear. Forty percent of the errors may be unavoidable even on a retrospective basis. One possible explanation is problems related to the use of arthroscopy as the standard of reference. Errors in the interpretation of knee MRI scans were categorized, including an assessment of discrepancies between MRI and diagnostic arthroscopy.

Methods.—The analysis included 561 patients who underwent both arthroscopy and MRI of the knee. The type and location of meniscal tears detected were established by prospective and retrospective readings. The criteria for a meniscal tear were an area of increased intrameniscal integrity that definitely touched a meniscal surface, contour irregularities with and without areas on increased signal intensity, and displaced meniscal fragments. Sixty-eight discrepancies were detected in 66 patients; these were analyzed for identification of error patterns.

Results.—Lateral meniscal tears were correctly diagnosed on a retrospective basis in 28% of patients with false negative results at prospective interpretation, and medial meniscal tears were detected retrospectively in 20% of patients with an initial false negative result. Seventy-five patients had arthroscopically proven tears of the anterior cruciate ligament (ACL). In the detection of tears of the medial meniscus, MRI was 92% sensitive in patients with an ACL tear and 97% in those without. In the detection tears of the lateral meniscus, sensitivity was 77% for patients with and 84% for those without an ACL tear. The most frequent error was the false negative finding of a tear of the middle portion and posterior horn of the lateral meniscus.

Conclusion.—As previously established, MRI is very accurate in detecting meniscal tears. Whereas most errors in the lateral meniscus involve false negative reports of tears in the middle and posterior horns, errors in the medial meniscus are equally divided between false negatives and false positives. Some false positive results may involve incomplete arthroscopic evaluation and confusion over the distinction between fraying and tearing.

▶ The reader is referred to paper by De Smet and Graf,[1] which comes to a slightly different conclusion. Another interesting article on the subject was published by De Smet et al.[2]

M.K. Dalinka, M.D.

References

1. De Smet AA, Graf BK: Meniscal tears missed on MR imaging: Relationship to meniscal tear patterns and anterior cruciate ligament tears. *AJR* 162:905–911, 1994.

2. De Smet AA, Tuite MJ, Norris MA, et al: MR diagnosis of meniscal tears: Analysis of causes of errors. *AJR* 163:1419–1423, 1994.

Bucket-Handle Tears of the Medial and Lateral Menisci of the Knee: Value of MR Imaging in Detecting Displaced Fragments

Wright DH, De Smet AA, Norris M (Univ of Wisconsin, Madison)
AJR 165:621–625, 1995 3–18

Background.—Magnetic resonance imaging is a useful diagnostic method in the detection of meniscal tears. Signs of a displaced meniscal fragment from a bucket-handle tear have been identified, but their sensitivity has not been investigated. The sensitivity of MRI for detecting these meniscal fragments and of the individual signs was assessed retrospectively in patients with arthroscopically diagnosed bucket-handle tears of the medial and lateral menisci.

Methods.—The MR images of 39 patients with arthroscopically proven bucket-handle tears (32 medial tears and 7 lateral tears) were reviewed by 2 independent examiners, with a third for arbitration of disagreements. The frequency of identification of a displaced meniscal fragment was determined as manifested by the following signs: a double posterior cruciate ligament (PCL) sign, a flipped meniscus sign, or a fragment within the intercondylar notch (Fig 6). The effect of an anterior cruciate ligament (ACL) tear on the sensitivity of MRI detection of meniscal fragments was evaluated in the 19 patients with concurrent ACL and meniscal tears.

Results.—Twenty-five of the 39 bucket-handle fragments were detected with MRI, for a sensitivity of 64%. Thirteen of these patients had all 3 signs, 6 had 2 signs, and 6 had 1 sign. The sensitivity of the individual signs was 44% for the double PCL sign, 41% for the flipped meniscus sign, and 61% for the fragment within the intercondylar notch. However, diagnosis was also possible based not on the identification of a displaced fragment but on signal extending to the meniscal surface in 9 patients, increasing the overall sensitivity of MRI to 87%. Sensitivity was significantly greater with larger than with smaller tears (84% vs. 40%). The flipped meniscus sign was detected in 44% of the medial tears and 29% of the lateral tears. A fragment in the intercondylar notch was detected in 66% of the medial tears and 43% of the lateral tears. The double PCL sign was detected in 53% of the medial tears and none of the lateral tears. The presence of an ACL tear did not significantly affect the sensitivity of MRI for detecting displaced meniscal fragments.

Conclusion.—Whereas MRI has good sensitivity for detecting bucket-handle tears involving the meniscus, it has much less sensitivity in detecting smaller bucket-handle tears. The fragment in the intercondylar notch and the flipped meniscus sign were seen with comparable frequency in tears of the medial and of the lateral menisci, but the double PCL sign was seen only with medial meniscal tears.

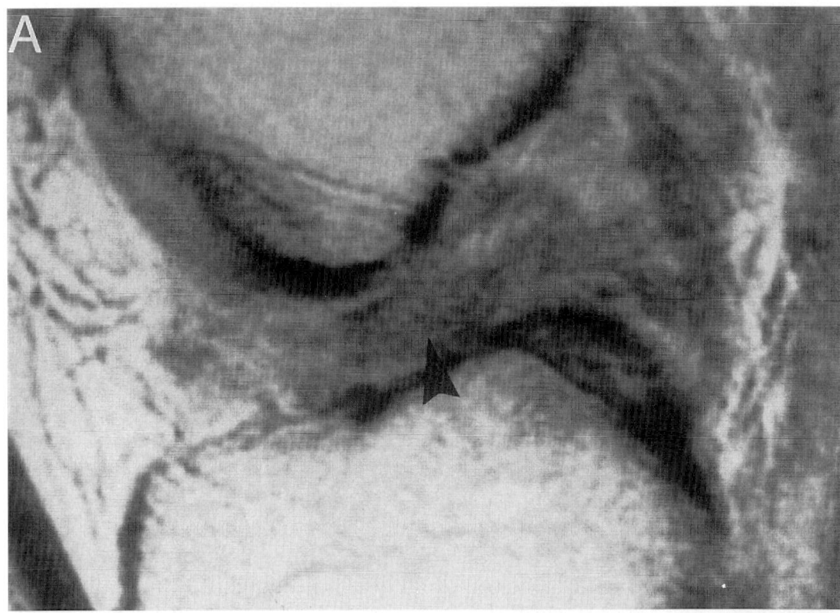

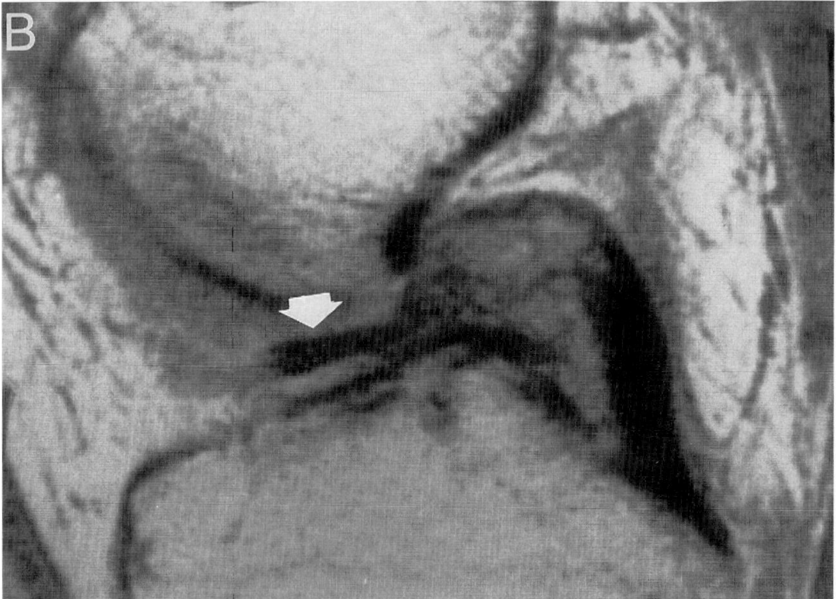

FIGURE 6.—Man, 24 years old, with arthroscopically proven displaced medial meniscal fragment and anterior cruciate ligament tear. The patient heard a pop and felt pain during a basketball game. **A,** sagittal proton density–weighted (recovery time 2,000 msec/echo time 20 msec) MR image shows acutely torn anterior cruciate ligament (*arrowhead*), with increased signal intensity. **B,** adjacent proton density–weighted (recovery time 2,000 msec/echo time 20 msec) MR image shows low-signal intensity band indicating displaced meniscal fragment (*arrow*) that was found in intercondylar notch at surgery. (Courtesy of Wright DH, De Smet AA, Norris M: Bucket-handle tears of the medial and lateral menisci of the knee: Value of MR imaging in detecting displaced fragments. *AJR* 165:621–625, 1995.)

▶ It is not surprising that larger fragments are easier to detect than smaller ones; what is surprising is that the overall sensitivity for detecting these fragments was only 0.64.

M.K. Dalinka, M.D.

Anterior Cruciate Ligament Tear: Prospective Evaluation of Diagnostic Accuracy of Middle- and High-Field-Strength MR Imaging at 1.5 and 0.5 T

Vellet AD, Lee DH, Munk PL, et al (Univ Hosp, London, Ont, Canada; Robarts Research Inst, London, Ont, Canada; Univ of Western Ontario, London, Ont, Canada)

Radiology 197:826–830, 1995 3–19

Background.—There is little information directly comparing the diagnosis of ligament tears on magnetic resonance scanners of different field strengths. Middle- and high–field-strength MRI scanners were compared for the diagnosis of anterior cruciate ligament tears.

Methods.—The analysis included 114 of a series of 230 patients referred for knee imaging in whom the diagnosis of torn or intact ACL was confirmed by surgery. All patients underwent MR imaging at field strengths of 0.5 and 1.5 tesla using state-of-the-art imagers. The sequences used were the same with both scanners, though a slightly longer imaging time and bandwidth optimization were used at 0.5 tesla. Radiologists interpreted the scans without knowledge of the patient's diagnosis or the field strength used. The sensitivity, specificity, and accuracy of middle-and high–field-strength MRI scanning were assessed.

Results.—An ACL tear was confirmed in 86 patients, and an intact ACL in 28. Both the middle- and high-field-strength scanners were about 90% accurate in diagnosing ACL tears. Neither was there any difference between the radiologists ability to diagnose meniscal tears or posterior cruciate ligament tears on the 2 magnets. Though the radiologists were usually able to identify the field strength used, they found no significant differences in image quality.

Conclusion.—Using a high–field-strength rather than a middle–field-strength MRI scanner does not improve the accuracy of diagnosis in patients with ACL tears. There are no differences in image quality, but the capital and operational costs of middle–field-strength scanners are significantly lower.

▶ This paper compares high– and middle–field-strength MRI units in the assessment of knee pathology. The authors identify a major issue that was not well addressed in similar papers that compared multiple field-strength magnets, i.e., the use of comparable software. The results are important and should be confirmed, as perhaps similar results could be achieved by less expensive magnets with more advanced software.

M.K. Dalinka, M.D

Tibial Stress Reaction in Runners: Correlation of Clinical Symptoms and Scintigraphy With a New Magnetic Resonance Imaging Grading System

Fredericson M, Bergman AG, Hoffman KL, et al (Stanford Univ, Calif)
Am J Sports Med 23:472–481, 1995 3–20

Objective.—Stress fractures are a common form of sports medicine injury that may be difficult to diagnose and manage. Traditionally runners with medial tibial pain have been regarded as having either a shin splint syndrome or a stress fracture. However, only about half of symptomatic patients will ever show radiographic evidence of a stress reaction. Magnetic resonance imaging may be able to document a progression of injury, from periosteal edema through progressive marrow involvement, and, finally, to frank cortical stress fracture. An MRI-based grading system for the evaluation of tibial stress injuries in runners was evaluated, including an attempt to identify clinical factors indicating more severe grades of stress injury.

Methods.—The analysis included 18 symptomatic legs in 14 runners who underwent clinical examination, bone scanning, and MRI, all performed within 10 days. The MRI findings were graded from 0 to 4: grade 0, a normal examination; grade 1, mild to moderate periosteal edema on T2-weighted images only; grade 2, more severe periosteal edema and bone marrow edema on T2-weighted images only; grade 3, moderate to severe periosteal and marrow edema on T1- and T2-weighted images; and grade 4, low-signal fracture line on all sequences, along with severe marrow edema on T1- and T2-weighted images. The MRI results were compared with the clinical and bone scan findings.

Results.—The MRI result was grade 0 in 11% of legs, grade 1 in 11%, grade 2 in 17%, grade 3 in 56%, and grade IV in 6%. Fourteen of the 18 legs had similar results on bone scanning; 2 had a more severe injury detected on MRI, and 2 had normal MRI findings but a grade 1 injury on bone scanning. According to MRI, the location of injury was the proximal tibia in 7 cases, the midtibia in 6, and the distal tibia in 3. All of the injuries were found along the compressive side of the tibia; 1 was found on the posteromedial border, which is subject to compressive forces during running. Eighty-eight percent of legs showed periosteal involvement. In most cases, the periosteal edema involved the bony insertions of the tibialis posterior, the flexor digitorum longus, and soleus muscles.

Conclusion.—Magnetic resonance imaging helps to define the location and extent of tibial stress reaction in runners. Physical findings such as localized tibial tenderness and pain on direct percussion over the involved area are linked with more involved marrow and cortical abnormalities. Tenderness to indirect percussion is a very specific indicator of grade 3 or 4 injury. There is good correlation between the results of bone scanning and MRI. Periosteal edema appears to represent the initial injury on a spectrum that can progress to a more serious bone injury. The article includes illustrations of the newly developed MRI grading system for runners with medial tibial pain.

► The authors show a spectrum of MRI abnormalities in patients with stress-related injury. A recent paper by Beck and Osternig[1] addresses the abnormality with respect to the muscles involved.

The factor of critical importance is when and for whom should an MRI be obtained in a patient with a suspected stress fracture. One is again referred to the appropriateness criteria of the American College of Radiology, which discusses this issue.

M.K. Dalinka, M.D.

Reference

1. Beck BR, Osternig LR: Medial tibial stress syndrome. The location of muscles in the leg in relation to symptoms. *J Bone Joint Surg (Am)* 76:1057–1061, 1994.

Foot and Ankle

Insufficiency Fracture of the Talus: Diagnosis With MR Imaging

Umans H, Pavlov H (Albert Einstein College, Bronx, NY; Hosp for Special Surgery, New York)

Radiology 197:439–442, 1995 3–21

Objective.—The clinical diagnosis of talar stress fracture, both insufficiency and fatigue, may be elusive mainly because of its extremely low prevalence and the frequently chronic and diffuse nature of the symptoms. The clinical setting and pattern of talar insufficiency fracture as diagnosed with MRI in 4 patients were studied in a retrospective review. The location and orientation of fractures and the presence of concomitant osseous and soft-tissue injury were noted on the MRI images.

Patients.—All 4 patients were women, aged 30 to 70. Of the 5 talar insufficiency fractures sustained, only 2 had typical features, occurring in the talar neck and oriented parallel to the talonavicular joint. The other 3 fractures were atypical in location and orientation. One fracture was oriented horizontally in the body of the talus; 2 occurred in the posteromedial talus, with 1 oriented vertically and the other oriented horizontally (Fig 2). Two patients had concomitant stress fractures, including a calcaneal stress fracture that occurred ipsilateral to a classically oriented talar neck fracture and a stress fracture of the distal tibia that occurred ipsilateral to an atypically oriented talar fracture.

Discussion.—Since 1965, only 11 talar stress fractures in 10 patients have been reported. Vertically and horizontally oriented insufficiency fractures of the talar body have not been previously reported. The atypically oriented talar insufficiency fractures may remain occult in plain radiographs due to overlap of osseous structures, particularly in the posterior subtalar joint and middle talocalcaneal facet. Concomitant or preexisting stress fracture of the distal tibia and calcaneus may occur in either the

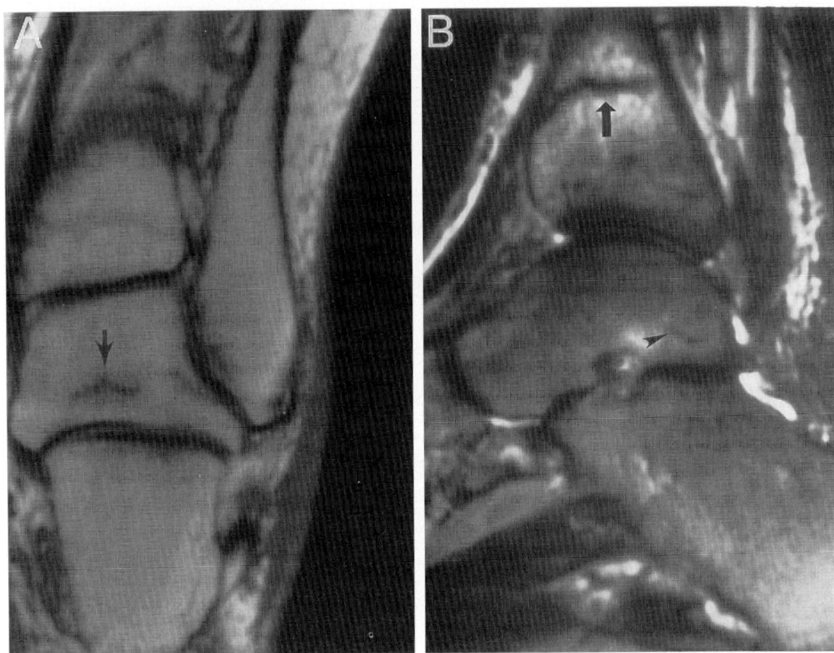

FIGURE 2.—Atypical orientation and location of an insufficiency fracture in the left talus of a 37-year-old woman. **A,** coronal T1-weighted spin-echo MR image (recovery time 400 msec/echo time 16 msec) demonstrates a horizontally oriented linear fracture of low-signal intensity in the posteromedial talus (*arrow*). **B,** sagittal T2-weighted fast spin-echo MR image (recovery time 4,000 msec/echo time 102 msec) demonstrates the talar fracture (*arrowhead*) and a concomitant stress fracture of the distal (*arrow*) surrounded by high-signal intensity marrow edema. (Courtesy of Umans H, Pavlov H: Insufficiency fracture of the talus: Diagnosis with MR imaging. *Radiology* 197:439–442, 1995; Radiological Society of North America.)

ipsilateral or contralateral limb. In addition to clinical familiarity with this entity, MRI provides early, specific diagnosis of talar insufficiency fracture and coexisting injuries to prevent delayed diagnosis and unnecessarily prolonged morbidity.

► This is another short paper illustrating another abnormality that can be specifically diagnosed on MRI.

M.K. Dalinka, M.D.

Cost-Effectiveness Analysis of the Ottawa Ankle Rules

Anis AH, Stiell IG, Stewart DG, et al (Univ of British Columbia, Vancouver, Canada; Univ of Ottawa, Ont, Canada; Ottawa Civic Hosp, Ont, Canada)
Ann Emerg Med 26:422–428, 1995 3–22

Objective.—Patients with ankle injuries are commonly seen in the emergency department (ED). Although less than 15% will prove to have an ankle fracture, almost all will have ankle or foot radiographs taken. The recently introduced Ottawa Ankle Rules provide a few simple clinical findings to promote more selective use of radiographs in patients with ankle injuries. Their implementation can reduce the use of ankle radiography and shorten patient waiting times without missing any fractures. The cost effectiveness of implementing the Ottawa Ankle Rules in U.S. and Canadian EDs was studied.

Implementation Study.—The incremental cost-effectiveness analysis was based on a controlled clinical trial examining the impact of teaching the Ottawa Ankle Rules to all physicians working in the ED of a university hospital. In this trial, patients seen after implementation of the Ottawa Ankle Rules had a 28% reduction in ankle radiographic series, a 14% reduction in foot radiographic series. There were no missed fractures, and patients were equally satisfied with their quality of care regardless of whether radiographs were ordered. Mean length of the ED visit was 36 minutes shorter for patients not having radiographs.

Cost-Effectiveness Analysis.—The current study used a decision analytic model to compare the implementation of the Ottawa Ankle Rules with current practice. There were differences in costs for the intervention and control groups because of differing probabilities of having radiographs, the decreased length of stay, the costs of re-evaluating patients with missed fractures, time lost from work, and litigation costs associated with missed fractures. Based on a survey of legal experts, a litigation rate of 5/10,000 patients with missed fractures was assumed for the United States; the estimated rate for Canada was about one fifth of the U.S. rate. Radiographs were assumed to be 100% sensitive and specific for the identification of ankle fractures.

Results.—The Ottawa Ankle Rules were cost effective under a range of different conditions. Depending on the charges for radiography, estimated savings in the United States ranged from $614,000 to $3,146,000 per 100,000 patients. The results were largely unaffected by varying assumptions regarding the missed fracture rate, the cost of radiography, and the probability and costs of lawsuits.

Conclusion.—Implementation of the Ottawa Ankle Rules would be a cost-effective measure, taking into account all direct and indirect costs and under reasonable assumptions about the likelihood of missing some fractures. Despite the high sensitivity in fracture prediction and the cost-saving potential, some physicians may still feel uncomfortable about using the Ottawa Ankle Rules. Fears about litigation related to missed fractures can be reduced if the rules are generally accepted as good clinical practice and endorsed by professional associations.

► The use of the Ottowa Ankle Rules and their cost savings are extremely important and pertinent for patient evaluation in the ED. This topic has also been covered in detail in the American College of Radiology appropriateness criteria handbook. The same authors have written extensively on this subject and have recently addressed similar criteria for the knee. The interested reader is referred to the *Academic Emergency Medicine*[1] and the *Annals of Emergency Medicine*[2] for further discussion of that subject.

M.K. Dalinka, M.D.

References

1. Stiell IG, Wells GA, McDowell I, et al: Use of radiography in acute knee injuries: Need for clinical decision rules. *Acad Emerg Med* 2:966–973, 1995.
2. Stiell IG, Greenberg GH, Wells GA, et al: Derivation of a decision rule for the use of radiography in acute knee injuries. *Ann Emerg Med* 26:405–413, 1995.

Imaging the Diabetic Foot

Gold RH, Tong DJF, Crim JR, et al (Univ of California, Los Angeles; Durham Radiology Associates, NC)

Skeletal Radiol 24:563–571, 1995 3–23

Background.—Successful management of infection and neuropathy in the diabetic foot relies on prompt, accurate diagnosis. Important considerations in the diagnostic imaging of the diabetic foot were reviewed.

Diabetic Angiopathy.—The ischemia caused by diabetic angiopathy combines with peripheral neuropathy to predispose the pedal skin to ulceration, which is the precursor to osteomyelitis. The soft-tissue disorder necrobiosis lipoidica diabeticorum results from a microangiopathy and may occur on the dorsum of the foot and the pretibial region.

Diabetic Neuropathy.—Spinal and peripheral nerve damage can result in diabetic neuroarthropathy, usually when patients are in their forties to sixties and after they have had diabetes for at least 15 years. Most cases involve the foot, especially the tarsal and tarsometatarsal joints and the metatarsophalangeal joints. Neuropathy may be atrophic, with osteoporosis, bone resorption, and dislocation, or hypertrophic, with osteophyte formation, sclerosis, eburnation, fragmentation, and dislocation. Which develops depends on whether the neuropathy involves the sympathetic, sensory, or motor fibers. Diabetic peripheral neuropathy refers to peripheral somatic or autonomic nerve damage caused solely by diabetes mellitus.

Forefoot abnormalities may result from infection or neuropathy alone or a combination of the 2 plus small-vessel disease. The initial radiographic signs of neuropathy in the intertarsal and metatarsophalangeal joints are joint swelling and laxity. Subluxation, subchondral fragmentation, new bone proliferation, and sclerosis follow, and relentless trauma can lead to rapid bony destruction.

Osteomyelitis.—Almost all cases of diabetic osteomyelitis of the foot stem from contiguous neurotrophic pedal ulcers. These ulcers generally occur at pressure sites over bony or joint prominences, most commonly below the metatarsal heads, at the tips of the toes, and over deformed interphalangeal joints. Diabetic patients may show atypical osteomyelitic changes. The diagnosis may be made more difficult by the absence of fever, bacteremia, or abnormalities of the erythrocyte sedimentation rate.

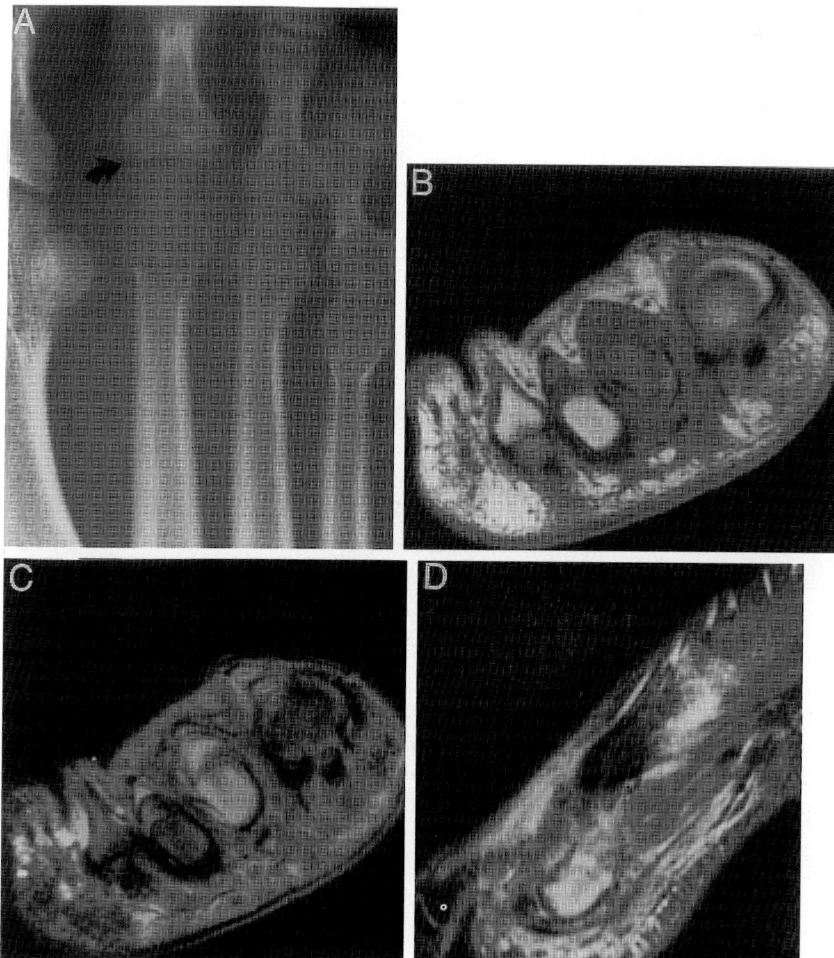

FIGURE 13.—Osteomyelitis in a 35-year old diabetic man. A radiograph (**A**) reveals marginal erosion, narrowing of the joint space (*arrow*), and juxta-articular osteoporosis. Exudate and edema in and around the bone are characterized on a T1-weighted spin-echo axial MR image (**B**; recovery time 500 msec/echo time 20 msec) by intermediate-signal intensity and on a T2-weighted image (**C**; recovery time 40,000 msec/echo time 104 msec) by bright signal intensity. A short-tau inversion recovery sagittal image features fat suppression (**D**; recovery time 2,366 msec/echo time 40 msec/inversion time 155 msec) and shows a bright signal emanating from the edematous soft tissue and the exudate-filled head of the second metatarsal. (Courtesy of Gold RH, Tong DJF, Crim JR, et al: Imaging the diabetic foot. *Skeletal Radiol* 24:563–571, 1995.)

Imaging Procedures.—The most frequent reason for ordering imaging studies of the diabetic foot is suspected osteomyelitis. Though plain radiographs are not sensitive for this purpose, they are at least as specific as technetium-99m–methylene diphosphonate (MDP) scanning. The 3-phase ^{99m}Tc-MDP scan is highly sensitive, but it has a high false positive rate; mean sensitivity is 85% and specificity 54%. A high false positive rate limits the usefulness of gallium-67 scintigraphy. The most sensitive of all radionuclide studies is indium-111 white blood cell (WBC) scanning; the absence of activity usually excludes active infection. However, these scans may be positive in many noninfected neuropathic joints.

Computed tomography may reveal sequestra, cortical destruction, periosteal new bone, and intraosseous gas that are undetected on MRI. Magnetic resonance imaging can, however, demonstrate ulcerations, edema, localized fluid collections, and evidence of osteomyelitis and neuroarthropathy. It is nearly 100% sensitive in diagnosing osteomyelitis and no less than 81% specific, and as such it can distinguish between cellulitis and soft-tissue ulceration (Fig 13). It is very helpful in patients with nondiagnostic radiographs or equivocal ^{99m}Tc-MDP bone scans. The MRI findings in patients with suspected osteomyelitis should be correlated with the clinical findings and other imaging studies.

Recommendations.—Patients with suspected osteomyelitis should first be screened with plain radiographs. If the films reveal osteolytic changes but no ulcer, neuropathy but not osteomyelitis is probably present. A patient with normal radiographs but a high clinical suspicion of osteomyelitis should undergo 3-phase ^{99m}Tc-MDP scanning or MRI. If the radiographs are positive, ^{111}In-WBC scanning should be performed to exclude osteomyelitis. Biopsy confirmation should be obtained if this scan is positive; the needle entry site should be beyond the edge of the associated ulcer.

▶ This is an excellent and balanced review article of imaging the diabetic foot. This issue is also covered in the American College of Radiology appropriateness criteria handbook, which was published in the last year.

M.K. Dalinka, M.D.

The Os Trigonum Syndrome: Imaging Features

Karasick D, Schweitzer ME (Thomas Jefferson Univ, Philadelphia)
AJR 166:125–129, 1996 3–24

Introduction.—Patients with os trigonum syndrome have ankle pain, tenderness, or swelling related to pathologic changes of the lateral tubercle of the posterior talar process. This syndrome is commonly associated with activities such as ballet, soccer, football, and downhill running that involve extreme plantar flexion, with compression of synovial and capsular tissue against the posterior tibia. Repetitive microtrauma and chronic inflammation lead to painful disruption of the cartilaginous synchondrosis between the os trigonum and lateral talar tubercle. Fracture of the trigonal process, tenosynovitis of the flexor hallucis longus, posterior tibiotalar impingement, and intra-articular loose bodies may also occur. The diagnosis of os trigonum syndrome can be difficult to make. The imaging findings of os trigonum syndrome were reviewed and illustrated.

Imaging Considerations.—The normal os trigonum appears on radiographs as triangular structure, usually solitary and less than 1 cm, with regular margins. The margins may become irregular with repetitive microtrauma, and hypertrophy of the ossicle or lateral tubercle may occur with continued impingement. Chronic chondro-osseous disruption between the os trigonum and talus may cause cystic and sclerotic changes along the synchondrosis; these changes can be distinguished from acute fractures by polydirectional tomography and CT. Several different types of posterior bony block can cause impingement pain in the posterior ankles. Pain may result from injury to the cartilaginous synchondrosis, which causes chondro-osseous microseparation and fibrosis. In another scenario, an acute fracture may result from forceful plantar flexion and pronation.

Technetium bone scans showing increased uptake in the os trigonum can help in diagnosing symptomatic os trigonum, as well as nonunited fractures of the posterior process. The MRI finding of fluid between the os trigonum and lateral talar process denotes disruption of the cartilaginous synchondrosis. Magnetic resonance imaging can also detect hallucis longus tenosynovitis, degenerative joint changes, and synovial osteochondromatosis. Arthrography can provide valuable information on the site of hindfoot pain and for surgical planning. On selective arthrography of the synchondrosis, pain relief after injection of local anesthetic confirms the diagnosis of symptomatic os trigonum.

Summary.—Information on the os trigonum syndrome was reviewed, with an emphasis on the imaging findings. Illustrations of the findings described can be found in the original article.

▶ This pictorial essay is a good review of the subject and should be seen in its entirety because of the high quality of the illustrations.

M.K. Dalinka, M.D

Magnetic Resonance Imaging of Plantar Plate Rupture

Yao L, Cracchiolo A, Farahani K, et al (Univ of California, Los Angeles)
Foot Ankle Int 17:33–36, 1996 3–25

Background.—The plantar ligament or plate is the weightbearing portion of the metatarsophalangeal joint (MTPJ) capsule. Rupture of the plantar plate affects the middle digits and plays an important role in the pathogenesis of hammertoe or clawtoe. A diagnosis of plantar plate rupture can be established with MTPJ arthrography. However, MRI has been useful in examining ligaments. The usefulness of MRI in evaluating the plantar plate with a small MRI receiver coil was determined.

Methods.—Thirteen patients with suspected plantar plate ruptures were examined with MRI of the MTPJ, using a 3-cm, flexible, receive-only surface coil placed horizontally over the symptomatic toe. For comparison, MRI was performed on the second MTPJ in 5 asymptomatic volunteers. The clinical features and MRI findings were compared.

Results.—In the volunteers, the plantar plate abutted the plantar aspect of the metatarsal head and attached to the proximal phalangeal base next to the joint surface. It was smooth, with low-intensity signal on T1-weighted images and had a higher-intensity signal than adjacent tendons on gradient-echo scans.

Eight of the 13 patients had MRI studies showing plantar plate ruptures. A tear appeared as an area of increased signal intensity extending beyond the plate attachment on the proximal phalangeal base. Plate derangement areas had the same signal intensity as synovium and joint fluid, and all occurred next to the metatarsal head, close to the plate's distal attachment. These MRI findings were significantly associated with clinical findings of MTPJ instability and ipsilateral hallux valgus.

Conclusion.—Magnetic resonance imaging is useful in the noninvasive diagnosis of plantar plate rupture and is particularly effective with the use of a small receiver coil and 3-dimensional image acquisition techniques.

▶ This article nicely shows that small, field of view, high-resolution images can accurately show small anatomical structures.

M.K. Dalinka, M.D.

Shoulder

Glenoid Labrum: MR Imaging With Histologic Correlation

Loredo R, Longo C, Salonen D, et al (Univ of Texas, San Antonio; Toronto Hosp; Ohio State Univ, Columbus; et al)

Radiology 196:33–41, 1995 3–26

Background.—Foci of MR high-signal intensity within the glenoid labrum have been ascribed to tears, degeneration, and normal variation. No data are available directly correlating the imaging findings with the histopathologic appearances. Even microscopic studies of this structure have yielded mixed findings.

Objective.—Magnetic resonance imaging was performed in 10 fresh-frozen shoulder joints from cadavers aged 58 to 92. The architecture of the glenoid labrum and the articular cartilage were evaluated in the same specimens.

Methods.—The specimens were imaged transaxially before and after intra-articular gadolinium injection and then were frozen and sectioned transversely for histologic analysis. The imaging techniques included T1-weighted, proton density-weighted, and T2-weighted spin-echo; multiplanar gradient-recalled echo; 3-dimensional Fourier transform gradient-recalled echo (GRE); spoiled gradient-recalled echo; and T1-weighted, fat-suppressed sequences.

Histology.—The labra consisted of moderately dense bundles of poorly vascularized fibrous connective tissue. Most shoulders had a sublabral band of tissue staining differently from the fibrous tissue and hyaline cartilage but continuous with adjacent cartilage. On the capsular side a transitional fibrous segment was present between the wedge-shaped fibrous labrum and the dense connective tissue of the capsule.

Correlations.—Normal labral tissue was of low-signal intensity on all images. Triangular areas of intermediate signal intensity corresponded to both degenerative changes and fibrovascular tissue. Round areas of altered signal intensity correlated variably with labral ossification, degeneration, and intralabral fibrovascular tissue. All but 1 of the shoulders had a complete or incomplete sublabral band of intermediate signal intensity that correlated with the transitional zone of fibrocartilage. Cartilage defects of varying extent were present in all shoulders.

Conclusion.—Altered signal intensity within the glenoid labrum may represent a variety of histopathologic processes. A sublabral band of uniformly increased signal intensity that is not associated with a blunted or frayed labrum is a normal finding.

► This is a nice study derived from a small number of cadavers in elderly patients but it is very well done.

M.K. Dalinka, M.D.

Acrominal Arch Shape: Assessment With MR Imaging

Peh WCG, Farmer THR, Totty WG (Washington Univ, St Louis)

Radiology 195:501–505, 1995 3–27

Background.—Neer[1] proposed that shoulder impingement syndrome results from pressure exerted by the curved undersurface of the acromion on the supraspinatus tendon and suggested that anterior acromioplasty be considered to widen the space and relieve symptoms. Subsequent observations associated an increased curvature of the undersurface of the acromial arch with rotator cuff disease.

Objective.—Parasagittal images through the acromion on routine MR study of the rotator cuff were compared with supraspinatus outlet view radiographs to see whether similar classification data could be obtained.

Methods.—Supraspinatus outlet-view radiographs were taken of a dried scapula in neutral position, as well as varying degrees of craniocaudal and anteroposterior angulation. Acromial shape was classified as flat (type 1), curved (type 2), or hooked (type 3), as demonstrated in Figure 3. Magnetic resonance imaging was performed in 39 patients with shoulder pain who were suspected on clinical grounds of having rotator cuff disease. Outlet

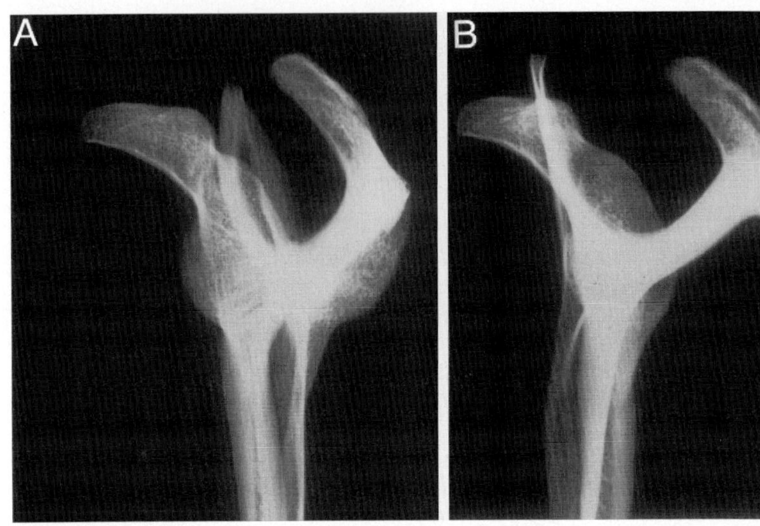

FIGURE 3.—Differnt appearances of the same dried scapular specimen with variation in angulation of the radiographic tube. **A,** image obtained at 5-degree anterior angulation without craniocaudal angulation. The acromion is flat, consistent with type 1 shape and type A thickness. **B,** image obtained at 5-degree posterior angulation without craniocaudal angulation. The acromion appears thicker than in **A** and is classified as type B. (Courtesy of Peh WCG, Farmer THR, Totty WGL: Acrominal arch shape: Assessment with MR imaging. *Radiology* 195:501–505, 1995: Radiological Society of North America.)

view radiographs also were available. In addition, MR images were acquired of 41 asymptomatic shoulders in healthy subjects.

Findings.—The apparent acromial shape and thickness varied in normal individuals depending on the particular MR section examined (Fig 4). Nearly 80% of control subjects exhibited a dependence of acromial shape with section position. A majority of symptomatic shoulders had a type 1 or type 2 acromial shape no more than 12 mm thick. The MR and radiographic findings correlated directly in only 14 of the 39 symptomatic shoulders. The shape of the arch correlated significantly with the appearance of the supraspinatus tendon on radiography but not on MRI.

Conclusion.—Supraspinatus outlet view radiography cannot at present be replaced by MRI for the purpose of detecting rotator cuff abnormality.

Reference

1. Neer CS II: Anterior acromioplasty for the chronic impingement syndrome in the shoulder: A preliminary report. *J Bone Joint Surg (Am)* 54A:41–50, 1972.

► The outline was incomplete. Not only was there a change in the apparent acrominal shape on MRI, but it also changed with respect to craniocaudal and anterior and posterior tube angulation.

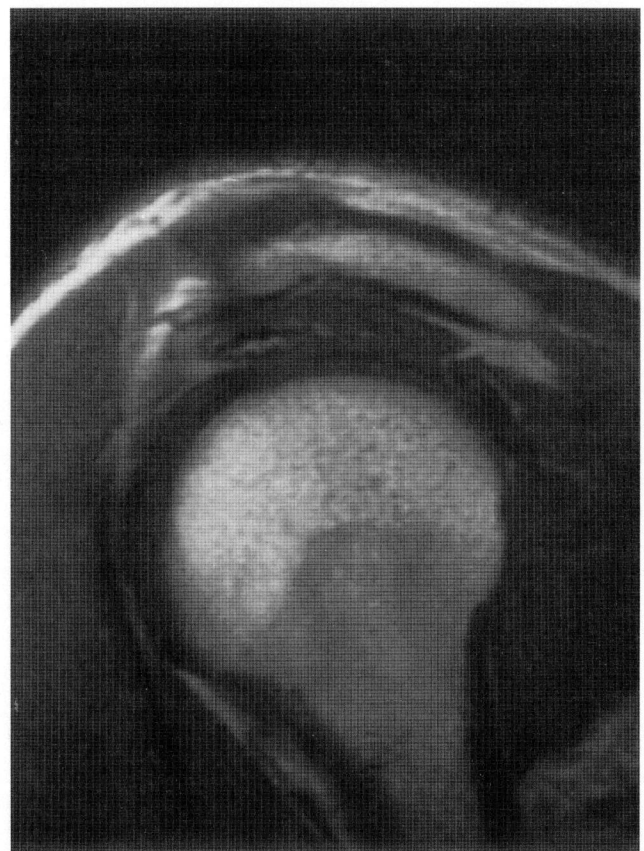

FIGURE 4.—Variation of shape and thickness of the acromion on oblique sagittal MR image (recovery time 500 msec/echo time 18 msec) of the same 22-year-old healthy man as in Figure 3. **B,** medial image demonstrates a hooked anterior end (type 3) and decreased thickness (type B). (Courtesy of Peh WCG, Farmer THR, Totty WGL: Acrominal arch shape: Assessment with MR imaging. *Radiology* 195:501–505, 1995; Radiological Society of North America.)

As opposed to what Bigliani reported (i.e., an increase of rotator cuff tears with type 3 acromions), the abnormalities occurred more frequently in patients with type 1 and 2 acromions. The outline of this paper should be modified.

M.K. Dalinka, M.D.

US Depiction of Partial-Thickness Tear of the Rotator Cuff

van Holsbeeck MT, Kolowich PA, Eyler WR, et al (Henry Ford Hosp, Detroit)
Radiology 197:443–446, 1995 3–28

Introduction.—Although ultrasound (US) has been used for the detection of complete rotator cuff tears for several years, different institutions have differing success rates. Part of the problem may be that it takes a long time to master the technique, though some researchers have achieved diagnostic sensitivities and specificities exceeding 90%. Partial rotator cuff tears are difficult to diagnose, which is 1 reason why few surgeons operate on patients with partial-thickness tears. Data from a previous study of rotator cuff abnormalities were used to evaluated sonographic criteria for the diagnosis of partial-thickness tears.

Methods.—Ultrasound was performed using a 7.5-MHz linear-array transducer in 52 patients with shoulder pain. Criteria for partial-thickness tears were a mixed hyperechoic and hypoechoic focus in the crucial zone of the supraspinatus tendon and a hypoechoic lesion seen in 2 orthogonal planes with articular or bursal extension.

Results.—The US results indicated partial-thickness tears in 17 lesions, 14 of which were confirmed at arthroscopy. There were 3 false positive results (all lesions that were predominantly hypoechoic in appearance) and 1 false negative result in a patient with a very small tear. Ultrasound had a diagnostic sensitivity of 93% and a specificity of 94% in detecting partial-thickness tears; positive predictive value was 82%, and negative predictive value was 98%. Twelve of the 14 patients had associated soft-tissue and bony abnormalities. All of the partial tears were in the supraspinatus tendon, and all but 2 were on the articular side of the tendon.

Conclusion.—Ultrasound is a potentially efficient technique for the detection of partial-thickness tears of the rotator cuff. The authors' hospital now uses US instead of MRI to evaluate the rotator cuff. Tendon scanning is best performed with electronically focused, high-frequency, linear-array transducers.

▶ The senior author is an outstanding musculoskeletal ultrostenographer, and this paper shows just how good this operator-dependent method of diagnosis can be. The reader is also referred to the paper by Farin and Jaroma.[1]

M.K. Dalinka, M.D.

Reference

1. Farin PU, Jaroma H: Acute traumatic tears of the rotator cuff: Value of sonography. *Radiology* 197:269–273, 1995.

Elbow

Ulnar Collateral Ligament Injury in the Throwing Athlete: Evaluation With Saline-Enhanced MR Arthrography

Schwartz ML, Al-Zahrani S, Morwessel RM, et al (Healthsouth Med Ctr, Birmingham, Ala; American Sports Medicine Inst, Birmingham, Ala; Univ of Virginia, Charlottesville; et al)
Radiology 197:297–299, 1995 3–29

Background.—Injuries to the ulnar collateral ligament (UCL) are common in athletes who throw. Lesions of the UCL are ususally diagnosed by history, physical examination, and imaging studies. However, sometimes no imaging study can depict the pathologic condition, so surgery is needed to demonstrate the abnormality. A saline-enhanced technique of MR arthrography was evaluated for its ability to demonstrate UCL abnormalities in throwing athletes.

Methods.—The study included 40 college- and professional-level throwing athletes. All had suspected UCL tears, based on the clinical findings of medial joint pain and opening of the medial joint space. An MR arthrographic technique was performed in which saline solution was injected into the elbow before imaging. Complete UCL tears were signaled by the presence of ligament discontinuity and extravasation of saline solution into the medial soft tissues. In partial tears, a small amount of saline solution extended past the distal attachment of the UCL without gross extravasation. The results were compared with the surgical findings in each patient.

Results.—The UCL was normal at MR arthrography and at surgery in 14 patients. Of the 26 patients who had UCL tears confirmed at surgery, all but 2 had positive findings on saline-enhanced MR arthrography. The imaging procedure correctly identified 18 of 19 complete and 6 of 7 partial UCL tears. Sensitivity was 92% for all UCL tears, 86% for partial tears, and 95% for complete tears.

Conclusion.—Saline-enhanced MR arthrography of the elbow is a useful technique for the depiction of UCL lesions in throwing athletes. The technique is especially valuable because it can demonstrate not only complete but also partial UCL tears. The ability to detect subtle UCL abnormalities at an early stage may enable the injured athlete to return to competition sooner.

▶ The authors obviously have considerable experience in the evaluation of this uncommon lesion. This paper will be helpful for those with experience in performing high-quality MRI of the elbow but is difficult to recommend to the novice.

M.K. Dalinka, M.D.

Lateral Epicondylitis: Correlation of MR Imaging, Surgical, and Histopathologic Findings

Potter HG, Hannafin JA, Morwessel RM, et al (Hosp for Special Surgery, New York)

Radiology 196:43–46, 1995 3–30

Purpose.—Lateral epicondylitis, or tennis elbow, is usually diagnosed clinically by physical examination and treated by conservative means. However, patients who fail to respond to conservative management may need further evaluation to identify the site of tendon injury and rule out frank rupture. The utility of MRI in the assessment of chronic refractory lateral epicondylitis was evaluated.

Patients.—Thirty-three patients with chronic lateral epicondylitis who had failed to respond to trials of conservative management were imaged with a gradient-recalled echo (GRE) MRI technique and axial and sagittal fast spin-echo sequences. Magnetic resonance images were evaluated for changes in intratendinous signal intensity and for morphologic alteration in tendon orientation. Twenty patients subsequently underwent surgical débridement with or without tendon repair. Three of them had elbow arthroscopy before undergoing open surgery. Surgical and histopathologic findings were compared with those from preoperative MRI.

Results.—Ten of the 20 operated patients had abnormal separation of the radial collateral ligament and extensor carpi radialis brevis tendon, which had been interpreted before operation as granulation tissue and inflammatory response. Tendon morphology was most easily seen on coronal GRE images. Frank ruptures of the extensor brevis origin and complete-thickness tears were seen on the scans of 7 patients. All 7 cases of frank tendon rupture were confirmed at operation.

Conclusion.—Magnetic resonance imaging to further investigate chronic lateral epicondylitis that does not respond to conservative management is highly recommended, because the findings on MR images correlate well with surgical and histologic findings.

▶ The authors show the value of MRI in this entity. Note that despite the term epicondylitis, there was no histopathologic evidence of either acute or chronic inflammation in any of the specimen examined. Mucoid degeneration and neovascularization were responsible for the long T2- and T2-weighted relaxation. We have found that fat-saturated, fast spin-echo or stir images are extremely sensitive in picking up these areas of high signal rather than the T2-weighted images used by the author.

M.K. Dalinka, M.D.

Hand and Wrists

The Natural History of Scaphoid Non-Union: Radiographical and Clinical Analysis in 102 Cases

Inoue G, Sakuma M (Nagoya Univ, Japan)

Arch Orthop Trauma Surg 115:1–4, 1996 3–31

Background.—Although earlier studies have reported few symptoms and limited disability in patients with scaphoid nonunion, recent reports suggest that this condition is associated with progressive osteoarthritis and the occurrence of symptoms over time. The patterns and sequence of degenerative arthritis of the wrist with symptomatic scaphoid nonunion were evaluated, and the clinical course of these wrists were documented.

Patients and Findings.—One hundred two symptomatic patients with 104 scaphoid nonunions of no less than 12-months duration were included in this retrospective radiographic and clinical analysis. At 5, 5–9, and 10 years duration or more, osteoarthritis was noted in 22%, 75%, and

100% of the nonunions, respectively. Overall incidence of osteoarthritis in the wrist was 55%. Osteoarthritic changes were initially noted at the scaphoid-radial styloid joint. These changes were characterized by radial styloid posting and/or dorsal radioscaphiod osteophyte formation. In patients with nonunion of 5 years duration or longer, the next radiographic irregularity observed was radioscaphiod joint narrowing. This subsequently progressed to narrowing of the midcarpal joint. A significant association between osteoarthritis at the scaphoid-radial styloid joint and dorsiflexed intercalated segment instability (DISI) deformity was observed. The overall incidence of DISI deformity of the wrist was 56%. The frequency of the DISI pattern paralleled increasing duration of nonunion.

Radiographic evidence of loss of trabeculation, sclerotic and cystic changes, and deformity of the proximal fragment were considered to be indicative of a true avascular necrosis; the relative radiodensity of the proximal fragment was not used to make this diagnosis. Avascular necrosis of the proximal fragment was observed in 8 nonunions in the proximal third, and 8 nonunions in the middle third of the scaphoid. The incidence of avascular necrosis of the proximal fragment increased with time, particularly in nonunions with greater than 20 years' duration.

Pain symptoms were not correlated with either arthritis severity or duration of nonunion. A good correlation between duration of nonunion and deceased grip strength or wrist motion was observed, however.

Conclusion.—Patients with symptomatic nonunion of the scaphoid are significantly likely to experience a predictable progression to osteoarthritis, with radiographic and clinical changes becoming worse over time.

▶ The authors have presented a long-term follow-up study of patients with ununited scaphoid fractures and identified the patterns and sequence of degenerative arthritis of the wrist with symptomatic nonunions. The paper is filled with interesting demographic data concerning ischemic necrosis, osteoarthritis, and collapse of the wrist.

M.K. Dalinka, M.D.

Comparison of the Findings of Triple-Injection Cinearthrography of the Wrist With Those of Arthroscopy

Weiss A-PC, Akelman E, Lambiase R (Brown Univ, Providence, RI)

J Bone Joint Surg (Am) 78A:348–356, 1996 3–32

Objective.—A prospective study was performed to determine the sensitivity, specificity, and accuracy of triple-injection cinearthrography of the wrist in detecting full-thickness tears of the scapholunate ligament, lunotriquetral ligament, and triangular fibrocartilage. Findings were compared with those obtained at subsequent arthroscopy of the wrist.

Patients and Methods.—Fifty consecutive patients (average age 36) were included in the study. All patients noted pain in the wrist with activities involving use of the wrist or with generalized motion of the wrist, and 19 also noted pain while at rest. The dominant hand was involved in 33 patients. Average symptom duration was 8 months. Arthrograms of the wrist were performed by the same radiologist using a standard triple-injection cinearthrogram protocol. Pressurized injections of 60% nonionic contrast medium were delivered to the radiocarpal, midcarpal, and distal radioulnar joints in a sequential fashion, after which exercise, followed by standard radiographic and cinefluorographic examinations, were performed. Before patients were injected, a static carpal series that included anteroposterior and lateral radiographs, radiographs with the wrist in radial and ulnar deviation, and an anteroposterior radiograph with the hand held in a grip were obtained. During the studies, fluoroscopic observation with cine-recording was used to evaluate dynamic carpal motion. All patients initially had 2.5 to 4.6 mL of contrast medium injected into the radiocarpal joint. Motion was evaluated with cinefluorography before and after at least 2 minutes of wrist exercise, after which a second complete series of 5 radiographs of the wrist was obtained. The contrast medium injected into the radiocarpal joint was given adequate time to disperse, after which 2 to 4 mL of contrast medium was injected into the midcarpal joints and 1 to 2 mL was injected into the distal radioulnar joints. Cinefluorographic assessment and static anteroposterior and lateral radiography were carried out after each injection. Subsequent arthroscopic evaluations of the wrist using the 3-portal technique were completed by 2 hand surgeons with previous knowledge of the arthrographic findings. Calculations of sensitivity, specificity, and accuracy of triple-injection cinearthrography were made according to whether all of the lesions that were seen on arthroscopy were detected during arthrographic examination as well.

Results.—Arthrography demonstrated 18 normal wrists, a single lesion in 21, and multiple lesions in 11 wrists. Tears of the scapholunate ligament were observed in 12 wrists, of the lunotriquetral ligament in 15, and of the triangular fibrocartilage in 18. On arthroscopic evaluation, 6 wrists were normal, a single lesion was noted in 25, and multiple lesions were seen in 19 wrists. Tears of the scapholunate ligament were observed in 22 wrists, of the lunotriquetral ligament in 15, and of the triangular fibrocartilage in 30.

The sensitivity, specificity, and accuracy of triple-injection cinearthrography in identifying full-thickness tears of the scapholunate ligament, lunotriquetral ligament and triangular fibrocartilage as a group were 56%, 83%, and 60%, respectively. A sensitivity of 60% and a specificity of 100% also were noted for both tears of the scapholunate ligament and the triangular fibrocartilage, and a 93% sensitivity and 97% specificity were found for tears of the lunotriquetral ligament. Accuracy of the arthrogram was 84% for tears of the scapholunate ligament, 76% for tears of the triangular fibrocartilage, and 96% for tears of the lunotriquetral ligament.

Conclusion.—In patients undergoing arthrography of the wrist, normal findings do not exclude the possibility of internal wrist derangement; thus, patients with negative arthrograms but persistent pain in the wrist should undergo arthroscopic evaluation. Primary arthroscopy also may be beneficial in patients with chronic wrist pain who have not undergone diagnostic imaging. The efficacy of this strategy remains to be determined, however.

► The authors studied 50 patients with both arthroscopy and MRI of the wrist and found arthroscopic abnormalities in 44 of these patients. Prior studies have discussed the lack of correlation between wrist pain and tears on arthrography, and, in addition, the frequency of bilateral tears in patients with a single painful wrist has been addressed by others but not in this paper.

The midcarpal joint injection consisted of 2 to 4 mL of contrast medium, which may not be sufficient. It is important that this injection be done with maximal distention, and although the authors reported distention or pain in the radiocarpal joint, they did not make this comment when they discussed the midcarpal joint.

In most centers, MRI is replacing arthrography in the evaluation of these cases. Of course, the major factor is the long-term patient outcome, and this has not been addressed. Please note that the arthroscopic charge was for the arthroscopic examination alone and did not include the other examination costs (operating room, anesthesia, etc.).

M.K. Dalinka, M.D

Evaluating Dorsal Wrist Pain: MRI Diagnosis of Occult Dorsal Wrist Ganglion

Vo P, Wright T, Hayden F, et al (Univ of Florida, Gainesville)

J Hand Surg (Am) 20A:667–670, 1995 3–33

Background.—Chronic wrist pain poses a difficult diagnostic and therapeutic challenge. Recalcitrant dorsal wrist pain has traditionally been evaluated surgically, although surgical exploration may fail to provide a specific diagnosis. Magnetic resonance imaging may offer an alternative and noninvasive means of evaluating patients with difficult to diagnose dorsal wrist pain. The efficacy of high-resolution MRI in evaluating patients with dorsal wrist pain was therefore investigated.

Patients and Methods.—Fourteen patients with chronic dorsal wrist pain of undetermined origin were included. In all patients, findings at physical and radiographic examination were negative, and no palpable masses were noted. The diagnosis of occult dorsal wrist ganglion was suspected, and MRI evaluation of the scapholunate region was carried out. Findings obtained at MRI were evaluated by an orthopedic radiologist and correlated with the patients' clinical or surgical results.

Results.—Ten of the 14 wrist MRIs were considered positive for occult dorsal wrist ganglion. The average greatest diameter of these lesions was 4.7 mm on T2-weighted images. Diagnoses were verified at surgery in 7 of the 10 patients and at follow-up evaluation in another patient, whose ganglion had subsequently become enlarged and clinically palpable. The remaining 2 patients underwent nonoperative treatment, and their MRI diagnoses were not verified by surgical or clinical evaluation. The positive predictive value of MRI among patients undergoing surgery was 100%.

Conclusion.—Properly formatted high-resolution MRI can effectively diagnose occult dorsal wrist ganglion among patients with chronic dorsal wrist pain of unknown etiology. This noninvasive modality also can be used to identify other lesions than may cause dorsal wrist pain in the scapholunate region, thereby reducing the need for and frequency of surgical exploration.

► This is another diagnosis that was frequently missed before the advent of MRI. Because these lesions are relatively common, care must be taken to exclude other causes of dorsal wrist pain before surgical treatment.

M.K. Dalinka, M.D.

Tumors

Chondrosarcoma: A Review

Springfield DS, Gebhardt MC, McGuire MH (Massachusetts Gen Hosp, Boston; Creighton Univ, Omaha, Neb)

J Bone Joint Surg Am 78A:141–149, 1996 3–34

Introduction.—Chondrosarcoma is a malignancy that arises from cartilage-producing cells. The tumors may be classified in a number of ways, which can be used to predict the risk of metastasis. The classification, clinical manifestation, and management of chondrosarcoma were reviewed.

Classification.—Histologic appearance determines the grade of the tumor. The tumors are graded 1 through 3, with 3 being the most likely to metastasize. A dedifferentiated chondrosarcoma, which has an even higher chance of metastasizing than the grade 3 chondrosarcoma, is surrounded by hyaline-cartilage matrix. This tumor has areas of malignant spindle cells different from recognizable cartilaginous cells and adjacent areas of neoplastic chrondrocytes. Premalignant chondrosarcomas also exist and may have atypical cellular appearance. Although there is no way to measure their risk of metastasizing, they have locally aggressive clinical behavior and may progress into chrondrosarcomas.

Chondrosarcoma may also be classified into primary (arising de novo) or secondary (arising from a benign cartilage lesion) types. Secondary chondrosarcomas are much less likely to metastasize than primary chondrosarcomas. Chrondrosarcomas can also be subdivided by their location, with central chondrosarcomas arising from within the medullary canal and peripheral chondrosarcomas arising from the bone surface.

Clinical Manifestation.—Chondrosarcomas affect predominantly middle-aged men. They can appear in any bone but are most common in the pelvis and the proximal femur. There is associated progressive but not debilitating pain, which may disrupt sleep and does not diminish with rest.

Physical abnormalities are typically subtle. The lesion is generally revealed on plain radiographs; it appears as a combination of bone destruction and a circumferential periosteal reaction. Typically there is irregular cortical thinning, and CT reveals intralesional calcifications.

Management.—A biopsy can confirm the clinical diagnosis or clarify a less obvious clinical picture. All chondrosarcomas should ideally be resected with wide margins. Magnetic resonance imaging can provide accurate preoperative information of the extent of disease. Irradiation has limited usefulness, usually only in situations where a wide operative margin cannot be obtained, as in the spine. Chemotherapy is not curative.

Conclusion.—Chondrosarcoma can be classified in several ways and has a varying prognosis. It can generally be recognized radiographically. Surgery is the mainstay of treatment.

▶ This paper is an excellent review of chondrosarcoma. It describes the classificiation of chondrosarcoma, including some of the less well-known types and discusses the treatment of the various subtypes of this lesion. The interested reader is referred to the paper on dedifferentiated chondrosarcoma by Mercuri et al. (Abstract 3–35) and the paper by Bauer et al.[1]

M.K. Dalinka, M.D.

Reference

1. Bauer HC, Brosjo O, Kriecbergs A, et al: Low risk of recurrence of enchondroma and low-grade chondrosarcoma in extremities. 80 patients followed for 2–25 years. *Acta Orthop Scand* 66:283–288, 1995.

Dedifferentiated Chondrosarcoma

Mercuri M, Picci P, Campanacci L, et al (Istituto Ortopedico Rizzoli, Bologna, Italy)

Skeletal Radiol 24:409–416, 1995 3–35

Introduction.—In 1971, Dahlin and Beabout described dedifferentiated chondrosarcoma (DDC) as "a high-grade non-cartilaginous sarcoma which arises within a pre-existing low-grade chondrosarcoma." A new neoplastic clone develops in this tumor that does not have the histologic characteristics of a cartilage tumor. The dedifferentiated component is more aggressive and can progress rapidly and obscure or eventually destroy the original cartilaginous tumor. Dedifferentiated chondrosarcomas may develop from the benign, necrotic, and calcified tissue of a latent chondroma.

This tumor occurs more frequently in older men. The most common tumor sites are the pelvis, femur, and proximal humerus. The typical clinical history is long-standing, mild pain that increases suddenly and rapidly. A concurrent soft-tissue mass or a pathologic fracture may be

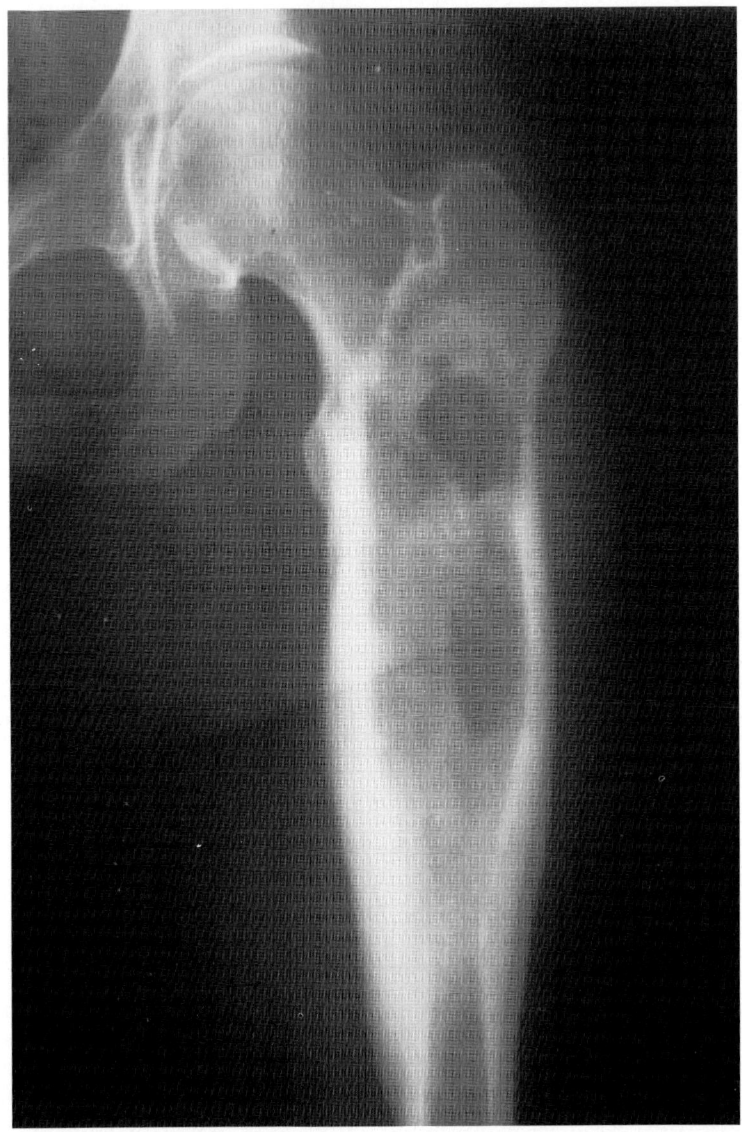

FIGURE 3.—Imaging of central dedifferentiated chondrosarcoma type 1. Radiograph of a dedifferentiated central chondrosarcoma in a 64-year-old woman. Benign calcified chondroma, low-grade central chondrosarcoma, and dedifferentiation can be seen. (Courtesy of Mercuri M, Picci P, Campanacci L, et al: Dedifferentiated chondrosarcoma. *Skeletal Radiol* 24:409–416, 1995.)

present. Medical records, histologic slides, and original imaging films of 74 patients with DDC were reviewed retrospectively.

Methods.—Criteria for inclusion included 1, presence of a well-differentiated cartilaginous tumor that was benign or low-grade malignant

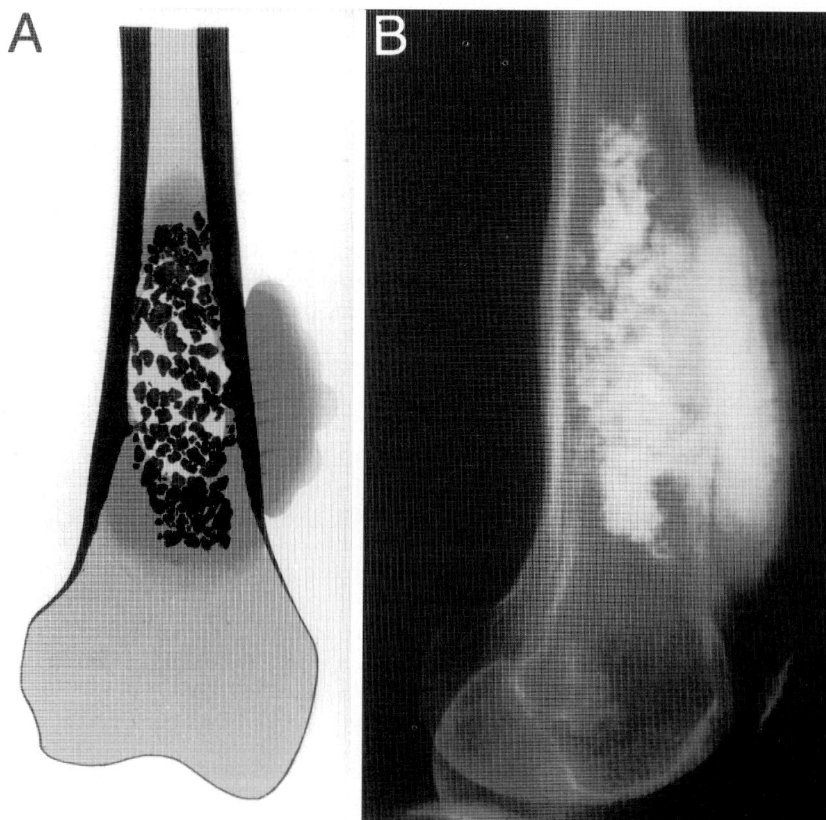

FIGURE 4.—Imaging of central dedifferentiated chondrosarcoma type 2. **A**, central chondrosarcoma dedifferentiated into grade 4 osteosarcoma. Superimposed onto a typical calcified chondroma or low-grade chondrosarcoma is osteosclerosis typical of osteosarcoma. **B**, a low-grade (grade 1) central chondrosarcoma dedifferentiated into grade 4 osteosarcoma in a 66-year-old woman, who had had pain for 6 months and swelling for 4 months. Diagnosis is possible with reasonable accuracy on the basis of imaging. (Courtesy of Mercuri M, Picci P, Campanacci L, et al: Dedifferentiated chondrosarcoma. *Skeletal Radiol* 24:409–416, 1995.)

(grades 1, 2),; 2, presence of a noncartilaginous high-grade sarcoma; 3, evidence of a clear-cut separation front between the 2 without any histologic transitional features.

Results.—The average age of 39 male and 35 female patients was 56. The most common tumor location was the femur, and the second most common location was the pelvis. The most common presenting symptom was pain in 85% of patients. There was a soft-tissue mass present in 29% of patients. Thirty-one percent of patients had a pathologic fracture. Onset of symptoms to diagnosis ranged from 1 month to 2 years in all except 2 patients. These patients experienced pain for 4 and 7 years before biopsy.

Imaging features were identical to those of a conventional sarcoma in some patients when the noncartilaginous high-grade component was small (Fig 3). In adult patients, the imaging studies may be suggestive of an osteolytic malignancy when the noncartilaginous component is predominant. In the majority of patients, imaging features provided evidence of both components of the dedifferentiated chondrosarcoma (Fig 4). The dedifferentiated component may be suspected in the presence of 1, a permeative osteolysis that rapidly destroys both previous cartilaginous lesion and bone; 2, a soft-tissue mass; 3, a pathologic fracture; and 4, angiographic evidence of a hypervascular tumor component.

Histologically tumors were grade 0 in 10 patients with enchondroma and grade 1 in 15, grade 2 in 26, and grade 3 in 13 patients with chondrosarcoma. The noncartilaginous component was malignant histiocytoma in 38 patients, osteosarcoma in 23 patients, fibrosarcoma in 2 patients, and angiosarcoma in 1.

Sixty of 74 patients underwent either local resection or amputation with a goal of cure. Surgical margins were related to the incidence of local recurrence. The local recurrence rate was 36% (22 patients). There were no local recurrences in 6 patients with radical margins. Recurrence was 29% (11/34) for patients with wide radical margins and (69%) (11/16) for patients with inadequate margins. The noncartilaginous component histologic pattern did not correlate with the local recurrence rate. Recurrence was 33% in patients with malignant fibrous histiocytoma and 30% in patients with osteosarcoma.

Conclusion.—It is possible that the entire histologic spectrum of benign chondroma, chondrosarcoma grades 1, 2, and 3, and the anaplastic noncartilaginous component can be represented in the transformation from chondroma to DDC. The predominant noncartilaginous component was malignant fibrous histocytoma or osteosarcoma. It was typically grade 4. A high incidence of skip metastases was likely because of the high incidence of local recurrence after wide resection of wide amputation. The overall 5-year survival rate of this cohort was 13%. Adjuvant chemotherapy and radiation therapy were not efficacious for these patients. Within the context of central cartilaginous tumors, DDC is not an infrequent lesion. It is rare in association with exostoses. The diagnosis of DDC can be made or suspected on the basis of imaging characteristics. However, histologic examination of the entire tumor is needed before confirmation of diagnosis of DDC.

Reference

1. Dahlin DC, Beabout JW: Dedifferentiation of low-grade chondrosarcomas. *Cancer* 28:461–466, 1971.

► This is a very large series of cases of this relatively uncommon tumor. The knowledge of this entity will enable us to come up with the correct diagnosis when we are evaluating routine radiographs.

M.K. Dalinka, M.D.

Parosteal Osteoma of Bones Other Than of the Skull and Face

Bertoni F, Unni KK, Beabout JW, et al (Mayo Clinic and Mayo Found, Rochester, Minn)

Cancer 75:2466–2473, 1995 3–36

Objective.—Osteomas rarely occur on any bone other than those of the skull and face. The clinical, radiographic, and histologic findings of a series of parosteal osteomas of other bones were reported.

Patients.—The experience included 14 patients with parosteal osteomas on bones other than those of the skull and face. Mean age of 8 men and 6 women was 45. Thirteen of the tumors occurred in long bones, and 1 occurred in the clavicle. In 7 patients, the mass had been present for a long time (18 months–31 years). Three patients were asymptomatic; the rest had symptoms of pain, a mass, or both. In their greatest dimension, the lesions ranged from 2.5 to 20 cm. On histologic examination, the lesions blended with the cortex without infiltrating the medullary cavity. They were made up of dense sclerotic lamellar bone with haversian systems, resembling the architecture of normal cortical bone. No spindle cell proliferations were found.

Treatment and Outcomes.—Resection was performed in 9 patients, biopsy in 4, and debulking in 1. Of the 11 patients for whom follow-up was available, none had recurrence or metastases at 1 to 23 years' follow-up.

Conclusion.—Parosteal osteoma of bones other than the skull and face is a very rare tumor that must be differentiated from the low-grade malignancy parosteal osteosarcoma. Parosteal osteoma may be diagnosed based on the absence of radiolucent areas on radiographs (Fig 3) and the absence of spindle cells on histologic sections. With close follow-up, these patients can avoid extensive, potentially debilitating treatment.

► This is a relatively large series concerning a very uncommon tumor. Judging by the illustrations, differentiating this benign entity from parosteal osteosarcoma would have to be performed by the pathologist because it is not possible to verify it by x-ray film.

M.K. Dalinka, M.D.

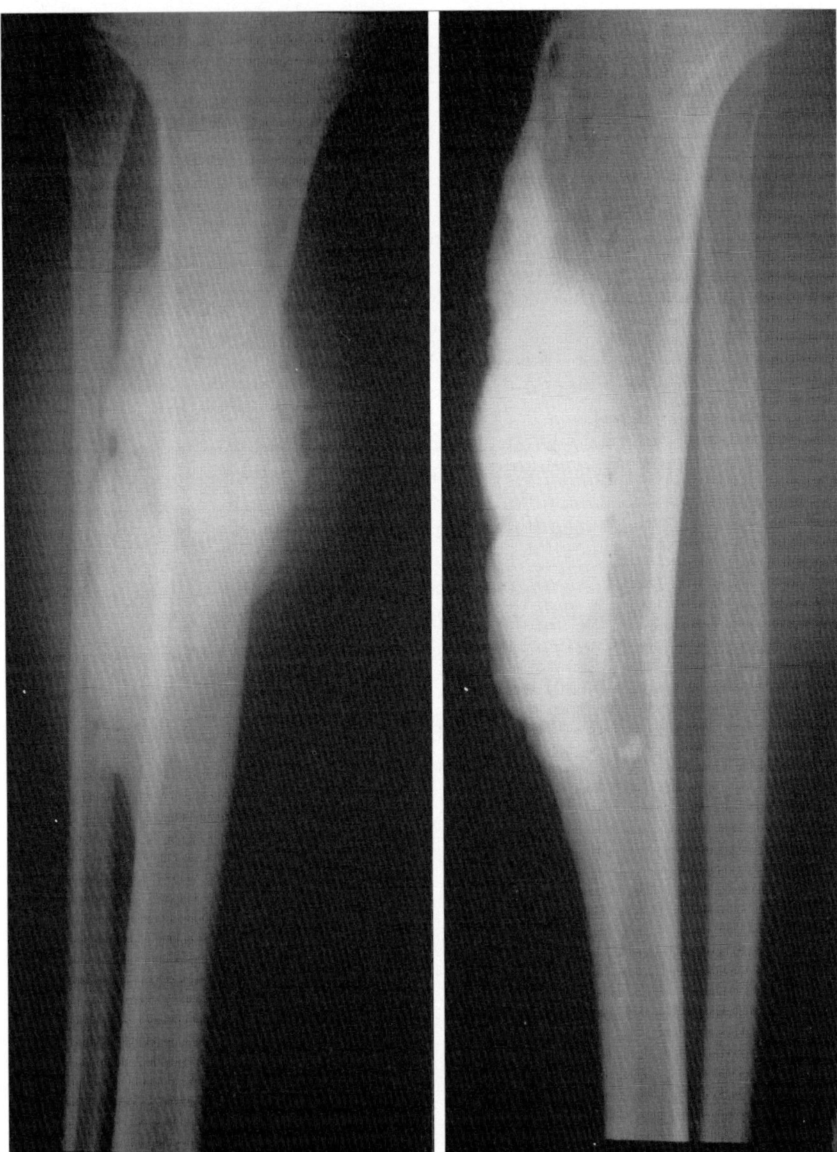

FIGURE 3.—Anteroposterior (**Left**) and lateral (**Right**) radiographs of tibia showing large metadiaphyseal osteoma involving medial, lateral, and anterior cortex and consisting of solid dense bone. The tubulation of the tibia is normal. A small area of medullary sclerosis distally appears unrelated to the osteoma. (Bertoni F, Unni KK, Beabout JW, et al: Parosteal osteoma of bones other than of the skull and face. *Cancer* 75:2466–2473, 1995; Copyright © 1995 American Cancer Society. Reprinted by permission of Wiley-Liss, Inc, a subsidiary of John Wiley & Sons, Inc.)

Musculoskeletal Neoplasm: Perineoplastic Edema Versus Tumor on Dynamic Postcontrast MR Images With Spatial Mapping of Instantaneous Enhancement Rates

Lang P, Honda G, Roberts T, et al (Univ of California, San Francisco)
Radiology 197:831–839, 1995 3–37

Introduction.—Patients undergoing limb-sparing procedures need accurate presurgical assessment of intraosseous and extraosseous extent of tumor. Conventional diagnostic testing has been limited in the delineation of the intraosseous, and particularly extraosseous, extent of tumor. Current MRI techniques, even those using paramagnetic contrast media, may also be limited in the evaluation of the extraosseous tumor margins. The ill-defined interface between the tumor and surrounding soft tissue may make it difficult to differentiate between extraosseous tumor and perineoplastic edema. Fourteen patients with primary neoplasms of the musculoskeletal system underwent sequential MRI to evaluate the ability of this procedure to differentiate between extraosseous tumor and perineoplastic edema.

Methods.—The average age of 8 male and 6 female patients was 19. The tumors consisted of 6 osteosarcomas, 1 Ewing sarcoma, 3 primary lymphomas of bone, 1 synovial sarcoma, 1 plasmacytoma, 1 aneurysmal bone cyst, and 1 unicameral bone cyst. The MRI was performed the evening before biopsy. The surgeon marked the site of intended biopsy with a permanent marker. Sequential MRI was performed after bolus injection of gadopentetate dimeglumine. The initial rates of enhancement were calculated on a pixel-by-pixel basis. They were displayed in a computer-generated "slope image" in which signal intensity reflected pixel slope value. Close correlation between slope images and large matching wedge-shaped biopsy specimens was done.

Results.—Twelve of 14 patients with malignant neoplasms had extraosseous tumor components that were detected on histologic examination. There was no histologic evidence of extraosseous tumor spread in the 2 patients with benign lesions. In 11 patients, histologic examination revealed areas that consisted of edematous muscle without microscopic evidence of tumor infiltration. Slope images were used to evaluate 18 areas of interest in these patients. The areas containing neoplastic tissue and the areas composed of nonneoplastic edematous muscle both demonstrated high-signal intensity on T2-weighted images and on conventional T1-weighted postcontrast images in all 14 patients. These images could not be distinguished clearly with signal intensity or morphologic features. Viable extraosseous tumor and infiltrated muscle indicated rapid, marked contrast enhancement, and edematous muscle was characterized by slower contrast enhancement on dynamic postcontrast MR images. Normal marrow, muscle, and subcutaneous fat tissues displayed gradual or no contrast enhancement. Slope image findings were as follows: Viable extraosseous tumor and infiltrated muscle demonstrated high-signal intensity because of their rapid enhancement, and edematous muscle without tumor infiltration exhibited intermediate intensity. Compared with viable neoplastic tissues, normal tissues had consistently lower mean linear slope values. Significant differences in initial slopes were determined between neoplastic and nonneoplastic tissues. More important, there were significant differences between viable extraosseous tumor and edematous muscle, as well as between infiltrated muscle and edematous muscle.

Conclusion.—Significant differences were detected between neoplastic and nonneoplastic tissues in initial slope values. Clear differences were detected between viable extraosseous tumor and muscle that was infiltrated by tumor and nonneoplastic edematous muscle. Overlap in initial slope values of these tissues was observed between different patients but never within the same patient. With dynamic MRI, absolute values should not be determined to be indicative of certain tissues for all patients. Rather, neoplastic and nonneoplastic tissue values need to be differentiated for each patient. Because the margins of lesions are defined accurately and tumor is clearly distinct from perineoplastic edema, slope images may be useful in preoperative planning of limb-sparing surgery.

► The authors have performed a very careful study on a small number of patients. I look forward to seeing confirmation of their findings in a larger study.

M.K. Dalinka, M.D.

MR Imaging of Soft-Tissue Masses: Diagnostic Efficacy and Value of Distinguishing Between Benign and Malignant Lesions

Moulton JS, Blebea JS, Dunco DM, et al (Univ of Cincinnati, Ohio; Children's Hosp Med Ctr, Cincinnati, Ohio)

AJR 164:1191–1199, 1995 3–38

Objective.—Generally soft-tissue masses are diagnostically evaluated histologically. The use of MRI to distinguish between benign and malignant lesions and to determine the pathologic character is controversial. Results of a retrospective study evaluating the efficacy of MRI in predicting the pathologic diagnosis and differentiating between neoplastic and nonneoplastic soft-tissue masses were presented.

Methods.—Magnetic resonance examinations using a 1.5-tesla system using various pulse sequences were conducted on 225 soft-tissue masses (179 benign and 46 malignant) from 86 male and 136 female patients aged 1 month to 90 years. Tumors were categorized as group I if a specific benign histologic diagnoses was predicted, group II if lesions were likely to be benign but nonspecific, or group III if the masses were likely to be malignant but nonspecific. Evaluations were compared with pathological results.

Results.—One hundred lesions categorized as benign were shown to be benign by other methods. There was no feature that distinguished benign from malignant tumors. Ten malignant tumors were misdiagnosed as

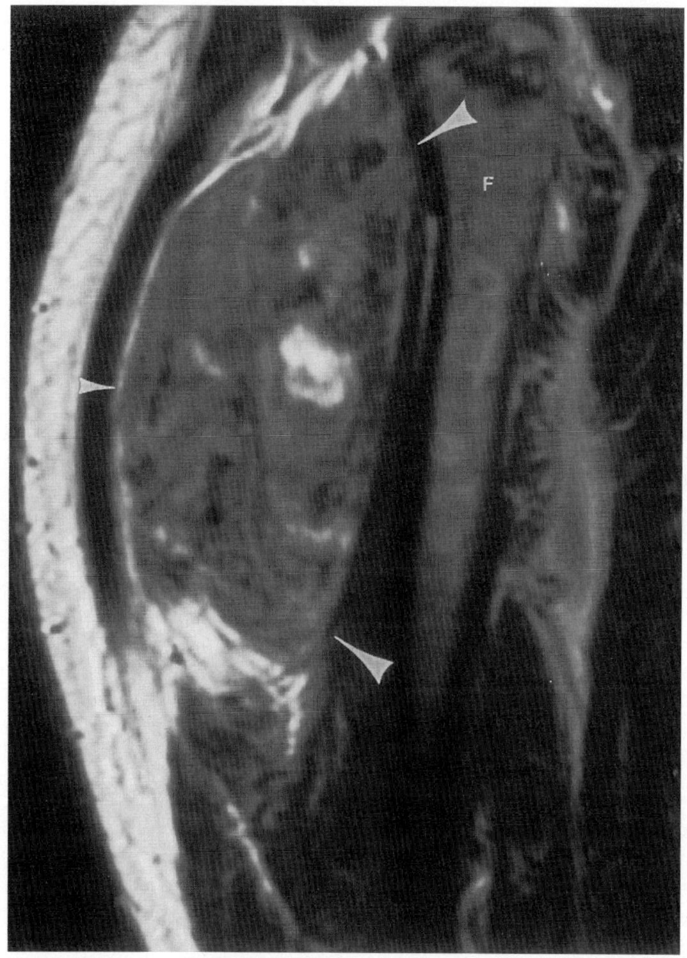

FIGURE 5.—Woman, 52, with a progressively enlarging mass in her thigh. Sagittal T2-weighted fast spin-echo (recovery time 4,000 msec/echo time 102 msec) MR image shows mass (*arrowheads*) to be partially poorly defined with markedly heterogeneous signal. Minimal low T2-weighted signal is present to suggest hemosiderin deposition. This was prospectively characterized as a probable malignant neoplasm (group III). Pathologic diagnosis was giant cell tumor of the tendon sheath. *Abbreviation: f*, proximal femur. (From Moulton JS, Blebea JS, Dunco DM, et al: MR imaging of soft-tissue masses: Diagnostic efficacy and value of distinguishing between benign and malignant lesions. *AJR* 164:1191–1199, 1995. Courtesy of Frank McWilliams, Cincinnati, Ohio.)

benign, and 19 benign tumors were misdiagnosed as malignant for a sensitivity of 78% and a specificity of 89%. The positive predictive value was 65%, and the negative predictive value was 94%.

Discussion.—Estimates of the ratio of benign to malignant tumors are as high as 100:1. Even though there is no MRI feature that consistently distinguished between neoplastic and nonneoplastic except for a homogeneous signal isointense with fat that is indicative of a benign lipoma, many benign lesions can be correctly diagnosed by MRI using a subjective approach that combines clinical and imaging data, characteristic homogenous T2-weighted signals, and location. Not all lesions will show characteristic features on imaging. (Fig 5).

In this study 44% of these characteristic lesions were correctly identified without biopsy. When these characteristic tumors were excluded, specificity fell to 76%, and sensitivity fell to 86%.

Conclusion.—Many soft-tissue masses can be diagnosed by MRI. Although most malignant tumors were identified by MRI, the technique was not able to stage the lesions. When the image is nonspecific, there is a significant chance that the tumor is malignant and a biopsy is indicated.

▶ This is a nice review of the subject. No mention is made, however, of the fact the histologic appearance (grade) of soft-tissue sarcomas is much more important prognostically than the specific diagnosis.

With the benign to malignant statistics quoted, a specificity of 68% and sensitivity of 86% are certainly not acceptable, because more than 90% of all soft-tissue tumors are benign. If the lesion is not characteristic, biopsy is mandatory.

M.K. Dalinka, M.D.

The Clinical Value of Prostate-Specific Antigen and Bone Scintigraphy in the Staging of Patients With Newly Diagnosed, Pathologically Proven Prostate Cancer

Rudoni M, Antonini G, Favro M, et al (Ospedale Maggiore, Novara, Italy)
Eur J Nucl Med 22:207–211, 1995 3–39

Objective.—Prostate-specific antigen (PSA) values are predictive of radionuclide bone scan results in prostate cancer patients who have had radical prostatectomies. Recently studies have shown that PSA values in patients with untreated prostate cancer can also predict bone scan results, thereby obviating bone scan staging in patients with low PSA values. These findings were confirmed in a retrospective study conducted to determine threshold negative predictive PSA values and to compare the bone scan predictive capability of PSA, prostatic acid phosphatase (PAP), and tumor grade (TG).

Methods.—Digital rectal examination (DREs), PSA concentration, and bone scan evaluation were conducted in 118 untreated prostate cancer patients (aged 50–90). Serum PAP concentrations were also measured in a subset of 79 patients.

Results.—Both PAP and PSA levels were significantly correlated with positive bone scan results. Fifty-four patients had a positive bone scan. No patients with a PSA level less than 10 ng/mL had a positive bone scan. A PSA value of 35 ng/mL on the receiver-operating characteristic curves separated normal from abnormal results and had a sensitivity of 83%, a specificity of 61%, and a negative predictive accuracy of 84% (Fig 2). Seven of 14 patients with PSA values between 10.1 and 20.0 ng/mL 7 of

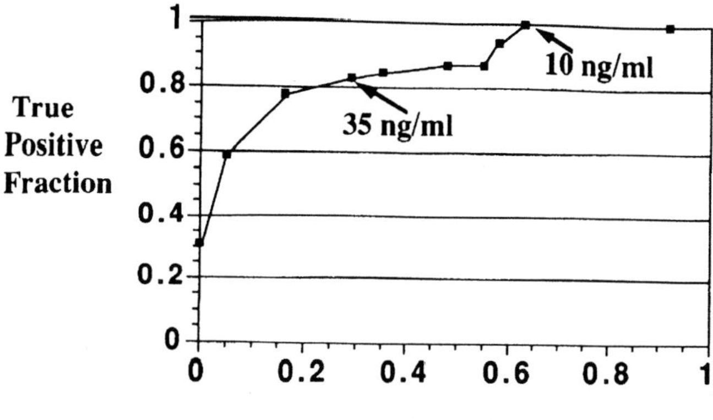

FIGURE 2.—Receiver-operating characteristic curve for serum prostate-specific antigen concentrations vs. bone scan results in 118 patients. (M Rudoni, Antonini G, Favro M, et al: The clinical value of prostate-specific antigen and bone scintigraphy in the staging of patients with newly diagnosed, pathologically proven prostate cancer. *Eur J Nucl Med* 22:207–211, 1995, copyright notice of Springer-Verlag.)

28 with PSA values between 20.1 and 50.0 ng/mL, 8 with PSA values between 50.1 and 100 ng/mL and 32 of 35 with PSA values greater than 100 ng/mL had a positive bone scan. A threshold PSA value of 20 ng/mL had a negative predictive value for a positive bone scan of 80%.

Conclusion.—These results indicate that patients with newly diagnosed prostate cancer and serum PSA concentrations of 10 ng/mL of less do not require bone scans for staging unless skeletal symptoms are present.

▶ Please note that the American College of Radiology appropriateness criteria published in 1995 came to the same conclusion and also discusses this issue with respect to other types of neoplasms.

M.K. Dalinka, M.D.

Bone Mineral Measurement

Anteroposterior Versus Lateral Bone Mineral Density of Spine Assessed by Dual X-ray Absorptiometry

Del Rio L, Pons F, Huguet M, et al (CETIR Centre Mèdic, Barcelona; Univ of Barcelona)

Eur J Nucl Med 22:407–412, 1995 3–40

Introduction.—Because lateral (LAT) dual-energy x-ray absorptiometry (DEXA) can allow the measurement of bone mineral density (BMD) in a predominantly trabecular area without posterior elements, it has been suggested that this projection may be more sensitive in the detection of vertebral bone loss than DEXA in the anteroposterior (AP) projection. The precision of LAT spine DEXA was evaluated in relation to standard BMD measurements, and its diagnostic sensitivity in detecting the loss of bone mass was assessed.

Methods.—Bone mineral density was measured in the lumbar spin and in 3 femoral sites with a DEXA absorptiometer, using AP and LAT projections. Measurement precision was evaluated by comparing the AP and LAT spine BMD 10 times within 1 month in 10 healthy volunteers and 5 osteoporotic women. Diagnostic sensitivity was prospectively evaluated by comparing the mean BMD values in 185 osteoporotic patients with vertebral fractures and 1554 patients with no risk factors that could affect bone metabolism.

Results.—In the patients without osteoporotic risk factors, BMD in the LAT projection showed stable bone mass between 20 and 40 years of age in both sexes, with significantly decreased bone mass after menopause, similar to the findings with AP projection, although the BMD values were lower with LAT than with AP projection. Absolute values for age-related spine bone loss was similar with both LAT and AP projections, but the percentage of bone loss was higher with the LAT than with the AP projection. There were significant correlations between LAT spin BMD and all the other BMD measurements, with the highest correlations with the AP projection BMD. The precision of the LAT projection was acceptable. The osteoporotic patients had clearly different BMD values than the control patients when BMD was assessed in the AP spine projection and Ward's triangle but were often similar to the control patients when BMD was assessed in the trochanter or LAT spine projection.

Conclusions.—The greater percentage age-related decrease in BMD detected in the LAT projection, compared with that detected in the AP projection, suggests that the trabecular bone of the vertebral body is more affected by aging and hormonal changes than is cortical bone. Lateral spine BMD measurement have acceptable precision, although the values are approximately twice those of the AP spine, which provides complementary information on the evolution of spine bone mass. However, spinal BMD measurements have less diagnostic sensitivity in the LAT than in the AP projection.

▶ The authors conclusions indicate that the AP projection is more sensitive in the diagnosis of osteoporosis than the lateral scan in addition to being more precise. All patients who have a lateral scan should also have an AP study.

M.K. Dalinka, M.D.

Axial Bone Mass in Older Women

Orwoll ES, Bauer DC, Vogt TM, et al (Kaiser Permanente Ctr for Health Research, Portland, Ore; Univ of California, San Francisco; Univ of Maryland, Baltimore)

Ann Intern Med 124:187–196, 1996 3–41

Background.—Substantial evidence indicates that bone mineral density (BMD) decreases in women with increasing age, particularly after menopause. This decrease in BMD is associated with an increased risk for fracture. Factors associated with axial BMD in the spine and proximal femur were evaluated.

Methods.—During a 2-year period, 9,704 nonblack women at least 65 years of age were studied. Bone mineral density of the lumbar spine, femoral neck, intertrochanteric region, trochanter, and the Ward triangle was measured with dual-energy x-ray absorptiometry. The women completed a questionnaire addressing family and reproductive history, medications, calcium intake, physical activity, weight, knee height, and height loss since the age of 25 years. They were also assessed for muscle strength and gait speed. The significance of associations between BMD and the assessed variables was studied.

Results.—A reduced BMD at all sites was associated with increasing age and was most strongly predicted by weight. There were positive associations between BMD and overall and knee height. Both spinal and femoral BMD increased with earlier menarche and later menopause and with current use of oral estrogen. The benefits of estrogen use decreased progressively after discontinuation of therapy. A family history of hip fracture was associated with reduced spine and femoral BMD. Calcium and vitamin D intake were positively associated with BMD, as were strength, walking speed, and the level of physical activity. Negative correlations were seen between BMD and tobacco use, caffeine intake, and glucocorticoid or anticonvulsant treatment; a positive association was seen between BMD and alcohol consumption and use of thiazide diuretics. The multivariable regression models explained 21% to 25% of the variation in femoral and spinal BMD.

Conclusions.—Several factors predict bone mass, including family and reproductive history, nutritional factors, medication use, and exercise. Examination of these factors can improve the estimation of fracture risk.

► In these changing economic times, the measurement of BMD has become an important issue; this paper is extremely pertinent. This complete review addresses many of the issues crucial to maintaining bone mineralization in older women and is necessary reading for those involved in ordering and interpreting bone mineral studies.

M.K. Dalinka, M.D.

Clinical Reproducibility of Dual Energy X-Ray Absorptiometry

Williams-Russo P, Healey JH, Szatrowski TP, et al (Mem Sloan-Kettering Cancer Ctr, New York; Cornell Multipurpose Arthritis Ctr, New York; Cornell Univ, New York)

J Orthop Res 13:250–257, 1995 3–42

Purpose.—Dual energy x-ray absorptiometry is widely recommended for use in measuring skeletal bone mass. However, its accuracy and precision in clinical patient populations have not been established. The short-term reproducibility of dual energy x-ray absorptiometry at various skeletal sites was assessed.

Methods.—Sixty-nine elderly patients with rheumatic diseases underwent dual energy x-ray absorptiometry for measurement of bone density twice on the same day. After an initial anteroposterior scan of the lumbar spine and proximal femur, the subjects got off the table and walked before being repositioned for the second scan. This process was performed once in all subjects at baseline and again at 6 months in 61 subjects, at 12 months in 54, at 16 months in 47, and at 24 months in 32. In addition, 38 patients underwent evaluation of the lumbar spine using the compare mode of the absorptiometer. For about one fourth of scans, the machine-generated region of interest was an obvious mismatch and had to be manually adjusted.

Results.—Correlation between the duplicate measurements of spinal bone density at baseline was excellent. Furthermore, the correlations remained stable over follow-up; the mean difference between duplicate baseline measurements was 1.82%, with a mean coefficient of variation of 1.29%. Reproducibility was much poorer at femoral sites but did not vary over time. The automated compare mode offered no advantage.

Conclusion.—Dual energy x-ray absorptiometry appears to offer good short-term reproducibility of bone mass measurements in the lumbar spine but less so in the hip. The documented levels of precision error have important ramifications for comparison of serial bone density measurements in individual patients. Clinically relevant statistical values include the mean difference between repeated measurements and the intraclass correlation coefficient, which can be adjusted for chance-expected agreement.

▶ The authors have shown that lateral dexa scans have less diagnostic sensitivity than scans in the anteroposterior projection, but there was no increase in the diagnostic sensitivity in osteoporosis. The lateral scan, when performed, should be performed in addition to the anteroposterior scan and not substitute for it.

M.K. Dalinka, M.D.

Miscellaneous Topics

Dialysis Arthropathy: Outcome After Renal Transplantation

Bardin T, Lebail-Darné JL, Zingraff J, et al (Clinque de Rhumatologie, Paris; Hôpital Lariboisière, Paris; Hôpital Necker, Paris; et al)

Am J Med 99:243–248, 1995 3–43

Objective.—A specific type of chronic arthropathy is common among patients receiving long-term maintenance hemodialysis. Dialysis arthropathy is strongly linked to β_2-microglobulin amyloid deposition and, to some extent, β_2-microglobulin retention. When these patients undergo successful renal transplantation, the rapid decline in serum β_2-microglobulin levels may permit the amyloid deposits to dissolve. The effects of successful renal transplantation were studied prospectively in patients with dialysis arthropathy.

Methods.—The 14 patients had been receiving hemodialysis for a mean of 195 months. All had a history of chronic joint pain before transplantation. When examined a mean of 54 months after renal transplantation, all patients were taking prednisone in a mean daily dose of 13.5 mg. Their rheumatologic manifestations from before and after transplantation were compared. Also, radiographs from before and after transplantation were analyzed in a blinded fashion by 3 separate observers. Amyloid deposits in articular samples were studied by Congo red staining and immunohistology.

Results.—Ten of the patients reported that their articular condition improved after renal transplantation. Three reported a worsening of their condition, and 1 noted no change. There was a significant reduction in the number of painful joints but no change in the number and size of subchrondral bone erosions. Two patients were found to have articular β_2-microglobulin amyloid deposits, 1 at 2 years and 1 at 10 years after transplantation.

Conclusion.—For patients with dialysis arthropathy, successful renal transplantation appears to halt progression of β_2-microglobulin amyloid. However, existing amyloid deposits do not dissolve, and the destructive arthropathies continue to progress. Though most patients report improvement of their joint symptoms, this is most likely the result of posttransplant corticosteroid treatment. Ideally renal transplantation should be performed before severe amyloid arthropathy has a chance to develop.

► Although many papers have addressed the radiologic appearance of amyloid arthropathy, this prospective study shows that renal transplantation does not reverse the process.

M.K. Dalinka, M.D.

Osteosclerosis in Intravenous Drug Abusers

Khosla S, Hassoun A, Heath H III (Mayo Clinic and Mayo Found, Rochester, Minn; Univ of Utah, Salt Lake City)
Endocrinologist 5:339–343, 1995 3–44

Purpose.—There are many different causes of acquired osteosclerosis, or increased bone density, and most are relatively easy to identify. However, there have been several reports of adult-onset acquired osteosclerosis occurring in IV drug abusers. These cases to not appear to be related to any of the previously known causes. Available information on the syndrome of osteosclerosis in IV drug abusers was reviewed.

Reported Patients and Findings.—Three cases were reported. The first patient, a woman with a long history of alcohol and IV drug abuse, presented with a 9-month history of bone pain in her legs, thighs, and hips. Increased skeletal bone density was noted on radiographs and progressed over 2 years' follow-up. The patient had a fivefold increase in her alkaline phosphatase level, which had been normal several years previously. A mild increase in serum parathyroid hormone levels and hypocalciuria were present as well, probably resulting from calcium flux into the skeleton.

Another report described 2 more IV drug abusers with osteosclerosis, who likewise had bone pain that was most severe in the lower extremities. Both patients had elevated serum hepatic transaminase activities and were seropositive for hepatitis C antibodies. Further serologic studies in the first patient also revealed hepatitis C antibodies. This prompted a search for skeletal osteosclerosis in a random series of hepatitis C–positive patients, but no affected patients were found. On the whole, the evidence suggests that acquired osteosclerosis in IV drug abusers with evidence of hepatitis C infection is a potentially important new syndrome, possibly related to some unidentified virus.

Discussion.—Acquired osteosclerosis may develop in IV drug abusers. These patients complain of worsening skeletal pain, especially in the lower extremities, and are found to have a primary increase in bone formation. They may also have mild secondary hyperparathyroidism resulting from hyperaccretion of calcium in the skeleton. Additional patients must be identified and further studies performed on their bone cells to identify the cause of this rare syndrome.

► This is a description of a new syndrome in which the diagnosis may be suggested by the radiologist.

M.K. Dalinka, M.D.

Study of Osteomyelitis: Utility of Combined Histologic and Microbiologic Evaluation of Percutaneous Biopsy Samples

White LM, Schweitzer ME, Deely DM, et al (Thomas Jefferson Univ Hosp, Philadelphia)

Radiology 197:840–842, 1995 3–45

Background.—False positive results for osteomyetitis occur in 40% to 65% of biopsies even when adequate tissue samples are obtained. The samples of many patients with suspected osteomyelitis will be culture negative, so some authors have recommended histologic examination of part of the biopsy specimen. However, this practice reduces the tissue sample available for microscopic evaluation. The necessity of performing both histologic and microbiologic examination of biopsy specimens in patients with suspected osteomyelitis was prospectively evaluated.

Methods.—The study included 25 adult patients with suspected osteomyelitis. Core and aspiration biopsy specimens were obtained with trephine techniques under radiologic guidance. The diagnosis of osteomyelitis was confirmed by either culture growth or characteristic histologic findings. All negative results were verified by documentation of nonprogression on clinical and radiologic examinations for 6 months, histopathologic evidence of tumor or other noninfectious disease, or negative results on open biopsy.

Results.—Histologic evidence of acute or chronic osteomyelitis was detected in 16 of 25 biopsy specimens. Culture results were also positive in 8 of 16. Culture was never positive unless histologic examination was positive as well. Nine patients had negative results on both histologic and microbiologic examination, and these results were true negative in 6 cases. These included 2 cases of metastatic disease, 2 of uncomplicated fracture, and 2 cases with no culture or histopathologic evidence of infection. Three patients with negative histologic and microbiologic results eventually proved to have osteomyelitis.

Conclusion.—Patients suspected of having osteomyelitis should receive both microbiologic and histologic evaluation of bone biopsy specimens. Though culture alone has a sensitivity of only 42%, this figure doubles when both culture and histologic examination are performed. Combined histologic examination and culture of bone biopsy specimens are necessary to reduce the number of repeat biopsies.

► This paper points out the importance of histologic evaluation of the core biopsy sample, which increases the sensitivity of culture in the diagnosis of osteomyelitis.

M.K. Dalinka, M.D.

Distribution of Calcification in the Triangular Fibrocartilage Region in 181 Patients With Calcium Pyrophosphate Dihydrate Crystal Deposition Disease

Yang B-Y, Sartoris DJ, Djukic S, et al (Veterans Affairs Med Ctr, San Diego, Calif)

Radiology 196:547–550, 1995 3–46

Introduction.—Calcium pyrophosphate dihydrate (CPPD) crystal deposition is a common disease of the elderly with clinical manifestations of crystal-induced synovitis, called pseudogout syndrome. Clinical signs and symptoms can mimic those of rheumatoid arthritis, osteoarthritis, and neuroarthropathy. Calcifications occur most frequently in the triangular fibrocartilage. The interosseous ligaments of the scapholunate and lunotriquetral areas and the hyaline cartilage of the midcarpal and carpometacarpal regions may be likewise affected. Radiographs of 316 wrists in 181 patients with definite or probable diagnosis of CPPD were reviewed retrospectively to determine the relative occurrence of calcification at specific sites around the ulnar aspect of the radiocarpal joint.

Methods.—The presence or absence of calcification in the following areas was documented: cartilage in the inferior radioulnar joint, triangular fibrocartilage, lunotriquetral ligament, lunotriquetral cartilage, and triquetral cartilage.

Results.—Calcifications occurred most frequently in the lunotriquetral ligament (49 wrists), not the triangular fibrocartilage (30 patients). The difference in frequency of calcification in these 2 sites was not significant. The occurrence of lunotriquetral ligament calcification was significantly more frequent in female than male patients.

Discussion and Conclusion.—The 2 major radiographic findings in patients with CPPD crystal deposition disease of the wrist were articular or periarticular calcification and pyrophosphate arthropathy. The latter is characterized by joint space narrowing in the metacarpophalangeal and radiocarpal areas, trapezoiscaphoid involvement, and relative sparing of the distal radioulunar joint. Incidence of CPPD has been reported to be from 27% to 94%. Although not significantly different, the lunotriquetral ligament was a more common site of calcification than the triangular fibrocartilage. Calcification in the lunotriquetral ligament and cartilage was seen to occur without simultaneous triangular fibrocartilage calcification. Increased occurrence of wrist calcification was associated with age only in patients with involvement of the lunotriquetral ligament. It was also more common in female patients.

▶ The authors have made an important observation in a large carefully performed study.

M.K. Dalinka, M.D.

Can Clinical Data Help to Screen Patients With Lymphoma for MR Imaging of Bone Marrow?

Tardivon AA, Munck J-N, Shapeero LG, et al (Institut Gustave Roussy, Villejuif, France; Univ of California, San Francisco)

Ann Oncol 6:795–800, 1995 3–47

Background.—The staging and treatment planning for patients with malignant lymphoma requires knowledge of the bone marrow status. This is usually accomplished with unilateral bone marrow aspiration or biopsy. However, MRI has been shown to be useful in the assessment of bone marrow disorders. Associations between MRI results and clinical and laboratory findings were studied to determine the characteristics of patients in whom bone marrow imaging would be useful.

Methods.—Forty consecutive patients with malignant lymphoma underwent bone marrow MRI, blind biopsy, and clinical examination. The MRI scans were interpreted by examiners blinded to the clinical data. The patients were followed for a mean of 23 months. During this time, positive bone marrow status was determined by positive blind biopsy in 6 patients, positive surgical biopsy in 2, positive bone scintigraphy in 2, positive CT study in 2, and MRI changes in 9.

Results.—The blind biopsy and MRI results were normal in 36%, abnormal in 16%, and discordant in 48%. Of the patients with discordant results, only 1 had an abnormal biopsy result with a normal MRI study. A positive MRI study was significantly predictive of subsequent bone marrow infiltration, with a sensitivity of 96.5%, specificity of 86%, and overall accuracy of 82%. Abnormal MRI studies were also significantly associated with constitutional symptoms, bone pain, or elevated alkaline phosphatase level. The treatment plan was altered in 3 patients on the basis of MRI findings.

Conclusion.—Magnetic resonance imaging can provide critical information predicting bone marrow involvement in patients with lymphoma. It is particularly useful in patients with normal biopsy results but with clinical symptoms associated with bone marrow involvement.

▶ The authors have shown that imaging of bone marrow is more accurate than bone biopsy. They suggest that its use should be limited to patients with normal bone biopsy results and clinical parameters associated with bone marrow involvement. Their data seem to show that it is rare to obtain a positive biopsy in the presence of a normal MRI. This would make me believe that MRI should be used in place of the biopsy rather than only in biopsy-negative patients.

M.K. Dalinka, M.D.

4 Pediatric Radiology

Introduction

The 1997 YEAR BOOK OF DIAGNOSTIC RADIOLOGY has fewer selections for "Pediatric Radiology" than in the 1996 YEAR BOOK that covered the Centennial Year of 1995, but the quality of the articles abstracted makes up for the decrease in quantity. I am confident that you will agree, although we know that this is but a sampling of the excellent "Pediatric Radiology" articles on mostly bread and butter topics that could have been abstracted.

In this year's sampling of abstracts from much of the 1996 pediatric radiology literature, you will find a balanced distribution among the major organ systems as follows:

1. The neuroendocrine section contains neurologic and endocrine abstracts, including calvarial frontal foramina, juvenile Huntington's disease, operculum syndrome, pontocerebellar hypoplasia, autoimmune thrombocytopenia, superior sagittal sinus thrombosis, extracorporeal membrane oxygenation (ECMO) effects on neural development, congenital hypothyroidism, and acute CNS injury assessed by MRS spectroscopy.
2. The musculoskeletal section contains a broad variety of pediatric bone disease abstracts, including Blount's disease, Legg-Calvé-Perthes' disease, MRI of thalassemia and lymphangiomatosis, vertebral osteoblastoma, distal humeral nonaccidental injury, systemic onset juvenile rheumatoid arthritis, and seronegative enthesopathy/arthropathy syndrome;
3. The cardiopulmonary section contains pediatric lung and heart abstracts, including internal mammary compartment window to the mediastinum, helical CT, pulmonary artery agenesis, anomalous right pulmonary artery, a rare vascular ring, double aortic arch/d-transposition, pericardial defects, aneurysmal pulmonary arteries, Perflubron liquid ventilation/ECMO, Lemierre's syndrome, thoracic percutaneous catheter drainage, myocardial scintigraphy in Kawasaki disease, high-resolution CT of allogenic marrow transplant/obstructive lung disease, and pulmonary plasma cell granuloma.
4. The gastrointestinal (GI) section contains abstracts of GI and abdominal/peritoneal organ topics, including congenital diaphragmatic hernia and midgut malfixation, single-photon emission CT of heterotaxy syn-

drome, MRI of anorectal anomalies, ultrasound (US) of jejunal intussusception, CT of ileocolic intussusception, color Doppler of appendicitis, peliosis hepatis, imaging of subperitoneal disease, MRI during hemangiomatosis therapy, AIDS-related lymphoma, acute pancreatitis, splenic injury, and liver transplant/portal hypertension Doppler imaging.

5. The genitourinary section contains mainly urinary tract abstracts but also a few genital tract abstracts, including juvenile nephronophthisis, ureterocele eversion and reflux, pyourachus, US vs. scintigraphy in urinary tract infections, congenital mesoblastic nephroma, ovarian torsion, posttraumatic arterial priapism, renovascular hypertension Doppler imaging, and systemic oxalosis.

Throughout this effort, focus has been on diagnostic imaging prioritized to the health and disease of children. To help children, we need to be informed. Children are the future.

Again I am grateful to the untiring secretarial assistance of Loretta Skinner, to time and requisite resources of the Division of Pediatric Radiology, Loma Linda University Medical Center and Children's Hospital, and to the tolerance of my spouse, Florence Young, for allowing me to bring home the clutter of stacks of articles and xeroxes and then to mentally dance with them. These abstracts and comments are the result.

Lionel W. Young, M.D.

Neuroendocrine System

Frontal Foramina in Pediatric Skull in Cases of Congenital Hydrocephalus

Sun JK, LeMay DR, Couldwell WT, et al (Univ of Southern California, Los Angeles; Los Angeles County Hosp, Calif)

Radiology 197:497–499, 1995 4–1

Background.—A number of different calvarial bone changes occur in patients with congenital hydrocephalus, including an increased craniofacial ratio, bulging anterior fontanelle, sutural diastasis, and macrocephaly with frontal bosselation. Frontal foramina may be present as well. The link between frontal calvarial foramina and congenital hydrocephalus secondary to CNS malformation was examined in a retrospective study.

Methods.—The study was prompted by the observation of frontal foramina on radiographs (Fig 1), CT scans (Fig 2), and 3-dimensional CT reconstructions (Fig 3) in 3 girls with Chiari II malformations. The axial head CT scans of 99 pediatric patients with hydrocephalus were reviewed to determine whether frontal foramina were present. Sixty-one of these children had Chiari II malformation, 23 had other diagnoses that may have contributed to their hydrocephalus, and 15 had no known cause of their hydrocephalus. The scans of 116 patients without hydrocephalus were reviewed as a control.

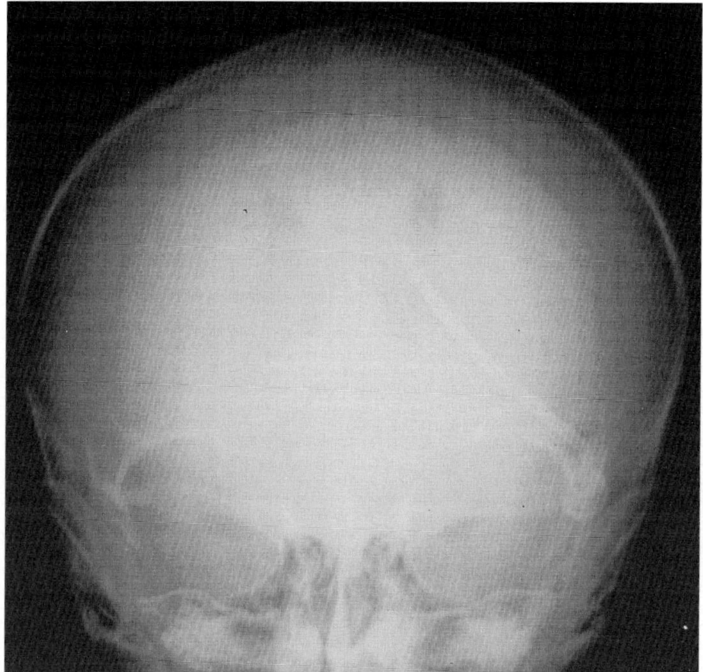

FIGURE 1.—Frontal skull radiograph depicts frontal foramina in a 6-year-old girl with Chiari II malformation. A ventriculoperitoneal shunt is present. (Courtesy of Sun JK, LeMay DR, Couldwell WT, et al: Frontal foramina in pediatric skull in cases of congenital hydrocephalus. *Radiology* 197:497–499, 1995; Radiological Society of North America.)

Results.—Thirteen percent of the children with Chiari II malformation had frontal foramina, as did 1 patient with Dandy-Walker malformation and 1 patient with occipital horn dilation. None of the control patients had frontal foramina. Three patients with frontal foramina underwent serial CT scanning, which depicted gradual closure of the foramina after ventriculoperitoneal shunting.

Conclusion.—Some patients with congenital hydrocephalus caused by CNS malformation have frontal calvarial foramina. The foramina can be demonstrated by palpation or plain skull or sinus radiographs, and they may help in recognizing undiagnosed congenital hydrocephalus with CNS malformation. The foramina may arise as a result of abnormal induction of bone formation caused by increased intracranial pressure; on their own, they have no direct pathologic consequences.

▶ Frontal foramina in association with congenital hydrocephalus were first observed by Naidich et al.[1] This nice retrospective study helps to establish the frequency of this condition. Frontal foramina are a form of craniolacuna (luckenshadel) that may be associated with congenital hydrocephalus. Perhaps there is a genetic basis for this finding, as with other conditions of delayed membranous ossification.[2]

L.W. Young, M.D.

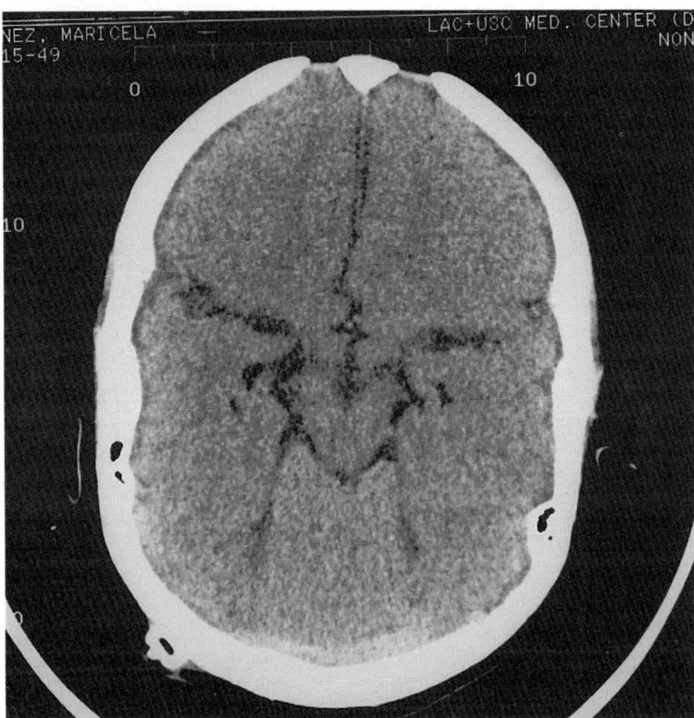

FIGURE 2.—Axial head CT scan of the same patient as in Figure 1 depicts frontal foramina without soft-tissue mass or extra-axial fluid collection. Typical features of Chiari II malformation are seen. (Courtesy of Sun JK, LeMay DR, Couldwell WT, et al: Frontal foramina in pediatric skull in cases of congenital hydrocephalus. *Radiology* 197:497–499, 1995; Radiological Society of North America.)

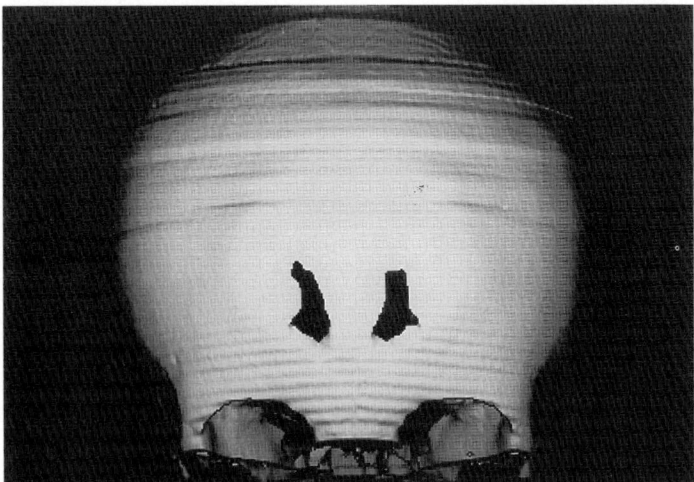

FIGURE 3.—Three-dimensional reconstruction of the skull shows frontal foramina in the same patient as in Figures 1 and 2. (Courtesy of Sun JK, LeMay DR, Couldwell WT, et al: Frontal foramina in pediatric skull in cases of congenital hydrocephalus. *Radiology* 197:497–499, 1995; Radiological Society of North America.)

References

1. Naidich TP, Pudlowski RM, Naidich JB, et al: Computed tomography signs of the Chiari II malformation: I. Skull and dural partitions. *Radiology* 134:65–71, 1980.
2. Gonzalez-del AA, Carnevale A, Takenaga R: Delayed membranous cranial ossification in a mother and child. *Am J Med Genet* 44:786–789, 1992.

Juvenile Huntington Disease: CT and MR Features

Ho VB, Chuang HS, Rovira MJ, et al (Madigan Army Med Ctr, Tacoma, Wash; Hosp for Sick Children, Toronto; Univ of Washington, Seattle; et al)
Am J Neuroradiol 16:1405–1412, 1995 4–2

Background.—The onset of Huntington disease (HD), a hereditary neurodegenerative disorder, usually occurs between 30 and 40 years of age. However, in 1% to 6% of the patients, the onset of HD occurs in childhood. The main radiologic feature of HD, documented mainly in adults, is caudate atrophy. This can seen on pneumoencephalography, CT, and MRI. The clinical and radiologic manifestations of juvenile HD were the subjects of this study.

Methods.—Six patients, aged 3–18 years, were included in the study. Three were girls. All 6 underwent CT, and 3 underwent MRI. The CT and MRI examinations were assessed for frontal horn distance to intercaudate distance and bicaudate ratios. The findings were compared with those of 24 age- matched healthy children and 12 age-matched patients with Leigh or Wilson disease.

Findings.—In all children with HD, atrophy of the caudate nuclei was identified. The frontal horn distance to intercaudate distance mean ratio was decreased to 1.64 (control:3.82) and mean bicaudate ratio was increased to 0.205 control:0.093 in the HD group. These ratios were significantly different from those in the 2 control groups. On MR images, increased proton density- and T2-weighted signal in the caudate nuclei and putamina was noted in the patients with HD.

Conclusion.—In both adults and children, the frontal horn distance to intercaudate distance and bicaudate ratios are useful for diagnosing HD. Children with HD also have increased proton density- and T2-weighted signal in the atrophic caudate nuclei and putamina on MR images.

► The CT and MRI measurement criteria for Huntington's disease in adults are validly applicable in childhood. Frontal horn/intercaudate ratio is decreased and bicaudate ratio is increased. Additional MRI findings of increased signal intensity in the basal ganglia are present in juvenile Huntington's disease. Other recent articles relate to genetic aspects of juvenile Huntington's disease,[1–3] as well as MRI.[4]

L.W. Young, M.D.

References

1. Telenius H, Kremer HP, Theilmann J, et al: Molecular analysis of juvenile Huntington disease; the major influence on (CAG) n repeat length is the sex of the affected parent. *Hum Mol Genet* 2:1535–1540, 1993.
2. Petit H, Pasquier F: Huntington disease. Current state of research. *Presse Medicale* 23:385–391, 1994.
3. Sharpe NF: Presymptomatic testing for Huntington disease: is there a duty to test those under the age of eighteen years? *Am J Med Genet* 46:250–253, 1993.
4. Comunale Jr. JP, Heier LA, Chutorian AM: Juvenile Form of Huntington's Disease: MR Imaging Appearance. *AJR* 165:414–415, 1995.

The Syndrome of Autosomal Recessive Pontocerebellar Hypoplasia, Microcephaly, and Extrapyramidal Dyskinesia (Pontocerebellar Hypoplasia Type 2): Compiled Data From 10 Pedigrees

Barth PG, Blennow G, Lenard H-G, et al (Univ Hosp, Amsterdam; Univ Hosp, Lund, Sweden; Univ of Düsseldorf, Germany; et al)

Neurology 45:311–317, 1995 4–3

Introduction.—Classification of pontocerebellar hypoplasia is based on 2 phenotypes. Pontocerebellar hypoplasia type 1 is characterized by spinal anterior horn degeneration and absence of extrapyramidal symptoms; pontocerebellar hypoplasia type 2 is characterized by progressive microcephaly, extrapyramidal dyskinesia, and normal spinal cord findings. Little is known about type 2, and a study was conducted to determine neurologic and neurodevelopmental follow-up, survival, and causes of death.

Methods.—Sixteen patients comprising 10 independent pedigrees were evaluated to determine intrafamilial and interfamilial variability in phenotype, including results of neuroimaging and geographical distribution. These patients demonstrated neurologic involvement from birth with near absence of cognitive and voluntary motor development, microcephaly, and pronounced extrapyramidal involvement with chorea or dystonia.

Results.—All 16 patients had an identical profile of early-onset severe chorea, microcephaly together with pontocerebellar hypoplasia, and virtually absent developmental milestones. Autosomal recessive transmission was found in the family distribution. Pregnancy was normal in all patients and ended at term in all except a patient who was born at 37 weeks. The disease was present in an all-or-none pattern, as nonhandicapped siblings and parents were symptom free. In all patients, extrapyramidal dyskinesia was manifested in the course of the first year. In all 11 patients who had MRI, severe pontocerebellar hypoplasia was present, involving the vermis and cerebellar hemispheres (Fig 2).

Conclusion.—Pontocerebellar hypoplasia type 2 phenotype is a distinct neurogenetic entity. Autosomal recessive transmission of the disease is supported by consanguinity found in some pedigrees, the absence of neurologic complaints by any of the parents, the all-or-none presentation within affected families, and affection of both sexes. So far, only white families have been identified. Magnetic resonance imaging findings are diagnostic of this disease. Extrapyramidal involvement is a marker for type

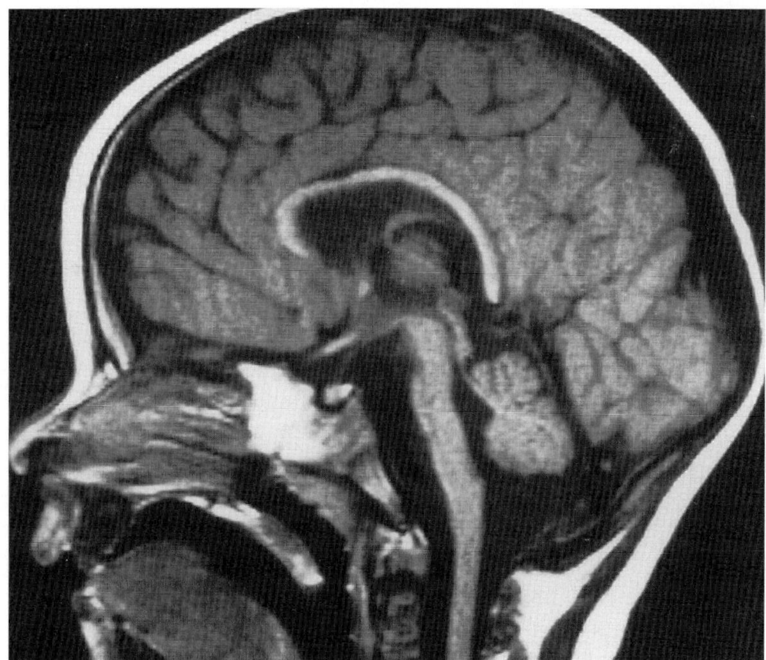

FIGURE 2.—Midsagittal T1-weighted MR image of a patient at age 0.9 year. Features include a hypoplastic pons; underdeveloped, atrophied image of the vermis; and a thin corpus callosum. (Reprinted from *Neurology* 45:311–317, 1995 by permission of Little, Brown and Company Inc.

2 pontocerebellar hypoplasia. Genetic linkage studies may lead to identifying the gene defect.

► The syndrome of pontocerebellar hypoplasia is well represented in this report on 16 patients. Pontine and cerebellar hypoplasia, as demonstrated by MRI, are the morphologic hallmarks of this neurogenetic entity. This report is unique in presenting a pedigree of 5 related families with this condition. Other recent articles indicate the use of CT and/or MRI to demonstrate the changes of pontine and cerebellar hypoplasia.[1–5]

L.W. Young, M.D.

References

1. Koskinen T, Valanne L, Ketonen LM, et al: Infantile-onset spinocerebellar ataxia: MR and CT findings. *Am J Neuroradiology* 16:1427–1433, 1995.
2. Pratap-Chand R, Gururaj AK, Dilip-Kumar S: A syndrome of olivopontocerebellar atrophy and deafness with onset in infancy. *Acta Neurol Scand* 91:133–136, 1995.
3. Al Shahwan SA, Bruyn GW, Al Deeb SM: Non-progressive familial congenital cerebellar hypoplasia. *J Neurol Sci* 128:71–77, 1995.
4. Riva A, Bradac GB: Primary cerebellar and spino-cerebellar ataxia: an MRI study on 63 cases. *J Neuroradiol* 22:71–76, 1995.
5. Pascual-Castroviejo I, Gutierrez M, Morales C, et al: Primary degeneration of the granular layer of the cerebellum. A study of 14 patients and review of the literature. *Neuropediatrics* 25:183–190, 1994.

Operculum Syndrome: Unusual Feature of Herpes Simplex Encephalitis
van der Poel JC, Haenggeli CA, Overweg-Plandsoen WCG (Academic Med Ctr, Amsterdam; Children's Hosp, Geneva)
Pediatr Neurol 12:246–249, 1995 4–4

Purpose.—Herpes simplex encephalitis (HSE) carries significant morbidity and mortality, which can be reduced by early recognition and treatment. The typical manifestation includes fever, convulsions, behavioral changes, focal neurologic signs, and deteriorating consciousness.

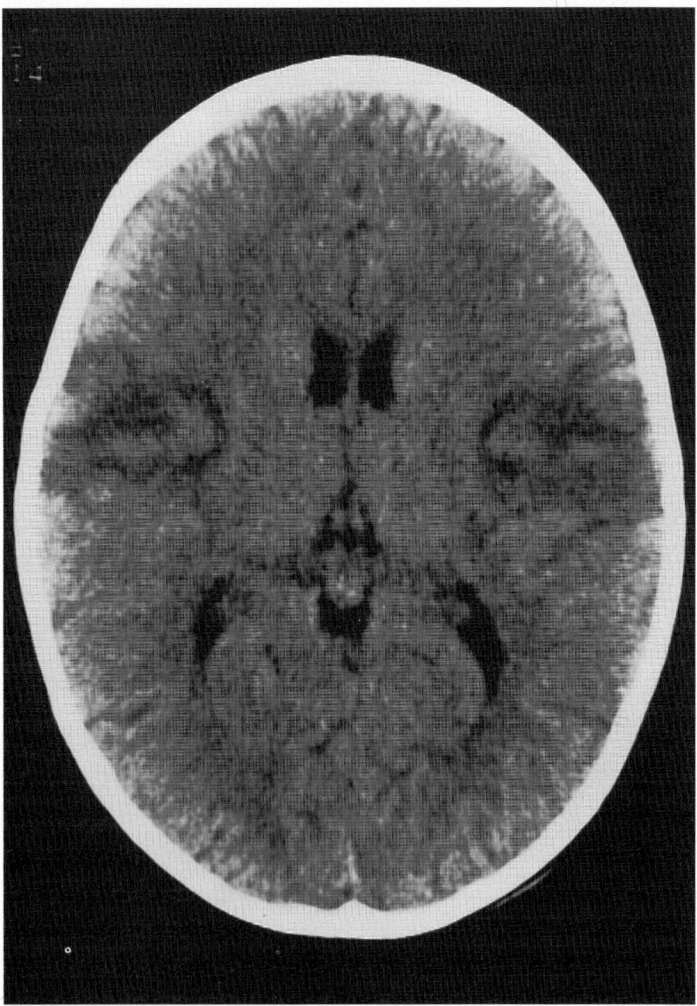

FIGURE 1.—Computed tomography scan obtained during the acute stage in patient 1. Note the bilateral hemispheric hypodensities in the opercular region. (Reprinted by permission of the publisher from Operculum syndrome: Unusual feature of herpes simplex encephalitis; by van der Poel JC, Haenggeli CA, Overweg-Plandsoen WCG; *Pediatr Neurol*; 12:246–249; Copyright 1995 by Elsevier Science Inc.)

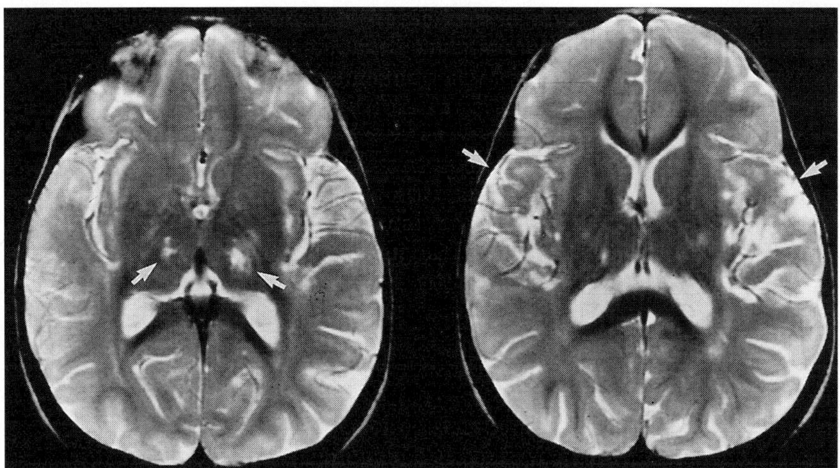

FIGURE 2.—Cerebral MR image 4 weeks after the acute illness of patient 2, documenting several lesions of increased signal intensity on T2-weighted images (recovery time 2,360 msec/echo time 100 msec), involving both thalami, the periventricular white matter around the atrium bilaterally, and both frontal opercular regions. (Reprinted by permission of the publisher from Operculum syndrome: Unusual feature of herpes simplex encephalitis; by van der Poel JC, Haenggeli CA, Overweg-Plandsoen WCG; *Pediatr Neurol*; 12:246–249; Copyright 1995 by Elsevier Science Inc.)

However, encephalitis may be difficult to recognize in children, particularly young children. Anterior operculum syndrome has been reported in children with encephalitic illness. The operculum syndrome manifests with anarthria and impaired mastication and swallowing, caused by focal, bilateral cortical damage in the anterior opercular regions. Two cases in children of HSE in which the operculum syndrome was a prominent feature were reported.

Patients.—The first patient was a 21-month-old boy in whom operculum syndrome was a presenting feature of HSE. He was admitted with fever and focal seizures involving both sides of the face. A cranial CT scan showed hypodense areas in both rolandic regions, with dense contrast enhancement. The hypodensities were increased on repeat CT scanning performed 3 days later (Fig 1). The second patient was a 24-month-old girl admitted with partial seizures of the left side of her face and her left arm. This patient underwent cerebral MRI, which showed increased signal intensity lesions on T2-weighted images. The lesions involved both thalami, the periventricular white matter near the atria of the left ventricles, and the right frontal operculum. At 4 weeks' follow-up, the right opercular lesion had grown larger, and a left opercular lesion had appeared (Fig 2).

In both patients, early recognition of the opercular syndrome permitted early acyclovir treatment. This may have been an important factor in the children's good general recovery. Both patients were left with persistent speech, mastication, and swallowing deficits. These problems were more pronounced in the second patient, whose clinical course was complicated by coma.

Discussion.—Operculum syndrome may be an underrecognized problem in patients with HSE. The pathophysiologic basis for this association may be the propensity of HSE to involve areas adjacent to the operculum (i.e., the inferomedial portions of the frontal and temporal lobe). It is essential to recognize operculum syndrome in HSE because of the potential for severe morbidity. Operculum syndrome may be a presenting manifestation in children with cortical dysplasia, meningitis, and encephalitis. In young children with HSE, operculum syndrome can have serious developmental consequences.

▶ Identification of HSE as early as possible is apparently dependent on recognition of clinical signs. They include supranuclear palsies of cranial nerves 5, 7, 9, and up to 12 that characterize the operculum syndrome. Children with the syndrome have severe impairment of voluntary motor control of the buccal and lingual musculature. Involuntary control may not be affected. The CT finding of hypodensity in the opercular regions and MRI T2-weighted hyperintensity in the opercula, the thalami, and atrial periventricular white matter are the major imaging signs that contribute to early recognition. An excellent recent background article on MR demonstration of the cerebral opercula[1] is listed with other pertinent recent references on herpes encephalitis.[2–4]

L.W. Young, M.D.

References

1. Chen C-Y, Zimmerman RA, Faro S, et al: MR of the cerebral operculum: Topographic identification and measurement of interopercular distances in healthy infants and children. *Am J Neuroradiol* 16:1677–1687, 1995.
2. Schlesinger V, Buller TS, Brunstrom JE, et al: Expanded spectrum of herpes simplex encephalitis in childhood. *J Pediatr* 126:234–241, 1995.
3. O'Reilly MAR, O'Reilly PMR, de Bruyn R: Neonatal herpes simplex type 2 encephalitis: Its appearances on ultrasound and CT. *Pediatr Radiol* 25:68–69, 1995.
4. Shanks DE, Blasco PA, Chason DP: Movement disorder following herpes simplex encephalitis. *Dev Med Child Neurol* 33:348–352, 1991.

Nature of the Brain Lesion in Fetal Allo-Immune Thrombocytopenia

Govaert P, Bridger J, Wigglesworth J (Gent Univ, Belgium; Hammersmith Hosp, London)
Dev Med Child Neurol 37:485–495, 1995 4–5

Introduction.—There are numerous reports of the diagnosis and management of fetal and neonatal intracranial manifestations of alloimmune thrombocytopenia. The literature includes a report of massive posthemorrhagic hydrocephalus in a stillborn girl at 33 weeks' gestation. In some patients, findings in life have suggested subpial hemorrhages. The cases of 3 neonates with pathologically confirmed brain damage are reported. In 2 cases, imaging in life allowed interpretation of the pattern of the initial lesion. In the third case, necropsy findings are presented.

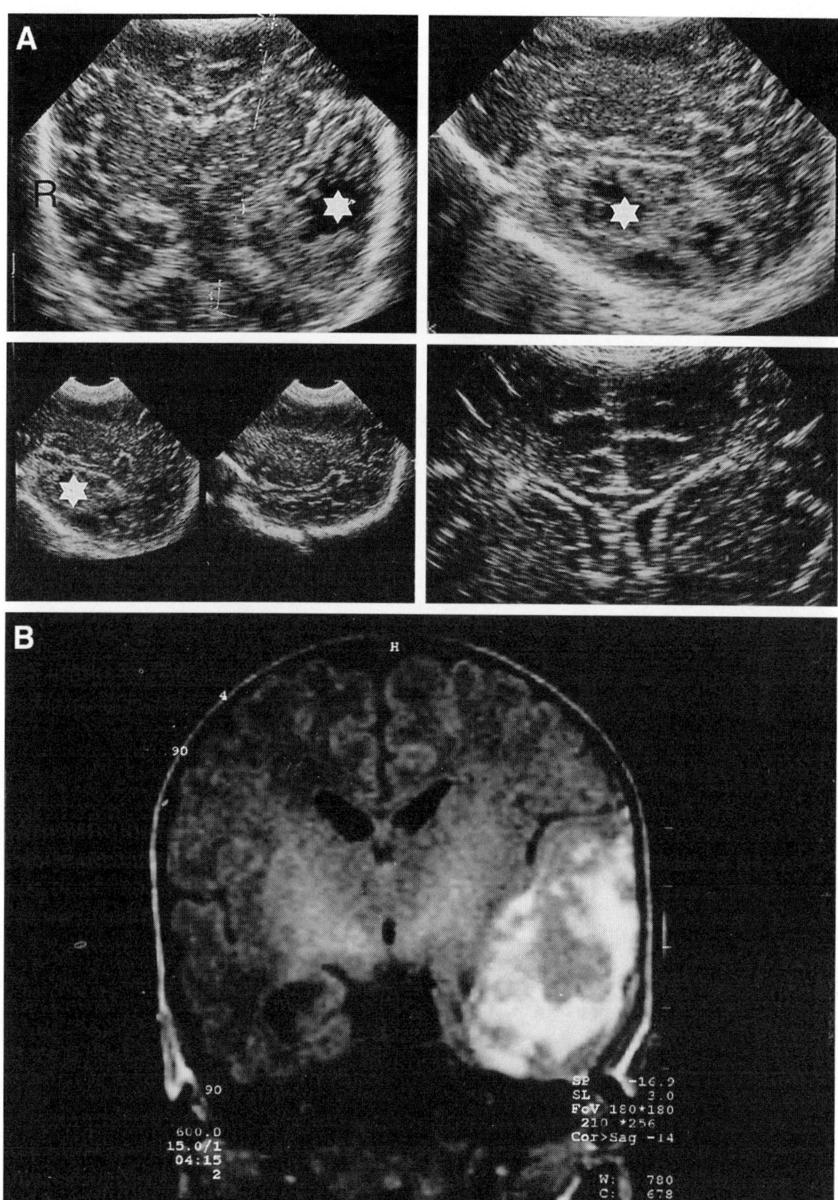

FIGURE 5.—**A**, ultrasound scan sections. **Top**, frontal view at foramen of Monro. **Bottom**, parasagittal view through injured and healthy temporal lobe. **B**, frontal MR image (T1 weighted) on day 7 in patient 3. Cystic necrosis and nonrecent hemorrhage (see *stars* in **A**) occupies whole of left temporal lobe and elevates compressed insular region; ependymal lining is accentuated due to posthemorrhagic changes. (Courtesy of Govaert P, Bridger J, Wigglesworth J: Nature of the brain lesion in fetal allo-immune thrombocytopenia. *Dev Med Child Neurol* 37:485–495, 1995.)

Patient 3.—A female infant was examined because severe thrombocytopenia and scarce truncal petechiae were inadvertently discovered. At 27 weeks' gestation, intra-uterine growth retardation was suspected. A partly cystic and partly hemorrhagic lesion encompassing the left temporal lobe was shown by sonography and MRI (Fig 5). The parenchymal lesion made occipital connection with the adjacent lateral ventricle. Results of imaging examinations indicated an onset of 1 week or more before delivery.

Discussion.—The incidence of fetal intracranial hemorrhage in alloimmune thrombocytopenia is roughly 7%; hemorrhage during delivery occurs in another 10%. Extensive subarachnoid haematoma formation often occurs with disseminated intravascular coagulation resulting from immune fetal hydrops and birth asphyxia, or associated with septicemia. These hemorrhages usually occur around the temporal lobe. Cystic encephaloclastic damage with porencephalic cavitation may occur. In prenatal hemorrhagic diathesis, it is unclear why the temporal lobe is particularly vulnerable to bleeding. Further research should address the recent suggestion that antibody-mediated vasculitis may play a major role.

▶ Fetal maternal alloimmune thrombocytopenia is a rare cause of spontaneous intracranial hemorrhage in utero. Neonatal imaging patterns of 2 of 3 infants with intracranial hemorrhage were demonstrated by sonographic and MRI findings. The authors propose a useful sequence of events involving antenatal brain hemorrhage and injury due to alloimmune thrombocytopenia. Other recent articles that corroborate the findings in this report are listed.[1, 2]

L.W. Young, M.D.

References

1. Dean LM, McLeary M, Taylor GA: Cerebral hemorrhage in alloimmune thrombocytopenia. *Pediatr Radiol* 25:444–445, 1995.
2. Glassman AB, Shieh WJ: Neonatal alloimmune thrombocytopenia: Current considerations. *Ann Clin Lab Sci* 24:407–411, 1994.

Doppler Imaging of Superior Sagittal Sinus Thrombosis

Lam AH (Royal Alexandra Hosp for Children, Sydney, Australia)

J Ultrasound Med 14:41–46, 1995 4–6

Background.—Although many reports on cerebral venous sinus thrombosis (CVST) in adults and older infants have been published, the imaging diagnosis of CVST in neonates is limited. Three neonates with superior sagittal sinus thrombosis (SSST) diagnosed by Doppler imaging with confirmation on CT, MRI, or digital subtraction angiography were presented. One infant died, and the other 2 recovered uneventfully.

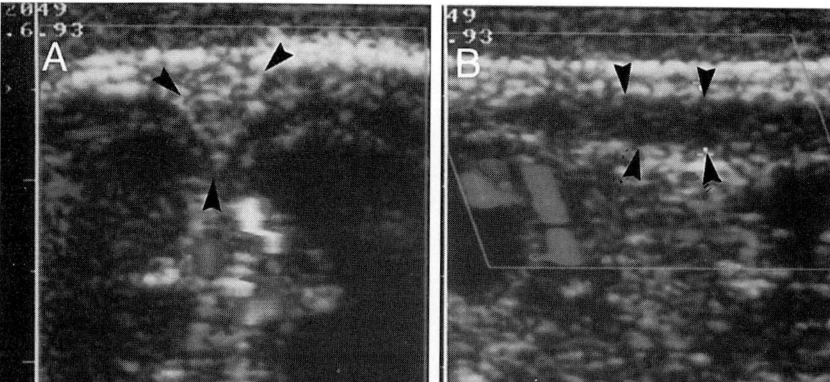

FIGURE 3.—Color Doppler sonography through the anterior fontanelle in coronal (**A**) and midline sagittal (**B**) sections shows absence of color-coded flow signal in the superior sagittal sinus in contrast to the adjacent cortical arterial flow. Note the hypoechoic, enlarged superior sagittal sinus with loss of normal concavity of the lower borders (*arrowheads*). (Courtesy of Lam AH: Doppler imaging of superior sagittal sinus thrombosis. *J Ultrasound Med* 14:41–46, 1995.)

Representative Case.—One patient was a 4-week-old boy, born at term, referred because of seizure. His perinatal history was normal. An episode of otitis media had been treated with antibiotics. Subsequently, the infant had a generalized truncal rash and diarrhea. The primary physician was present during a focal seizure with twitching of both eyes and pallor. The boy was hospitalized, and phenobarbitone was given. A CT scan demonstrated a left intraventricular hemorrhage (IVH). Cranial sonography with Doppler imaging showed the left IVH and an echogenic SSS with loss of the normal concavity of the inferior borders. Color and duplex imaging showed absence of venous flow (Fig 3). On an MR scan obtained 2 days later, a hyperintense SSS was observed in T1-weighted and long recovery time sequences. Medical treatment effectively controlled the focal seizure, and the patient was discharged. One month later, follow-up cranial sonography and Doppler sonography showed recanalization of the SSS, normal venous flow, and resolution of the IVH.

Conclusion.—Neonates with SSST rarely undergo diagnostic imaging. This condition is underdiagnosed because of the nonspecificity of its clinical manifestation and physicians' desire to avoid invasive radiologic procedures that may prove unnecessary. Although not always available or practical, MRI provides a sensitive, noninvasive method for diagnosing neonatal SSST. Doppler imaging proved diagnostic in the patients described in the current report. It should be used in the initial evaluation of this condition, as it is the most convenient and least invasive diagnostic technique.

▶ Doppler sonography is the appropriate imaging modality in the initial assessment for SSST. Magnetic resonance imaging is the ideal corroborative imaging method, and it also facilitates recognition of other locations of cerebral venous thrombosis. Other recent articles on Doppler imaging and MRI of cerebral venous thrombosis are listed.[1–6]

L.W. Young, M.D.

References

1. Bezinque SL, Slovis TL, Touchette AS, et al: Characterization of superior sagittal sinus blood flow velocity using color flow Doppler in neonates and infants. *Pediatr Radiol* 25:175–179, 1995.
2. Wasenko JJ, Holsapple JW, Winfield JA: Cerebral venous thrombosis demonstration with magnetic resonance angiography. *Clin Imaging* 19:153–161, 1995.
3. Uziel Y, Laxer RM, Blaser S, et al: Cerebral vein thrombosis in childhood systemic lupus erythematosus. *J Pediatr* 126:722–727, 1995.
4. Garcia DJ, Baker AS, Cunningham MJ, et al: Lateral sinus thrombosis associated with otitis media and mastoiditis in children. *Pediatr Infect Dis J* 14:617–623, 1995.
5. Dormont D, Anxionnat R, Evard S, et al: MRI in cerebral venous thrombosis. *J Neuroradiol* 21:81–99, 1994.
6. Confavreux C, Brunet P, Petiot P, et al: Congenital protein C deficiency and superior sagittal sinus thrombosis causing isolated intracranial hypertension. *J Neurol Neurosurg Psychiatry* 57:655–657, 1994.

MR Angiography in Pediatric Neurological Disorders

Lee BCP, Park TS, Kaufman BA (Washington Univ, St Louis; St Louis Children's Hosp)
Pediatr Radiol 25:409–419, 1995 4–7

Objectives.—The value of MR angiography and conventional MRI in diagnosing intracranial abnormalities in children was compared, the sensitivity of MR angiography and conventional angiography was compared, and the value of MR angiography in surgical planning was determined.

Background.—Magnetic resonance angiography is commonly used to assess vascular abnormalities in adults, but its use in children is limited. Noninvasive techniques for assessing intracranial vessels are preferred in children because the risks of conventional angiography are higher. The clinical role of MR angiography in children has not been determined.

Methods.—In children younger than 16 years with neurologic disorders, 103 MR arteriography examinations and 83 MR venography examinations were performed. Conventional cerebral angiography was performed in 30 patients. Both MR arteriography and MR venography were compared with MRI and conventional angiography. In MR angiography, 3- and 2-dimensional time-of-flight techniques were used.

Results.—In 63 patients, MR arteriography examinations were abnormal. In 45 patients, MR venography examinations were abnormal. Magnetic resonance arteriography showed the relation of intracranial arteries to meningomyeloceles in 3 cases (Fig 1). Magnetic resonance venography showed the relation of the sinus to the encephaloceles in 3 cases (Fig 12). Magnetic resonance arteriography was useful in detecting arterial narrow-

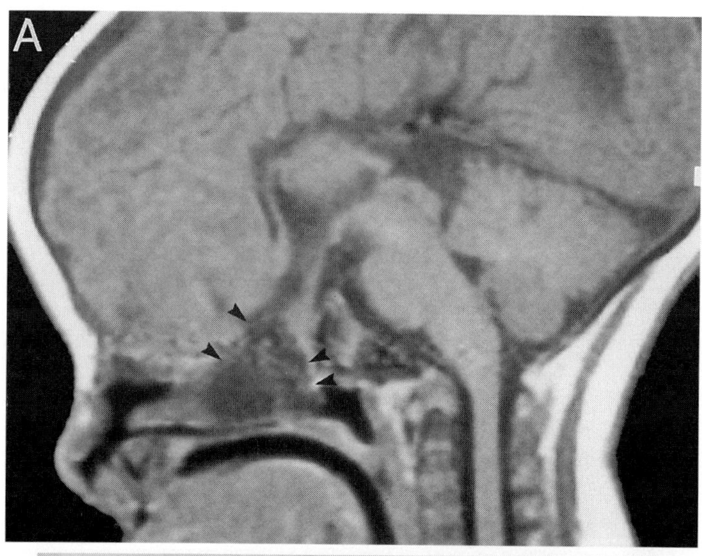

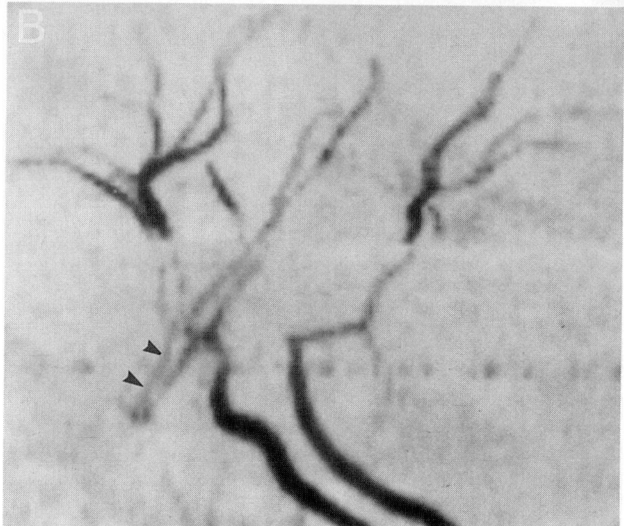

FIGURE 1.—Sphenoid encephalocele. **A**, sagittal T1-weighted image shows encephalomeningocele extending into the sphenoid sinus (*arrowheads*). **B**, lateral MR angiogram (double slabs) shows displacement of the proximal segment of the anterior cerebral arteries inferiorly into the encephalocele (*arrowhead*). (*Pediatr Radiol*; MR angiography in pediatric neurological disorders; Lee BCP, Park TS, Kaufman BA; 25:409–419; Fig 1; 1995; Copyright notice of Springer-Verlag.)

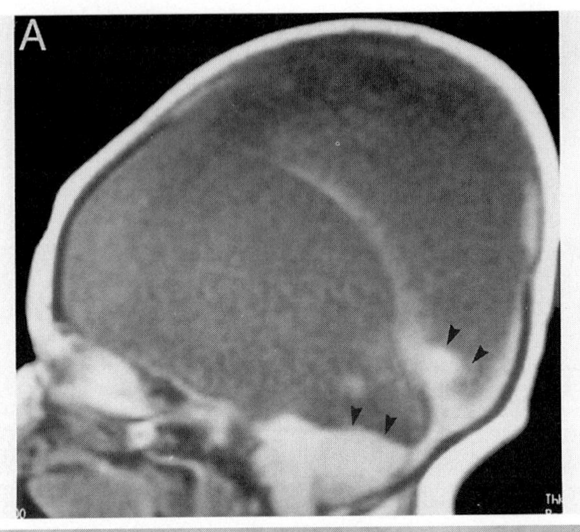

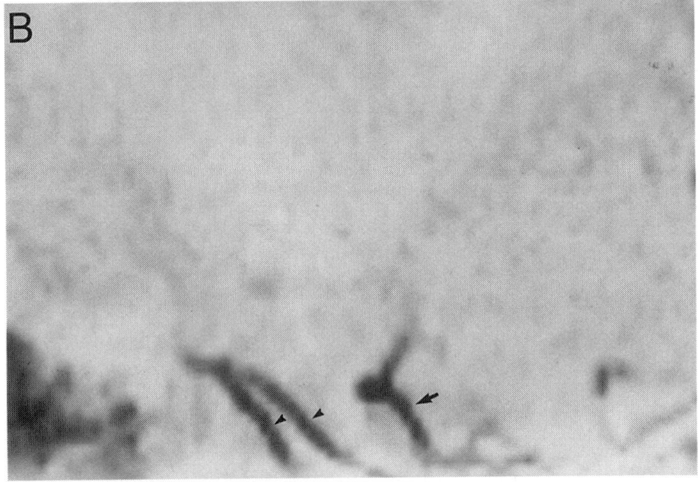

FIGURE 12.—Encephalocele. **A**, sagittal TW-weighted image shows encephalocele. **B**, off-lateral MR venogram shows interruption of the sagittal sinus st the site of encephalocele (*arrowheads*). (*Pediatr Radiol*; MR angiography in pediatric neurological disorders; Lee BC, Park TS, Kaufman BA: 25:409–419; Fig 12; 1995; Copyright notice of Springer-Verlag.)

ing, but the degree of stenosis was overestimated compared with conventional angiography.

Conclusion.—Assessment of vascular distortions related to congenital brain malformations and intracranial tumors was best done with MR arteriography and MR venography. However, MR venography was preferred for evaluating dural sinus and cerebral venous thrombosis and compression. Magnetic resonance arteriography had almost no role in surgical planning of vascular malformations and aneurysms and was not accurate in evaluating tumor vascularity or lesions in small arteries and arteritis.

▶ Magnetic resonance arteriography and MR venography are excellent adjuncts to MRI. Each can give additional information about vascular irregularities due to congenital CNS malformations and neoplasms. The authors accurately point out shortcomings of both MR angiographic methods in assessing vascular malformations for surgical planning. Accuracy and morphologic detail of conventional angiography is not supplanted. Other recent articles on the use of MRA arteriography in children recommend its screening capability and its value in assessing the carotid artery after extracorporeal membrane oxygenation.[1–3] Magnetic resonance arteriography and venography may be sustituted for conventional angiography to avoid its associated greater morbidity.

L.W. Young, M.D.

References

1. Koelfen W, Wentz U, Freund M, et al: Magnetic resonance angiography in 140 neuropediatric patients. *Pediatr Neurol* 12:31–38, 1995.
2. Vogl TJ, Balzer JO, Stemmler J, et al: MR angiography in neuropediatric problems: The technic and the clinical results. *Rofo. Fortschritte auf dem Gebiete der Rontgenstrahlen und der Neuen Bildgebenden Verfahren* 156:112–119, 1992.
3. Allison JW, Glasier CM, Start JE, et al: Head and neck MR angiography in pediatric patients: A pictorial essay. *Radiographics* 14:795–805, 1994.

Local Vascular CO2 Reactivity in the Infant Brain Assessed by Functional MRI

Toft PB, Leth H, Lou HC, et al (Danish Research Ctr of Magnetic Resonance, Hvidovre, Denmark)

Pediatr Radiol 25:420–424, 1995 4–8

Background.—Functional MRI (fMRI) is sensitive to increased cerebral blood flow (CBF) during brain activation and CO_2 inhalation in the adult brain, with a spatial resolution of about 2 mm. This imaging modality was used in the detection of local deficits in vascular CO_2 reactivity in brains of respiratory distressed infants.

Methods and Findings.—Five respiratory distressed, intubated infants underwent T2-sensitive gradient-echo MRI at 1.5 tesla to assess local cerebral vascular response to hyperventilation. Two adults who were hyperventilating voluntarily were also examined. The signal change during hyperventilation was sparse in 1 preterm infant. In the other 4 infants, who were born at term, the mean signal of the brain slice examined declined by 1.2% to 2.6% per kPa change in P_{CO_2}, reflecting reduced CBF during hyperventilation. In a pixel-wise analysis, vascular response was absent in the basal ganglia, thalamus, and occipital region. In the adults, the vascular reactivity was homogeneously distributed primarily over the gray matter.

Conclusion.—Functional MRI can demonstrate local impairment of vascular CO_2 reactivity in brains of respiratory distressed infants. A wide range of reactivity patterns was observed in the 4 term infants, in accordance with different patterns of locally impaired CBF regulation. Thus, it appears that the normal term brain can regulate CBF locally, most likely through musculated channels.

▶ The results of these experiments are a successful foray into functional MRI in the infant brain. By using a gradient-echo T2-weighted sequence, locally impaired cerebral CO_2 reactivity was shown, a particular advantage over the cumbersome xenon-133 method. Functional MRI is an advance in MRI technique that previously depended on correlation of morphologic MRI with other functional imaging methods, such as positron emission tomography.[1] Other recent articles that relate to perinatal asphyxia and MR brain imaging are listed.[2–7]

L.W. Young, M.D.

References

1. Kuenzle Ch, Baenziger O, Martin E, et al: Prognostic value of early MR imaging in term infants with severe perinatal asphyxia. *Neuropediatrics* 25:191–200, 1994.
2. Andersson JL, Sundin A, Valind S: A method for coregistration of PET and MR brain images. *J Nucl Med* 36:1307–1315, 1995.
3. Naruse S, Takaya K, Yoshioka H: Metabolic and functional magnetic resonance imaging of the brain: clinical application to pediatric brain diseases. *No To Hattatsu* 27:138–145, 1995.
4. Goplerud JM, Delivoria-Papadopoulos M: Nuclear magnetic resonance imaging and spectroscopy following asphyxia. *Clin Perinatol* 20:345–367, 1993.
5. De Reuck J, Decoo D, Vienne J, et al: Significance of white matter lucencies in posthypoxic-ischemic encephalopathy: Comparison of clinical status and of computed and positron emission tomographic findings. *Eur Neurol* 32:334–339, 1992.
6. Graham SH, Meyerhoff DJ, Bayne L, et al: Magnetic resonance spectroscopy of N-acetylaspartate in hypoxic-ischemic encephalopathy. *Ann Neurol* 35:490–494, 1994.

Neonates Treated With ECMO: Predictive Value of Early CT and US Neuroimaging Findings on Short-Term Neurodevelopmental Outcome

Bulas DI, Glass P, O'Donnell RM, et al (Children's Research Inst, Washington, DC; Children's Natl Med Ctr, Washington, DC; George Washington Univ, Washington, DC)

Radiology 195:407–412, 1995 4–9

Objective.—The predictive value for developmental outcome of neuroimaging findings in infants treated with extracorporeal membrane oxygenation (ECMO) was determined.

Background.—Some full-term neonates with cardiopulmonary failure are treated with ECMO. Such neonates are often in severe respiratory distress and are affected by hypoxia, acidosis, hypotension, or hyperventilation-induced alkalosis. With ECMO, however, there is increased risk of intracranial hemorrhage and infarction because of unilateral ligation of the carotid artery and jugular vein, alteration of cerebral blood flow, and administration of heparin.

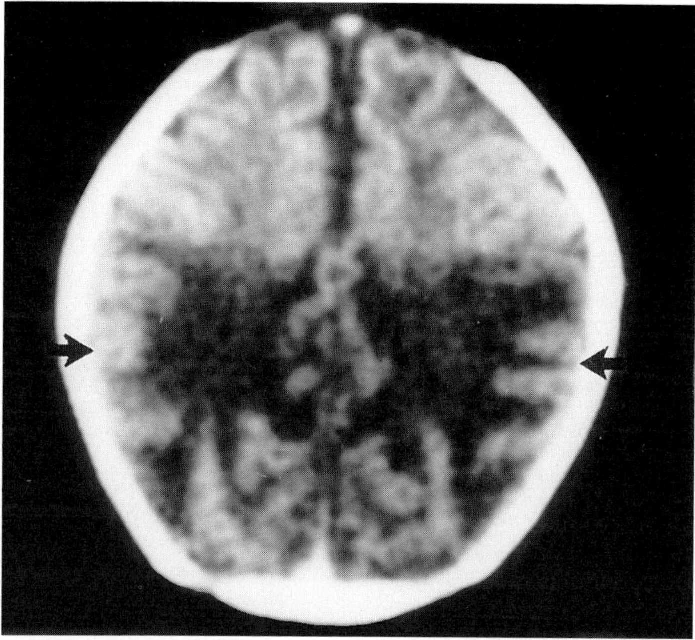

FIGURE 2.—Computed tomography scan obtained in a 2-week-old female infant who had undergone extracorporeal membrane oxygenation for treatment of meconium aspiration. Image demonstrates bilateral large occipitoparietal infarcts (*arrows*) consistent with a major nonhemorrhagic abnormality. (Courtesy of Bulas DI, Glass P, O'Donnell RM, et al: Neonates treated with ECMO: Predictive value of early CT and US neuroimaging findings on short-term neurodevelopmental outcome. *Radiology* 195:407–412, 1995; Radiological Society of North America.)

Methods.—Cranial ultrasonography was performed in neonates before venoarterial cannulation, and sonograms were obtained each day during treatment with ECMO. Cranial (CT) scans were obtained within 3 weeks of decannulation. Findings from CT scans and sonograms were categorized as major or minor hemorrhagic abnormalities or as major or minor nonhemorrhagic abnormalities (Fig 2). Neuroimaging examinations were assigned a score (Table 1), and findings were correlated with developmental outcome.

Results.—There were 183 surviving infants who were evaluated at 1 or 2 years. In 85 infants, there were neuroimaging abnormalities. In 105 infants, development was normal. Development was suspect in 37 infants and delayed in 41 infants. The incidence of delayed development in infants with normal imaging scores was 11% (Fig 4). Mean imaging scores were significantly worse in infants with delayed development. The sensitivity of normal imaging findings for predicting normal outcome was 65%, and specificity was 63%. Infants with nonhemorrhagic abnormalities were at higher risk for delayed development than infants with isolated hemorrhagic abnormalities.

TABLE 1.—Neuroimaging Scores

Abnormality	Score
Ventricular dilatation (relative weight = 1)	
Minimal	1.0
Moderate	2.0
Marked	3.0
Subarachnoid-space dilatation (relative weight = 1)	
Wide interhemispheric fissure	0.5
Large subarachnoid space	1.0
Hemorrhage (relative weight = 2)	
Sinus thrombosis	0.5
Subependymal	0.5
Single petechial	0.5
Scattered petechial	1.0
Intraventricular	1.0
Parenchymal	
Small (≤1 cm)	1.5
Large (>1 cm)	3.0
Extraaxial	
Small	0.5
Large	1.0
Parenchymal lesions (relative weight = 3)	
Focal atrophy	0.5
Periventricular leukomalacia or area of low attenuation	
Focal	0.5
Patchy	2.0
Diffuse	3.0
Generalized atrophy	
Mild	2.0
Moderate	3.0
Infarct	3.0

(Courtesy of Bulas DI, Glass P, O'Donnell RM, et al: Neonates treated with ECMO: Predictive value of early CT and US neuroimaging findings on short-term neurodevelopmental outcome. *Radiology* 195:407–412, 1995; Radiological Society of North America.)

Conclusion.—Neuroimaging scores can help establish risk categories for developmental outcome, but should not be used alone to predict outcome. The chance of survival for infants with a major intracranial hemorrhage is decreased, but those who survive have a better neurologic outcome than infants who survive major nonhemorrhagic injuries. Neuroimaging scores may improve with the use of MRI.

▶ The neuroimaging score from cranial ultrasound and CT examinations of infants placed on ECMO for general cardiopulmonary failure helped to predict developmental outcome in full and near-term neonates. The surprising greater risk in survivors from nonhemorrhagic lesions compared with hemorrhagic lesions is correlated with neurodevelopmental outcome. However, placement of an infant in a risk category should be done with caution because imaging findings alone do not offer high enough sensitivity and specificity percentages to generalize. Recent articles on ECMO correlation with cerebral injury and outcome and listed.[1–5] Brain single-photon emission is also being used to evaluate ECMO patients,[1] as well as MRI[2–4] and color Doppler.[5]

L.W. Young, M.D.

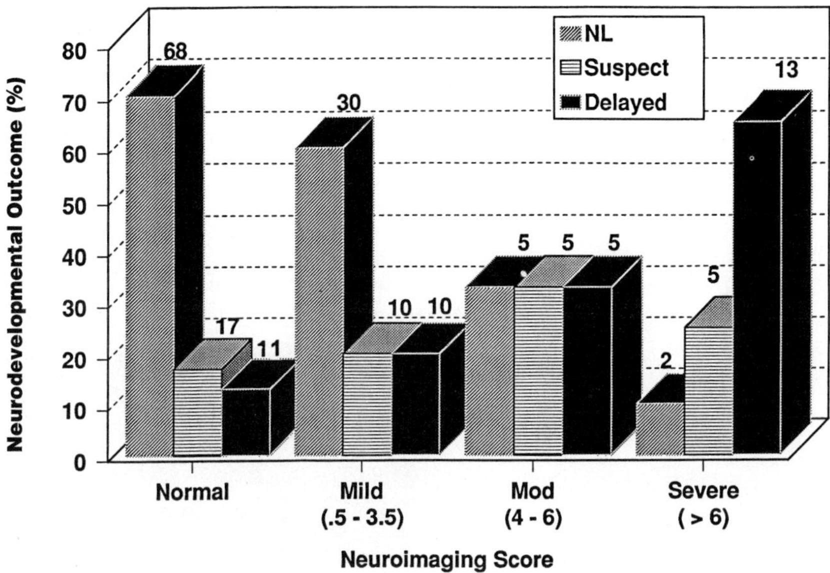

FIGURE 4.—Graph relates neurodevelopmental outcome to degree of abnormality at neuroimaging in neonates treated with extracorporeal membrane oxygenation. *Abbreviations*: *NL*, normal development; *Mod*, mederate. (Courtesy of Bulas DI, Glass P, O'Donnell RM, et al: Neonates treated with ECMO: Predictive value of early CT and US neuroimaging findings on short-term neurodevelopmental outcome. *Radiology* 195:407–412, 1995: Radiological Society of North America.)

References

1. Park CH, Spitzer AR, Desai HJ, et al: Brain SPECT in neonates following extracorporeal membrane oxygenation: Evaluation of technique and preliminary results. *J Nucl Med* 33:1943–1948, 1992.
2. Lazar EI, Abramson SJ, Weinstein S, et al: Neuroimaging of brain injury in neonates treated with extracorporeal membrane oxygenation: Lessons learned from serial examinations. *J Pediatr Surg* 29:186–190, 1994.
3. Griffin MP, Minifee PK, Landry SH, et al: Neurodevelopmental outcome in neonates after extracorporeal membrane oxygenation: Cranial magnetic resonance imaging and ultrasonography correlation. *J Pediatr Surg* 27:33–35, 1992.
4. Lago P. Rebsamen S, Clancy RR, et al: MRI, MRA, and neurodevelopmental outcome following neonatal ECMO. *Pediatr Neurol* 12:294–304, 1995.
5. Baumgart S. Streletz LJ, Needleman L, et al: Right common carotid artery reconstruction after extracorporeal membrane oxygenation: Vascular imaging, cerebral circulation, electroencephalographic, and neurodevelopmental correlates to recovery. *J Pediatr* 125:295–304, 1994.

Proton Magnetic Resonance Spectroscopy in Children With Acute Central Nervous System Injury

Auld KL, Ashwal S, Holshouser BA, et al (Loma Linda Univ, Calif; Huntington Med Research Insts, Pasadena, Calif; California Inst of Technology, Pasadena)

Pediatr Neurol 12:323–334, 1995 4–10

Background.—The biochemical state of the CNS can be examined noninvasively with proton MR spectroscopy (^{1}H-MRS). When performed carefully, nonquantitative ^{1}H-MRS can provide useful additional informa-

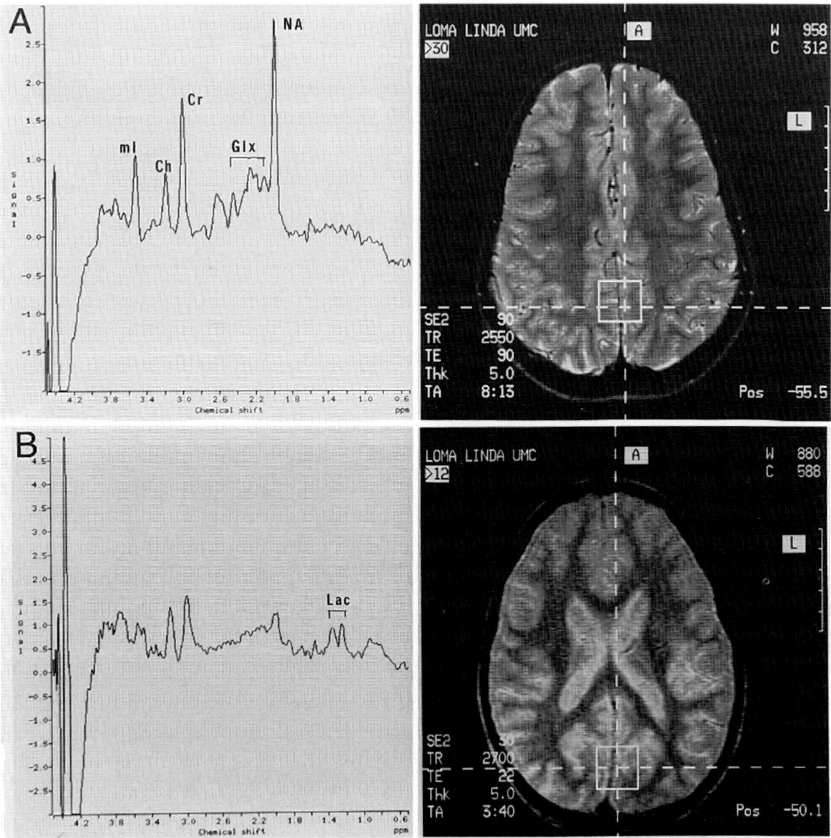

FIGURE 3.—Proton magnetic resonance spectroscopy (^{1}H-MRS) spectra in older children. **A,** Spectra of occipital gray matter obtained in a normal boy, 8 years (echo time 30 msec, recovery time, 3 s). **B,** ^{1}H-MRS from a girl, 4 years (Patient 11) who is in a persistent vegetative state secondary to hypoxic–ischemic injury displaying decreased *N*-acetylaspartate (NA) and creatinine (Cr) peaks and the presence of lactate compared with control (echo time 20 msec, recovery time, 3 s) and the recovery time–weighted MRI within 24 hours displaying edema. In this patient the NA/Cr and NA/choline–containing compound ratios are also decreased. (Reprinted by permission of the publisher from Proton magnetic resonance spectroscopy in children with acute central nervous system injury; Auld KL, Ashwal D, Holshouser BA, et al; *Pediatr Neurol* 12:323–334; Copyright 1995 by Elsevier Science Inc.)

tion. It is particularly useful in the assessment of a wide range of acute severe neuronal disturbances in children in ICUs.

Methods.—Thirty infants and children with acute CNS injuries underwent ^{1}H-MRS to determine whether changes in specific metabolite ratios can predict outcome. The mean patient age was 38 months. The mean time of study after the insult was 7 days. The occipital gray and parietal white matter were studied.

Findings.—When patients with good or moderately good outcomes were compared with those with bad outcomes, significant differences were found. The ratios of *N*-acetylaspartate (NA) to creatinine and phosphocreatinine and the ratio of NA to choline-containing compounds were significantly lower among patients with bad outcomes. Eighty percent of the children with bad outcomes and none with good or moderate outcomes showed the presence of lactate. The outcomes of 94% of the patients could be classified correctly based on linear discriminant analysis and the combinations of 4 clinical variables. The outcomes of 81% were correctly classified through spectroscopic variables alone. All outcomes could be classified correctly by the combination of clinical and ^{1}H-MRS variables (Fig 3).

Conclusions.—Proton magnetic resonance spectroscopy may be useful in conjunction with clinical evaluation in determining neurologic outcomes in children with serious acute CNS injuries. Additional research on this emerging technology is needed to determine which patient populations benefit most from it, the optimal timing and number of studies required to obtain valid and reliable data, metabolite quantitation, and the relationship between ^{1}H-MRS and other noninvasive measures of cerebral function for predicting outcome.

▶ Proton MR spectroscopy combined with clinical findings, as attested in this and other recent articles,[1–5] has substantial promise in predicting outcomes and possibly influencing management strategies of acute CNS injuries in children.

L.W. Young, M.D.

References

1. Harada M, Tanouchi M, Aral K, et al: Therapeutic efficacy of a case of pyruvate dehydrogenase complex deficiency monitored by localized proton magnetic resonance spectroscopy. *Magn Reson Imaging* 14:129–133, 1996.
2. Duncan DB, Herholz K, Kagel H, et al: Positron emission tomography and magnetic resonance spectroscopy of cerebral glycolysis in children with congenital lactic acidosis. *Ann Neurol* 37:351–358, 1995.
3. Holzbach U, Hanefeld F, Helms G, et al: Localized proton magnetic resonance spectroscopy of cerebral abnormalities in children with carbohydrate-deficient glycoprotein syndrome. *Acta Paediatr (Germany)* 84:781–786, 1995.
4. Shevell MI, Matthews PM, Scriver CR, et al: Cerebral dysgenesis and lactic acidemia: An MRI/MRS phenotype associated with pyruvate dehydrogenase deficiency. *Pediatr Neurol* 11:224–229, 1994.
5. McConnell JR, Swindells S, Ong CS, et al: Prospective utility of cerebral proton magnetic resonance spectroscopy in monitoring HIV infection and its associated neurological impairment. *AIDS Res Hum Retroviruses* 10:977–982, 1994.

Thyroid Scintigraphy and Perchlorate Discharge Test in the Diagnosis of Congenital Hypothyroidism

El-Desouki M, Al-Jurayyan N, Al-Nuaim A, et al (King Saud Univ, Riyadh, Saudi Arabia; Ministry of Health, Riyadh, Saudi Arabia)

Eur J Nucl Med 22:1005–1008, 1995 4–11

Introduction.—Congenital hypothyroidism (CH) may be caused by an absent or hypoplastic thyroid gland, an ectopic gland, or a congenital error of thyroid hormone metabolism. Determining the presence and location of the thyroid gland in hypothyroid children is crucial in planning for genetic counselling and determining prognosis. Thyroid scintigraphy has been recommended in the evaluation of these children. The scintigraphic findings in infants evaluated for CH were reviewed.

Methods.—Over a 5-year period, 147 infants with clinically diagnosed CH underwent a technetium-99m pertechnetate thyroid scan, followed by a perchlorate discharge test (PDT) 24 to 48 hours later. Thyroid uptake of potassium perchlorate was measured every 15 minutes for 1 hour and every 30 minutes for an additional hour. A discharge of more than 50% indicated a complete organification defect, and a discharge of 20% to 50% indicated a partial organification defect. The scans were reviewed without knowledge of other laboratory test results and were classified as indicating no thyroid activity, ectopic location, or normal location with normal or increased size and uptake.

Results.—Of the 147 infants, 32 (21.8%) were found to be athyrotic, 62 (42.2%) had an ectopic thyroid, and 53 (36%) had a normally located thyroid gland with increased uptake. Ectopic glands, seen in either the lingual or the sublingual position, were either large or small and demonstrated either decreased or increased uptake. Among the patients with ectopic glands, high uptake was associated with an enlarged gland, in which the PDT showed an organification defect (Fig 3).

Discussion.—Thyroid scintigraphy and perchlorate discharge testing revealed the full spectrum of possible gland anatomy, location, and size in children with congenital hypothyroidism. Therefore, quantitative ^{99m}Tc pertechnetate and PDT play an important role in obtaining etiologic, genetic, and prognostic information in the clinical evaluation of hypothyroid infants.

▶ Use of thyroid scintigraphy and the perchlorate discharge test are worthwhile for determining etiologic, genetic, and prognostic information about CH. The ectopic thyroid is a frequent cause of CH. It may have an inborn error of thyroid hormone metabolism that can cause dysmorphogenesis that may be demonstrated by the perchlorate discharge test. Application of the perchlorate test to determine defects in organification is valuable in any milieu but especially in Saudi Arabia where the incidence of thyroid dysmorphogenesis in CH is higher. Other recent articles on thyroglobulin newborn screening for congenital hypothyroidism and correlation with scintigraphy

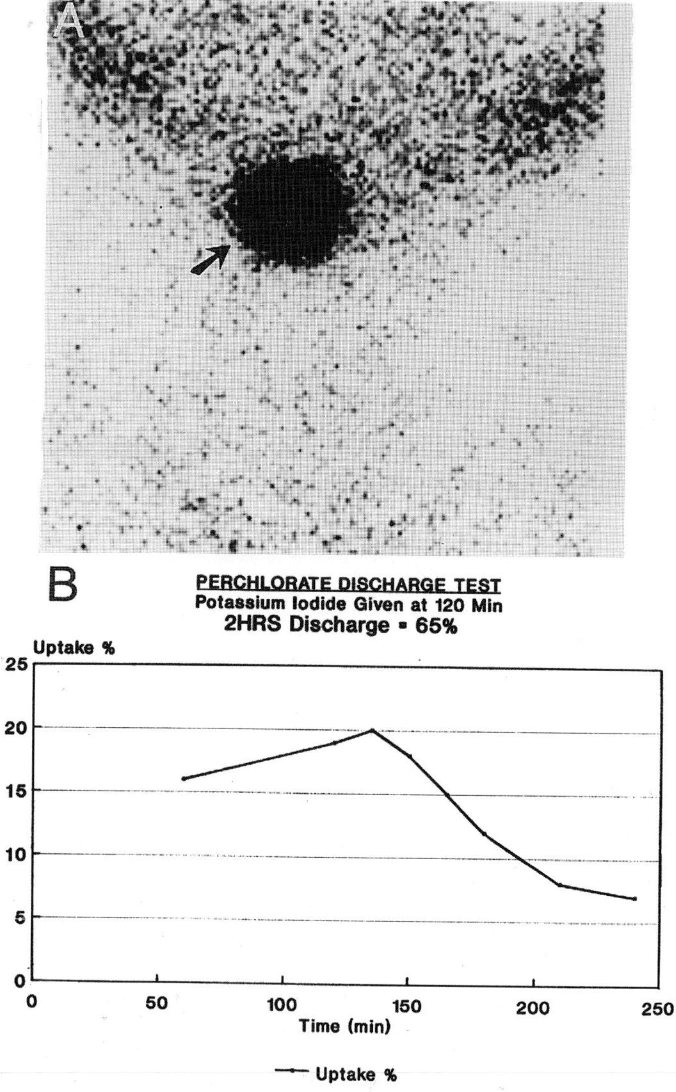

FIGURE 3.—A, technetium-99m–pertechnetate thyroid scintigraphy, revealing a large sublingual gland (*arrow*), which is demonstrating increased activity. The perchlorate discharge test result (**B**) was strongly positive. (*Eur J Nucl Med*; Thyroid scintigraphy and perchlorate discharge test in the diagnosis of congenital hypothyroidism; El-Desouki M, Al-Jurayyan N, Al Nuaim A, et al; 22:1005–1008; Fig 3; 1995; Copyright notice of Springer-Verlag.)

are listed.[1,2] Ultrasonography has been reported in recent articles [3,4] to be useful, especially in identifying either a small eutopic thyroid gland or an ectopic thyroid gland.

L.W. Young, M.D.

References

1. Mitchell ML, Hermos RJ: Measurement of thyroglobulin in newborn screening specimens from normal and hypothyroid infants. *Clin Endocrinol* 42:523–527, 1995.
2. Nadel HR: Where are we with nuclear medicine in pediatrics? *Eur J Nucl Med* 22:1433–1451, 1995.
3. Takashima S, Nomura N, Tanaka H, et al: Congenital hypothyroidism: Assessment with ultrasound. *Am J Neuroradiol* 16:1117–1123, 1995.
4. Wakamoto H, Miyazaki M, Tatsumi K, et al: Thyroid ultrasonography in congenital isolated thyroid stimulating hormone deficiency. *Arch Dis Child* 72:439–440, 1995.

Musculoskeletal System

Physiological Bowlegs or Infantile Blount's Disease. Some New Aspects on an Old Problem

Eggert P, Viemann M (Universitäts-Kinderklinik, Kiel, Germany)
Pediatr Radiol 26:349–352, 1996 4–12

Background.—Differentiating between physiologic bowlegs and infantile Blount's disease is very difficult in children aged 11–30 months. The current study investigated whether the metaphyseal/diaphyseal angle is suitable for distinguishing one diagnosis from the other.

Methods.—Fourteen children with severe bowing of the legs were studied retrospectively. The patients were examined, and the tibiofemoral and metaphyseal/diaphyseal angles on radiographs obtained at the initial evaluations were measured (Fig 1).

Findings.—As expected, the tibiofemoral angles varied substantially, making it impossible to differentiate between Blount's disease and physiological bowing using this parameter. The variable findings about metaphyseal/diaphyseal angle measurement were unexpected. Contrary to previous results by Levine and Drennan, measures of the metaphyseal/diaphyseal angle apparently do not differentiate between tibia vara and physiological bowing. In the current series, some of these angles fell in a range that seemed to indicate physiologic bowlegs according to Levine and Drennan, which was likely because the bowlegging disappeared in these children during the next months. However, many metaphyseal/diaphyseal angles fell in a range definitely indicating Blount's disease, which was clearly incorrect because bowlegging in these children also disappeared in the following months (Fig 3).

Conclusion.—Even with the measurement of the metaphyseal/diaphyseal angle, it is impossible to safely differentiate physiologic bowlegging and early manifestations of infantile Blount's disease in 11- to 30-month-old children. The authors question whether infantile Blount's disease is a diagnosis in its own right.

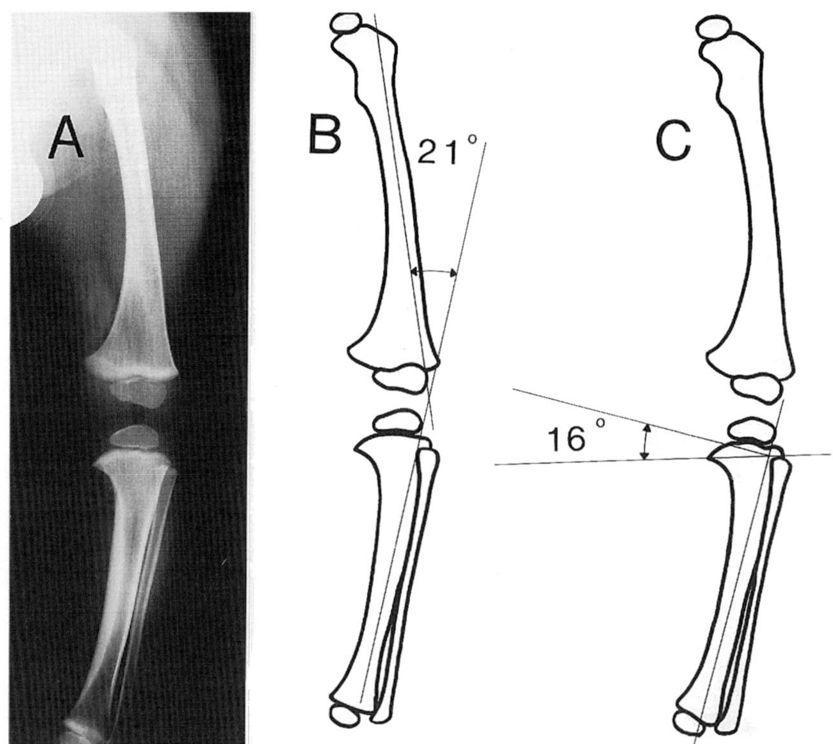

FIGURE 1.—**A**, radiograph of the left leg of a girl aged 18 months showing considerable bowing. **B**, the tibiofemoral angle is measured between the axes of the femur and the tibia. C, the metaphyseal/diaphyseal angle is defined as the angle between a line perpendicular to the axis of the tibia and a line through the most distal ossified beak of the medial and lateral beak of the tibial metaphysis. (*Pediatr Radiol*; Physiological bowlegs or infantile Blount's disease. Some new aspects on an old problem; Eggert P, Viemann M; 26:349–352; Fig 1; 1996; Copyright notice of Springer-Verlag.)

► This article presents clarifying if not specific diagnostic aspects on the problem of physiologic bowlegs versus infantile Blount's disease. The lack of any specificity of the tibiofemoral angle is clearly shown. The tibial metaphyseal/diaphyseal angle similarly has substantial overlap with physiologic bowing[1]. Perhaps Dr. John Caffey's emphasis on the differences in configurations of the medial metaphyseal margins of the proximal tibias in physiologic bowing and Blount's disease are possibly better in differentiating physiologic bowing from infantile Blount's disease than any measurements are.

L.W. Young, M.D.

Reference

1. Ducou le Pointe H, Mousselard H, Rudelli A, et al: Blount's disease: Magnetic resonance imaging. *Pediatr Radiol* 25:12–14,1995.

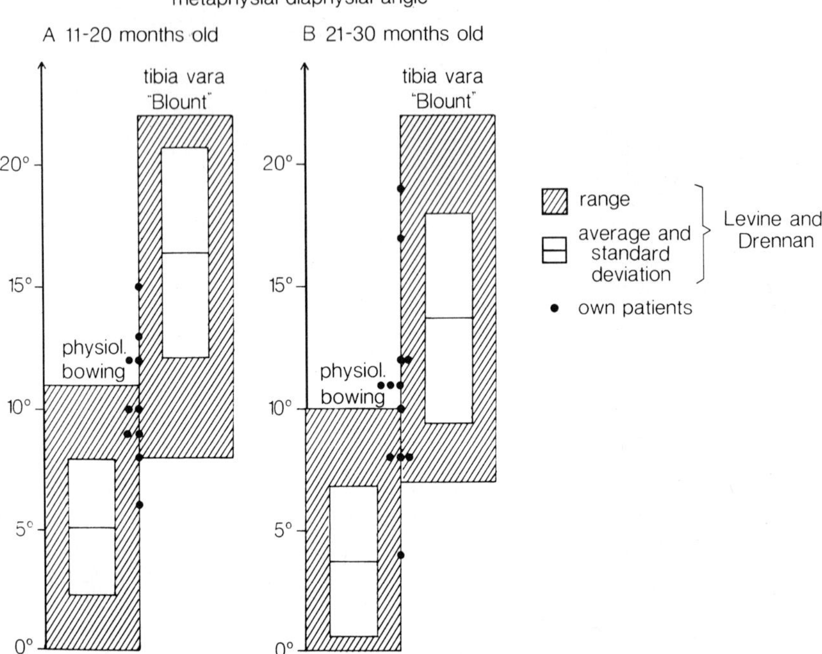

FIGURE 3.—A and B. A diagram showing the age-dependent metaphyseal/diaphyseal angle of our patients compared with data published by Levine and Drennan (see original article for complete reference information). (*Pediatr Radiol*; Physiological bowlegs or infantile Blount's disease. Some new aspects on an old problem; Eggert P, Viemann M; 26:349–352; Fig 3; 1996; Copyright notice of Springer-Verlag.)

Blount's Disease: Magnetic Resonance Imaging

Ducou le Point H, Mousselard H, Rudelli A, et al (Hôpital d'enfants, Paris)

Pediatr Radiol 25:12–14, 1995 4–13

Background.—Blount's disease is characterized by a tibia vara caused by a growth disturbance of the medial tibial plate. The cause is unknown. Although the radiologic findings of Blount's disease have been extensively reported; changes on MR images have been less well described.

Methods.—The radiographic and MR images of 9 patients treated for idiopathic tibia vara were reviewed. Six patients were affected unilaterally, and 3 bilaterally. Initial radiographs were staged according to Cantonne's criteria (Fig 1). A 0.5- or 1.5-tesla apparatus was used for MR imaging.

Findings.—In all patients, bony epiphyses were poorly developed. The cartilaginous component of the epiphyses compensated partly for the collapse of the physes in 6 tibiae and completely in the other 6. Two tibiae showed an abnormal area between the medial meniscus and cartilaginous part of the epiphysis. The medial meniscus was abnormally large in 4 cases, and the signal in the medial meniscus was abnormal in 2 (Fig 4).

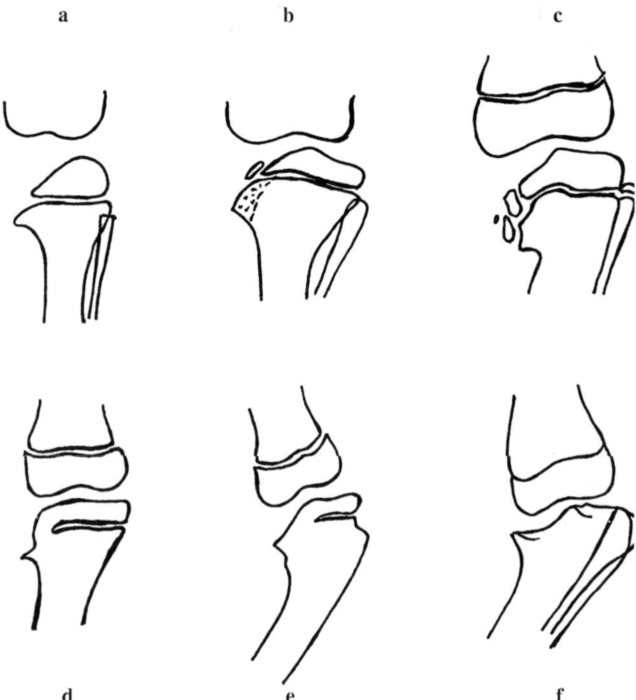

FIGURE 1.—Cantonne's classification. **A**, stage I (2–3 years old): asymmetry of the tibial epiphysis. Note the medial metaphyseal break. **B**, stage II (3–5 years old): sloped epiphysis (oblique, downward and medial) and uneven metaphyseal shape. **C**, stage III (5–8 years old): vertical medial epiphysis and metaphysis, medial calcifications. **D**, stage IV (8–11 years old): small medial bony bridge. **E**, stage V: medial bony bridge. **F**, stage VI: adult aspect of the physis. (*Pediatr Radiol*; Blount's disease: Magnetic resonance imaging; Ducou le Point H, Mousselard H, Rudelli A, et al; 25:12–14; Fig 1; 1995; Copyright notice of Springer-Verlag.)

Conclusion.—In patients with Blount's disease, the shape of the ossified and cartilaginous epiphysis affects treatment. Metaphyseal valgus osteotomy is done when the epiphysis is normally shaped, and elevation of the medial tibial plateau is performed to correct an abnormal epiphyseal shape, such as a pagoda roof. Magnetic resonance imaging demonstrates the shape of the ossified and cartilaginous epiphysis as well as meniscal and physeal abnormalities. Thus it may affect treatment choice. Early treatment improves prognosis.

► Cartilaginous and fibrous imaging by MRI gives additional information to help plan surgery in Blount's disease. This report represents an encouraging initial analysis of abnormal findings shown by MRI in Blount's disease. Certainly the differentiation between physiologic bowlegs and infantile Blount's disease presents a problem that may not be resolved by measurement of angles, as addressed by Eggert.[1] The best results of surgery before

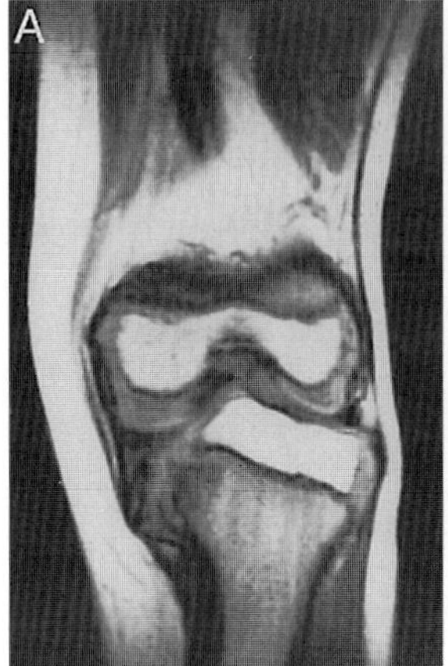

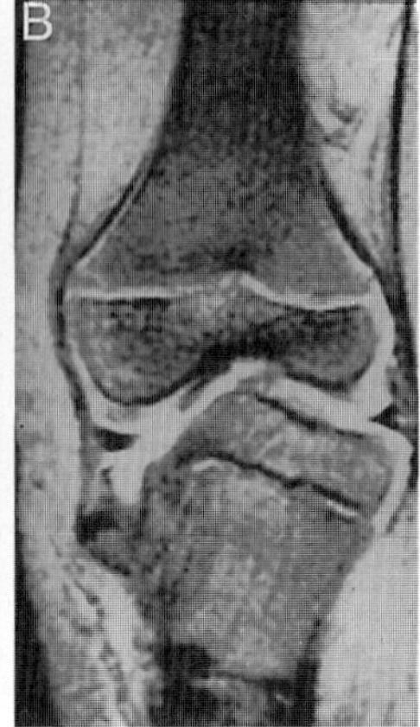

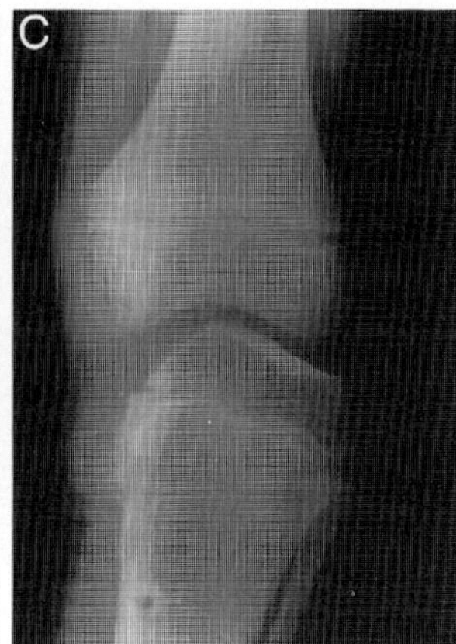

FIGURE 4.—Blount's disease in the left knee of a 5-year-old girl, Cantonne's stage III. **A**, coronal T1-weighted image (recovery time 600 msec/echo time 27 msec): sloped epiphysis. The physis ends medially at the same level as the ossified epiphysis. An abnormal area of low signal intensity is seen below the medial meniscus. **B**, coronal T2-weighted image (recovery time 500 msec/echo time 30 msec/15 degrees) 1 year after surgery: the abnormal area is still of low spinal intensity; a localized bony bridge is now clearly visible. **C**, plain radiograph 1 year after surgery shows the same localized bony bridge. (*Pediatr Radiol*; Blount's disease: Magnetic resonance imaging; Duco le Point H, Mousselard H, Rudelli A, et al; 25:12–14; Fig 4; 1995; Copyright notice of Springer-Verlag.)

age 9 years have been reported recently by Catonne.[2] Another article discusses the importance of defining femoral varus in late onset Blount's disease.[3]

L.W. Young, M.D.

References

1. Eggert P, Viemann M: Physiological bowlegs or infantile Blount's disease. Some new aspects on an old problem. *Pediatr Radiol* 26:349–352, 1995.
2. Catonne Y, Dubousset J, Seringe R, et al: Coxa vara in children. Apropos of 28 cases. *Revue de Chirurgie Orthopedique et Reparatrice de l Appareil Moteur* 78:153–163, 1992.
3. Kline SC, Bostrum M, Griffin PP: Femoral varus: an important component in late-onset Blount's disease. *J Pediatr Orthop* 12:197–206, 1992.

Legg-Calvé-Perthes Disease: Comparison of Conventional Radiography, MR Imaging, Bone Scintigraphy and Arthrography

Kaniklides C, Lönnerholm T, Moberg A, et al (Univ Hosp, Uppsala, Sweden)
Acta Radiol 36:434–439, 1995 4–14

Background.—In patients with Legg-Calvé-Perthes disease (LCPD), the most important prognostic factors are the extent to which the femoral head is involved and the presence of lateral subluxation of the hip. These factors are less sensitively assessed by conventional radiographs, so additional studies such as arthrography, bone scintigraphy, and MRI are often

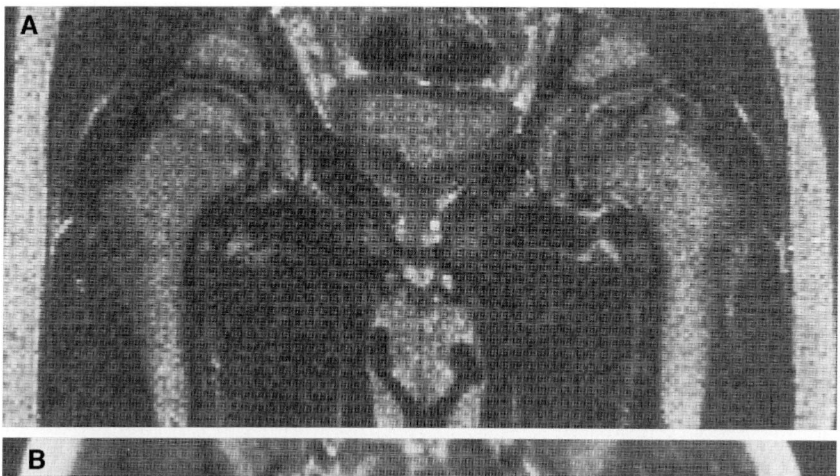

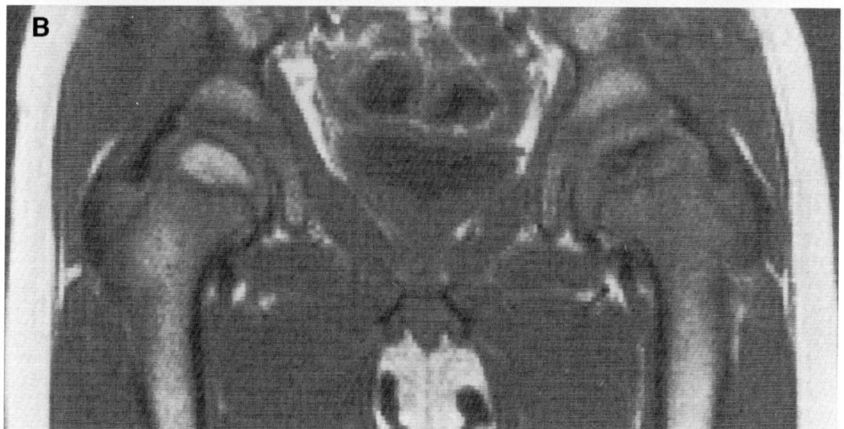

FIGURE 1.—Boy, 4 years, with Legg-Calvé-Perthes disease of the left hip. **A,** T2-weighted MR image shows structures with increased signal intensity located medially in the epiphysis, suggestive of revascularization on the left side. The cartilaginous capital epiphysis is poorly covered by the acetabulum. The right hip is normal. **B,** corresponding T1-weighted image shows a large avascular lesion with low-signal intensity, classifed as Catterall group 3. (Courtesy of Kaniklides C, Lönnerholm T, Moberg A, et al: Legg-Calvé-Perthes disease: Comparison of conventional radiography, MR imaging, bone scintigraphy and arthrography. *Acta Radiol* 36:434–439, 1995.)

needed. Examinations by these 4 radiologic modalities were compared for their facility to show the size of the necrosis, the degree of lateral subluxation, and the disease stage in patients with LCPD.

Methods.—The prospective study included 24 hips of 22 patients with LCPD. All hips were evaluated by all 4 modalities within a 1-month period at the time of diagnosis. Conventional radiography included anteroposterior and Lauenstein projections of both hips. The MRI scans included coronal views of both hips and sagittal views of the affected hip. The bone scintigrams, also performed in anteroposterior and Lauenstein projections, were obtained 2 hours after injection of hydroxydiphosphonate, and bilateral arthrography was performed with the use of general anesthesia. Three radiologists evaluated each of the imaging studies independently.

Results.—The best technique for evaluating the extent of involvement of the femoral head—better than conventional radiography or bone scintigraphy—was MRI. However, arthrography was at least as good as MRI in depicting the shape of the articular surfaces and in determining whether lateral subluxation was present. The conventional radiographs were not very sensitive in determining the degree of lateral subluxation and the extent of femoral head necrosis. Valuable anatomical and pathophysiologic information about the extent and location of femoral head involvement, as well as about the degree of lateral subluxation, was provided by MRI. Magnetic resonance imaging was also better than bone scintigraphy at showing revascularization (Fig 1, A and B).

Conclusion.—Conventional radiography remains an important technique for the diagnosis of LCPD. Magnetic resonance imaging findings can establish or exclude this diagnosis, as well as demonstrate revascularization or loss of containment, and may provide important information about the extent and location of necrosis. For patients with advanced deformity, significant lateral subluxation, or extremely restricted abduction, dynamic arthrography may be needed to tell whether containment of the femoral head is surgically achievable.

► The comparative values of the currently available imaging modalities for the diagnosis of LCPD are aptly addressed in this article. Since a previous YEAR BOOK reference,[1] the superior contribution of MRI is better understood. Magnetic resonance imaging detects the extent and location of femoral head necrosis, the presence of revascularization, and the loss of acetabular containment. Each of the other modalities—radiography, arthrography, and scintigraphy—may contribute to these findings. Not any of the other modalities alone is as specific as MRI. Demonstration on MRI of early marrow edema, as well as extent of necrosis in the epiphysis, is considered the most important indicator of the disease's prognosis.[2] Bone scintigraphy for LCPD has been compared with MRI.[3] Scintigraphic cross-sectional imaging by single-photon emission CT approaches MRI's facility in demonstrating extent of disease.[4]

L.W. Young, M.D.

References

1. 1995 YEAR BOOK OF DIAGNOSTIC RADIOLOGY, p 442.
2. Ranner G, Fotter R, Linhart W, et al: Radiologic diagnosis of Perthes disease [review]. *Radiologe* 34:21–29, 1994.
3. Uno A, Hattori T, Noritake K, et al: Legg-Calvé-Perthes disease in the evolutionary period: Comparison of magnetic resonance imaging with bone scintigraphy. *J Pediatr Orthop* 15:362–367, 1995.
4. Oshima M, Yoshihasi Y, Ito K, et al: Initial stage of Legg-Calvé-Perthes disease: Comparison of three-phase bone scintigraphy and SPECT with MR imaging. *Eur J Radiol* 15:107–112, 1992.

MRI Marrow Observations in Thalassemia: The Effects of the Primary Disease, Transfusional Therapy, and Chelation

Levin TL, Sheth SS, Ruzal-Shapiro C, et al (Babies and Children's Hosp, New York; Columbia-Presbyterian Med Ctr, New York; Mem Sloan-Kettering Cancer Ctr, New York)

Pediatr Radiol 25:607–613, 1995 4–15

Background.—Thalassemia is characterized by ineffective erythropoiesis, intramedullary hemolysis, and bone marrow expansion. Treatment consists of hypertransfusions to maintain hemoglobin greater than 9 to 10 g/dL to suppress marrow expansion. Chelation with deferoxamine decreases the heavy iron load associated with repeated transfusions. The MR appearance of bone marrow in untreated, hypertransfused but not chelated, and hypertransfused and well-chelated patients was reported.

Methods.—Images of the spine, pelvis, and femurs were obtained on T1- and T2-weighted images in 13 patients. Three patients, aged 2.5 to 3 years, were not treated. Another 3 patients, aged 6 months to 8 years, were hypertransfused but not chelated because of their age. The remaining 7 patients, aged 12 to 35 years, were hypertransfused and chelated. The signal appearance of marrow and that of surrounding muscle and fat were compared. Fatty marrow—isointense with subcutaneous fat—and red marrow—hypointense to fat and slightly hyperintense to muscle—were

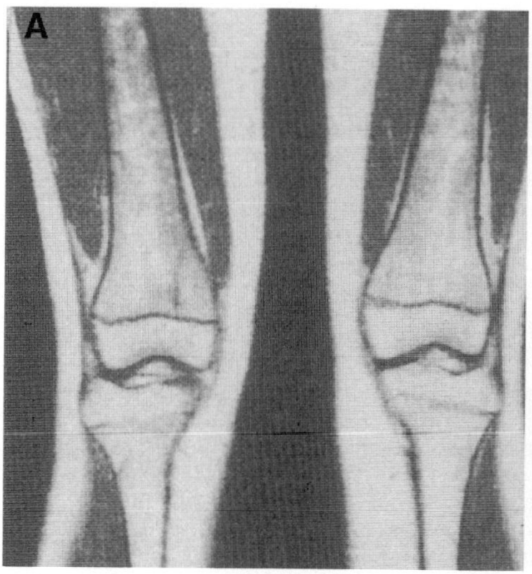

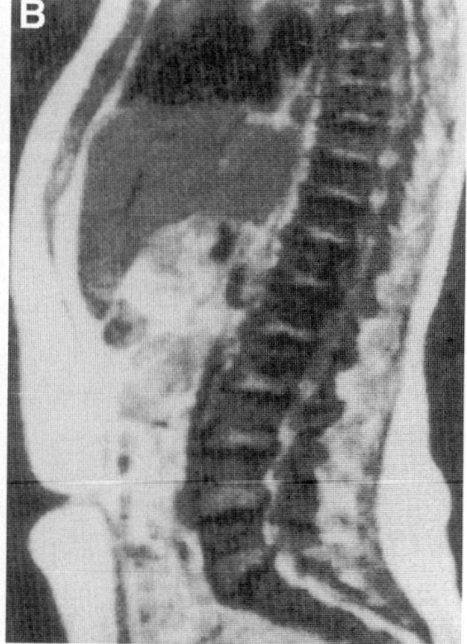

FIGURE 6.—**A,** transfused and well-chelated 15-year-old patient: Coronal T1-weighted (recovery time 516 msec/echo time 30 msec) image of the knees demonstrates heterogeneous signal consistent with both red and fatty marrow in the femurs. Modeling deformity of the femurs is present. **B,** sagittal T1-weighted (recovery time 560 msec/echo time 30 msec) image of the spine in the same patient demonstrates low signal in the vertebral bodies consistent with iron deposition in the central marrow. Vertebral body flattening reflects early treatment with deferoxamine. (*Pediatr Radiol;* MRI marrow observations in thalassemia: The effects of the primary disease, transfusional therapy, and chelation; Levin TL, Sheth SS, Ruzal-Shapiro C, et al; 25:607–613; Fig 6; 1995; Copyright notice of Springer-Verlag.)

also compared. Iron deposition within red marrow was interpreted as indicating marrow hypointense to muscle.

Findings.—The appearance of the signal in untreated patients indicated red marrow through the central and peripheral skeleton. Marked iron deposition in the central and peripheral skeleton was noted in patients hypertransfused but not chelated. Patients who were hypertransfused and well chelated had iron deposition in the central skeleton and a mixed appearance of marrow in the peripheral skeleton (Fig 6).

Conclusion.—A patient's transfusion and chelation therapy determines the MR appearance of bone marrow in thalassemia. Despite chelation treatment, iron is deposited in sites of active red marrow. Red marrow retreats centrally with age and affects the iron deposition pattern. The biological effects of iron deposition in the long-term have not been established.

▶ The use of MRI for observation of treatment of patients with thalassemia is of substantial value, as shown by this article. Magnetic resonance imaging also has value in corroborating findings in sickle cell anemia.[1, 2] Magnetic resonance imaging findings in the normal, age-related conversion of bone marrow are a requisite template for better appreciating the thalassemia and sickle cell anemia findings.[3, 4] Magnetic resonance imaging of bone marrow findings in osteosarcoma and in Ewing's sarcoma were also recently reported.[5–7]

L.W. Young, M.D.

References

1. Fernandez M, Slovis TL, Whitten-Shurney W: Maxillary sinus marrow hyperplasia in sickle cell anemia. *Pediatr Radiol* 25:209S–211S, 1995.
2. Hernigou P, Bernaudin F: Course of bone tissue after bone marrow allograft in adolescents with sickle cell disease. *Rev Chir Orthop Reparatrice Appar Mot* 80:138–143, 1994.
3. Yamada M, Matsuzaka T, Uetani M: Normal age-related conversion of bone marrow in the mandible: MR imaging findings. *AJR* 165:1223–1228, 1995.
4. Taccone A, Oddone M, Occhi M, et al: MRI "road-map" of normal age-related bone marrow. *Pediatr Radiol* 25:588–595, 1995.
5. Kauffman WM, Fletcher BD, Hanna SL, et al: MR imaging findings in recurrent primary osseous ewing sarcoma. *Magn Reson Imaging* 12:1147–1153, 1994.
6. Ryan SP, Weinberger E, White KS, et al: MR imaging of bone marrow in children with osteosarcoma: Effect of granulocyte colony-stimulating factor. *AJR* 165:915–920, 1995.
7. Harris AC, Todd WM, Hackney MH, et al: Bone marrow changes associated with recombinant granulocyte-macrophage and granulocyte colony-stimulating factors. Discrimination of granulocytic regeneration. *Arch Pathol Lab Med* 118:624–629, 1994.

Value of RARE-MRI Sequences in the Diagnosis of Lymphangiomatosis in Children

Stöver B, Laubenberger J, Hennig J, et al (Univ of Freiburg, Germany; Charité Humboldt Univ, Berlin)

Magn Reson Imaging 13:481–488, 1995 4–16

Objective.—Three patients with extensive cavernous lymphangiomatosis were examined with MRI using both conventional spin-echo sequences

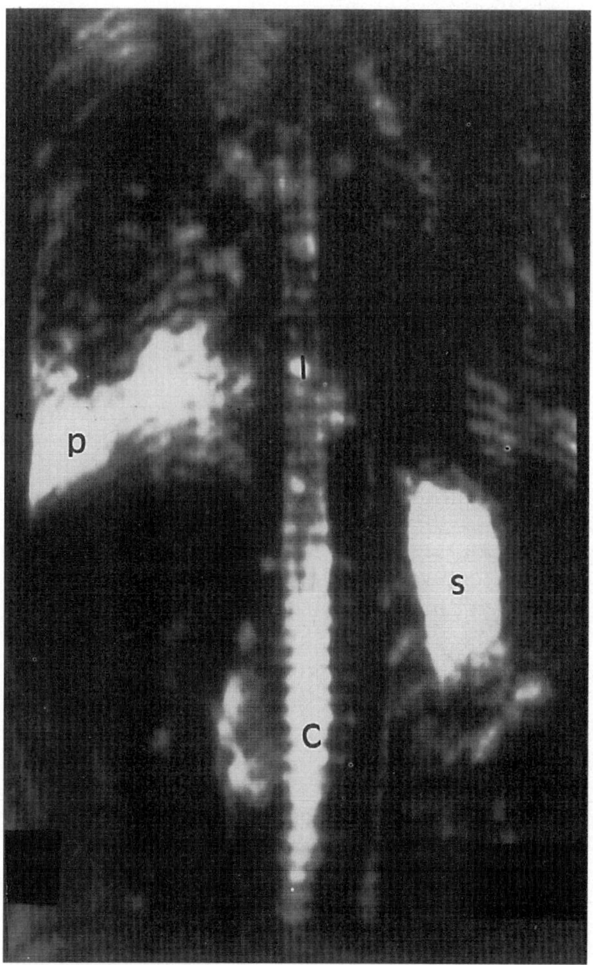

FIGURE 1.—Girl, 7 years. B, rapid acquisition with relaxation enhancement–hydrography (recovery time 10 sec/echo time 25 msec) including the thorax and abdomen in 1 coronal view. *Abbreviations: p,* pleural effusion (i.e., chylothorax predominantly right sided); *C,* cerebrospinal fluid; *L,* 1 of the spinal lesions located in the tenth thoracic vertebral body; in addition, 1 above the seventh and eighth, 2 below the first and third vertebral body of the lumbar spine; *S,* liquid in the stomach. (Reprinted from *Magn Reson Imaging*; vol 13; Stöver B, Laubenberger J, Hennig J, et al; Value of RARE-MRI sequences in the diagnosis of lymphangiomatosis in children; pp 481–488, Copyright 1995; with kind permission from Elsevier Science Ltd, The Boulevard, Langford Lane, Kidlington OX5 1GB, UK.)

and rapid acquisition with relaxation enhancement (RARE)–MR hydrography. These cases demonstrate the value of RARE-MR hydrography in detecting multiple lesions and excluding the diagnosis of hemangiomatosis.

Patients and Methods.—The patients, all female, were aged 7, 9, and 22 years. The whole skeleton was involved in the 7-year-old girl and the left gluteal and pelvic region in the 9-year-old girl. Surgery was performed 3 times in the remaining patient, at 4 years for removal of lymphangioma in the neck; at 11 years for removal of a large lymphatic mass involving the neck, the axilla, and the right thoracic wall; and at 22 years to remove a 2 by 2 cm mass of the right greater lip of the pudendum. All 3 patients underwent RARE hydrography in the coronal, sagittal, and axial planes.

Results.—Multiple skull lesions were revealed at MRI examination in the 7-year-old girl. Two lesions were located in the right frontal bone and others were present in the tabula interna of the right occipital bone. Vertebral lesions were detected as well, and a chylothorax was observed (Fig 1, B). In the 9-year-old girl, RARE-MR hydrography revealed the full extent of the mass, which aided removal of the whole mass macroscopically. In the young woman, RARE-MR hydrography showed that the lymphangiomatosis had invaded the retroperitoneum, as well the entire pelvis. When displacement of both kidneys was apparent, the surgeon planned removal of the retroperitoneal mass to maintain kidney function. In addition, RARE sequences were used for follow-up investigations.

Conclusion.—Sequences of RARE allow isolated depiction of water and can be used as a screening method for the whole body in patients with lymphangiomatosis. Regions without positive findings in RARE-MR hydrography require no further investigation, and the examination time for the entire body is considerably shortened. Spin-echo sequences can thus be restricted to regions with fluid-filled cystic spaces. Sequences of RARE are also valuable in differentiating lymphangiomas from hemangiomas and from hemangiolymphangiomas.

▶ Generalized lymphangiomatosis in childhood may affect many organ areas, but frequently its involvement produces symptoms mainly in 1 organ system. Magnetic resonance imaging has the capability of detecting most, if not all, of the lesions. The MR investigation time is shortened by the use of RARE sequences. Additional spin-echo sequences may follow as needed. Other recent articles on lymphangioma and lymphangiomatosis, some of which use MRI, CT, and ultrasonography, are listed.[1–6]

L.W. Young, M.D.

References

1. Tazelaar HD, Kerr D, Yousem SA, et al: Diffuse pulmonary lymphangiomatosis. *Hum Pathol* 24:1313–1322, 1993.
2. Canil K, Fitzgerald P, Lau G: Massive chylothorax associated with lymphangiomatosis of the bone. *J Pediatr Surg* 29:1186–1188, 1994.
3. Ko S-E, Ng S-H, Shieh C-S, et al: Mesenteric cystic lymphangioma with myxoid degeneration: Unusual CT and MR manifestations. *Pediatr Radiol* 25:525–527, 1995.

4. Borecky N, Gudinchet F, Laurini R, et al: Imaging of cervico-thoracic lymphangiomas in children. *Pediatr Radiol* 25:127–130, 1995.
5. Swensen SJ, Hartman TE, Mayo JR, et al: Diffuse pulmonary lymphangiomatosis: CT findings. *J Comput Assist Tomogr* 19:348–352, 1995.
6. Morgenstern L, Bello JM, Fisher BL, et al: The clinical spectrum of lymphangiomas and lymphangiomatosis of the spleen. *Am Surg* 58:599–604, 1992.

CT and MR Imaging of Vertebral Osteoblastoma: A Report of Two Cases

Özkal E, Erongun U, Çakir B, et al (Selçuk Univ, Konya, Turkey)

Clin Imaging 20:37–41, 1996 4–17

Background.—Benign osteoblastomas, comprising about 1% of all primary bone tumors, tend to affect the vertebral column. The CT and MR findings of 2 patients with spinal osteoblastoma were reported.

Case Report.—Girl, 10 years, evaluated for a 1-year history of cervical pain. Physical examination and plain radiographic findings were normal. A methylene diphosphate bone scan showed increased nodal osteoblastic activity at the right side of C3. CT showed an expansile lytic lesion on the right pedicle of C3 extending to the inferior articular process with inhomogeneous matrix ossification peripherally, surrounded by a discontinuous thin shell of bone. An inhomogeneous and hyperintense lesion was seen on T1-weighted MR images. The signal intensity of the tumor was reduced on proton-density and T2-weighted images. No bone shell was seen on the tumor borders on spin-echo sequences.

Case Report.—Man, 53, with a 5-year history of pain near the lower part of his neck and left shoulder. On plain radiographs, a partially calcified lytic lesion on the left transverse process of C7 was seen. On CT, a tumoral mass with amorphous calcifications was found originating from the transverse process, extending to the pedicle, and obliterating a C6-7 neural foramen. An inhomogeneous isointense lesion was shown on T1-weighted MR images; the lesion had a higher signal intensity on T2-weighted images. A thin rim of signal void at the outer margin of the bone tumor was observed on T2-weighted gradient-echo sequences.

Conclusion.—Computed tomography is the best modality for diagnosing bone tumors that are poorly shown on conventional radiographs. Although CT is better than MRI in characterizing the morphology and matrix of a tumor, MRI is very useful for detecting tumor extension and for differentiating soft-tissue tumor from reactive edema.

▶ The superiority of imaging osteoblastoma with CT over MRI is well shown in these cases. CT demonstrates the matrix ossification and surrounding bony shell to best advantage. In another recent article, MRI is shown not to be diagnostic in the related lesion of vertebral osteoid osteoma in three children.[1] The substantial role of high-resolution planar and pinhole skeletal scintigraphy in osteoid osteoma has also recently been addressed.[2] Other recent reports on osteoblastoma and osteoid osteoma are listed.[3–7]

L.W. Young, M.D.

References

1. van Rhijn LW, Ramos LMP, Verbout AJ: Misleading magnetic resonance imaging in spinal osteoid osteomata. *Acta Orthop Scand* 67:81–83, 1996.
2. Roach PJ, Connolly LP, Zurakowski D, et al: Osteoid osteoma: Comparative utility of high-resolution planar and pinhole magnification scintigraphy. *Pediatr Radiol* 26:222–225, 1996.
3. Bremer R, Niethard F, Ewerbeck V: Benign bone tumors in the growth years—osteoid osteoma and osteoblastoma. *Orthopade* 24:24–28, 1995.
4. Jundt G: Pathologic-anatomic characteristics of benign bone tumors. *Orthopade* 24:2–14, 1995.
5. Zambelli PY, Lechevallier J, Bracq H, et al: Osteoid osteoma or osteoblastoma of the cervical spine in relation to the vertebral artery. *J Pediatr Orthop* 14:788–792, 1994.
6. Loizaga JM, Calvo M, Lopez Barea F, et al: Osteoblastoma and osteoid osteoma. Clinical and morphological features of 162 cases. *Pathol Res Pract* 189:33–41, 1993.
7. Raskas DS, Graziano GP, Herzenberg J, et al: Osteoid osteoma and osteoblastoma of the spine. *J Spinal Disorders* 5:204–211, 1992.

Pediatric Skeletal Age: Determination With Neural Networks

Gross GW, Boone JM, Bishop DM (Thomas Jefferson Univ, Philadelphia; Univ of California, Sacramento)

Radiology 195:689–695, 1995 4–18

Introduction.—Skeletal age in children is usually assessed by taking a posteroanterior radiograph of the left hand and wrist and comparing that film with a standard atlas. If the skeletal age differs by more than 2 standard deviations from the chronologic age, a skeletal growth abnormality is diagnosed. An automated, computer-based technique, i.e., a neural network for calculating skeletal age in children, was developed and tested.

Results.—The neural network was developed using a database of 521 hand radiographs from healthy children and adolescents. All were emergency department patients with trauma to the hand or wrist region but no fracture and no known or suspected endocrine disorders. The radiographs were digitized for calculation of 4 ratios from 7 linear measurements (Fig 2). These data were used to train the neural network, by the jackknife method, to calculate skeletal age. The neural network's calculation for each patient was compared with estimates made by an experienced pediatric radiologist using the standard atlas technique.

Results.—The neural network's calculations and the radiologist's estimates of skeletal age were very similar. The mean difference between skeletal and biologic age was −0.262 years for the neural network and

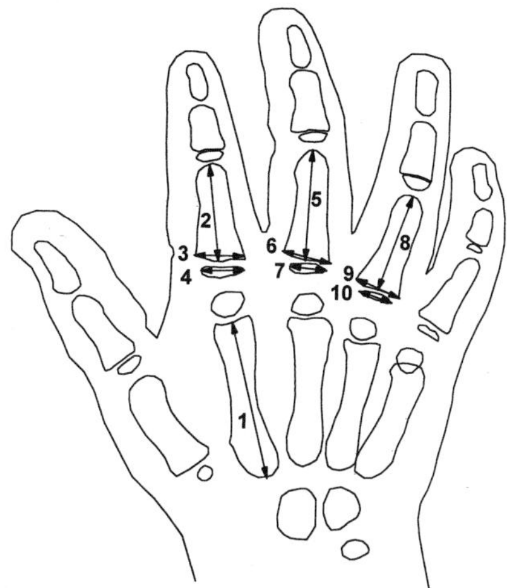

FIGURE 2.—Diagram of a hand radiograph demonstrates the 10 measurements that were acquired manually from the digitized images. Of these 10 measurements, 7 were used to form the inputs to the neural network. Because of scale variations between the digital images in the database, the 7 measured values were expressed as 4 ratios (therefore canceling out scale factors) before input to the neural network. Parameter *1*, m_4/m_3; parameter *2*, m_7/m_6; parameter *3*, m_{10}/m_9; parameter *4*, m_4/m_1. (Courtesy of Gross GW, Boone JM, Bishop DM: Pediatric skeletal age: Determination with neural networks. Radiology 195:689–695, 1995; Radiological Society of North America.)

−0.232 years for the radiologist (Fig 6). However, in nearly half of cases, the neural network's calculation of skeletal age was closer to the child's actual biological age than the radiologist's estimate. The mean error was greater for the white children than for the black children in this study.

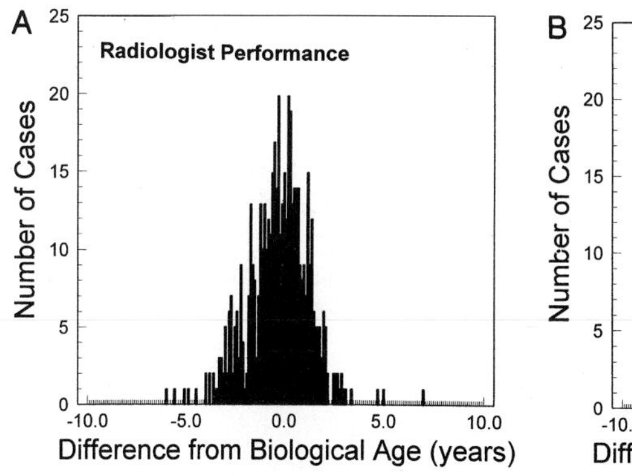

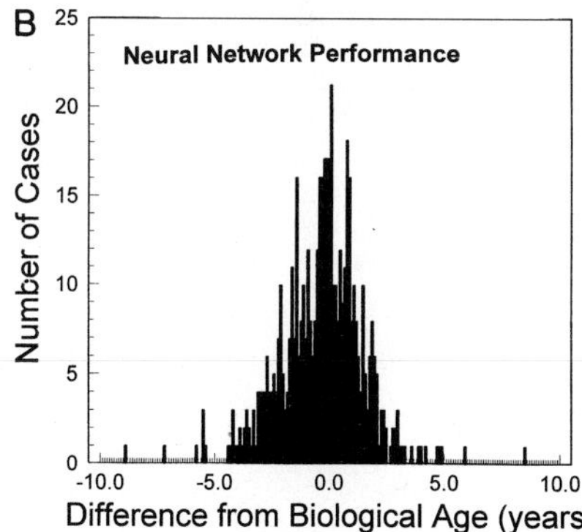

FIGURE 6.—**A**, the difference between the radiologists' skeletal age determination and biological age is shown as a histogram. The mean error was −0.232 year ± 0.54. **B**, the difference between the neural network calculation and biological age is shown, with a mean error of −0.262 year ± 1.82. (Courtesy of Gross GW, Boone JM, Bishop DM: Pediatric skeletal age: Determination with neural networks. *Radiology* 195:689–695; Radiological Society of North America.)

Conclusion.—A neural network for the calculation of skeletal age in children is presented. This simple, computer-based technique may help to improve the diagnostic accuracy, reliability, and consistency of pediatric skeletal age assessments. However, the findings of the neural network should always be cross-checked against the standard atlas images by an experienced radiologist.

▶ Recent developments of automated computer-based techniques to assist in determination of skeletal age are noteworthy. The simple neural network described by these authors uses 7 measured values (expressed as ratios) to arrive at an assessment not significantly different from assessment of standard images by radiologists. The methodology is used as an additional check to the standard method when a radiologist may not be familiar with the details of skeletal age assessment. The standard method is assessment of radiographic images by a radiologist who has learned to use the Greulich and Pyle or some other visual skeletal age assessment method. Other recent articles on computer methods are listed,[1–4] including computer assisted techniques with the Tanner skeletal age assessment method.[3,4] The applicability of the Greulich and Pyle method to all ethnoracial and economic population groups has also been recently addressed.[5]

L.W. Young, M.D.

References

1. Sun YN, Ko CC, Mao CW, et al: A computer system for skeletal growth measurement. *Comput Biomed Res* 27:2–12, 1994.
2. Pietka E: Computer-assisted bone age assessment based on features automatically extracted from a hand radiograph. *Comput Med Imaging Graph* 19:251–259, 1995.
3. Drayer NM, Cox LA: Assessment of bone ages by the Tanner-Whitehouse method using a computer-aided system. *Acta Paediatr* 406(suppl):77–80, 1994.
4. Tanner JM, Gibbons RD: Automatic bone age measurement using computerized image analysis (review). *J Pediatr Endocrinol* 7:141–145, 1994.
5. Loder RT, Estle DT, Morrison K, et al: Applicability of the Greulich and Pyle skeletal age standards to black and white children of today. *Am J Dis Child* 147:1329–1333, 1993.

Distal Humeral Physeal Injuries in Child Abuse: MR Imaging and Ultrasonography Findings

Nimkin K, Kleinman PK, Teeger S, et al (Univ of Massachusetts, Worcester)
Pediatr Radiol 25:562–565, 1995 4–19

Objective.—The 3 cases presented here demonstrate the role of US and MRI in evaluating distal humeral physeal injury in suspected child abuse. Such injuries, particularly fracture-separation of the distal humeral epiphysis, are seen in cases of abuse involving infants and toddlers.

Methods.—The patients were a 3-month-old boy, a 12-month-old boy, and a 23-month-old girl. All had plain films of the elbow, followed by

MRI; elbow sonography was performed in 1 case. Magnetic resonance images were obtained with a 1.5-tesla unit using a surface coil. The sedated children had sagittal and coronal T1-weighted and magnification-prepared gradient-echo images; 2 children had an additional axial MPGR or T2-weighted sequence. Elbow ultrasound was performed in the sagittal and coronal planes.

Results.—In the 3-month-old boy, radiography showed posterior displacement of the proximal left ulna and radius, together with numerous other metaphyseal fractures typical of abuse. At MRI, a Salter II fracture-separation of the distal left humerus without fracture extension into unossified epiphysis was identified, together with posterior displacement of the distal humeral epiphysis. Ultrasound demonstrated posterior displacement of the distal left humeral epiphysis and fluid in the olecranon fossa (Fig 1). Abuse by the infant's grandmother was later confirmed. The other children also had Salter II fracture-separation of the distal left humerus, confirmed in both cases to have resulted from abuse. Abuse was not considered, however, until distal humeral physeal injury was identified.

Discussion.—Distal humeral fracture-separation occurs in abused infants who have been subjected to violent twisting or pulling of the arm. This type of injury may be underdiagnosed in such cases because detection is difficult with plain film. Radiographic clues include an associated distal humeral metaphyseal fragment, a displaced metaphyseal fragment, a displaced medial epicondyle, or a displaced capitellar ossification center. The nature of the injury is well delineated at MRI, and the use of ultrasound and MRI may obviate the need for intraoperative arthrography.

► Correlative imaging contributes to more complete demonstration of the abnormal findings of child abuse. Ultrasonography and MRI especially and effectively display findings at the elbow. Ultrasonography may identify an abnormality not demonstrated at radiography.[1–3] Although sonography is easier to perform, MRI findings usually show the normal and abnormal morphology more exquisitely.[4] A recent excellent article on patterns of inflicted skeletal injury features postmortem correlation of radiologic and histopathologic findings in 31 mortalities from child abuse.[5]

L.W. Young, M.D.

References

1. Davidson RS, Markowitz RI, Dormans J, et al: Ultrasonographic evaluation of the elbow in infants and young children after suspected trauma. *J Bone Joint Surg* 76:1804–1813, 1994.
2. Bar-On E, Howard CB, Porat S, et al: The use of ultrasound in the diagnosis of atypical pathology in the unossified skeleton. *J Pediatr Orthop* 15:817–820, 1995.
3. Strait RT, Siegel RM, Shapiro RA: Humeral fractures without obvious etiologies in children less than 3 years of age: When is it abuse? *Pediatrics* 96:667–671, 1995.
4. Beltran J, Rosenberg ZS, Kawelblum M, et al: Pediatric elbow fractures: MRI evaluation. *Skeletal Radiol* 23:277–281, 1994.
5. Kleinman PK. Marks Jr. SC, Richmond JM, et al: Inflicted skeletal injury: A postmortem radiologic-histopathologic study in 31 infants. *AJR* 165:647–650, 1995.

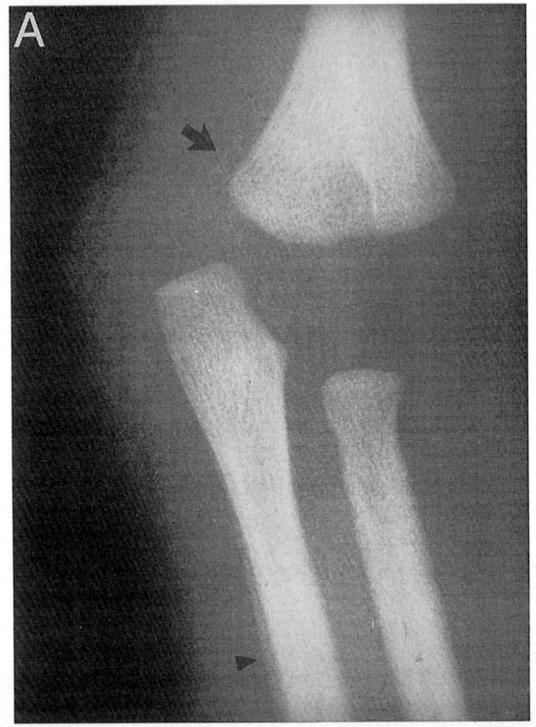

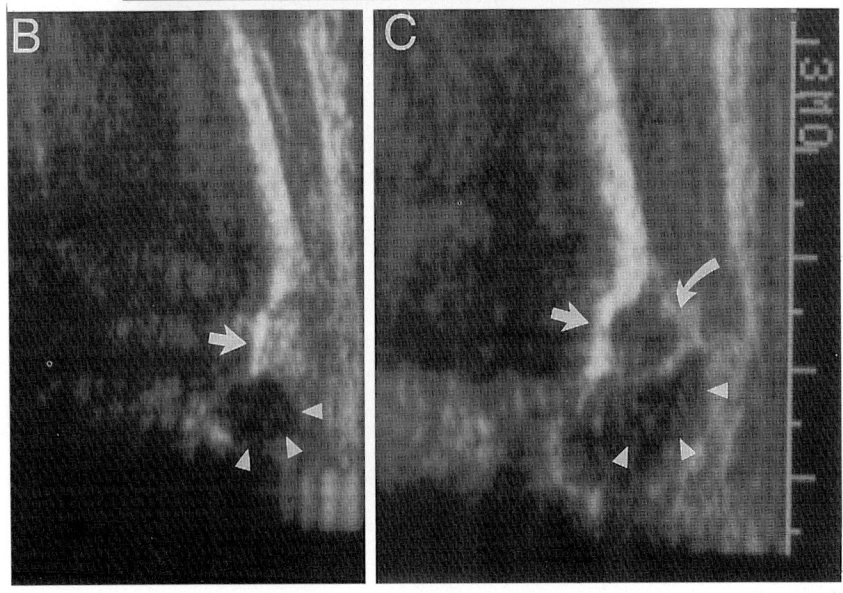

(*Continued*)

FIGURE 1 (cont.)

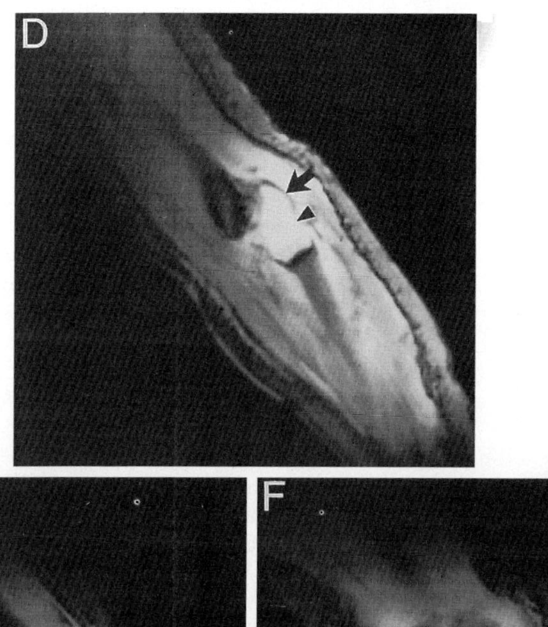

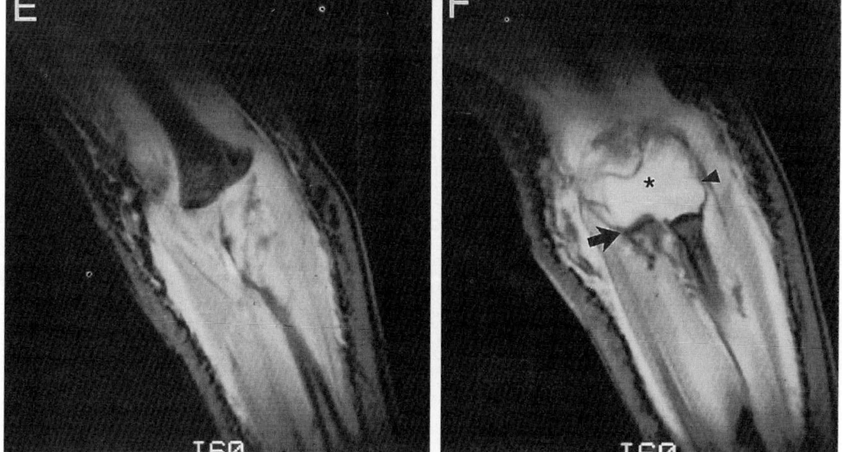

FIGURE 1.—Male infant, 3 months, was admitted with left arm swelling without a history of trauma. **A,** external oblique view of the left elbow reveals posteromedial displacement of the proximal ulna and radius relative to the distal humerus. A tiny bony fragment (*arrow*) is adjacent to the distal medial humeral metaphysis. Periosteal reaction is also noted along the shaft of the ulna (*arrowhead*). The anteroposterior view was normal. **B,** sagittal ultrasound image, obtained from the posterior aspect of the normal elbow, reveals a normal relationship between the distal humeral metaphysis (*arrow*) and epiphysis (*arrowheads*). **C,** sagittal ultrasound image of the abnormal elbow reveals posterior displacement of the distal humeral epiphysis (*arrowheads*) relative to the metaphysis (*arrow*). Fat pad is displaced posteriorly by fluid in the olecranon fossa (*curved arrow*). **D,** sagittal magnification-prepared gradient-echo image (recovery time 500 msec/echo time 21 msec/flip angle 30 degrees) confirms posterior displacement of the distal humeral epiphysis (*arrow*) and a normal relationship between the epiphysis and the radius (*arrowhead*). **E,** coronal magnification-prepared gradient-echo image (recovery time 500 msec/echo time 17 msec/flip angle 30 degrees) through the distal humerus shows a "naked" metaphysis with no contact between the metaphysis and the epiphysis. **F,** a more posterior image shows the normal relationship between the radius (*arrowhead*), ulna (*arrow*), and distal humeral epiphysis (*asterisk*). (*Pediatr Radiol;* Distal humeral physeal injuries in child abuse: MR imaging and ultrasonography findings; Nimkin K, Kleinman PK, Teeger S, et al; 25:562–565; Fig 1;1995; Copyright notice of Springer-Verlag.)

Radiologic Features of Systemic Onset Juvenile Rheumatoid Arthritis
Lang BA, Schneider R, Reilly BJ, et al (Dalhousie Univ, Halifax, NS, Canada; Univ of Toronto)
J Rheumatol 22:168–173, 1995 4–20

Background.—Juvenile rheumatoid arthritis (JRA) has varied clinical patterns of disease and prognosis. In contrast with patients with the subtype of rheumatoid factor–positive JRA, early destructive joint changes are not emphasized in patients with systemic onset JRA (SOJRA). However, there has been little study of the radiographic abnormalities in patients with SOJRA. The radiologic manifestations in patients with SOJRA were reviewed, with particular attention to early changes.

Methods.—The medical records of 42 patients with a diagnosis of SOJRA who were seen over a 7-year period and radiographs were reviewed. The radiographs were reviewed by an experienced radiologist blinded to the clinical course.

Results.—The patients were observed for a mean of 3 years. The most common site of early radiologic changes was the wrist, followed by the ankles, knees, tarsal joints, hips, and metacarpophalangeal joints. The most common radiologic abnormalities were soft tissue swelling and/or osteopenia (in 81%), followed by subchondral changes, growth abnormalities, joint space narrowing, erosions, subluxation, and ankylosis (Fig 2). Of the 29 patients with radiographs obtained within 1 year of the onset of disease, polyarthritis developed in 24 within 3 months after the onset of systemic symptoms and pauciarticular arthritis developed in 5. Of the 36

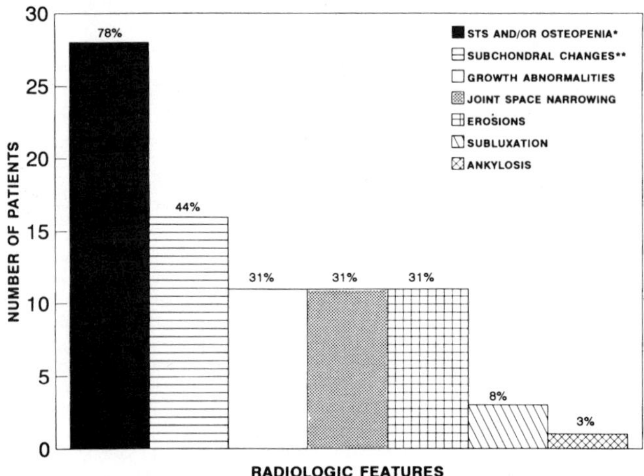

FIGURE 2.—Frequency of radiologic abnormalities detected in patients with systemic onset juvenile rheumatoid arthritis within 2 years of disease onset (N = 36). (Courtesy of Lang BA, Schneider R, Reilly BJ, et al: Radiologic features of systemic onset juvenile rheumatoid arthritis. *J Rheumatol* 22:168–173, 1995.)

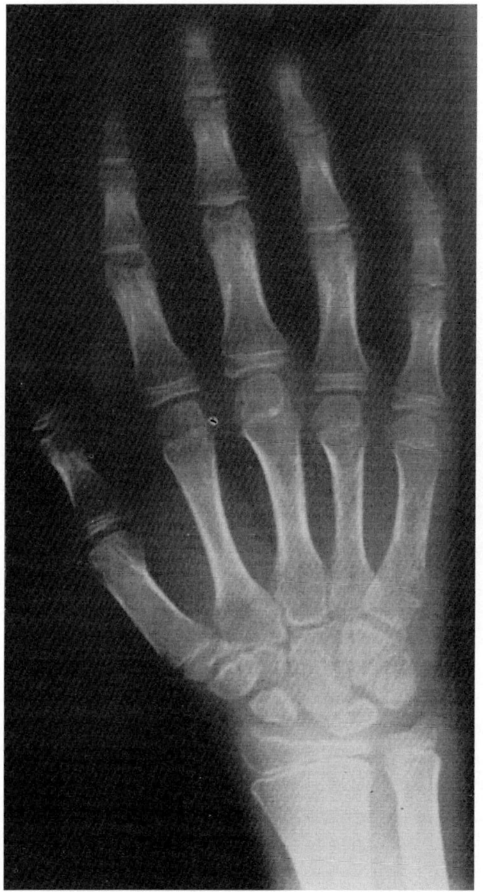

FIGURE 3.—Boy with SOJRA that began at the age of 10 years. Right hand and wrist. Series of radiographs showing progressive joint space narrowing and erosions within the carpus and at the metacarpophalangeal, proximal interphalangeal, and distal interphalangeal joints. **B**, 12 years of age. (Courtesy of Lang BA, Schneider R, Reilly BJ, et al: Radiologic features of systemic onset juvenile rheumatoid arthritis. *J Rheumatol* 22:168–173, 1995.)

patients with radiographs obtained within 2 years of disease onset, 11 (31%) had erosions and 5 had progressive joint space narrowing (Figs 3, B and 4, B). There were advanced radiologic abnormalities in 24% of the patients, which included joint ankylosis, subluxation, protrusio acetabuli, and complete joint destruction. Five patients had joint ankylosis of the apophyseal joints of the cervical spine (Fig 5). Other unusual radiologic abnormalities included soft tissue calcification localized to the tissue around the wrist and hips in the absence of intraarticular steroid treatment and large cystic lesions in the shoulders. Clinical disease and radiologic damage correlated well, with persistent systemic disease activity and active arthritis more likely in patients with either joint space narrowing or bone erosions.

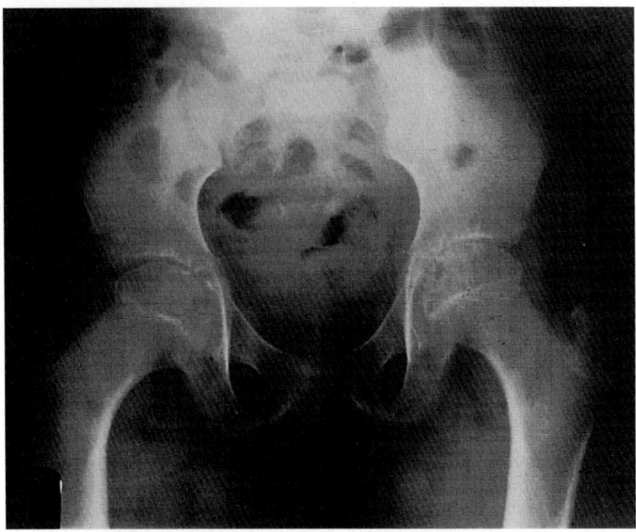

FIGURE 4.—Girl with systemic onset juvenile rheumatoid arthritis since the age of 7 years. Bilateral hips. Series of radiographs showing osteopenia followed by early cartilage loss and subchondral irregularity and finally protrusio acetabuli with destruction of the femoral heads. B, age 9½ years. (Courtesy of Lang BA, Schneider R, Reilly BJ, et al: Radiologic features of systemic onset juvenile rheumatoid arthritis. *J Rheumatol* 22:168–173, 1995.)

Discussion.—Early erosive damage and joint space narrowing were common radiologic findings in patients with SOJRA, occurring within 2 years of disease onset in 33%. These early radiographic changes in patients with SOJRA have not been reported previously. This course of radiologic disease is similar to that seen in patients with rheumatoid factor–positive JRA. This subgroup of patients with SOJRA are at increased risk of severe joint damage and may benefit from early, more aggressive treatment.

► The development within 2 years of radiographically substantial arthritic changes that progressed to severe arthritis occurred in a subgroup of children with SOJRA. Temporomandibular joint involvement also seems to be more severe early in the SOJRA subgroup.[1] These findings of severe arthritis should stimulate prospective analyses of children with SOJRA for development of radiologically or MRI demonstrable abnormalities. Contrary to earlier suggestions, the gross morphologic manifestations of arthritic disease and their speed of occurrence in SOJRA are not unlike those expected of rheumatoid factor–positive polyarticular JRA. Another recent article indicates that bone mineral content is reduced even earlier in SOJRA than in rheumatoid factor–positive JRA.[2] Rapid onset of radiologic findings in a migrating monoarticular form of JRA was recently reported in children of Assyrian ancestry.[3] Rapid onset has also been observed in an infantile form of JRA.[4] A relatively recent general review article on JRA is also listed.[5]

L.W. Young, M.D.

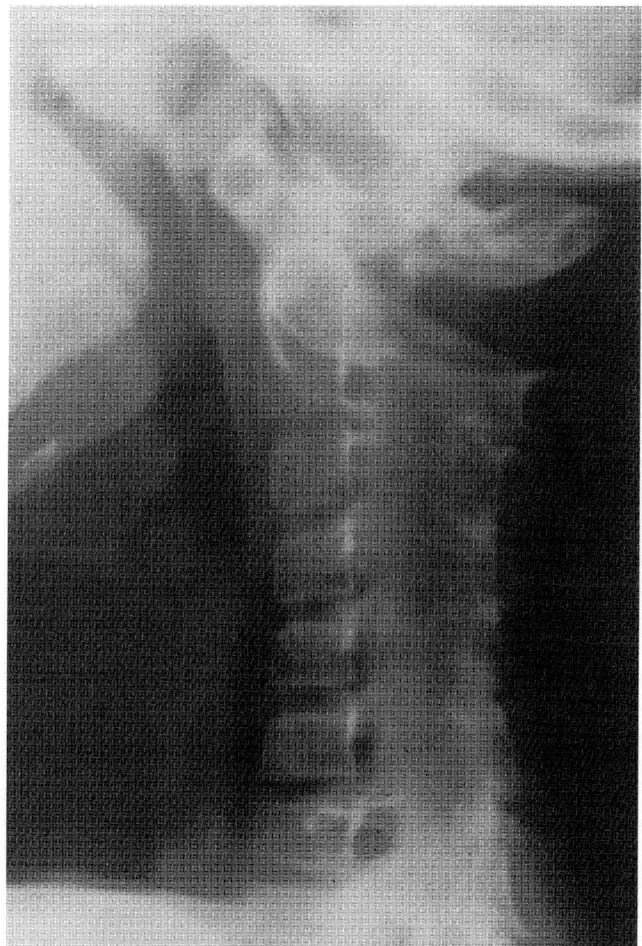

FIGURE 5.—Boy with systemic onset juvenile rheumatoid arthritis since the age of 3½ years. Cervical spine radiograph taken 5 years after diagnosis at the age of 8½ years. There is fusion of the apophyseal joints of the cervical spine (C2–C7). (Courtesy of Lang BA, Schneider R, Reilly BJ, et al: Radiologic features of systemic onset juvenile rheumatoid arthritis. *J Rheumatol* 22:168–173, 1995.)

References

1. Hu Y-S, Schneiderman ED: The temporomandibular joint in juvenile rheumatoid arthritis: I. Computed tomographic findings. *Pediatr Dent* 17:46–54, 1995.
2. Polito C, Strano CG, Rea L, et al: Reduced bone mineral content and normal serum osteocalcin in non-steroid–treated patients with juvenile rheumatoid arthritis. *Ann Rheum Dis* 54:193–196, 1995.
3. Miller III JR, Emery HM: Migrating monopredominant arthritis in children of Assyrian ancestry. *J Rheumatol* 178–180, 1996.
4. Maeno N. Imanaka H, Takei S, et al: Clinical features of infantile patient with juvenile rheumatoid arthritis. *Ryumachi* 34:901–907, 1994.
5. Tucker LB: Juvenile rheumatoid arthritis (review). *Curr Opin Rheumatol* 5:619–628, 1993.

Atlantoaxial Subluxation in Children With Seronegative Enthesopathy and Arthropathy Syndrome: 2 Case Reports and a Review of the Literature

Foster HE, Cairns RA, Burnell RH, et al (Univ of British Columbia, Canada; British Columbia's Children's Hosp, Canada; Univ of Adelaide, Australia; et al)

J Rheumatol 22:548–551, 1995 4–21

Objective.—In juvenile ankylosing spondylitis (JAS), peripheral arthritis is the typical presentation. Axial spine involvement is usually a later manifestation, and cervical involvement typically does not occur until after lumbar involvement. The risk of definite JAS or another spondyloarthropathy is high in HLA-B27–positive children with seronegative enthesopathy and arthropathy (SEA) syndrome. Two cases of early, nontraumatic atlantoaxial subluxation in children with SEA syndrome were reported.

Case Report.—Boy, 13, came to medical attention with arthritis of the left knee and tenderness of the left sacroiliac joint and both Achilles tendon entheses, as well as other tendon insertions. Anterior flexion of the lumbar spine was restricted, and the neck was flexed forward and to the right, with limitation of movement because of painful spasms of the paracervical muscles. The patient's erythrocyte sedimentation rate was 90 mm/hour and he was positive for HLA-B27. Shoulder, knee, and hip radiographs were normal. The patient was significantly disabled, requiring treatment with sulfasalazine and low-dose prednisone. He did not meet the criteria for JAS but was considered to have SEA syndrome.

Though the patient's peripheral arthritis soon improved, he still had severe pain and limited movement in his neck. Cervical spine radiographs showed an anterior atlantodental interval (AADI) of 3 mm in extension, increasing to 8 mm in forward flexion; the normal flexion AADI value in children is less than 5 mm. Extensive thickened synovium was noted on an MRI scan. Though the patient's symptoms resolved, his AADI continued to increase to 11 mm in forward flexion. Synovial thickening between the odontoid and anterior arch of C1 continued as well, though there was no spinal cord compression nor any neurologic abnormality. The patient underwent elective posterior cervical fusion about 1 year later.

Discussion.—Two cases of children with atlantoaxial subluxation associated with SEA syndrome were reported. All children with inflammatory arthropathy should have a careful evaluation of neck symptoms, as well as cervical spine radiographs in flexion and extension. Magnetic resonance imaging with gadolinium enhancement can depict the synovial mass and any spinal cord compression in patients with atlantoaxial subluxation. Improvement in the symptoms of neck pain and stiffness may actually increase the risk of neurologic complications because of increased movement. Surgical stabilization may be indicated in this situation.

▶ The authors report patients with SEA syndrome who demonstrate the unusual early occurrence of atlantoaxial subluxation. Early manifestation of juvenile cervical spondyloarthropathy before sacroiliac manifestations is common in SEA syndrome. An excellent recent review article on juvenile spondyloarthropathies is listed.[1]

L.W. Young, M.D.

Reference

1. Azouz ME, Duffy CM: Juvenile spondyloarthropathies: Clinical manifestations and medical imaging. *Skeletal Radiol* 24:399–408, 1995.

Cardiopulmonary System

Internal Mammary Compartment: Window to the Mediastinum
Kuzo RS, Ben-Ami TE, Yousefzadeh DK, et al (Univ of Chicago)
Radiology 195:187–192, 1995 4–22

Background.—Ultrasonography (US) can be used to examine the mediastinum and is especially useful in children. This report describes the authors' experience with US of the internal mammary compartment of children as a method of evaluating the mediastinum.

Methods.—The internal mammary compartment was examined by spectral and color Doppler US as part of a comprehensive evaluation of the mediastinum in patients referred because of suspicion of a central vascular abnormality or mediastinal mass. Sixty-six patients were included in this study group, with an age range of 2 days to 18 years.

Findings.—Of the 66 patients, 5 had abnormal internal mammary arterial flow. This flow was actually reversed in 1 patient (Fig 2). The internal mammary venous flow was reversed or absent in 10 patients with vein obstruction or Glenn shunts. In patients with shunts, this retrograde flow in the internal mammary vein can reflect adequate shunt function. Forty-four patients underwent US for a suspected mediastinal mass. In 23 patients this mass was lymphoma. Seventeen patients were diagnosed with non-Hodgkin's lymphoma and 5 had internal mammary lymphadenopathy. Six patients were diagnosed with Hodgkin's disease and 3 had internal mammary lymph node involvement. In 1 patient the nodal mass involved 1 interspace, whereas in the other 7 it involved multiple interspaces. None of the 6 patients with infectious adenopathy and none of the patients with benign mediastinal masses or vascular abnormalities had internal mammary nodes that could be visualized.

Conclusion.—These results demonstrate that US of the internal mammary compartment is easily performed in children and should be part of the examination of the mediastinum when central vascular abnormality or a mediastinal mass is suspected. Reversal of internal mammary venous

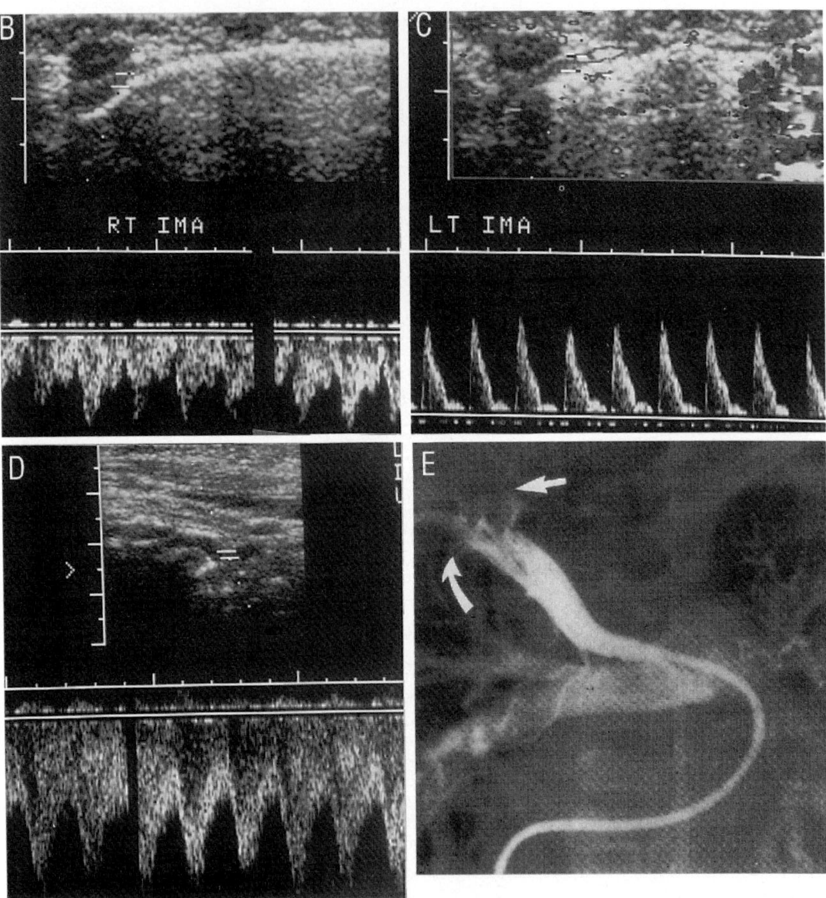

FIGURE 2 .—Images obtained in a 4-month-old girl admitted for ligation of patent ductus arteriosus. Her blood pressure was lower in the right arm than in other extremities. **B**, Doppler spectrum of right internal mammary artery shows reversal of flow and high diastolic flow velocity. **C**, Doppler spectrum shows antegrade flow in left internal mammary artery and a normal flow pattern. **D**, Doppler spectrum of enlarged tortuous right vertebral artery also shows reversal of flow and high diastolic velocity. **E**, angiogram obtained during cardiac catheterization, with catheter through right pulmonary artery into the anomalus right subclavian artery that arises from it, demonstrates washout from reversed flow in vertebral (*straight arrow*) and internal mammary (*curved arrow*) arteries. (Courtesy of Kuzo RS, Ben-Ami TE, Yousefzadeh DK, et al: Internal mammary compartment: Window to the mediastinum. *Radiology* 195:187–192, 1995; Radiological Society of North America.)

flow usually is indicative of central venous stenosis or occlusion. Alteration of the normal waveform or flow reversal is indicative of arterial collateral flow. Internal mammary lymphadenopathy is more common with lymphoma than with infection. Normal internal mammary lymph nodes are not visualized by US scans.

► The authors nicely demonstrate the value of US and Doppler imaging in a variety of conditions of mediastinal lymphatic and vascular disease in children. Recent or basic articles relevant to this usage are listed.

L.W. Young, M.D.

References

1. Betsch B: Color Doppler ultrasound of the mediastinum: Examination technique and sectional anatomy of the image. *Radiologe* 34:599–604, 1994.
2. Scatarige JC, Hamper UM, Sheth S, et al: Parasternal sonography of the internal mammary vessels: Technique, normal anatomy, and lymphadenopathy. *Radiology* 172:453–457, 1989.
3. Wernecke K, Potter R, Peters PE, et al: Parasternal mediastinal sonography: Sensitivity in the detection of anterior mediastinal and subcarinal tumors. *AJR* 150:1021–1026, 1988.

Invited Article: Helical/Spiral CT Scanning: A Pediatric Radiology Perspective

White KS (Primary Children's Med Ctr, Salt Lake City, Utah)

Pediatr Radiol 26:5–14, 1996 4–23

Background.—The use of helical/spiral CT scanning may be useful in the assessment of children. The advantages of this modality are decreased sedation rates and radiation exposure with scanning at extended pitch, improved image quality, and better 3-dimensional and reformatted images. The technical and clinical considerations in the helical/spiral CT scanning of children were reviewed.

Technical Considerations.—Helical CT data are obtained while the table is in continuous motion. Before reconstruction, the data are interpolated. Continuously sampling the data permits reconstruction of overlapping slices. Also, the scan speed is increased with helical CT, which reduces the scan time by at least 50%. The collimation thickness and pitch determine scanning speed in a particular anatomical area. In helical scanning, the radiation dose can be decreased if the pitch is increased. Also, because images may be reconstructed retrospectively at any position along the scan interval, the number of recuts needed may be reduced. When 2 contiguous slices do not clearly show a small anatomical structure because of partial volume effects, the intermediate scan can be reconstructed retrospectively, which obviates the need for rescanning.

Clinical Considerations.—With helical CT, the sedation requirements in children are reduced. Complete data sampling, overlapping reconstructions, and the possibility of reducing slice thickness potentially increase lesion detection with helical CT. With overlapping image reconstruction, the detectability of hepatic and pulmonary lesions in patients with cancer is increased. Because the faster scan speed may reduce motion-related artifacts and vascular enhancement may be more uniform, image quality may be improved with helical CT. Little information is available on vas-

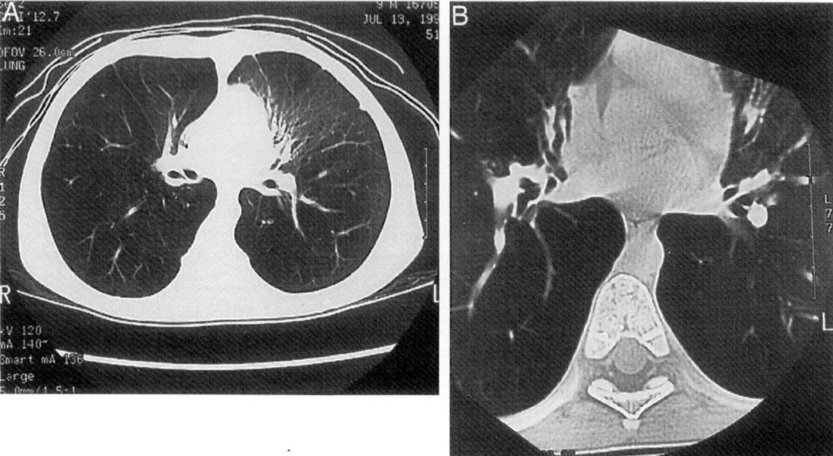

FIGURE 3.—Images of the chest in a boy, 9 years, with a history of meconium aspiration and ongoing symptoms of airway occlusive disease. The survey image (**A**) obtained with 5-mm collimation demonstrates vascular crowding and mixed central interstitial and alveolar opacities in the lingula. The remainder of the lung is hyperinflated and shows wide separation of the pulmonary vasculature. A high-resolution 3-mm-thick image of the central airways (**B**) demonstrates marked fibrosis and crowding of mildly dilated segmental and subsegmental bronchi in the right middle and left upper lobes. Note the excellent detail of the encasing fibrosis in the right middle lobe and the nodule thickening of lingular subsegmental bronchi. (Invited article: Helical/spiral CT scanning: A pediatric radiology perspective; White KS *Pediatr Radiol;* 26:5–14; Fig 3; 1996; Copyright notice of Springer-Verlag.)

cular contrast enhancement in pediatric CT. Hand injection was used, which resulted in variations in cc/kg-min injection rates. Rather than setting a delay from the time of injection initiation, the delay is set relative to the completion of contrast infusion. Specific protocols for helical CT imaging of the head, paranasal sinuses, temporal bone, neck, chest (Fig 3), abdomen, and pelvis were outlined.

Conclusion.—Helical imaging has several potential advantages over conventional CT in the assessment of children. Images are produced faster, thereby lowering radiation exposure, reducing the sedation requirement, and improving image quality.

► The pertinent and clinical considerations for the use of helical/spiral CT in the field of pediatrics are well presented in this article. Other noteworthy recent articles on the use of helical/spiral CT in children are listed.[1-6]

L.W. Young, M.D.

References

1. Ambrosino MM, Roche KJ, Genieser NB, et al: Application of thin-section low-dose chest CT (TSCT) in the management of pediatric AIDS. *Pediatr Radiol* 25:393–400, 1995.
2. White KS: Reduced need for sedation in patients undergoing helical CT of the chest and abdomen. *Pediatr Radiol* 25:344–346, 1995.
3. Cox TD, White KS, Weinberger E, et al: Comparison of helical and conventional chest CT in the uncooperative pediatric patient. *Pediatr Radiol* 25:347–349, 1995.

4. Mooney DP, Sargent SK, Pluta D, et al: Spiral CT: Use in the evaluation of chest masses in the critically ill neonate. *Pediatr Radiol* 26:15–18, 1996.
5. Gavant ML, Menke PG, Fabian T: Blunt traumatic aortic rupture: Detection with helical CT of the chest. *Radiology* 197:125–133, 1995.
6. van der Bruggen-Bogaarts BA, Broerse JJ, Lammers JW: Radiation exposure in standard and high-resolution chest CT scans. *Chest* 107:113–115, 1995.

The Varied Manifestation of Pulmonary Artery Agenesis in Adulthood

Bouros D, Pare P, Panagou P, et al (Univ of Crete, Greece; Univ of British Columbia, Vancouver, Canada; Army Gen Hosp, Athens, Greece; et al)

Chest 108:670–676, 1995 4–24

Background.—The rare congenital anomaly unilateral pulmonary artery agenesis (UPAA), which is often associated with other cardiovascular anomalies, is usually diagnosed and treated during the first year of life. However, isolated UPAA may have a benign clinical course and so may go unrecognized until adulthood, when it is detected incidentally on a chest radiograph. Six patients with UPAA that was not detected until adulthood are described.

Findings.—The diagnosis of UPAA was made according to the history, clinical examination, and imaging studies, which included chest radiography, ventilation-perfusion scanning, digital subtraction angiography (DSA), CT, and MRI. Plain chest radiographs showed ipsilateral cardiac and mediastinal displacement, smaller hemithorax, absent pulmonary artery shadow, ipsilateral hemidiaphragm elevation, ipsilateral absent or diminished pulmonary vascular markings, and contralateral lung hyperinflation and "herniation." Three patients had a right aortic arch, though none had air trapping on the expiratory chest radiograph. Four patients had a mildly restrictive pattern on pulmonary function studies. Ipsilateral mixed-type bronchiectasis was detected by selective bronchography in 2 of 4 patients. The definitive diagnosis was made by DSA (Fig 3) in all patients. Though CT and MRI were also diagnostic, they provided no useful additional information.

Discussion.—Diagnosis of UPAA may be elusive in patients whose abnormality is unsuspected until adulthood. The chest radiographic features in these patients are more extensive than indicated by the relatively benign clinical course. If the diagnosis of UPAA is suspected, an inspiratory and expiratory posteroanterior radiograph and lung ventilation-perfusion scan should be performed. If the diagnosis is still in doubt, DSA is indicated. The differential diagnosis and pathogenesis of UPAA are discussed, along with the relative merits of MRI and CT scanning.

► Don't let the title of this article confuse you! Pulmonary artery agenesis is a congenital anomaly pediatric disease. The clinical problem may not manifest itself until adulthood, but most cases in the literature have been in children. The youngest patient in this report was diagnosed at age 17 years (see Fig 3). A 3-month-old infant in whom echocardiography and cardiac

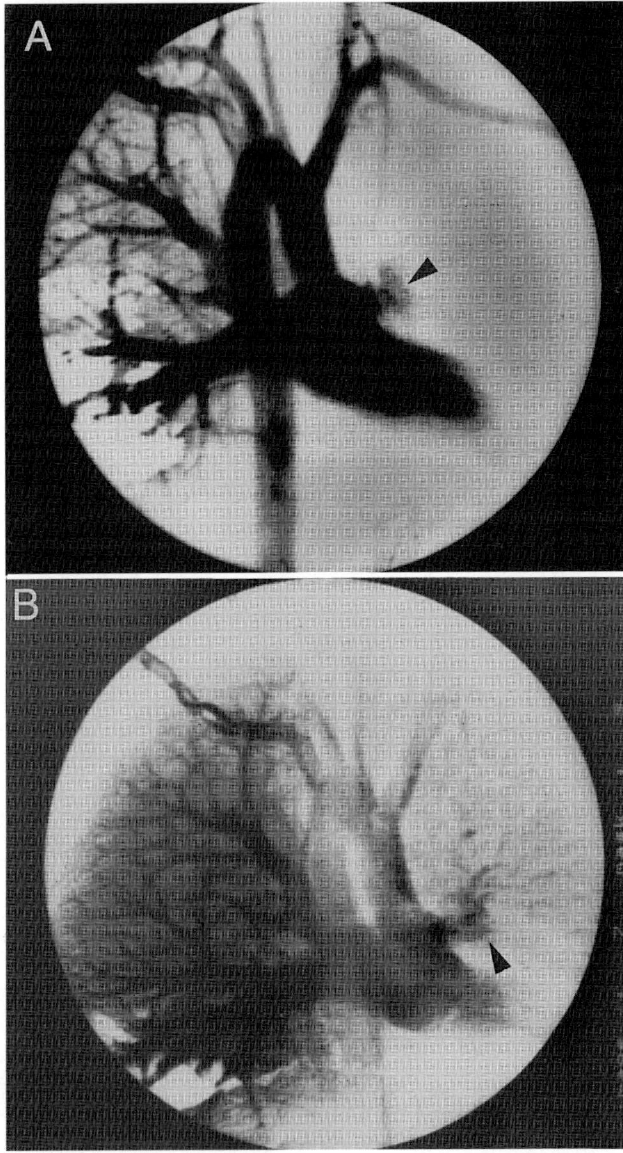

FIGURE 3.—Digital subtraction angiography of a patient with left unilateral pulmonary artery agenesis. *Top*, proximal interruption of the left pulmonary artery (*arrowhead*). Both sides of the heart are filled with the contrast media at the same time due to ventricular septal defect. *Bottom*, collateral circulation on the affected lung is shown (*arrowhead*). (Courtesy of Bouros D, Pare P, Panagou P, et al: The varied manifestation of pulmonary artery agenesis in adulthood. *Chest* 108:670–676, 1995.)

catheterization were diagnostic was recently reported.[1] Differential diagnosis based only on the chest radiographic findings may include several other unilateral small lung possibilities. Associated congenital anomalies of the cardiovascular system may produce signs and symptoms of UPAA. Although

MRI is probably the diagnostic modality of choice for UPAA, initial workup is usually radiography and lung ventilation-perfusion scintigraphy. Digital subtraction angiography and conventional pulmonary arteriography[2] may also be used.

L.W. Young, M.D.

References

1. Serino W, Argento G, Fiorilli R, et al: The isolated agenesis of a branch of the pulmonary artery. A case report: its diagnosis and therapy (review). *Cardiologia* 38:531–534, 1993.
2. Herraiz SI, Gonzalez PW, Rodriguez VF, et al: Unilateral agenesis of the pulmonary artery. Experience with 4 cases (review). *Anales Espanoles de Pediatria* 38:139–144, 1993.

Anomalous Origin of the Right Pulmonary Artery From the Ascending Aorta: Diagnosis By Magnetic Resonance Imaging

Kim TK, Choe YH, Kim HS, et al (Seoul Natl Univ Hosp, Korea; Sejong Gen Hosp, Korea)

Cardiovasc Intervent Radiol 18:118–121, 1995 4–25

Background.—Anomalous origin of the right pulmonary artery from the ascending aorta, a congenital anomaly, is rare. The diagnosis relies on cardiovascular imaging. Although echocardiography and CT have been reported, the role of MRI in such patients is still uncertain. Magnetic resonance imaging findings in 3 patients with anomalous origin of the right pulmonary artery from the ascending aorta were reported.

Case Report.—Boy, 6 months old, was brought for medical attention because of a 1-month history of irritability and vomiting. Heart auscultation showed a grade 3/6 systolic murmur at the left sternal border. Right ventricular hypertrophy was demonstrated on the ECG. Subsequently angiocardiography demonstrated an anomalous origin of the right pulmonary artery from the posterior aspect of the ascending aorta 1.5 cm above the aortic valve, as well as the patent ductus arteriosus, and ECG-gated, T1-weighted, spin-echo MRI was performed. The axial and right anterior oblique sagittal image clearly demonstrated the anomalous origin of the right pulmonary artery from the posterior aspect of the ascending aorta (Fig 1). Treatment consisted of reimplantation of the right pulmonary artery to the main pulmonary artery, ligation of the patent ductus arteriosus, and lung biopsy specimens of both upper lobes. Pathologic assessment showed mild medial hypertrophy, Health-Edwards grade I, identical in the 2 specimens. At the 1-year follow-up, the patient was doing well.

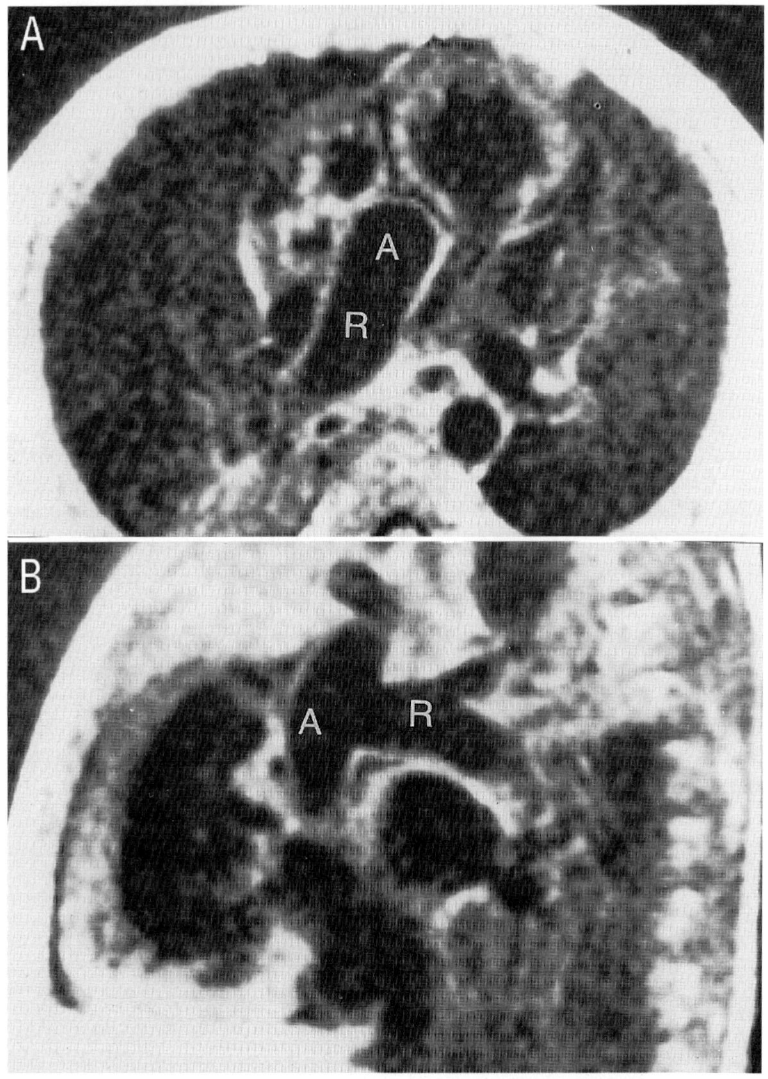

FIGURE 1.—Boy, 6 months. Axial (**A**) and right anterior oblique sagittal (**B**) MRIs show the origin of the right pulmonary artery (*R*) from the posterior aspect of the ascending aorta (*A*). (*Cardiovasc Intervent Radiol*; Anomalous origin of the right pulmonary artery from the ascending aorta: Diagnosis by magnetic resonance imaging; Kim TK, Choe YH, Kim HS, et al; 18:118–121; Fig 1; 1995; Copyright notice of Springer-Verlag.)

Conclusion.—Anomalous origin of the right pulmonary artery from the posterior aspect of the ascending aorta was clearly visible on MRI. Combined anomalies such as patent ductus arteriosus, aortopulmonary window, and interruption of the aortic arch were also shown in all 3 patients studied. Thus, MRI appears to be an accurate imaging modality in the diagnosis of anomalous origin of the right pulmonary artery from the ascending aorta. It obviates the need for angiocardiography.

▶ These 3 cases of anomalous origin of the right pulmonary artery from the ascending aorta are noteworthy because they are excellent examples of definitive findings of MRI that obviate the need of angiocardiography. Cardiac catheterization with angiocardiography,[1] although also diagnostic, is invasive and relatively risky in patients with severe pulmonary hypertension. Echocardiography did not demonstrate this anomaly in any of the 3 patients.

L.W. Young, M.D.

Reference

1. Siy LL, Chen MR, Chiu IS, et al: Right pulmonary artery arising from ascending aorta: Report of a successfully treated case. *J Formosan Med Assoc* 92:751–754, 1993.

Left Aortic Arch With Right Descending Aorta and Right Ligamentum Arteriosum Associated With d-TGA and Large VSD: Surgical Treatment of a Rare Form of Vascular Ring

Watanabe M, Kawasaki S, Sato H, et al (Juntendo Univ, Tokyo)
J Pediatr Surg 30:1363–1365, 1995 4–26

Background.—Pulmonary hypertension develops quickly in infants with d-loop transposition of the great arteries (d-TGA) and a large ventricular septal defect (VSD). An infant with severe respiratory distress undergoing pulmonary artery (PA) banding surgery who later needed intubation and mechanical respiration for respiratory failure was described.

Case Report.—Boy, born at term after an uncomplicated delivery (birth weight was 3,430 g), had a heart murmur, retractions, and peripheral cyanosis detected at 1 month of age. On echocardiography, d-TGA, a large VSD, and a huge PA were observed. A chest radiograph demonstrated cardiomegaly and increased pulmonary markings. When the patient was 41 days old, PA banding surgery was performed. Though the surgery improved respiratory distress, an upper respiratory tract infection developed 40 days postoperatively, and respiratory failure recurred. The boy's airway was intubated, and he was placed on a respirator. At 8 months of age, a contrast esophagogram revealed compression of the posterosuperior esophagus (Fig 1, B). On a chest radiograph, hazy infiltration in the lower right lung and upper left lung was observed (Fig 2). On ECG-gated spin-echo MRI, the left aortic arch passed halfway around the trachea and esophagus. A huge PA was also seen. At 9 months of age, the boy underwent a right posterolateral thoracotomy. A short, thick ligamentum was discovered between the

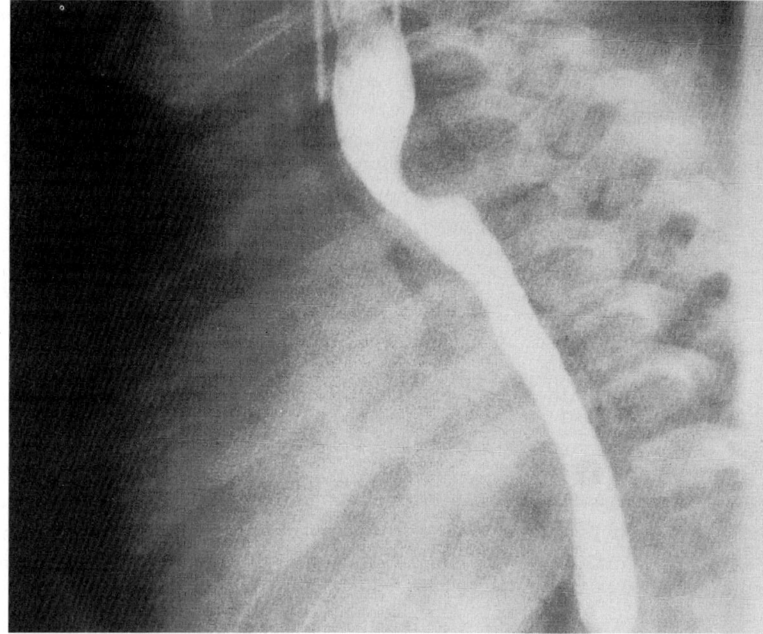

FIGURE 1.—B, lateral view of the esophagus with Gastrografin injection. Note the posterior indentation and the anterior tapering. (Courtesy of Watanabe M, Kawasaki S. Sato H, et al: Left aortic arch with right descending aorta and right ligamentum arteriosum associated with d-TGA and large VSD: Surgical treatment of a rare form of vascular ring. *J Pediatr Surg* 30:1363–1365, 1995.)

descending aorta and right PA. Division of the ligamentum relieved esophageal and tracheal constriction. The boy's respiratory distress improved gradually. About 1 month later, his airway was extubated. Stridor and wheezing resolved. A chest radiograph demonstrated remarkable improvement.

Conclusion.—In this patient, diagnostic imaging depicted a left aortic arch, right descending aorta, and effective PA banding. After right-sided thoracotomy and division of the ligamentum arteriosum, respiratory distress resolved gradually, and the patient's airway was extubated.

► The circumflex aorta or left aortic arch with right descending aorta was demonstrated in a generic way by the esophagram examination. The definitive diagnosis was made at surgery. Although MRI is the preferable modality in such a case, the demonstration of the atretic ductus arteriosus is unlikely and may not be possible. However, a double aortic arch with both arches patent is capable of MRI demonstration. In a recent similar case reported by Schlesinger et al.[1], the MRI examination shows findings of a right aortic arch, and the authors effectively interpreted the additional findings. Interesting dialogue about the findings is found in a letter to the editor.[2] Even though MRI offers cross-sectional imaging in multiple planes, specific demonstra-

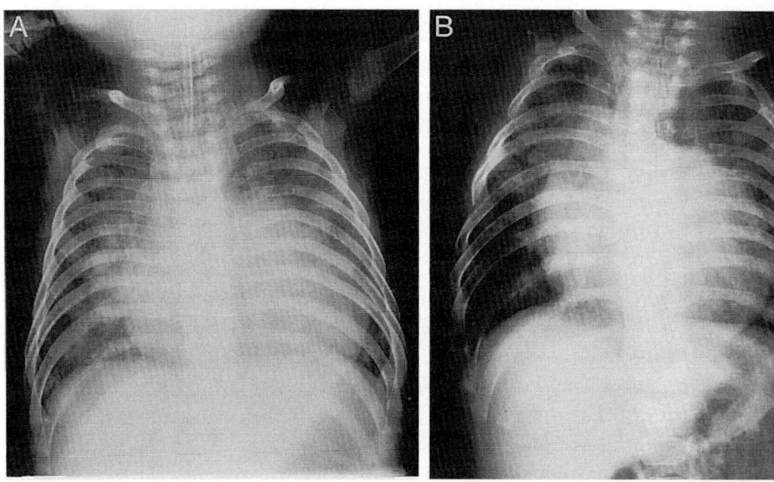

FIGURE 2.—Chest x-ray film before and after the second surgical procedure. **A**, before surgery to release the vascular ring, there was hazy infiltration in both fields (7/26/93). **B**, 1 month after surgery, there was remarkable improvement in lung field findings. Cardiomegaly is still obvious (9/4/93). (Courtesy of Watanabe M, Kawasaki S, Sato H, et al: Left aortic arch with right descending aorta and right ligamentum arteriosum associated with d-TGA and large VSD: Surgical treatment of a rare form of vascular ring. *J Pediatr Surg* 30:1363–1365, 1995.)

tion of an atretic aortic segment or a ligamentum arteriosum may not be possible. Imaging can go just so far. Operative visualization often is necessary for definitive clarification of the vascular ring components especially when imaging shows a "vascular ring" with either a right aortic arch or left aortic arch, but no double aortic arch. This exact scenario is demonstrated in the accompanying selected article by Tuma.[3]

L.W. Young, M.D.

References

1. Schlesinger AE, Mendeloff E, Sharkey AM, et al: MR of right aortic arch with mirror-image branching and a left ligamentum arteriosum: An unusual cause of a vascular ring. *Pediatr Radiol* 25:455–457, 1995.
2. Newman B: MR of right aortic arch. *Pediatr Radiol* 26:367–369, 1996.
3. Tuma S, Slavik Z, Tax P, et al: Double aortic arch in d-transposition of the great arteries complicated by tracheobronchomalacia. *Cardiovasc Intervent Radiol* 18:115–117, 1995.

Double Aortic Arch in d-Transposition of the Great Arteries Complicated by Tracheobronchomalacia

Tůma S, Slavík Z, Tax P, et al (Univ Hosp Motol, Prague, Czech Republic)
Cardiovasc Intervent Radiol 18:115–117, 1995 4–27

Background.—The co-occurrence of d-transposition of the great arteries and malformations of the aortic arch is very rare. One patient—the fourth reported in the literature to date—was described.

Case Report.—A severely cyanotic boy was born after a complicated term delivery. Systolic regurgitant murmur and right ventricular hypertrophy were detected, and echocardiography showed visceral situs solitus with atrioventricular concordance and ventriculoarterial discordance, which was consistent with transposition of the great arteries. Also noted were a small ventricular septal defect, patent foramen ovale, and patent ductus arteriosus. Balloon atrial septostomy was done at 24 hours. Angiocardiography at this time confirmed the diagnosis but also revealed a double aortic arch. The aortic anomaly was clearly shown on repeat echocardiogram and esophagogram. Mild mixed stridor progressed quickly. At 3 weeks of age, the infant underwent resection of the left-sided aortic arch distal to the origin of the left subclavian artery and resection of the bilateral ducts. Ventilation difficulty necessitated a tracheostomy 5 weeks after birth. Tracheobronchography done after the second procedure demonstrated severe bilateral tracheobronchomalacia. The infant could not be weaned from the ventilator. Six months later, he died of severe pneumonia caused by pseudomonas infection.

Conclusion.—This infant had simultaneous d-transposition of the great arteries and malformations of the aortic arch. Despite successful surgery, the patient died from tracheobronchomalacia at 7 months of age.

▶ Double aortic arch produces the same esophagram findings as left aortic arch with right ascending aorta, or right aortic arch with left ascending aorta. Angiography or MRI is capable of confirming double aortic arch of a single arch and a diverticulum of Kommerell. Recent articles on vascular rings, aortic arches, and associated cardiac anomalies are thought provoking and interesting and are listed.[1–8]

L.W. Young, M.D.

References

1. Paquet M, Williams RL: Origin of the right subclavian artery from the right pulmonary artery in a newborn with complete transposition of the great arteries. *Can J Cardiol* 10:932–934, 1994.
2. Burrows PE, MacDonald CE: Magnetic resonance imaging of the pediatric thoracic aorta. *Semin Ultrasound CT MR* 14:129–144, 1993.

3. Anand R, Dooley KJ, Williams WH, et al: Follow-up of surgical correction of vascular anomalies causing tracheobronchial compression. *Pediatr Cardiol* 15:58–61, 1994.
4. Sakurai M, Ito T, Togo T, et al: Surgical management of vascular ring in 5 cases. *Kyobu Geka—Japanese J Thoracic Surg* 48:841–844, 1995.
5. van Son JA, Starr A: Demonstration of vascular ring anatomy with ultrafast computed tomography. *Thorac Cardiovasc Surg* 43:120–121, 1995.
6. van Son JA, Julsrud PR, Hagler DJ, et al: Imaging strategies for vascular rings. *Ann Thorac Surg* 57:604–610, 1994.
7. van Son JA, Julsrud PR, Hagler DJ, et al: Surgical treatment of vascular rings: the Mayo Clinic experience. *Mayo Clinic Proc* 68:1056–1063, 1993.
8. Chun K, Colombani PM, Dudgeon DL, et al: Diagnosis and management of congenital vascular rings: A 22-year experience. *Ann Thorac Surg* 53:597–602, 1992.

Diagnosis of Congenital Pericardial Defects, Including a Pathognomic Sign for Dangerous Apical Ventricular Herniation, on Magnetic Resonance Imaging

Gassner I, Judmaier W, Fink C, et al (Univ of Innsbruck, Austria)
Br Heart J 74:60–66, 1995 4–28

Objective.—Four children having congenital pericardial defects were examined by MRI in an attempt to develop criteria for distinguishing between various forms of defect and to detect potentially fatal partial apical defects at an early stage.

Case Report.—Boy, 12 years, had become progressively less physically fit in the past 9 months. He had marked stinging retrosternal pain extending to the left shoulder and arm after swimming and drinking a carbonated beverage. There were ECG signs of anterolateral myocardial infarction, and cardiac enzyme levels were increased. On chest radiographs, lung tissue was interposed between the nearly spherical heart and the diaphragm (Fig 5). Echocardiography indicated a hypokinetic anterior wall. Magnetic resonance tomography showed marked elevation of the cardiac apex, well away from the diaphragmatic surface (Fig 7), and an indentation of the outer margin of the left ventricle. Pericardial fat abutted on this sulcus (Fig 8). Cineangiography confirmed a partial left-sided pericardial defect with herniation of the left ventricle and diastolic compression of the left coronary artery by the free pericardial edge. Exploration showed no left-sided pericardium in the apical region. The myocardium was deeply indented along the free rim of the defect, and subepicardial hemorrhage was noted.

Discussion.—Seven deaths caused by ventricular herniation through an apical pericardial defect have been reported. Complete laterodorsal displacement of the heart into the left hemithorax in the supine position is a pathognomonic finding of complete left-sided pericardial defect. Bulging

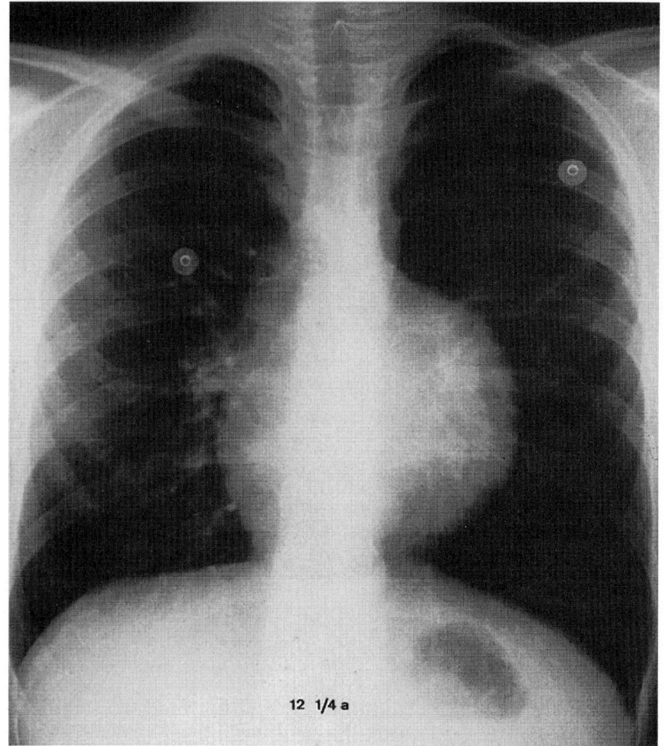

FIGURE 5.—Chest radiograph when patient was aged 12 years showing a spherical heart and interposition of lung between inferior cardiac surface and left hemidiaphragm. (Courtesy of Gassner I, Judmaier W, Fink C, et al: Diagnosis of congenital pericardial defects, including a pathognomonic sign for dangerous apical ventricular herniation, on magnetic resonance imaging. *Br Heart J* 74:60–66, 1995; published by BMJ Publishing Group.)

of the left atrial appendage without gross displacement of the heart indicates a partial left-sided atrial pericardial defect. A partial defect at the cardiac apex may threaten life.

▶ Magnetic resonance imaging demonstrates various forms of congenital left-sided pericardial defects. It is the modality of choice for this diagnosis because of its multiplanar capability combined with specific imaging of cardiac chambers at each phase of the cardiac cycle. Echocardiographic and chest radiographic findings may be suggestive but are not conclusive for this condition. The life-threatening aspect of ventricular herniation into a partial pericardial defect must not be lost sight of when only a bulge at the atrial level is shown radiographically. Computed tomography[1, 2] and angiography[3] are also reliable diagnostic imaging methods that can demonstrate pericardial defects.

L.W. Young, M.D.

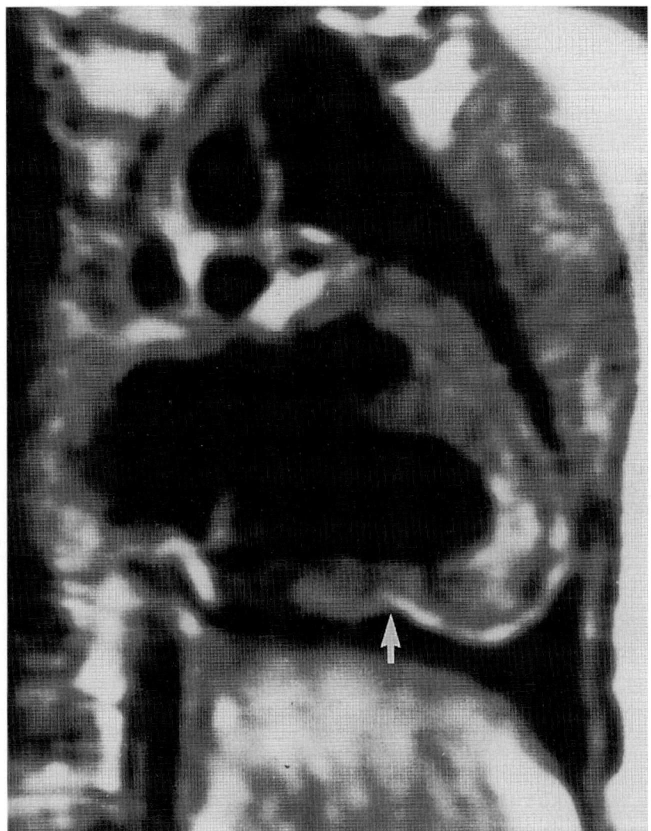

FIGURE 7.—Coronal MR tomogram (T1 weighted, spin echo) showing lung tissue separating the diaphragm and the heart. A groove is noted in the diaphragmatic portion of the left ventricular myocardium (*arrow*). (Courtesy of Gassner I, Judmaier W, Fink C, et al: Diagnosis of congenital pericardial defects, including a pathognomonic sign for dangerous apical ventricular herniation, on magnetic resonance imaging. *Br Heart J* 74:60–66, 1995; published by BMJ Publishing Group.)

References

1. Jacob JLB, Souza AS Jr, Parro A Jr: Absence of the left pericardium diagnosed by computed tomography. *Int J Cardiol* 47:293–296, 1995.
2. Kornyei V, Kiss A, Kamaras J: Congenital absence of the left pericardium. Case report and review of the literature. *Orvosi Hetilap* 134:1703–1707, 1993.
3. Rees AP, Risher W, McFadden PM, et al: Partial congenital defect of the left pericardium: angiographic diagnosis and thoracoscopic pericardiectomy: Case report. *Cathet Cardiovasc Diagn* 28:231–234, 1993.

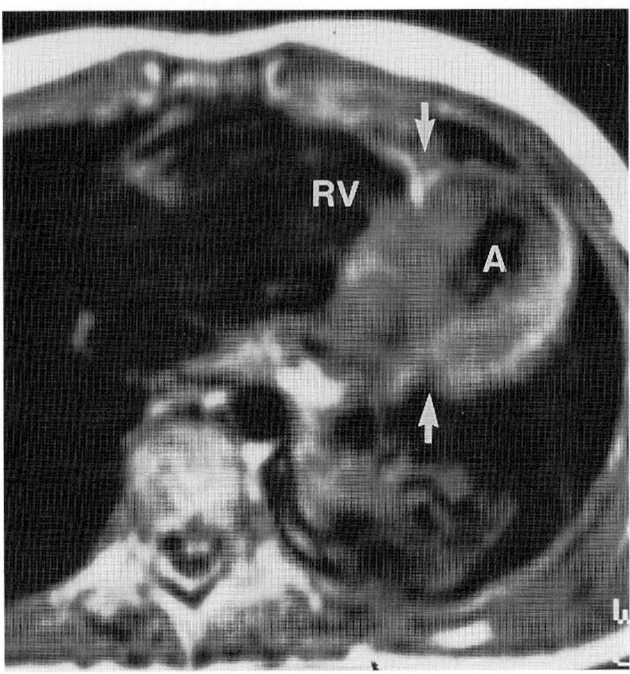

FIGURE 8.—Axial MR tomogram at the apical level of the heart. *Abbreviations: RV,* right ventricle; *A,* apex of the left ventricle. (Courtesy of Gassner I, Judmaier W, Fink C, et al: Diagnosis of congenital pericardial defects, including a pathognomonic sign for dangerous apical ventricular herniation, on magnetic resonance imaging. *Br Heart J* 74:60–66, 1995; published by BMJ Publishing Group.)

Assessment of Airways Compression by MR Imaging in Children With Aneurysmal Pulmonary Arteries

Ditchfield MR, Culham JAG (British Columbia's Children Hosp, Vancouver, Canada)

Pediatr Radiol 25:190–191, 1995 4–29

Background.—Magnetic resonance imaging obviates the need for angiography in the assessment of airways compression by congenital vascular rings and pulmonary artery slings. The role of MRI can be expanded to encompass other vascular compressive lesions as well. Two patients with aneurysmal pulmonary arteries—1 congenital and 1 acquired—were presented.

Case Reports.—Girl, 13 months, with a small ventricular septal defect (VSD) and mild pulmonary stenosis (PS), was admitted to the ICU with pneumococcal septicemia. Although the girl's condition improved after 5 days of IV antibiotic therapy, cardiomegaly developed. A pericardial effusion was diagnosed and drained. However, the fever persisted. A repeat echocardiogram obtained at

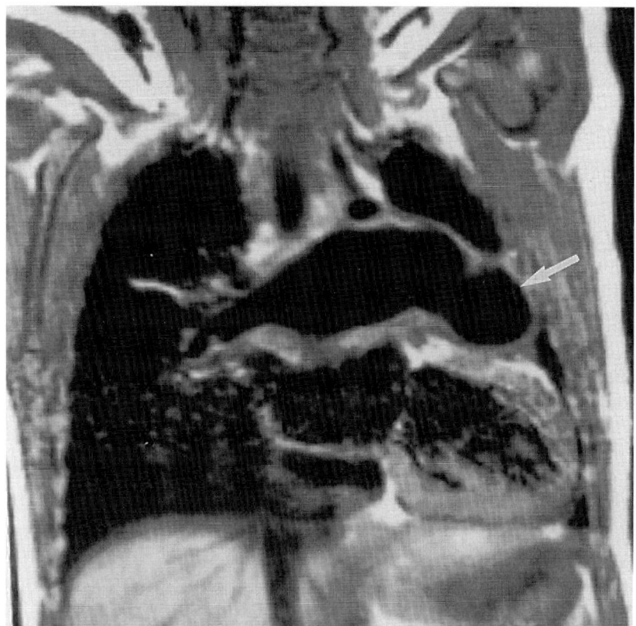

FIGURE 1.—Coronal spin-echo MRI demonstrating a massively dilated right pulmonary artery elevating the aortic arch and compressing the superior aspect of the left atrium. An additional saccular component of the aneurysm projects inferiorly and to the left off the main pulmonary artery (*arrow*). (*Pediatr Radiol*; Assessment of airways compression of MR imaging in children with aneurysmal pulmonary arteries; Ditchfield MR, Culham JAG; 25:190–191: Fig 1; 1995; Copyright notice of Springer-Verlag.)

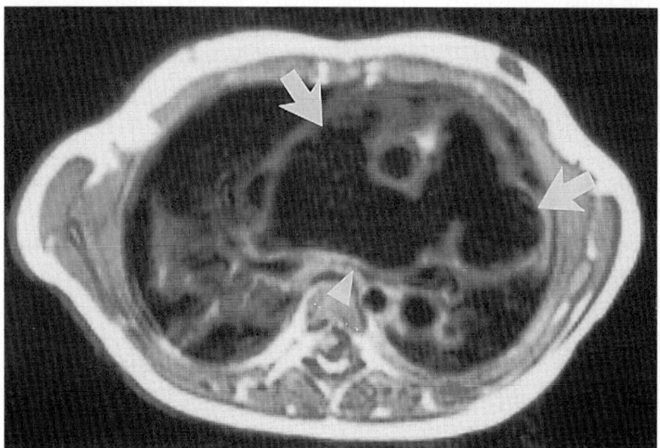

FIGURE 2.—Axial spin-echo MRI demonstrating a dilated right pulmonary artery compressing the right main bronchus and obliterating the proximal portion of the left main bronchus (*arrowhead*). Additional saccular components of the aneurysm project laterally on the left and anteriorly on the right (*arrows*). (*Pediatr Radiol;* Assessment of airways compression by MR imaging in children with aneurysmal pulmonary arteries; Ditchfield MR, Culham JAG: 25:190–191; Fig 2; 1995; Copyright notice of Springer-Verlag.)

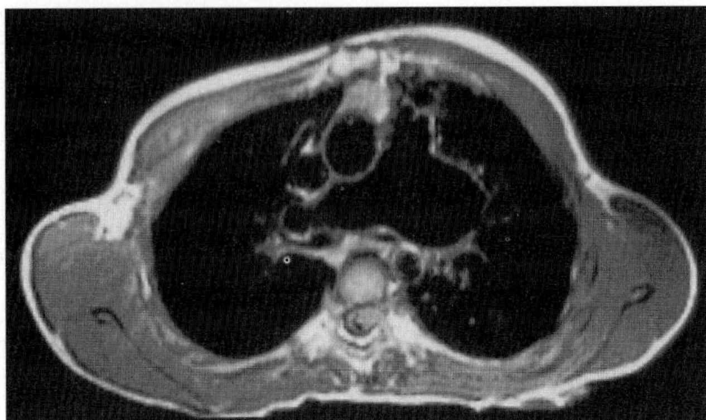

FIGURE 3.—Axial spin-echo MRI demonstrating the grossly dilated main, right, and left pulmonary arteries, which reduce in size rapidly distal to the hila. The left bronchus is narrow (*arrow*) and was obliterated on the next slice. (*Pediatr Radiol;* Assessment of airways compression by MR imaging in children with aneurysmal pulmonary arteries; Ditchfield MR, Culham JAG: 25:190–191; Fig 3; 1995; Copyright notice of Springer-Verlag.)

20 days showed a massively dilated pulmonary artery. Mycotic pulmonary artery aneurysm was diagnosed. After another 6 weeks of antibiotic treatment, the fever was gone, but echocardiography showed the aneurysm had not changed. During the next 2 years, the girl's respiratory symptoms recurred, despite maximal conservative treatment. She was also failing to thrive, her height and weight being well below the fifth percentile. Further investigation with spin-echo cardiac-gated MRI showed the extent of markedly aneurysmal pulmonary arteries. The main and right pulmonary arteries were diffusely enlarged, and additional saccular components projected anteriorly on the right and inferiorly on the left. The pulmonary arteries compressed the trachea at the level of the carina, obliterating the proximal part of the left main bronchus (Figs 1 and 2). In addition, compression was observed superiorly on the aortic arch, anteriorly on the chest wall, laterally on the superior vena cava, and inferiorly on the right and left atria as well as possibly on the left upper pulmonary vein. After pulmonary arterioplasty, the resected tissue showed thickening, focal calcification, and changes from old inflammation with no acute infection or vasculitis.

Boy, 9, with tetralogy of Fallot and absent-pulmonary-valve syndrome was diagnosed in the neonatal period. At that time, echocardiography showed grossly enlarged main, left, and right pulmonary arteries. At the age of 2 years, VSD was repaired with a Dacron patch and a homograft pulmonary valve was inserted. Persistent wheeze and cough and recurrent respiratory tract infections necessitated hospital admission. A grossly dilated main and left pulmonary artery was observed on a chest radiograph. The left main bronchus was narrow, and left lung perfusion was reduced, particularly in the upper lobe. Grossly dilated main, right, and left pulmonary arteries, which decreased in size rapidly distal to the hila, were defined on spin-echo, cardiac-gated MRI with the patient in a body coil. Compression of both main bronchi was observed, more markedly on the left (Fig 3).

Conclusion.—With spin-echo MRI, anatomic assessment of the great arteries can be done accurately and noninvasively. Thin, contiguous, or overlapping slices in axial and coronal planes should be obtained. Unlike echocardiography and angiography, MRI enables accurate assessment of the airways, depicting the exact relationship of the great arteries to any area of airway narrowing. Though sedation may be necessary, MRI is otherwise noninvasive and does not require any radiation or IV contrast medium.

► Congenital aneurysmal dilatation of pulmonary arteries[1] and mycotic pulmonary artery aneurysms have the propensity to compress and obstruct the airway causing lobar overinflation or atelectasis. This article nicely demonstrates MRI findings in a patient with tetralogy of Fallot and absent pulmonary valve/congenital avalvular pulmonary artery, as well as a patient with a mycotic pulmonary artery aneurysm. Other recent noteworthy articles on absent pulmonary valve syndrome, including airway compression and mycotic aneurysm of the pulmonary artery are listed.[2–6]

L.W. Young, M.D.

References

1. Borg SA, Young LW, Roghair GD: Congenital avalvular pulmonary artery and infantile lobar emphysema. *AJR* 125:412–421, 1995.
2. Siwik ES, Preminger TJ, Patel CR: Association of systemic to pulmonary collateral arteries with tetralogy of Fallot and absent pulmonary valve syndrome. *Am J Cardiol* 77:547–549, 1996
3. Godart F, Rey C, Breviere GM, et al: Agenesis of the pulmonary valves. Experience over 20 years. *Archives des Maladies du Coeur et des Vaisseaux* 88:673–679, 1995.
4. Mulla N, Paridon SM, Pinsky WW: Cardiopulmonary performance during exercise in patients with repaired tetralogy of Fallot with absent pulmonary valve. *Pediatr Cardiol* 16:120–126, 1995.
5. Ram SP, Lim MK, Mazeni A: Absent pulmonary valve syndrome—A case report. *Med J Malaysia* 49:93–95, 1994.
6. Kumar RV, Roughneen PT, de Leval MR: Mycotic pulmonary artery aneurysm following pulmonary artery banding. *Eur J Cardiothorac Surg* 8:665–666, 1994.

Use of Liquid Ventilation With Perflubron During Extracorporeal Membrane Oxygenation: Chest Radiographic Appearances

Gross GW, Greenspan JS, Fox WW, et al (Thomas Jefferson Univ, Philadelphia; Univ of Pennsylvania, Philadelphia; Temple Univ, Philadelphia)
Radiology 194:717–720, 1995 4–30

Introduction.—Most newborn infants undergoing extracorporeal membrane oxygenation (ECMO) improve progressively and need to be treated

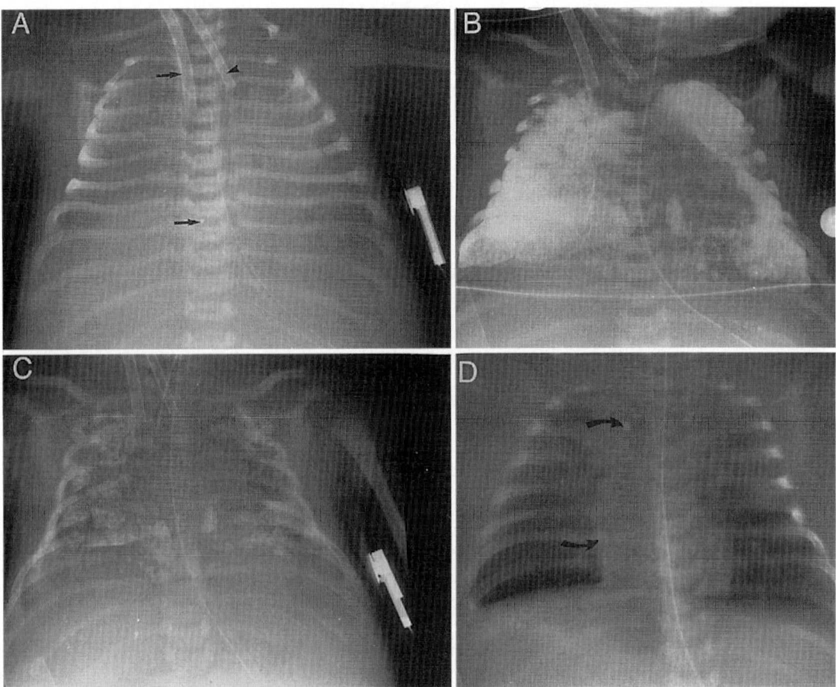

FIGURE 1.—Effect of instillation of perflubron. **A,** radiograph (anteroposterior view) shows ECMO support with venous (*arrows*) and arterial (*arrowhead*) bypass cannulas, which are judged to be in a good position. The end of the venous cannula is marked by the opaque dot (*lower arrow*). The lungs are nearly completely opaque, a common finding during ECMO bypass. The patient's airway is intubated, and ventilatory pressure settings are low, as is customary during ECMO bypass. **B,** radiograph (anteroposterior view) obtained 6 days after commencement of ECMO (because there was no clinical improvement at this point, 40 mL of Perflubron was instilled via the endotracheal tube) shows diffuse but nonhomogeneous distribution of the highly radiopaque perflubron in both lungs. The uneven distribution of perflubron may be attributed to airway obstruction and microatelectasis. The heart produced a zone of relative radiolucency in the left hemithorax. **C,** radiograph (anteroposterior view) obtained 5 days later, with no introduction of additional perflubron into the lungs, shows a marked reduction in the amount of intrapulmonary perflubron. Note the patchy and uneven distribution of residual perflubron. Progressive clinical improvement accompanied this change. **D,** radiograph (anteroposterior view) obtained 15 days after instillation of perflubron, when ECMO bypass was no longer being performed, shows only a few isolated collections of perflubron still in the lungs (*arrows*). Although there is diffuse accentuation of interstitial lung markings, which reflect persistent pulmonary parenchymal disease, the patient's clinical status had markedly improved. *Abbreviation: ECMO,* extracorporeal membrane oxygenation. (Courtesy of Gross GW, Greenspan JS, Fox WW, et al: Use of liquid ventilation with perflubron during extracorporeal membrane oxygenation: Chest radiographic appearances. *Radiology* 194:717–720, 1995; Radiological Society of North America.)

for no longer than 10 to 14 days. In the occasional infant who does not respond adequately to ECMO bypass support, systemic oxygenation may be improved by liquid ventilation with perfluorochemicals.

> *Two Case Reports.*—Infant, 1 month, and newborn with respiratory failure underwent ECMO in conjunction with perflubron ventilation. The material was instilled slowly via endotracheal tube. The neonate died shortly after ECMO was withdrawn, but the infant survived and had breathed room air since age 6 months. The chest radiographic appearances associated with instillation orf 40 mL of perflubron in about 1 hour are shown in Figure 1.

Conclusion.—In addition to offering a means of salvaging small infants who fail to respond adequately to ECMO, liquid ventilation with perflubron is an effective means of demonstrating neonatal pulmonary abnormalities.

► This article documents the use of liquid ventilation with perflubron during extracorporeal membrane oxygenation (ECMO). Perflubron is increasingly being used in ECMO patients. The physiologic advantages of potential respiratory salvage therapies of such respiratory distressed infants do not usually offer the added advantage of contrast medium opacity that perflubron does. Perfluorochemicals, such as perflubron, are excellent solvents for oxygen and carbon dioxide. The radiopaque perflubron clears within 24 to 48 hours. Additional recent articles on ECMO and liquid ventilation with perfluorochemicals are listed.[1–5]

L.W. Young, M.D.

References

1. Hirschl RB, Tooley R, Parent AC, et al: Improvement of gas exchange, pulmonary function and lung injury with partial ventilation. A study model in a setting of severe respiratory failure. *Chest* 108:500–508, 1995.
2. Wolfson MR, Stern R, Kechner N, et al: Utility of a perfluorochemical liquid for pulmonary diagnostic imaging. *Artif Cells Blood Substit Immobil Biotechnol* 22:1409–1420, 1994.
3. Jackson JC, Standaert TA, Truog WE, et al: Full-tidal liquid ventilation with perfluorocarbon for prevention of lung injury in newborn non-human primates. *Artif Cells Blood Substit Immobil Biotechnol* 22:1121–1132, 1994.
4. Paulson TE, Spear RM, Peterson BM: New concepts in the treatment of children with acute respiratory distress syndrome (review). *J Pediatr* 127:163–175, 1995.
5. Sedin G: Ventilatory techniques in the treatment of newborn infants (review). *J Perinat Med* 22:557–563, 1994.

Jugular Thrombophlebitis Complicating Bacterial Pharyngitis (Lemierre's Syndrome)

De Sena S, Rosenfeld DL, Santos S, et al (UMDNJ-Robert Wood Johnson Med School, New Brunswick, NJ)
Pediatr Radiol 26:141–144, 1996 4–31

Background.—Lemierre's syndrome, a rare entity characterized by *Fusobacterium* septicemia, internal jugular vein thrombosis, and septic emboli, affects previously healthy teenagers after a primary oropharyngeal infection. Two patients with this relatively obscure clinical entity were described.

Case Report.—Girl, 14, with a history of recurrent streptococcal pharyngitis was brought for medical care with a 3-day history of sore throat, dysphagia, and fever. Initial treatment consisted of intramuscular Decadron and oral prednisone. However, the patient had progressive dysphagia, dysarthria, trismus, and left ear pain with continued fever. On a contrast-enhanced CT scan of the neck, a left peritonsillar phlegmon was noted, but there was no evidence of internal jugular vein thrombosis (Fig 1). Intravenous ticarcillin-clavulanate and vancomycin were begun. Later that day, increasing dysphagia, drooling, and tachycardia developed, and the patient was taken to the pediatric ICU. Findings on chest radiograph obtained at transfer were grossly normal. Left-eye pain with ptosis

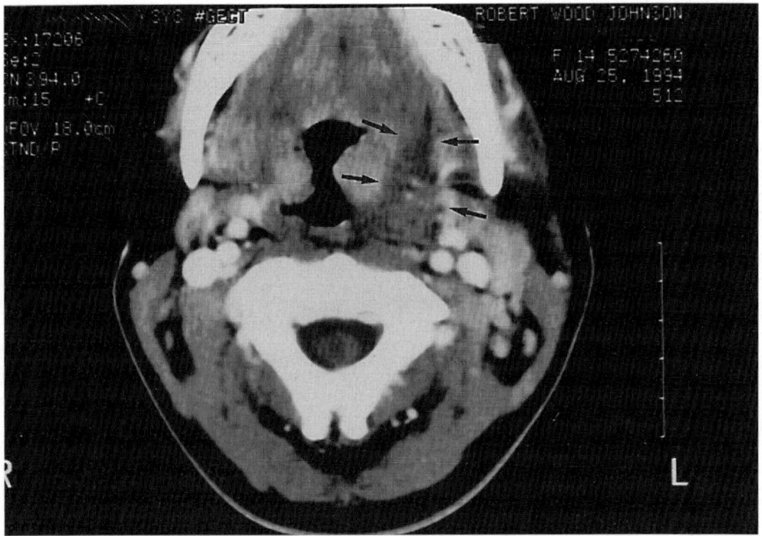

FIGURE 1.—Contrast-enhanced CT scan of the neck in a 14-year-old girl with a 3-day history of sore throat, dysphagia, and fever demonstrates a left parapharyngeal phlegmon (*arrows*). (*Pediatr Radiol;* Jugular thrombophlebitis complicating bacterial pharyngitis (Lemierre's syndrome); de Sena S, Rosenfeld DL, Santos S, et al: 26:141–144; Fig 1; 1996; Copyright notice of Springer-Verlag.)

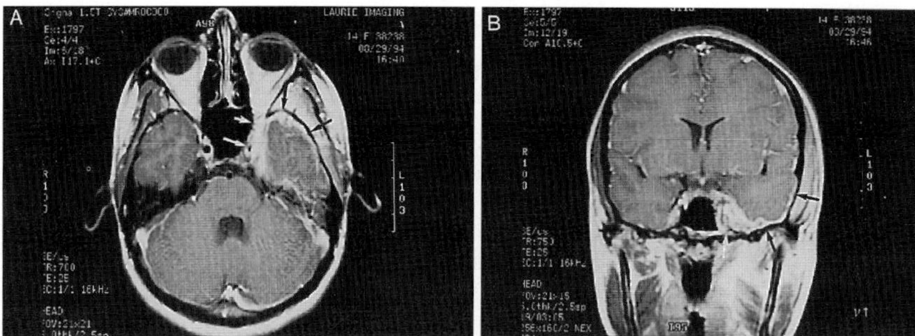

FIGURE 2.—Axial (**A**) and coronal (**B**) T1-weighted MRI scan of the brain following gadolinium administration. Thick, focally enhancing dura along the surface of the temporal lobe (*black arrows*) extends to the dura propria of the left cavernous sinus (*white arrow*). Note the mass effect on the left cavernous internal carotid artery, as evidenced by attenuation of its flow void on the axial image (*curved white arrow*). (*Pediatr Radiol;* Jugular thrombophlebitis complicating bacterial pharyngitis (Lemierre's syndrome); de Sena S, Rosenfeld DL, Santos S, et al; 26:141–144; Fig 2; 1996; Copyright notice of Springer-Verlag.)

and temporal swelling developed the following day. *Fusobacterium nucleatum* grew in blood cultures. No abnormalities were found on a contrast-enhanced CT brain scan. On an MR image of the brain, inflammatory changes involving the left temporal fossa with extension into the left cavernous sinus were seen (Fig 2). Four days after admission, a repeat contrast-enhanced CT neck scan showed improvement in the left peritonsillar phlegmon and new left internal jugular vein thrombosis (Fig 3). Intravenous heparin was begun;

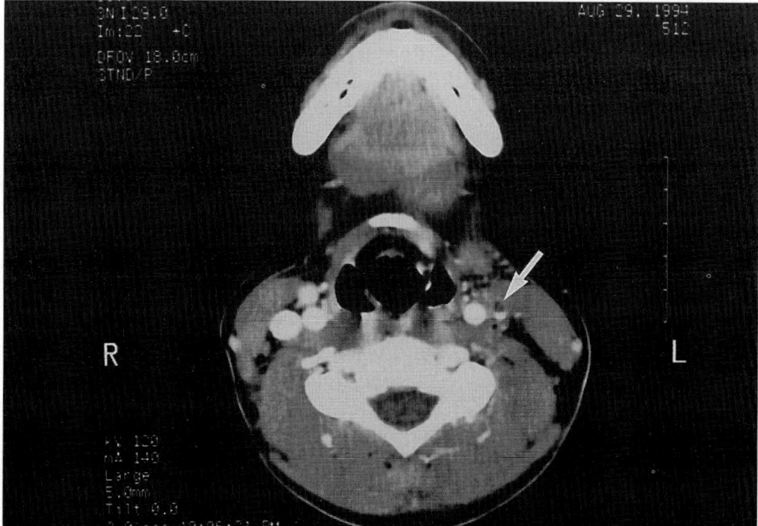

FIGURE 3.—Contrast-enhanced CT scan of the neck demonstrates left internal jugular vein thrombosis (*arrow*). (*Pediatr Radiol*; Jugular thrombophlebitis complicating bacterial pharyngitis (Lemierre's syndrome); de Sena S, Rosenfeld DL, Santos S, et al; 26:141–144; Fig 3; 1996; Copyright notice of Springer-Verlag.)

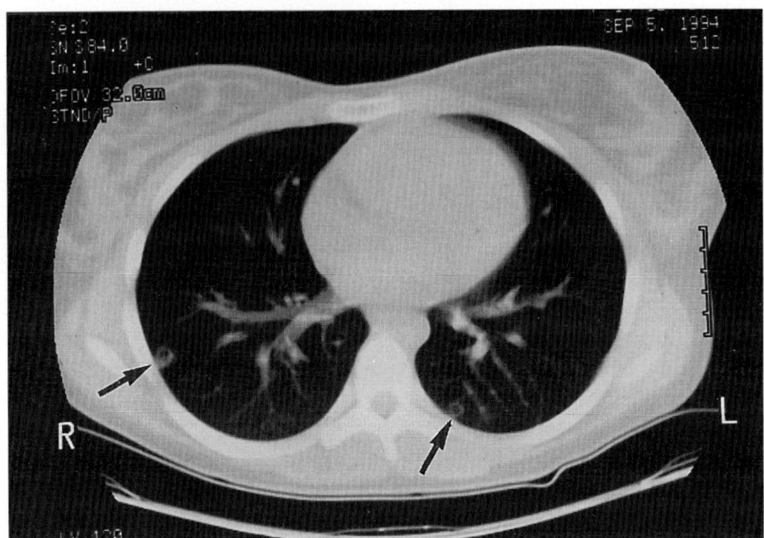

FIGURE 4.—Computed tomography scan of the thorax demonstrates bilateral hypodensities at lung bases representing septic emboli (*arrows*). (*Pediatr Radiol;* Jugular thrombophlebitis complicating bacterial pharyngitis (Lemierre's syndrome); de Sena S, Rosenfeld DL, Santos S, et al; 26:141–144; Fig 4; 1996; Copyright notice of Springer-Verlag.)

later the anticoagulant was changed to oral Coumadin. On hospital day 11, an abdominal CT scan was obtained for severe flank pain. Bilateral microabscesses of the lung bases were observed (Fig 4). The patient's condition continued to improve. Serial Doppler ultrasound (US) examinations demonstrated gradual resolution of the thrombosis. She was discharged home after 22 days in the hospital, with IV ticarcillin-clavulanate to complete a 6-week course. Oral Coumadin was continued for 3 months.

Conclusion.—Internal jugular vein thrombosis and evidence of metastatic infections are the radiologic hallmarks of Lemierre's syndrome. Internal jugular vein thrombosis is usually diagnosed on US or contrast-enhanced CT. On CT, it typically appears as a low-attenuating intraluminal filling defect within a distended vessel with enhancing walls. Surrounding soft tissues may be inflamed. On US, the vein looks distended, nonpulsatile, and noncompressible, with intraluminal echoes reflecting thrombus. Ultrasound has been proposed for the initial imaging of suspected internal jugular vein thrombosis. Parenchymal infiltrates and effusions suggesting septic pulmonary emboli are adequately shown on regular chest radiographs. Thoracic CT more accurately demonstrates the size and extent of such emboli and is useful in assessing smaller lesions that are not demonstrated adequately on conventional radiographs.

► Lemierre's syndrome has received recent attention, mainly because it represents a clinically compelling constellation of jugular thrombophlebitis, bacterial pharyngitis, and septic emboli. Computed tomography is the method of choice for demonstrating each of these associated abnormalities. Some additional recent articles on Lemierre's syndrome are listed.[1–5]

L.W. Young, M.D.

References

1. Alvarez A, Schreiber JR: Lemierre's syndrome in adolescent children-anaerobic sepsis with internal jugular vein thrombophlebitis following pharyngitis: Part 1. *Pediatrics* 2:354–359, 1995.
2. Hughes CE, Spear RK, Shinabarger CE, et al: Septic pulmonary emboli complicating mastoiditis: Lemierre's syndrome revisited. *Clin Infect Dis* 18:633–635, 1994.
3. Ahkee S, Srinath L, Huang A, et al: Lemierre's syndrome: Postanginal sepsis due to anaerobic oropharyngeal infection. *Ann Otol Rhinol Laryngol* 103:208–210, 1994.
4. Carlson ER, Bergamo DF, Coccia CT: Lemierre's syndrome: Two cases of a forgotten disease. *J Oral Maxillofac Surg* 52:74–78, 1994.
5. Blok WL, Meis JF, Gyssens IC: Postanginal sepsis caused by *Fusobacterium necrophorum*: Lemierre syndrome. *Ned Tijdschr Geneeskd* 137:1013–1016, 1993.

Percutaneous Catheter Drainage of Tension Pneumatocele, Secondarily Infected Pneumatocele, and Lung Abscess in Children

Zuhdi MK, Spear RM, Worthen HM, et al (Children's Hosp of San Diego, Calif)

Crit Care Med 24:330–333, 1996 4–32

Background.—The development of a lung pneumatocele can complicate bacterial pneumonia in children. However, to date there have been no reports of percutaneous catheter drainage of a tension pneumatocele or secondarily infected pneumatoceles in children.

Methods.—Five patients, aged 2 to 21 years, had 7 pneumatoceles and lung abscesses drained percutaneously. A chest CT scan was obtained to localize the optimal site for drainage, and a modified Seldinger method was used to insert a no. 8.5 French soft catheter percutaneously into the cyst or cavity. The catheter was left in place until drainage ceased.

Findings.—Within 24 hours of drainage, all patients showed improvement clinically and radiologically, and none was febrile. Aerobic bacteria grew in culture from 3 cysts or cavities, anaerobic bacteria from 1, and mixed bacteria from 3. Three pneumatoceles infected secondarily were found in 1 patient. In 2 mechanically ventilated patients, 4 of 5 secondarily infected pneumatoceles were under tension. The trachea was extubated in both patients within 24 hours of drainage after prolonged mechanical ventilation. Catheters were in place from 1 to 20 days (Figs 1 and 2).

Conclusions.—Percutaneous catheter drainage is safe and effective in children with tension pneumatocele, secondarily infected pneumatocele, and lung abscess. Early drainage is a useful diagnostic and therapeutic

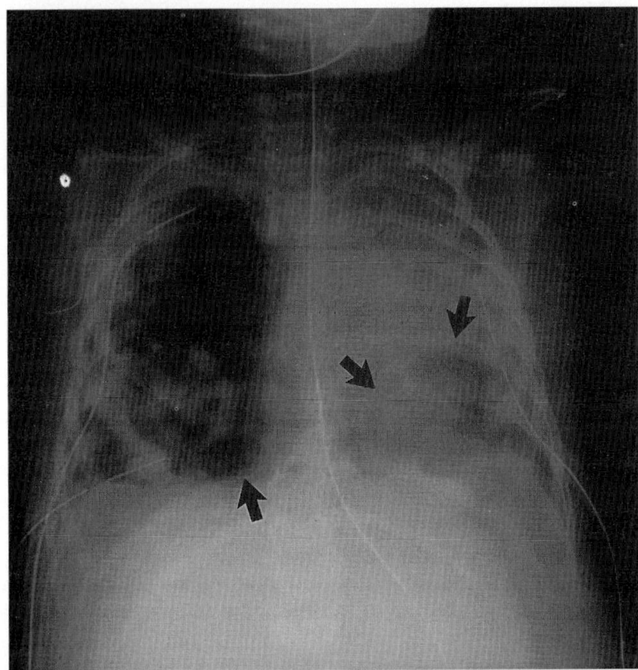

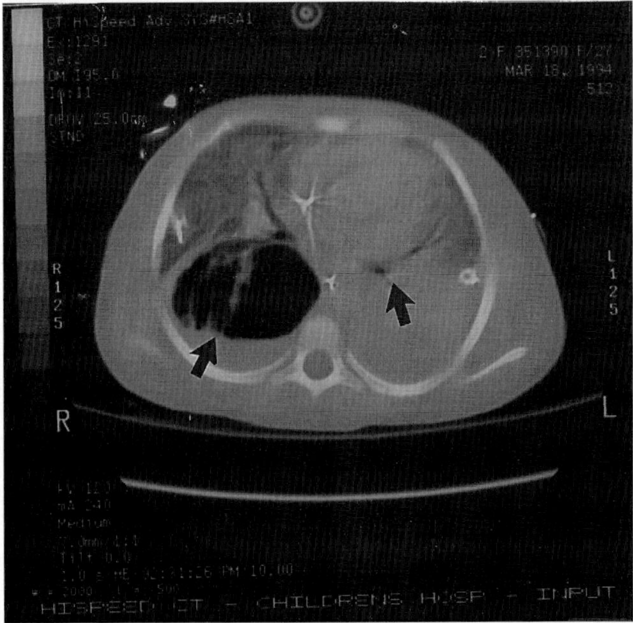

FIGURE 1.—Top, bilateral tension pneumatoceles (*arrows*) in a 2-year-old child with pneumococcal pneumonia. Tube thoracostomies were performed previously to treat pyopneumothoraces. **Bottom,** CT of the same patient shows tension pneumatoceles containing fluid (*arrows*). (Courtesy of Zuhdi MK, Spear RM, Worthen HM, et al: Percutaneous catheter drainage of tension pneumatocele, secondarily infected pneumatocele, and lung abscess in children. *Crit Care Med* 24[2]:330–333, 1996.)

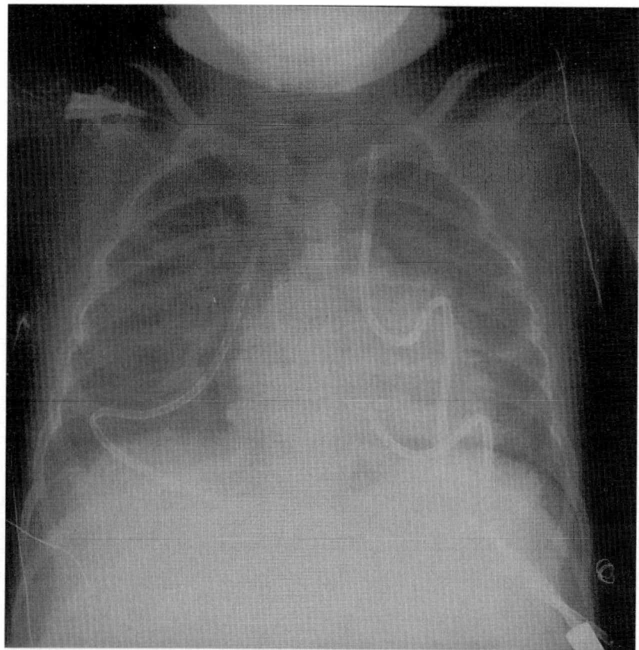

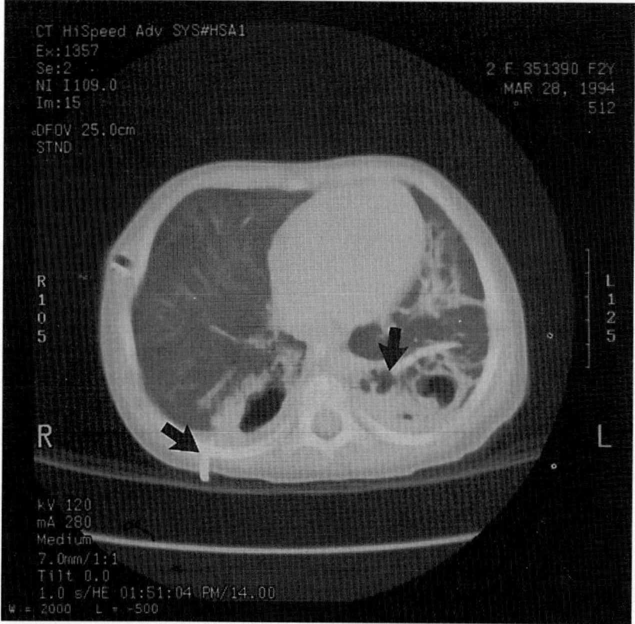

FIGURE 2.—**Top,** chest radiograph shows 3 soft catheters percutaneously inserted to drain the pneumatoceles in the same patient as in Fig 1. **Bottom,** CT shows the drainage catheters entering the pneumatoceles (*arrows*). Note the dramatic change in the size of the pneumatoceles in comparison with Fig 1. (Courtesy of Zuhdi MK, Spear RM, Worthen HM, et al: Percutaneous catheter drainage of tension pneumatocele, secondarily infected pneumatocele, and lung abscess in children. *Crit Care Med* 24[2]:330–333, 1996.)

procedure. Tension pneumatocele drainage may be helpful in weaning from mechanical ventilation. Chest CT is useful in defining the optimal site for percutaneous drainage.

► The interventional imaging technique of percutaneous catheter placement and drainage was effectively used for tension pneumatocele, secondarily infected pneumatocele, or lung abscess. Computed tomography provided imaging for determining the optimum site of intervention to effect decompression, drainage, and weaning of a child from mechanical ventilation. Other recent articles relevant to lung abscess and percutaneous catheter placement and drainage are listed.[1–3]

L.W. Young, M.D.

References

1. Bruckheimer E, Dolberg S, Shlesinger Y, et al: Primary lung abscess in infancy. *Pediatr Pulmonol* 19:188–191, 1995.
2. Klein JS, Schultz S, Heffner JE: Interventional radiology of the chest: Image-guided percutaneous drainage of pleural effusions, lung abscess, and pneumothorax. *AJR* 164:581–588, 1995.
3. Ha HK, Kang MW, Park JM, et al: Lung abscess. Percutaneous catheter therapy. *Acta Radiol* 34:362–365, 1993.

Myocardial Scintigraphy With ^{99m}Tc-Sestamibi in Children With Kawasaki Disease

Schillaci O, Banci M, Scopinaro F, et al (Univ "la Sapienza," Rome)
Angiology 46:1009–1014, 1995 4–33

Background.—Kawasaki disease (KD) is a multisystem vasculitis affecting children. Its prognosis is largely dependent on the extent of coronary artery abnormalities. Echocardiography can detect coronary aneurysms but may not be useful in assessing their progression. Coronary angiogra-

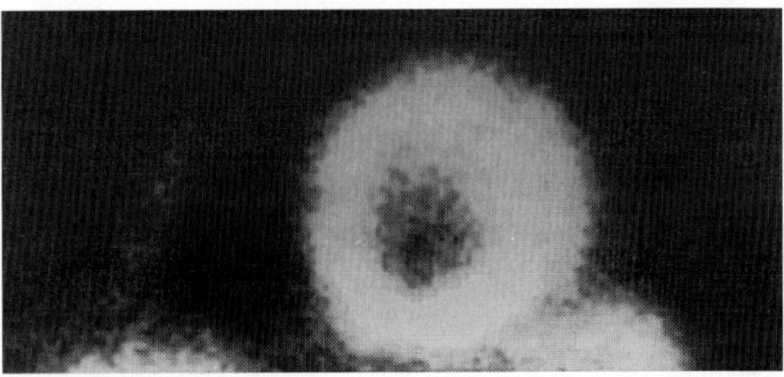

FIGURE 2.—Left anterior oblique 45-degree, rest scan. (Courtesy of Schillaci O, Banci M, Scopinaro F, et al: Myocardial scintigraphy with ^{99m}Tc-Sestamibi in children with Kawasaki disease. *Angiology* 46:1009–1014, 1995.)

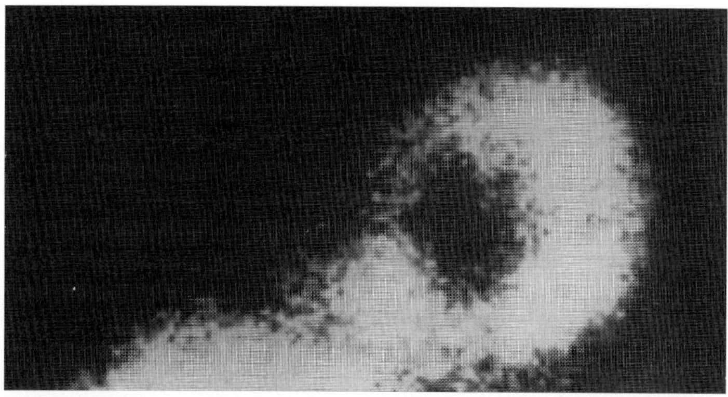

FIGURE 3.—Left anterior oblique 45-degree after dipyridamole infusion; reversible defect in the anteroseptal wall. (Courtesy of Schillaci O, Banci M, Scopinaro F, et al: Myocardial scintigraphy with ^{99m}Tc-Sestamibi in children with Kawasaki disease. *Angiology* 46:1009–1014, 1995.)

phy yields complete diagnostic information but is invasive and cannot be repeated for monitoring. The use of scintigraphy with technetium ^{99m}–Sestamibi (^{99m}Tc-MIBI) was assessed in the noninvasive evaluation of myocardial perfusion in patients with KD.

Methods.—Fifteen patients with KD and cardiovascular complications underwent evaluation with echocardiography, electrocardiography, and ^{99m}Tc-Sestamibi imaging. Both stress and rest myocardial scintigraphy was performed, and regional perfusion within 5 segments of the left ventricles was evaluated. Eight patients also underwent cardiac catheterization. The accuracy of myocardial scintigraphy in detecting coronary lesions was analyzed.

Results.—Electrocardiography demonstrated an abnormal Q wave in 2 patients. Echocardiography depicted 14 aneurysms in 12 patients. Abnormal uptake of ^{99m}Tc-MIBI appeared on the myocardial scintigraphies of 12 patients, including 10 of the patients with coronary aneurysms and 2 children without aneurysms (Figs 2 and 3). One of these children without aneurysms had more than 75% narrowing of the left anterior descending artery on coronary angiography.

Conclusion.—Myocardial scintigraphy with ^{99m}Tc-Sestamibi has a sensitivity of 88% and a specificity of 93% in detecting coronary lesions. This method of coronary imaging is safe and has considerable clinical utility in monitoring cardiac involvement in infants and children with KD.

► The higher-energy photon advantage of ^{99m}Tc-Sestamibi over thallium-201 scintigraphy is the rationale for preferring this noninvasive method of assessment of infants with KD. Rest/dipyridamole ^{99m}Tc-Sestamibi has respectable sensitivity and specificity that justifies continuance of its use. In the midchildhood to adolescent age groups, ^{99m}Tc-Sestamibi has been used with stress exercise and at rest with similar substantial results.[1] Technetium 99m–pertechnetate is another radionuclide that has been used with success in conjunction with echocardiography to evaluate the cardiac status of children with KD.[2] Ultimately angiography may be necessary to define severe cardiac sequelae.[3]

L.W. Young, M.D.

References

1. Paridon SM, Galioto FM, Vincent JA, et al: Exercise capacity and incidence of myocardial perfusion defects after Kawasaki disease in children and adolescents. *J Am Coll Cardiol* 25:1425–1427, 1995.
2. Kao C-H, Hsieh K-S, Chen Y-C, et al: Labeled WBC cardiac imaging and two-dimensional echocardiography to evaluate high-dose gamma globulin treatment in Kawasaki disease. *Clin Nucl Med* 20:813–816, 1995.
3. Takahashi N, Fukushige J, Hijii T, et al: Occlusion of the right coronary artery as sequelae of Kawasaki disease: The clinical features of 9 cases. *Cardiology* 86:207–210, 1995.

Obstructive Lung Disease in Children After Allogeneic Bone Marrow Transplantation: Evaluation With High-Resolution CT

Sargent MA, Cairns RA, Murdoch MJ, et al (British Columbia's Children's Hosp, Vancouver, Canada)

AJR 164:693–696, 1995 4–34

Introduction.—Pulmonary function tests are difficult to perform in children suspected of having chronic obstructive lung disease as a complication of bone marrow transplantation. High-resolution CT findings were evaluated to determine the value of CT as a diagnostic test in this setting.

Patients and Methods.—A review of records between 1980 and 1992 at the study institution identified 10 children in whom symptoms of chronic obstructive lung disease developed after bone marrow transplantation. All 10 had chronic graft-vs.-host disease. Ten high-resolution CT scans of the lungs were obtained in 7 of these children. Spirometry, performed before CT in 5 cases and after CT in 2, confirmed airflow obstruction. The CT scans were examined blindly with similar images from 5 controls. A retrospective study of the scans of children with obstructive lung disease analyzed parenchymal hypoattenuation, bronchial dilatation, bronchial wall thickening, and abnormal parenchymal opacity.

Results.—Normal scans of the controls were correctly identified by all 3 observers. Observer diagnoses were abnormal for 17 initial scans and equivocal for 4 in the patients with obstructive lung disease. All 3 follow-up scans were rated as abnormal by the observers. Scans of all 7 patients had areas of parenchymal hypoattenuation (Fig 1). Expiratory air-trapping was identified in these areas in 3 cine high-resolution CT studies (Fig 2). Twenty-three of 25 lobes in 5 patients showed bronchial dilatation. No bronchial abnormalities were apparent in the 2 youngest children. The CT abnormalities observed in these cases were similar to those reported in cases of bronchiolitis obliterans.

Conclusion.—Obstructive lung disease is a significant complication of pediatric allogenic bone marrow transplantation. Whereas chest radiographs showed little abnormality in these patients, high-resolution CT

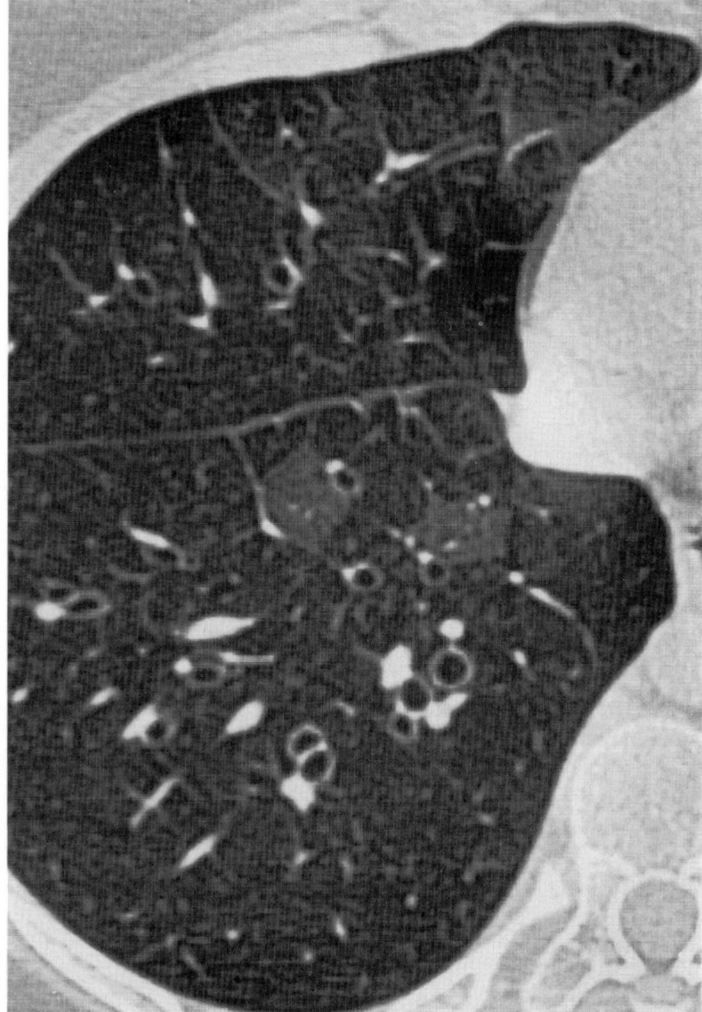

FIGURE 1.—Hypoattenuation and bronchial dilatation in obstructive lung disease in an 11-year-old boy. Obstructive lung disease was diagnosed on spirometry 11 months after bone marrow transplantation for leukemia. High-resolution CT scan at the time of diagnosis of obstructive lung disease shows diffuse hypoattenuation and thin-walled dilated bronchi. Two small polygonal areas of normal attenuation are seen anteromedially in the lower lobe. (Courtesy of Sargent MA, Cairns RA, Murdoch MJ, et al: Obstructive lung disease in children after allogeneic bone marrow transplantation: Evaluation with high-resolution CT. *AJR* 164:693–696, 1995.)

demonstrated extensive morphologic changes. The characteristic features seen at CT can assist in diagnosis, particularly in young children unable to cooperate with spirometry.

► This article documents the development of obstructive lung disease after chronic graft-vs.-host disease, a "bronchiolitis obliterans" complication of

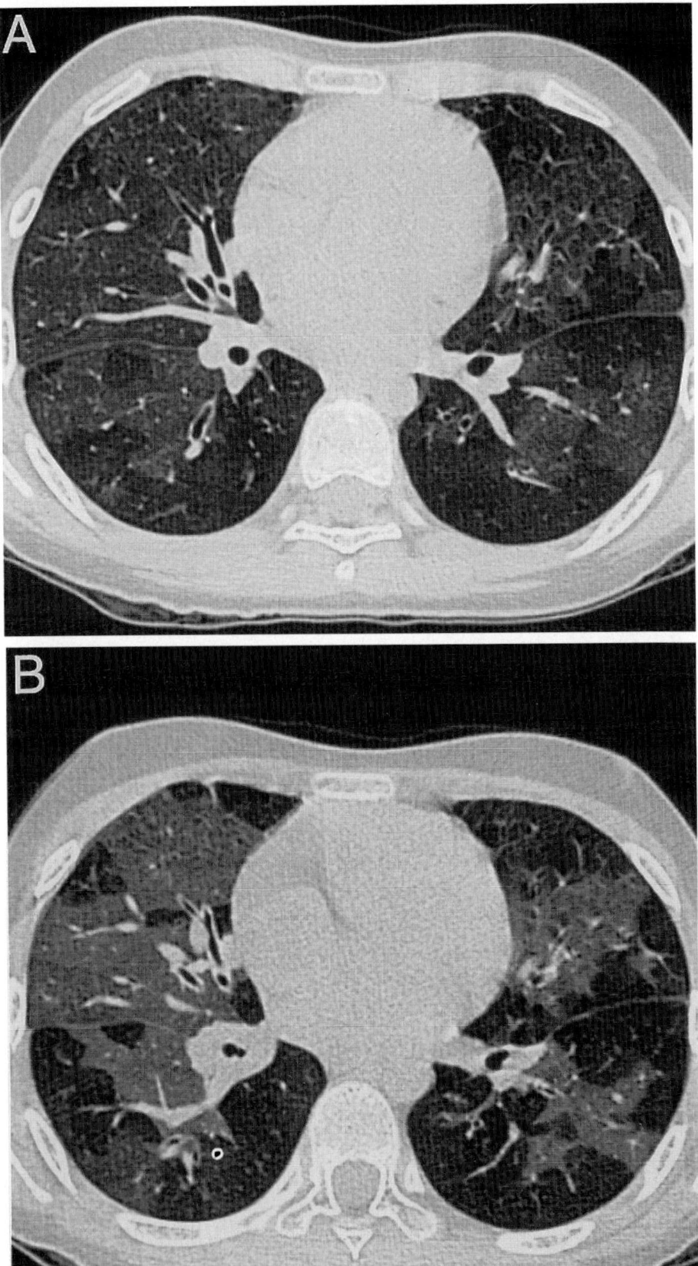

FIGURE 2.—Expiratory air trapping on cine high-resolution CT scans in an 11-year-old boy. Obstructive lung disease was diagnosed on spirometry 6 months after bone marrow transplantation for aplastic anemia. **A,** inspiratory high-resolution CT scan obtained 9 months later shows multiple areas of reduced parenchymal attenuation. **B,** cine high-resolution Ct scan at same level as in **A** shows expiratory air trapping in areas of hypoattenuation. The density difference between the normal and abnormal (hyperlucent) lung is accentuated. (Courtesy of Sargent MA, Cairns FA, Murdoch MJ, et al: Obstructive lung disease in children after allogeneic bone marrow transplantation: Evaluation with high-resolution CT. *AJR* 164:693–696, 1995.)

pediatric allogeneic bone marrow transplantation. Noninvasive high-resolution CT findings may effectively demonstrate this childhood disease when chest radiographic findings may not. Other noteworthy recent articles on obstructive lung disease from this cause are listed.[1–3] Gastroesophageal reflux has also been implicated as a cause of obstructive lung disease in bone marrow transplant patients.[1]

L.W. Young, M.D.

References

1. Schultz KR, Fernandez CV, Israel DM, et al: Association of gastroesophageal reflux with obstructive lung disease in children after allogeneic bone marrow transplantation (letter). *Blood* 85:3763–3765, 1995.
2. Schultz KR, Green GJ, Wensley D, et al: Obstructive lung disease in children after allogeneic bone marrow transplantation. *Blood* 84:3212–3220, 1994.
3. Philit F, Wiesendanger T, Archimbaud E, et al: Post-transplant obstructive lung disease ("bronchiolitis obliterans"): A clinical comparative study of bone marrow and lung transplant patients. *Eur Respir J* 8:551–558, 1995.

Plasma Cell Granuloma of the Lung in Childhood: Atypical Radiologic Findings and Association With Hypertrophic Osteoarthropathy

Estellés EM, Andrés V, Vallcanera A, et al (Hosp Infantil La Fé, Valencia, Spain)

Pediatr Radiol 25:369–372, 1995 4–35

Introduction.—Plasma cell granuloma (PCG) is the most frequent of the rare primary lung tumors of childhood. It is a benign, pseudotumoral lesion that has been included among the benign lymphoid disorders of the lung, probably representing hyperplasia of the pulmonary lymphoid system in response to chronic antigenic stimulation. It is detected incidentally in three fourths of cases. Previous reports have identified no way of making the exact diagnosis of PCG before surgery. Three cases of PCG in children were reported.

Case Report.—Girl, 5, complained of abdominal pain. She had mucocutaneous pallor and adenopathy in the axillary, cervical, and inguinal areas. Her erythrocyte sedimentation rate was elevated, and she had marked anemia. A right parahilar intrapulmonary mass was seen on chest radiography and CT (Fig 2). This mass was adherent to the mediastinum, had no calcifications, and showed irregular enhancement. The mass appeared mediastinal in origin at surgery and was closely adherent to the pericardium and visceral pleura. Plasma cell granuloma of the lung with infiltration of adjacent mediastinal structures was diagnosed.

Discussion.—Two of the 3 cases of PCG of the lung in children described in this study were associated with infiltration of the adjacent

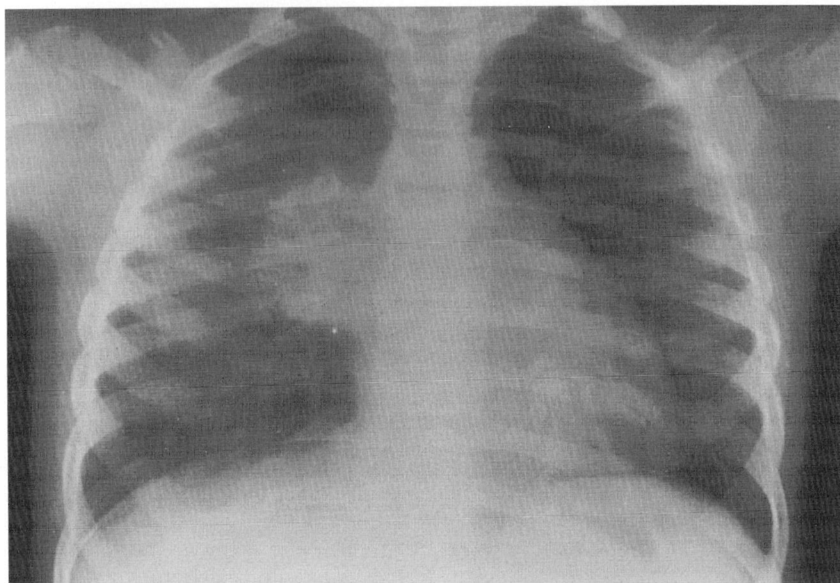

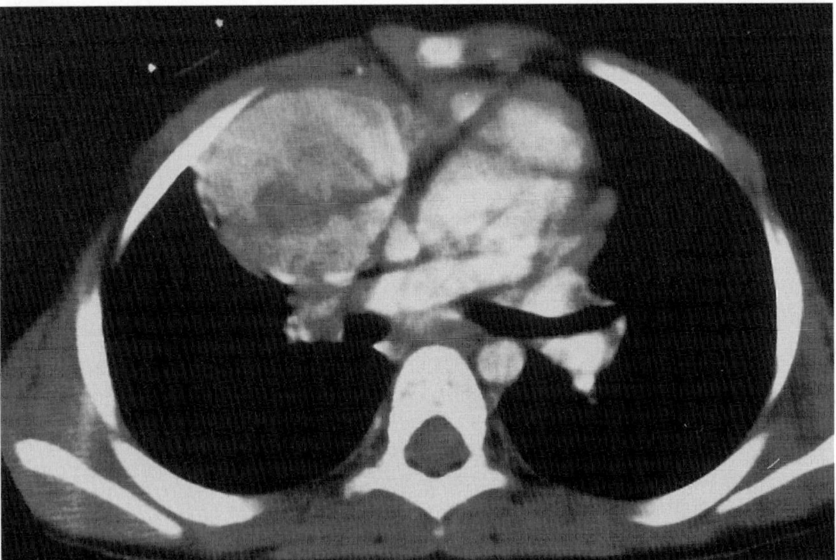

FIGURE 2.—Girl, 5 years, with plasma cell granuloma. Posteroanterior chest plain film (**A**) and contrast-enhanced CT (**B**) show right parahilar pulmonary mass. (*Pediatr Radiol*; Plasma cell granuloma of the lung in childhood: Atypical radiologic findings and association with hypertrophic osteoarthropathy; Estellés EM, Andrés V, Vallcanera A, et al; 25:369–372; Fig 2; 1995; Copyright notice of Springer-Verlag.)

mediastinal structures and diaphragm. This type of invasion may be more common in children than adults. The third case of PCG was associated with hypertrophic osteoarthropathy; this link has not been reported previously. The usual radiologic appearance of PCG is a round, well-defined, peripherally located pulmonary mass. It has no pathognomic features on CT scanning.

► Considering the pathogenesis of this inflammatory pseudotumor and its histology, including lack of a capsule, close adherence of pulmonary PCG to adjacent structures may not be as unusual as the authors suggest. The association with hypertrophic osteoarthropathy certainly isn't either. In another recent article, demonstration of plasma elevations of interleukin-6 and interleukin-1β in a 10-year-old boy who developed a pulmonary PCG supports the causation theory of cytokine production dysregulation.[1] In that article, MRI with and without IV gadolinium showed a central area of calcification in the discrete mass. Computed tomography has demonstrated calcification in this lesion.[2] Plasma cell granuloma is not specific to the respiratory tract,[3] but it occurs most commonly there.[4]

L.W. Young, M.D.

References

1. Rohrlich P, Peuchmaur M, de Napoli Cocci S, et al: Interleukin-6 and Interleukin-1β production in a pediatric plasma cell granuloma of the lung. *Am J Surg Pathol* 19:590–595, 1995.
2. Kushihashi T, Munechika H, Satou S, et al: CT findings of pulmonary inflammatory pseudotumors (plasma cell granulomas). *Nippon Igaku Hoshasen Gakkai Zasshi* 54:13–19, 1994.
3. Shedden AI, Narla LD: Plasma cell granuloma presenting as an iliopsoas mass—mimicking a rhabdomyosarcoma. *Pediatr Radiol* 21:444, 1991. .
4. Laufer L, Mares AJ, Shulman H, et al: Plasma cell granuloma of the chest and lung in childhood. *Harefuah* 126:497–500, 1994.

Gastrointestinal Systems

Midgut Malfixation in Patients With Congenital Diaphragmatic Hernia: What Is the Risk of Midgut Volvulus?

Levin TL, Liebling MS, Ruzal-Shapiro C, et al (Babies and Children's Hosp, New York; Montefiore Med Ctr, Bronx, NY; Columbia-Presbyterian Med Ctr, NY)

Pediatr Radiol 25:259–261, 1995 4–36

Background.—Anomalies of intestinal rotation and fixation have been associated with congenital diaphragmatic hernia (DH), especially with herniation developing early in fetal development. However, midgut volvulus is a rare complication of DH repair. Intestinal rotation and fixation after DH repair were assessed using 1 series that was reviewed retrospectively.

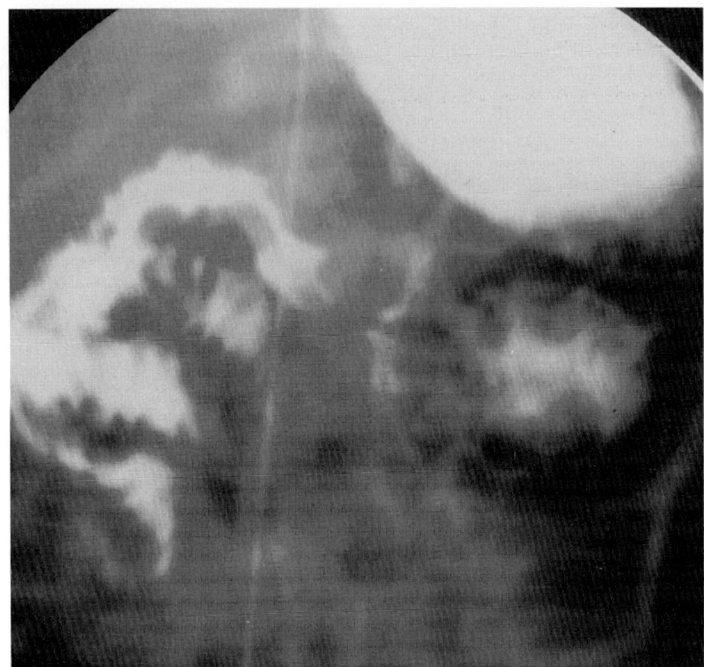

FIGURE 1.—An upper gastrointestinal series demonstrates obvious malifixation of the bowel in an infant with repaired right-sided diaphragmatic hernia; with no normal duodenojejunal junction or proximal jejunal loops in the right upper guadrant. (*Pediatr Radiol;* Midgut malfixation in patients with congenital diaphragmatic hernia: What is the risk of midgut volvulus?; Levin TL, Liebling MS, Ruzal-Shapiro C, et al; 25:259–261; Fig 1; 1995; copyright notice of Springer-Verlag.)

Methods and Findings.—Twenty-four patients with repaired DH underwent an upper GI series for evaluation of the rotation and fixation of the bowel. All 7 patients with repaired right-sided hernias with a radiographically abnormal duodenojejunal junction (DJJ) had an obvious anomaly of fixation. In this group, the right upper quadrant showed duodenal and jejunal loops (Fig 1). None of these patients had a small bowel with a corkscrew appearance. Gastroesophageal reflux was noted in all 7 patients, primarily to the level of the cricopharyngeal muscle. In 17 infants with left-sided DH repair, the DJJ was malpositioned. However, the findings in these patients were less pronounced. Twelve patients with left-sided hernia repairs had gastroesophageal reflux.

Conclusion.—These patients demonstrated a spectrum of rotational abnormalities. Midgut volvulus did not develop in any of the patients, despite malfixation. The occurrence of volvulus is probably limited by postoperative adhesions.

▶ This analysis of 24 patients with repaired DH in whom midgut volvulus is unusual brings to mind other conditions of malrotation and fixation that also are usually not complicated by midgut volvulus, specifically, gastroschisis and omphalocele. Postmanipulation adhesions probably do limit the occurrence of volvulus in these conditions. In another recent article concerning DH, it is suggested that inadequate muscle differentiation in the primitive mesenchyme might contribute to the occurrence of congenital hernia at the esophageal hiatus and nonrotation of the midgut.[1] However, intrathoracic intestinal volvulus has been reported.[2] A recent comprehensive general article on childhood intestinal malrotation may also be of interest.[3]

L.W. Young, M.D.

References

1. Chandraraj S, Briggs CA: Congenital diaphragmatic hernia through the oesophageal hiatus with nonrotation of the midgut. A case report. *J Anat* 178:265–272, 1991.
2. Nunez R, Rubio JL, Pimentel J, et al: Congenital diaphragmatic hernia and intrathoracic intestinal volvulus. *Eur J Pediatr Surg* 3:293–295, 1993.
3. Ford EG, Senac MO Jr., Srikanth MS, et al: Malrotation of the intestine in children. *Ann Surg* 215:172–178, 1992.

Technetium-99m-Sulfur Colloid SPECT Imaging in Infants With Suspected Heterotaxy Syndrome

Oates E, Austin JM, Becker JL (New England Med Ctr, Boston; Tufts Univ, Boston)

J Nucl Med 36:1368–1371, 1995 4–37

Background.—Single-photon emission CT (SPECT) complements planar technetium 99m–sulfur colloid liver/spleen imaging in the assessment of a variety of hepatosplenic disorders. Imaging with SPECT isolates small, ectopic, or poorly functioning spleen from overlying or adjacent liver, thus facilitating the detection of splenic tissue in infants suspected of having heterotaxy syndrome. The diagnostic value of adjunctive SPECT imaging in infants and children thought to have polysplenia/asplenia syndrome was investigated.

Methods.—Ten planar-only and 9 planar plus SPECT (planar-SPECT) liver/spleen scans were obtained from 15 infants during a 10-year period. Thirteen patients were less than 1 month old at initial examination. Four infants undergoing planar-only studies had follow-up planar-SPECT imaging. Scintigraphic impressions were correlated with clinical diagnoses.

Findings.—Splenic tissue was identified in 13 infants. Two were asplenic. Planar-only scintiscans correctly depicted 4 infants with spleens and the 2 without spleens but was equivocal in another 4. In all patients undergoing planar-SPECT imaging, the results were positive. Furthermore splenic tissue was documented by SPECT imaging only in 4 of 13 patients (Fig 2).

Conclusion.—Single-photon emission CT is invaluable for identifying and localizing functioning splenic tissue in infants with possible heterotaxy syndrome, especially when planar views are not conclusive. Imaging with SPECT is practical and easily performed without sedation.

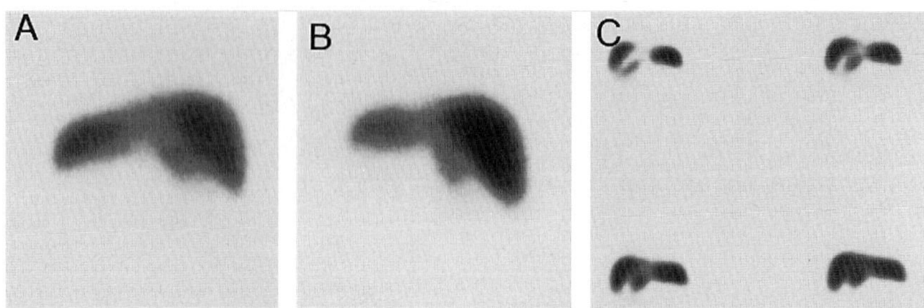

FIGURE 2.—Ectopic spleen identified only on single-photon emission CT images. Right posterior oblique (**A**) and posterior planar (**B**) views do not clearly show the spleen. Coronal single-photon emission CT images (**C**) define the spleen (*arrows*) inferoposterior to the right hepatic lobe near the midline. (Reprinted by permission of the Society of Nuclear Medicine from Oates E, Austin JM, Becker JL: Technetium-99m-sulfur colloid SPECT imaging in infants with suspected heterotaxy syndrome. *J Nucl Med* 36:1368–1371, 1995; Fig 2.)

► Single-photon emission CT selectively complements planar scintigraphy in localizing functional renal tissue in infants suspected of having heterotaxy syndrome. It is superior to planar imaging alone because of the pitfall of overlapping signals with planar imaging.[1] Ultrasonography and CT were done in too small a number of patients for any valid correlations compared with SPECT. Imaging using SPECT seems to be ideal for examining the status of the spleen in suspected heterotaxy syndrome where identification of functioning splenic tissue is critical. Another recent article of interest concerning visceral heterotaxy and the spleen is listed.[2]

L.W. Young, M.D.

References

1. Bakir M, Bilgic A, Ozmen M, et al: The value of radionuclide splenic scanning in the evaluation of asplenia in patients with heterotaxy. *Pediatr Radiol* 24:25–28, 1994.
2. Uemura H, Ho SY, Devine WA, et al: Analysis of visceral heterotaxy according to splenic status, appendage morphology, or both. *Am J Cardiol* 76:846–849, 1995.

Pre-Operative MRI of Anorectal Anomalies in the Newborn Period

McHugh K, Dudley NE, Tam P (John Radcliffe Hosp, Oxford, England)
Pediatr Radiol 25:33–36, 1995 4–38

Background.—Anorectal atresias are common congenital malformations, which can present diagnostic challenges, in that radiography and CT both have limitations in determining the true level of the levator sling musculature in neonates. The value of MRI findings in the evaluation of neonates with anorectal atresia was assessed retrospectively.

Methods.—Over a 1-year period, 9 newborns with anorectal atresias underwent MRI examinations 1 to 4 days after birth. The level of the atresia and the levator sling were determined, with particular reference to images obtained in the plane through the symphysis pubis and coccyx (PC plane) and in the plane passing through the ischial rami (I plane). High anomaly was determined when the lower limit of the rectal pouch ended above the PC plane. Intermediate anomaly was defined by the rectum ending at the PC, but not within the I plane. Low anomaly was determined by the presence of the distal rectum in both the PC and the I planes (Fig 1). The size of the puborectal and external anal sphincter (EAS) muscles was also assessed.

Results.—In 8 of the 9 infants, there was agreement between the MRI determinations of the level of atresia and muscle development and the operative findings. The MRI findings indicated 3 high, 1 intermediate, and 5 low anomalies in the 9 infants. Surgery revealed that 1 of the infants with a low anomaly on MRI had a high anomaly with a rectourethral fistula. All of the infants had uniformly hyperintense T1-weighted signal (Fig 2, A), with more variable T2-weighted signal.

Discussion.—Magnetic resonance imaging, because it can directly depict the distal rectum and the related musculature in multiple planes, can

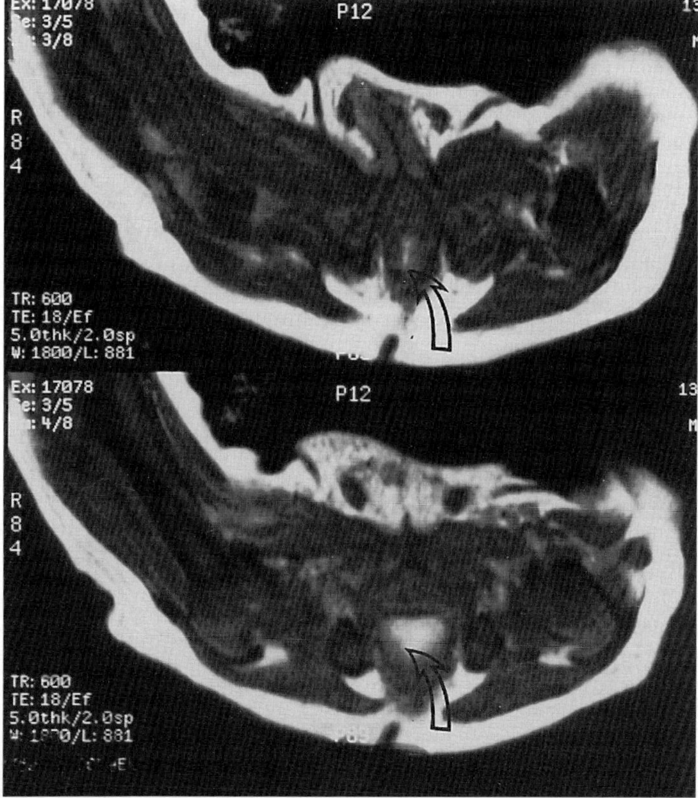

FIGURE 1.—Axial T1-weighted image showing increased T1-weighted signal meconium (*curved open arrow*) within the distal rectum in both the I (**A**) and the PC (**B**) planes, indicating a low anorectal anomaly. (*Pediatr Radiol;* Pre-operative MRI of anorectal anomalies in the newborn period; McHugh K, Dudley NE, Tam P; 25:33–36; Fig 1; 1995; Copyright notice of Springer-Verlag.)

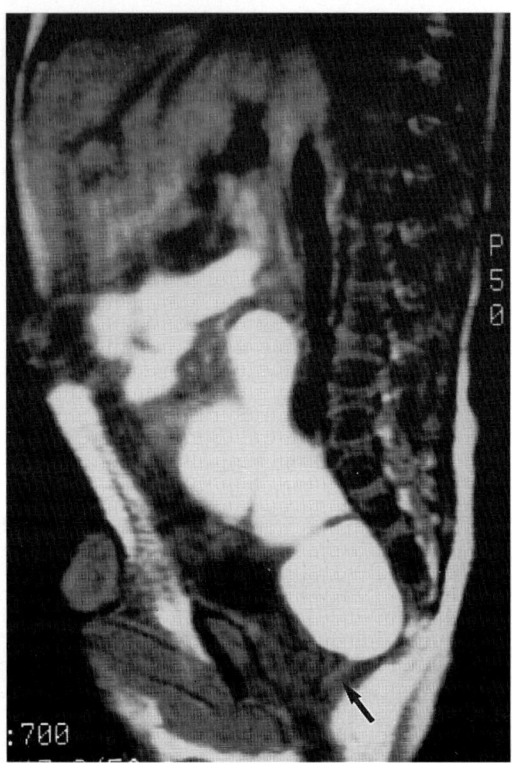

FIGURE 2.—A, hyperintense T1 signal of meconium distending the rectosigmoid in a newborn boy with a low anorectal malformation and duodenal atresia. Note the fistulous tract (*arrow*). (*Pediatr Radiol;* Pre-operative MRI of anorectal anomalies in the newborn period; McHugh K, Dudley NE, Tam P; 25:33–36; Fig 2; 1995; Copyright notice of Springer-Verlag.)

provide valuable diagnostic information in the evaluation of neonates with anorectal malformations. The MRI findings can be used to guide the surgical management and predict likely future continence. Because MRI can be performed soon after birth, the risk of overdistention and perforation is reduced.

▶ Preoperative MRI is valuable in showing the presence and relative size of the puborectalis and the external anal sphincter of the anorectal malformation complex in the neonate. The hyperintense signal of meconiun also helps. The ability of MRI to depict associated genitourinary and spinal abnormalities is a worthwhile bonus. Other recent articles on anorectal malformations of related interest are listed.[1–6]

L.W. Young, M.D.

References

1. Poenaru D, Uroz-Tristan J, Leclerc S, et al: Imperforate anus, malrotation and Hirschsprung's disease: A rare association. *Eur J Pediatr Surg* 5:187–189, 1995.

2. Tsakayannis DE, Shamberger RC: Association of imperforate anus with occult spinal dysraphism. *J Pediatr Surg* 30:1010–1012, 1995.
3. Beek FJA, Boemers TML, Witkamp TD, et al: Spine evaluation in children with anorectal malformations. *Pediatr Radiol* 25:28S–32S, 1995.
4. Ueno S, Yokoyama S, Soeda J, et al: Three-dimensional display of the pelvic structure of anorectal malformations based on CT and MR images. *J Pediatr Surg* 30:682–686, 1995.
5. Ahmad MZ-M, Brereton RJ, Huskisson L: Rectal atresia and stenosis. *J Pediatr Surg* 30:1546–1550, 1995.
6. Walton M, Bass J, Soucy P: Tethered cord with anorectal malformation, sacral anomalies and presacral masses: An under-recognized association. *Eur J Pediatr Surg* 5:59–62, 1995.

Ultrasonography of Jejunal Intussusception in Children

Jéquier S, Argyropoulou M, Bugmann P (Clinique de pédiatrie, Genève; Hôpital cantonal universitaire de Genève)

Can Assoc Radiol J 46:285–290, 1995 4–39

Background.—Jejunal intussusception is a rare condition that occurs in 2 forms. Either an underlying lesion acts as the lead point, or intussusception is idiopathic postoperatively. The ultrasound (US) findings in 3 children with these different forms of jejunal intussusception were reported.

Methods.—Two children had hamartomatous polyps of the jejunum acting as lead points for antegrade jejunoileocolic intussusception and retrograde jejunoduodenogastric intussusception. The third child had idiopathic postoperative intussusception.

Findings.—Ultrasonographic features were different and abnormal in each patient, depending on the underlying condition and direction of the

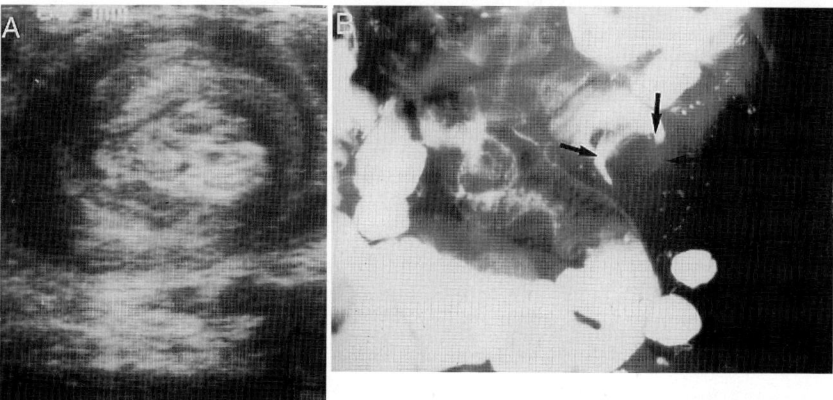

FIGURE 1.—Boy, 8 months. **A**, transverse ultrasonography examination of the right lower quadrant shows a large, complex, soft-tissue mass with a hypoechoic border, concentric layers of alternating hypoechogenicity and hyperechogenicity, and a hypoechoic center. **B**, barium meal with follow-through shows a large intraluminal mass (*arrows*) in the proximal small bowel. (Reprinted from Jéquier S, Argyropoulou M, Bugmann P: Ultrasonography of jejunal intussusception in children. *Can Assoc Radiol J* 46:285–290, 1995 by permission of the publisher.)

intussusception. The hamartomatous polyps appeared as hyperechoic solid masses, which could not be diagnosed more precisely on US. The patient with idiopathic postoperative intussusception was found to have a target lesion. The findings of US prompted the next imaging procedure—air enema in the patient with colonic involvement and preoperative barium meal in all 3 (Fig 1). Surgical delays were successfully avoided.

Conclusion.—Ultrasonography should be used to assess patients with possible jejunal intussusception. The use of this modality enables appropriate diagnostic GI studies and timely diagnosis.

▶ Imaging is frequently used to confirm the diagnosis of ileocolic intussusception. This is because reduction is possible in conjunction with the imaging diagnosis. Comparatively less is written about imaging of jejunal small bowel intussusception. Jejunal intussusceptions usually do not extend into the colon. Jejunal intussusception may be suggested by findings on ultrasonography. When antegrade (prograde) intussusception is demonstrated on its proximal or cephalic end, it has a funnel appearance leading into the narrowed central portion of the antegrade caudal-propelled intussusceptum. The convex lead point of the intussusceptum causes a "claw sign" on its caudal margin during retrograde barium enema examination. Thus, in retrograde intussusception, the "reversed claw sign" may be produced.[1] The advantage of ultrasonography is that it can demonstratea bull's eye target or donut sign on transverse views or a "hayfork" or pseudo–kidney sign on longitudinal views. Other noteworthy recent articles on small bowel intussusception are listed.[2–4]

L.W. Young, M.D.

References

1. Radhakrishna K, Das PC, Rao PLNG: Retrograde intussusception: A lead-point for prograde intussusception. *J Pediatr Surg* 29:1609–1610, 1994.
2. Kaste SC, Williams J, Rao BN: Postoperative small-bowel intussusception in children with cancer. *Pediatr Radiol* 25:21–23, 1995.
3. Choi SO, Park WH, Km SP: Enteric duplications in children—an analysis of 6 cases. *J Korean Med Sci* 8:482–487, 1993.
4. Couture A, Veyrac C, Baud C, et al: Evaluation of abdominal pain in Henoch-Schonlein syndrome by high frequency ultrasound. *Pediatr Radiol* 22:12–17, 1992.

CT of Intussusception in the Pediatric Patient: Diagnosis and Pitfalls

Cox TD, Winters WD, Weinberger E (Univ of Washington, Seattle)

Pediatr Radiol 26:26–32, 1996 4–40

Background.—When the typical signs and symptoms of intussusception in young children are present, the clinical diagnosis is not difficult to make. However, some children with intussusception have an atypical clinical manifestation, with a location outside the ileocecal region, a pathologic lead point, transient occurrence, or underlying systemic disease. In this situation, CT may be used. The CT findings of 5 children with intussusception were reviewed.

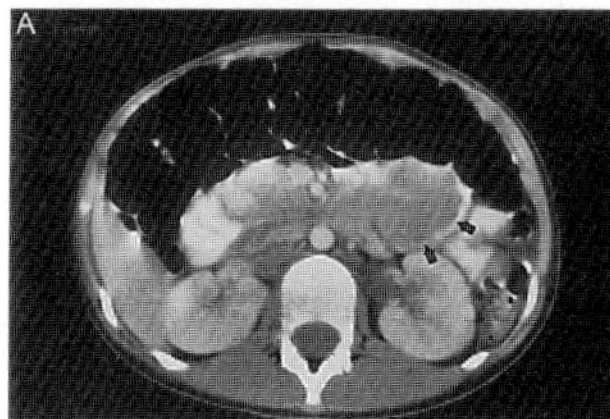

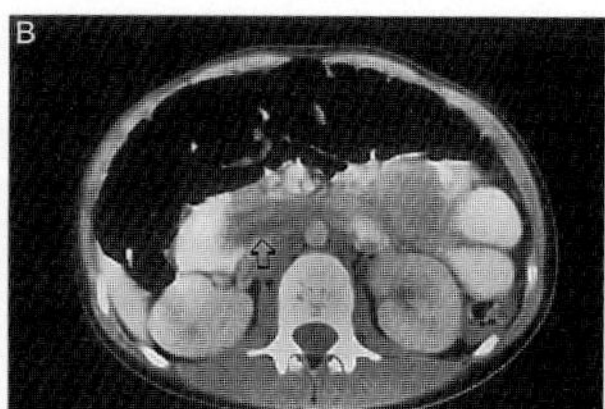

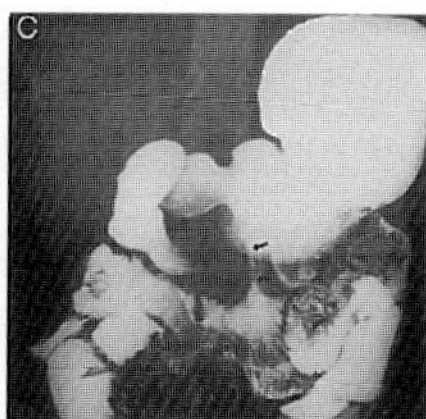

FIGURE 1.—Duodenal intussusception in Peutz-Jeghers syndrome. This 10-year-old girl had a history of recurrent pancreatitis and CT was performed after luminal narrowing of the descending duodenum (presumed to be caused by a mural or extrinsic mass) was seen at endoscopy. **A,** contrast-enhanced CT demonstrates an intraluminal mass in the ascending limb of the duodenum (*arrows*). **B,** layering of different tissue attenuations is seen in the third portion of the duodenum (*arrow*). The alternating bands of low and high density likely relate to layers of muscularis and mucosa/submucosa that are adjacent to one another. **C,** an upper gastrointestinal series showed the intussusception beginning in the third portion of the duodenum, with barium coating the dilated intussuscipiens (*arrows*). Hamartomatous polyps were found in the third and fourth portions of the duodenum at surgery, with no necrosis of involved bowel. (*Pediatr Radiol*; CT of intussusception in the pediatric patient: Diagnosis and pitfalls; Cox TD, Winters WD, Weinberger E; 26:26–32; Fig 1; 1996; Copyright notice of Springer-Verlag.)

Patients.—The patients were 3 boys and 2 girls, aged 5 to 13 years. Some of the children had had symptoms for weeks or even months. These symptoms may have been related to the children's underlying systemic diseases, which included lymphoma and Peutz-Jeghers syndrome. In each case, the diagnosis of intussusception was made by CT.

Findings.—Computed tomography demonstrated an intraluminal mass in all 5 patients (Fig 1). Most patients had intraluminal, eccentrically located fat, with the target sign of alternating layers of high and low attenuation. Fluid-distended loops, inflammation, and loss of tissue planes were found in patients with a longer-standing process. These findings correlated with the surgical findings of necrosis and nonviable bowel. Two additional false positive for intussusception cases were identified; in these the target appearance of intussusception eventually proved to be caused by other processes.

Conclusion.—Computed tomography may aid in making the diagnosis of intussusception in children with atypical signs and symptoms. The CT findings are similar to those in adults and depend on the location and duration of the intussusception and the presence of a lead point. There is the potential for diagnostic error, however, and the presence of a target sign must be correlated with other CT findings.

► In children with complicated manifestations of abdominal disease, CT is frequently used to examine for abnormality. Intussusception is usually not suspected, and its discovery is unexpected. The target sign is a characteristic, if not pathognomonic, CT finding of intussusception. Other conditions may produce a target sign. Ultrasonographic findings may be corroborative[1] or lend additional interpretive insight. Sometimes a mass of intussusception may be identifiable on plain radiography.[2] Another provocative article contends that the important additional finding of a mass as a lead point may not be demonstrated on air enema but may be shown on radiopaque contrast enema.[3] What apparently is important is the correlation of findings by different imaging modalities, including ultrasound and CT. Other noteworthy recent articles aptly portray new approaches to intussusception.[4, 5] The comparisons between air vs. radiopaque contrast for intussusception examination/reduction, the relationship of air or liquid pressure to perforation,[6, 7] the differences in air and liquid radiation doses, and other aspects of preferences in the management of intussusception continue unabated.

L.W. Young, M.D.

References

1. Lim JH, Ko YT, Lee DH, et al: Determining the site and causes of colonic obstruction with sonography. *AJR* 163:1113–1117, 1994.
2. Sargent MA, Babyn P, Alton DJ: Plain abdominal radiography in suspected intussusception: a reassessment. *Pediatr Radiol* 24:17–20, 1994.
3. Miller SF, Landes AB, Dautenhahn LW, et al: Intussusception: Ability of fluoroscopic images obtained during air enemas to depict lead points and other abnormalities. *Radiology* 197:493–496, 1995.
4. Connolly B, Alton DJ, Ein SH, et al: Partially reduced intussusception: when are repeated delayed reduction attempts appropriate? *Pediatr Radiol* 25:104–107, 1995.
5. Rohrschneider WK, Troger J: Hydrostatic reduction of intussusception under US guidance. *Pediatr Radiol* 25:530-534, 1995.
6. Daneman A, Alton DJ, Wesson D, et al: Perforation during attempted intussusception reduction in children—a comparison of perforation with barium and air. *Pediatr Radiol* 25:81–88, 1995.
7. Zambuto D, Bramson RT, Blickman JG: Intracolonic pressure measurements during hydrostatic and air contrast barium enema studies in children. *Radiology* 196:55–58, 1995.

Diagnosis of Appendiceal Abscess in Children With Acute Appendicitis: Value of Color Doppler Sonography

Quillin SP, Siegel MJ (Mallinckrodt Inst of Radiology, St Louis)
AJR 164:1251–1254, 1995 4–41

Background.—The detection of appendiceal perforation before surgery is important, because it can change clinical management. Children with acute appendicitis underwent color Doppler imaging of the right lower quadrant to determine which characteristics indicate appendiceal perforation and whether this imaging modality is beneficial for diagnosing appendiceal abscesses.

Methods.—Forty-seven children underwent color Doppler sonography along with gray-scale sonography. All had surgically proved appendicitis. At pathologic assessment, nonperforating appendicitis was confirmed in 27 children and perforating appendicitis in 20. Seven patients in the latter group had abscesses, and 10 had phlegmon. The color Doppler sonograms were reviewed for the presence or absence of appendiceal hyperemia, hyperemic periappendiceal or pelvic fluid collections, and hyperemic soft tissues.

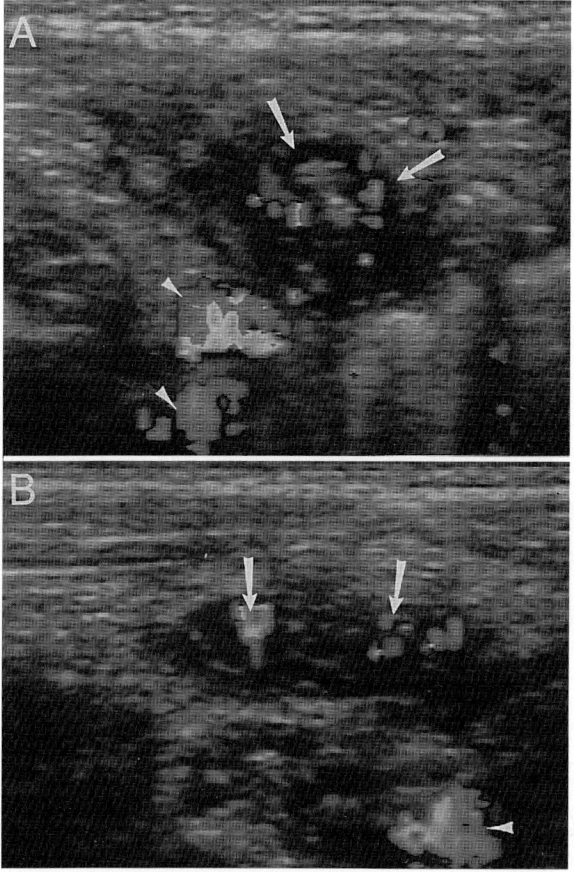

FIGURE 1.—Boy, 8 years, with surgically proven acute perforating appendicitis. Transverse (**A**) and longitudinal (**B**) images of appendix reveal scattered blood flow (*white arrows*). *White arrowheads* are the iliac vessels. (Courtesy of Quillin SP, Siegel MJ: Diagnosis of appendiceal abscess in children with acute appendicitis: Value of color Doppler sonography. *AJR* 164:1251–1254, 1995.)

Findings.—On color Doppler sonography, appendiceal hyperemia was observed in 78% of the patients with nonperforating appendicitis and in 40% of those with perforating appendicitis. Hyperemia was scattered in 67% of the patients with no perforation and in 75% of those with perforation (Fig 1). Focal appendiceal hyperemia was present in the rest of the patients with blood flow identifiable on color Doppler sonography. Thirty-five percent of the patients with perforating appendicitis had hyperemic, loculated periappendiceal or pelvic fluid collections, later proved to be abscesses surgically, on color Doppler assessment. None of the children with nonperforating appendicitis had a hyperemic, loculated periappendiceal or pelvic fluid collection. Increased color Doppler signal in the adjacent right lower quadrant bowel loops and soft tissues, indicating phlegmon or peritonitis, was observed in 10 patients with perforating appendicitis.

Conclusion.—A hyperemic periappendiceal or pelvic fluid collection and periappendiceal soft-tissue hyperemia are the best indicators of appendiceal perforation on color Doppler sonography. The finding of a hyperemic, loculated fluid collection is apparently specific for abscess.

▶ Supportive evidence is presented for the use of color Doppler sonography as an adjunct to gray-scale sonography in children suspected to have acute appendicitis. Noninvasive color Doppler sonography is specifically valuable for demonstrating findings of perforating appendicitis. Other recent articles concerning the use of adjunctive imaging to examine for acute appendicitis in children are listed,[1–4] including a classification of the imaging findings[2] and data on why such imaging need not be routine.[3]

L.W. Young, M.D.

References

1. Wang YJ, Shian WJ, Chu HY, et al: Leukemoid reaction in a child with appendiceal abscess: A case report. *Chung Hua I Hsueh Tsa Chih* 53:311–314, 1994.
2. Perale R, Talenti E, Toffolutti T, et al: Ruolo diagnostico dell'ecografia nell' appendicite acuta del bambino. *Radiol Med* 81:849–856, 1991.
3. Sarfati MR, Hunter GC, Witzke DB, et al: Impact of adjunctive testing on the diagnosis and clinical course of patients with acute appendicitis. *Am J Surg* 166:660–664, 1993.
4. Malnati R, Capasso G, Stagni S, et al: Current diagnostic-therapeutic trends in treatment of pediatric appendicitis. *Minerva Pediatr* 46:117–121, 1994.

MR Findings in Peliosis Hepatis

Saatci I, Coskun M, Boyvat F, et al (Hacettepe Univ, Ankara, Turkey)
Pediatr Radiol 25:31–33, 1995 4–42

Introduction.—In the rare condition of peliosis hepatis (PH), blood-filled cavities or cystic spaces are found in the liver. The cause of PH is unknown, but it is found in patients with a variety of diseases such as tuberculosis, cancer, and AIDS, as well as in patients taking androgenic steroids. The MRI findings of PH in a steroid-treated child with Fanconi anemia were reported.

Case Report.—Boy, 9, was diagnosed as having Fanconi anemia, which was treated with packed red blood cell transfusions, steroids, and androgens. His aplastic anemia remained in remission for 3 years. About 3½ years after the diagnosis of Fanconi anemia, the patient was hospitalized with fever and severe pancytopenia. Liver function studies were normal, but abdominal ultrasound showed diffuse, mixed echogenic masses in the liver. Magnetic resonance imaging was performed to further investigate the liver condition, which was suspected to be PH. The liver was enlarged and heterogeneous and had multiple foci of varying signal intensity.

All sequences showed increased signal intensity of the right hepatic lobe. Multiple foci of brighter signal located throughout the liver, particularly in the right lobe, were consistent with subacute blood. Some nodules became more intense on postcontrast images. A chronic hematoma cavity was indicated by the presence of a cystic mass with an enhancing rim. The spleen was normal. The patient died of sepsis, and the presence of PH was confirmed at autopsy.

Conclusion.—The MRI findings of PH were described. This diagnosis should be considered when a steroid-treated patient is found to have complex lesions within an enlarged liver. Confirming the diagnosis of PH is essential because PH may be reversible after treatment is stopped.

► Peliosis hepatis as proven in this boy is an uncommon but highly perplexing condition. It is demonstrable by MRI, ultrasound, and CT. It should be recognized as an indication of some underlying potentially treatable but possibly fatal condition. Other fatalities have been reported.[1–2] Other recent articles on peliosis hepatis are listed.[3–6]

L.W. Young, M.D.

References

1. Makdisi WJ, Cherian R, Vanveldhuizen PJ, et al: Fatal peliosis of the liver and spleen in a patient with agnogenic myeloid metaplasia treated with danazol. *Am J Gastroenterol* 90:317–318, 1995.
2. Engel P, Jacobsen GK: An unusual case of retroperitoneal seminoma and fatal peliosis of the liver. *Histopathology* 22:379–382, 1993.
3. Selby DM, Stocker JT: Focal peliosis hepatis, a sequela of asphyxial death? *Pediatr Pathol Lab Med* 15:589–596, 1995.
4. Calvacanti R, Pol S, Carnot F, et al: Impact and evolution of peliosis hepatis in renal transplant recipients. *Transplantation* 15:315–316, 1994.
5. Bracero LA, Gambon TB, Evans R, et al: Ultrasonographic findings in a case of congenital peliosis hepatis. *J Ultrasound Med* 14:483–486, 1995.
6. Jamadar DA, D'Souza SP, Thomas EA, et al: Case report: Radiological appearances in peliosis hepatis. *Br J Radiol* 67:102–104, 1994.

Direct Spread of Subperitoneal Disease Into Solid Organs: Radiologic Diagnosis

Oliphant M, Berne AS, Meyers MA (Crouse Irving Mem Hosp, Syracuse, NY; State Univ of New York)

Abdom Imaging 20:141–147, 1995 4–43

Introduction.—The continuous potential space connecting the peritoneum, retroperitoneum, and abdominal organs is known as the subperitoneal space (SS). The SS is known to play an important pathogenetic role in the direct spread of inflammatory, infectious, traumatic, and neoplastic disease. The potential for direct extension of disease through the SS into the solid abdominal viscera and its radiologic diagnosis were discussed.

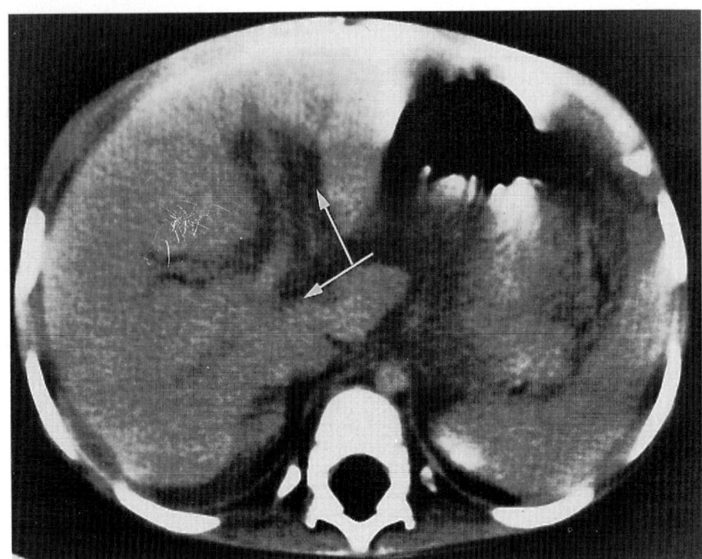

FIGURE 2.—Case 2. Burkitt's lymphoma extending into the liver. Computed tomography scan shows the tumor extending along the celiac axis and hepatic artery into the porta hepatis and more deeply in the liver (*arrow*). (Courtesy of Oliphant M, Berne AS, Meyers MA: Direct spread of subperitoneal disease into solid organs: Radiologic diagnosis. *Abdom Imaging* 20:141–147, 1995.)

Case 2.—Boy, 2 years, underwent CT examination of a large abdominal mass. The scan showed a large suprarenal mass spreading along the upper abdominal aorta and small mesentery. The mass tracked to the porta hepatis along the celiac axis before passing into the left hepatic lobe (Fig 2). The pathologic diagnosis was Burkitt's lymphoma.

Case 3.—Boy, 18 months, was seen with abdominal distention, poor appetite, and weight loss. His CT scan showed a large, complex mass in the right suprarenal area with aortic spread. This patient also had direct extension along the celiac axis to the porta hepatis and liver; the left renal hilum was involved as well (Fig 3). Neuroblastoma was diagnosed.

Case 4.—Boy, 2 years, underwent evaluation of an abdominal mass of suspected renal origin. Imaging studies revealed a mass in the right kidney that was continuous with a right suprarenal lesion that extended, along the aorta, into the SS to the right renocrural area. The small intestine mesentery was also involved with this tumor, which proved to be neuroblastoma (Fig 4).

Comment.—The cases illustrate how abdominal disease can spread through the SS to involve the liver and kidneys. Once the tumor has entered the SS, it can extend along the vessels and bile ducts within the hepatoduodenal ligament to reach the porta hepatis. From there, it can reach the liver by following the areolar connective tissue and portal canals.

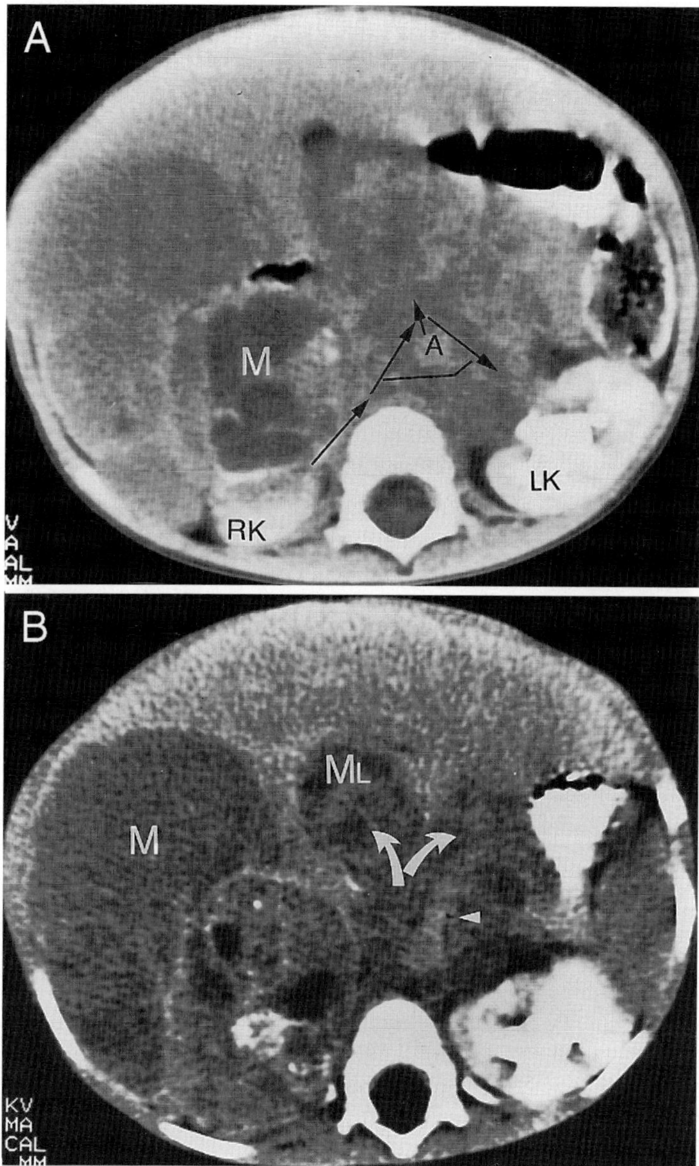

FIGURE 3.—Case 3. Direct extension of neuroblastoma into the liver. **A,** computed tomography scan shows a complex mass (*M*) with calcifications extending along the renal vasculature to encase and spread along the aorta (*A*) and extending medially to the left renal hilum (*arrows*). The right kidney (*RK*) is displaced inferiorly and posteriorly. Note the posterolateral displacement of the left kidney (*LK*) and partial obstruction of the ureteropelvic junction. **B,** CT cephalad to **A** shows tumor spreading along the celiac axis (*arrowhead*) and hepatoduodenal ligament into the liver. Spread is also along the gastrohepatic ligament (*arrows*). *, normal liver wedged between uplifted right lobe of liver by complex mass (*M*) and tumor that spread into the liver. (Courtesy of Oliphant M, Berne AS, Meyers MA: Direct spread of subperitoneal disease into solid organs: Radiologic diagnosis. *Abdom Imaging* 20:141–147, 1995.)

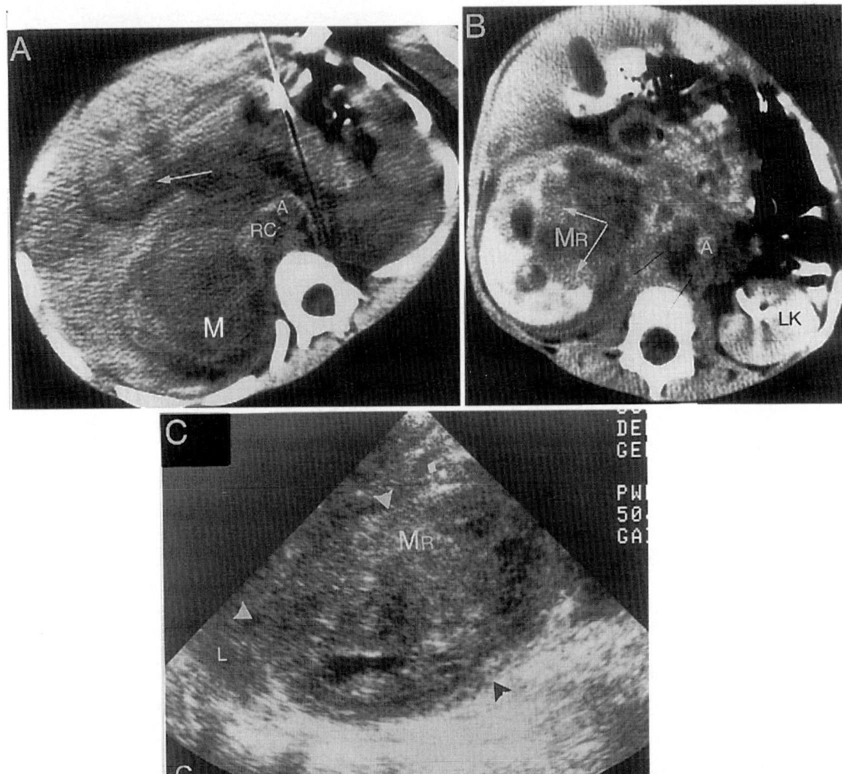

FIGURE 4.—Case 4. Direct extension of neuroblastoma manifesting as a primary renal mass. **A,** CT scan of the upper half of the abdomen shows a mass (*M*) that extends into the liver through the porta hepatis (*arrow*). Note the retrocrural mass on the right (*RC*). *A* is the aorta. **B,** CT scan at the level of the kidneys. The tumor grows into the right kidney (*arrows*), forming an intrarenal mass in the central portion of the kidney (M_R) and extends to the renal cortex. The right kidney is displaced, and its collecting system is obstructed. Note the tumor encases the aorta (*A*) and extends toward the left kidney (*LK*). **C,** ultrasound of right kidney (*arrowheads*). Poorly marginated echogenic mass (M_R) within the central portion of the kidney extends to its periphery and causes obstruction to the collecting system. (Courtesy of Oliphant M, Berne AS, Meyers MA: Direct spread of supperitoneal disease into solid organs: Radiologic diagnosis. *Abdom Imaging* 20:141–147, 1995.)

Discussion.—The natural pathways between the SS and the abdominal viscera provide a direct path for the spread of disease, such as tumors and inflammation. The imaging findings of disease spread via the SS to the liver, kidney, and spleen were described. Direct extension via the SS provides a unifying concept for understanding the clinical manifestation of abdominal disease at a distance from its site of origin.

► This is an excellent demonstration of the spread of pathologic processes of hemorrhage, inflammation, infection, and cancer via the SS into solid organs in pediatric and adult patients. Related articles, some by the same authors, provide additional insight.[1–6] This information is particularly applicable to cross-sectional imaging.

L.W. Young, M.D.

References

1. Obaro RO, Lata A: Journey through the abdominal underpass: The subperitoneal pathway of disease spread revisited. *Can Assoc Radiol J* 46:353–362, 1995.
2. Oliphant M, Berne AS, Meyers MA: Bidirectional spread of disease via the subperitoneal space: The lower abdomen and left pelvis. *Abdom Imaging* 18:117–125, 1993.
3. Oliphant M, Berne AS, Meyers MA: Spread of disease via the subperitoneal space: The small bowel mesentery. *Abdom Imaging* 18:109–116, 1993.
4. Oliphant M, Berne AS, Meyers MA: The subperitoneal space: Normal and pathologic anatomy, in Meyers MA (ed): *Dynamic Radiology of The Abdomen: Normal and Pathologic Anatomy, ed 4*. New York, Springer-Verlag, 1994, pp 455–476.
5. Arenas AP, Sanchez LV, Alibillos JM, et al: Direct dissemination of pathologic abdominal processes through perihepatic ligaments: Identification with CT (review). *Radiographics* 14:515–527, 1994.
6. Auh YH, Lim JH, Kim KW, et al: Loculated fluid collections in hepatic fissures and recesses: CT appearance and potential pitfalls (review). *Radiographics* 14:529–540, 1994.

Haemangiomatosis in Children: Value of MRI During Therapy

Stöver B, Laubenberger J, Niemeyer C, et al (Humboldt Univ, Berlin; Univ of Freiburg, Germany)

Pediatr Radiol 25:123–126, 1995 4–44

Background.—Magnetic resonance imaging has become the method of choice for imaging extended hemangiomas, especially in infants with hemangiomatosis of the liver and lung. To date, there have been no reports of MRI monitoring of hemangioma or hemangiomatosis during interferon treatment.

Methods.—Five children with hemangiomatosis, 1 with capillary hemangioma, and 1 with extended arteriovenous malformation underwent 18 MR examinations. The children's ages ranged from 1 month to 12 years.

Findings.—The liver, liver and lung, periorbital area, and thigh were involved. The extent of the lesions and size of the hemangiomas on MR images could be measured. Coronal views clearly demonstrated the involved structures in liver and lung hemangiomas (Fig 1). The response to interferon was documented in 2 children, who showed decreases in lesion size and, subsequently, in number. T2-weighted images showed slightly reduced signal intensity. However, no definitive fibrotic zones were observed during treatment. Signal intensity of the liver parenchyma was homogeneous in both weightings after complete regression of disease, and there were no fibrotic areas visible 18 months after interferon was begun. Two children did not respond to treatment, 1 of whom died of congestive heart failure. The size of the periorbital hemangioma was decreased. The thigh lesion could be classified as an arteriovenous malformation.

Conclusion.—Magnetic resonance imaging can confirm hemangioma' sis as suggested by signs of congestive cardiac failure and an enlarged ' of mixed echogenicity on ultrasound scans in children. Magnetic

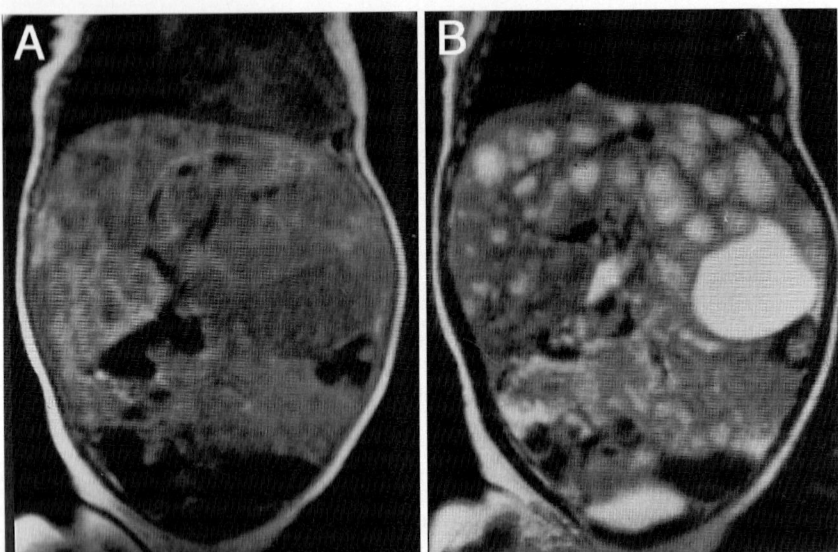

FIGURE 1.—Four-month-old girl. (A) T1-weighted (recovery time 520 mesc/echo time 20 mesc) coronal sequence, including thorax and abdomen: evident enlargement of the liver because of multiple hemangiomas of intermediate-signal intensity, decreased (relative to normal liver parenchyma) and enlarged vessels. (B) Identical position of the slice, T2 weighted (recovery time 3,200 mesc/echo time 125 msec). The hyperintense signal of the hemangiomatosis allows precise delineation of each hemangioma from the normal liver. Most of the multiple lesions show a rim but no evident capsule. Each lesion itself reveals homogeneous signal intensity. (*Pediatr Radiol;* Hemangiomatosis in children: Value of MRI during therapy; Stöver B, Laubenberger J, Niemeyer C, et al; 25:123–126; Fig 1; 1995; Copyright notice of Springer-Verlag.)

nance imaging is a reliable technique that enables characterization of liver, lung, and peripheral lesions. This modality is also useful in monitoring the response to interferon treatment.

▶ Magnetic resonance imaging is the method of choice for imaging extended hemangiomas and hemangiomatosis. The authors also make a good case for using MRI monitor interferon therapy of hemangiomatosis in children. Fibrotic transformation MRI findings were not depicted in the MRI examinations, as might have been expected. Maybe fibrosis does not always occur. Other noteworthy recent articles on hemangiomatosis or hemangioendothelioma are listed.[1–7]

L.W. Young, M.D.

References

1. Pobiel RS, Bissett GS III: Pictorial essay: Imaging of liver tumors in the infant and child. *Pediatr Radiol* 25:495–496, 1995.
2. Wong DC, Masel JP: Infantile hepatic haemangioendothelioma. *Aust Radiol* 39:140–144, 1995.

3. al-Fawaz IM, al Mobaireek KF, al-Suhaibani M, et al: Pulmonary capillary hemangiomatosis: A case report and review of the literature. *Pediatr Pulmonol* 19:243–248, 1995.
4. Berger TM, Berger MF, Hoffman AD, et al: Imaging diagnosis and follow-up of infantile hepatic haemangioendothelioma: A case report. *Eur J Pediatr* 153:100–102, 1994.
5. Tazelaar HD, Kerr D, Yousem SA, et al: Diffuse pulmonary lymphangiomatosis. *Hum Pathol* 24:1313–1322, 1993.
6. Hamdi F, Cuny JF, Truchetet F, et al: Diffuse neonatal hemangiomatosis. A case with tetralogy of Fallot. *Ann Pediatr* 40:625–627, 1993.
7. Park CH, Hwang HE, Hong J, et al: Giant infantile hemangioendothelioma of the liver scintigraphic diagnosis. *Clin Nucl Med* 21:293–295, 1996.

AIDS-Related Lymphoma: Radiologic Features in Pediatric Patients

Siskin GP, Haller JO, Miller S, et al (State Univ of New York, Brooklyn; Long Island College Hosp, Brooklyn)

Radiology 196:63–66, 1995 4–45

Objective.—Lymphoma is the most frequently encountered AIDS-related tumor in children, though it represents only part of the range of AIDS-associated B-cell proliferative disorders. The findings of AIDS-related lymphoma were compared in pediatric and adult patients.

Methods.—The retrospective study included 9 children and adolescents with AIDS-related lymphoma. In each patient, neoplastic changes were noted that were not consistent with hyperplastic lymphoid tissue. The

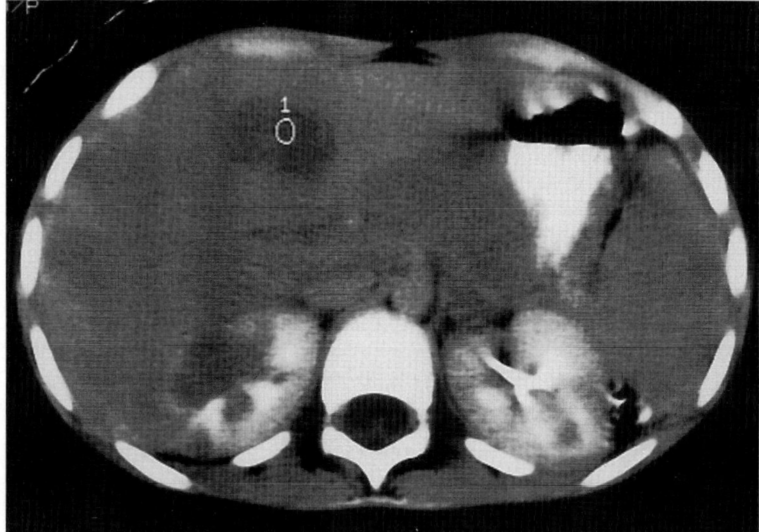

FIGURE 1.—Contrast material–enhanced CT scan shows well-circumscribed, low-attenuation lesions in the liver and 1 spleen. (Courtesy of Siskin GP, Haller JO, Miller S, et al: AIDS-related lymphoma: Radiologic features in pediatric patients. *Radiology* 196:63–66, 1995; Radiological Society of North America.)

clinical, pathologic, and radiologic findings were compared with published findings of adult patients with AIDS-related lymphoma.

Results.—At least 2 sites were involved with lymphoma in 8 of the 9 pediatric patients. The liver was involved in 7 patients, the spleen and chest in 5 each, and the bone and kidneys in 4 each. The liver, spleen, and kidneys were the only sites of intra-abdominal involvement. Lymphomas in these organs, whether solitary or multiple, appeared as well-circumscribed, low-attenuation lesions (Fig 1). The children's symptoms depended on the disease site but included seizures, respiratory distress, testicular swelling, and increased abdominal girth.

Conclusion.—The features of AIDS-related lymphoma in pediatric patients were described. Lymphoma and other B-cell proliferative disorders are common in children with AIDS, and their pathogenesis is linked to Epstein-Barr virus. The lymphomas can occur in almost any site. Intra-abdominal lymphomas may be detected in the liver, spleen, and kidneys; the differential diagnosis for lesions in these locations would include mycobacterial infection and Kaposi's sarcoma. Pediatric AIDS patients with lymphomas tend to have site-specific symptoms in contrast to the systemic B-type symptoms reported in adults.

▶ Although almost any site may be symptomatic and involved with AIDS-related lymphoma in the pediatric patient, the most frequent sites in this study's group of patients were liver and spleen. Lymphoma in patients with AIDS is a neoplastic complication that may be intra-abdominal,[1] intrathoracic,[2] or intracranial.[3] The clinical findings in children reflect specific sites of involvement, whereas in adults the clinical findings are usually systemic. Airway obstructive symptoms and cystic thymic hyperplasia in a child with AIDS is the subject of another recent report.[4]

L.W. Young, M.D.

References

1. Haller JO, Cohen HL: Gastrointestinal manifestations of AIDS in children (review). *AJR* 162:387–393, 1994.
2. Ambrosino MM, Roche KJ, Genieser NB, et al: Application of thin-section low-dose chest CT (TSCT) in the management of pediatric AIDS. *Pediatr Radiol* 25:393–400, 1995.
3. Dickson DW, Llena JF, Nelson SJ, et al: Central nervous system pathology in pediatric AIDS (review). *Ann NY Acad Sci* 693:93–106, 1993.
4. Mercado-Deane M-G, Sabio H, Burton EM, et al: Cystic thymic hyperplasia in a child with HIV infection: Imaging findings. *AJR* 166:171–172, 1996.

Acute Pancreatitis in Children: CT Findings of Intra- and Extrapancreatic Fluid Collections

King LR, Siegel MJ, Balfe DM (Washington Univ, St Louis)

Radiology 195:196–200, 1995 4–46

Background.—The CT findings associated with pancreatitis have been well documented in adults, in whom extrapancreatic fluid collections are most commonly seen in the lesser sac, the anterior pararenal space, and the posterior pararenal spaces. The CT appearance of pancreatitis and the locations of fluid collections were studied in children in a retrospective investigation.

Methods.—The CT scans of 28 children with clinical diagnoses of acute pancreatitis were reviewed. Pancreatic abnormalities were classified as enlargement, irregularity of contour, or areas of decreased attenuation. In addition, extrapancreatic fluid collections were classified as peritoneal, retroperitoneal, mesenteric, or ligamentous.

Results.—Twenty of the 28 children had pancreaata of a normal size and 8 (29%) demonstrated diffuse pancreatic enlargement. Two of these 8 children also had areas of low attenuation, indicating multiple fluid collections within the pancreatic parenchyma. Fourteen children had extrapancreatic fluid collections, including the 8 patients with pancreatic enlargement. The extrapancreatic fluid collections were classified as peritoneal in 9 (64%), retroperitoneal in 10 (71%), mesenteric in 10 (71%), and ligamentous in 10 (71%). The most common sites of extrapancreatic fluid collections were the anterior pararenal space, the lesser sac, the lesser omentum, and the transverse mesocolon (Fig 5).

Discussion.—Compared with adults, children with pancreatitis are significantly less likely to have intrapancreatic fluid collections and more likely to have extrapancreatic fluid collections in the peritoneal, retroperitoneal, or mesenteric spaces. Understanding these CT patterns has clinical utility in confirming the diagnosis of pancreatitis.

► Because of the unique anatomical position of the pancreas and its lack of a well-defined fibrous capsule, it is not surprising that pancreatic inflammatory or traumatic injury may be associated with a variety of intrapancreatic and extrapancreatic fluid collections. Some of these liquid collections lack containment and have no precise configuration. Most pancreatic liquid collections diminish spontaneously, but some may be complicated by the formation of troublesome pseudocysts. Several recent additional articles of interest on acute pancreatitis are listed.[1–5]

L.W. Young, M.D.

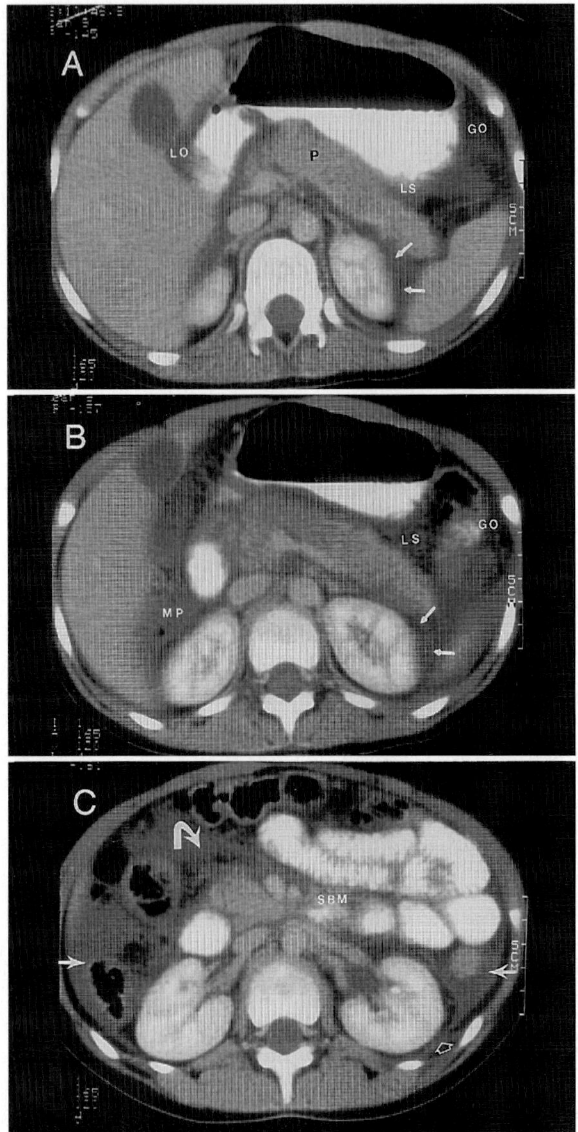

FIGURE 5.—Acute pancreatitis in a 7-year-old girl. **A,** CT scan shows mild diffuse enlargement of the pancreas (*P*) with fluid collections in the lesser sac (*LS*), the lesser omentum (*LO*), the greater omentum (*GO*), and the left anterior pararenal space (*arrows*). **B,** CT scan obtained at a more caudal level shows inflammatory changes involving the Morison pouch (*MP*), the lesser sac (*LS*), the anterior pararenal space (*arrows*), and the greater omentum (*GO*). **C,** CT scan of the midabdomen demonstrates thickening of the small bowel wall. Fluid is located in the small bowel mesentery (*SBM*), the paracolic gutters (*straight solid arrows*), the transverse mesocolon (*curved arrow*), and the posterior renal fascia (*open arrow*). (Courtesy of King LR, Siegel MJ, Balfe DM: Acute pacreatitis in children: CT findings of intra- and extrapancreatic fluid collections. *Radiology* 195:196–200, 1995; Radiological Society of North America.)

References

1. Haddock G, Coupar G, Youngston GG, et al: Acute pancreatitis in children: A 15-year review. *J Pediatr Surg* 29:719–722, 1994.
2. Sanada Y, Yoshizawa Y, Chiba M, et al: Ventral pancreatitis in a patient with pancreas divisum. *J Pediatr Surg* 30:665–667, 1995.
3. Sivit CJ, Eichelberger MR: CT diagnosis of pancreatic injury in children: Significance of fluid separating the splenic vein and the pancreas. *AJR Am J Roentgenol* 165:921–924, 1995.
4. Hilfer CL, Holgersen LO: Massive chylous ascites and transected pancreas secondary to child abuse: Successful non-surgical management. *Pediatr Radiol* 25:117–119, 1995.
5. Ohno Y, Ohgami H, Nagasaki A, et al: Complete disruption of the main pancreatic duct: A case successfully managed by percutaneous drainage. *J Pediatr Surg* 30:1741–1742, 1995.

Splenic Injury From Blunt Abdominal Trauma in Children: Follow-Up Evaluation With CT

Benya EC, Bulas DI, Eichelberger MR, et al (George Washington Univ, Washington, DC)
Radiology 195:685–688, 1995 4–47

Objective.—Most children with hemodynamically stable splenic injuries after blunt abdominal trauma can be treated successfully without surgery. The time course of splenic healing with follow-up CT in these children was evaluated to determine if the initial CT grade of splenic injury could help predict rate of healing.

Methods.—Thirty-seven children, aged 12 months to 16 years, with splenic injury graded at emergent CT were prospectively followed-up with nonenhanced and contrast material–enhanced CT at 2 weeks to 11 months after injury. Based on a modified classification of Mirvis, initial CT was classified as grade 1 in 3 patients with superficial laceration or subcapsular hematoma less than 1 cm in diameter; grade 2 in 12 patients with parenchymal lacerations 1 to 3 cm deep or central or subcapsular hematoma less than 3 cm in diameter; grade 3 in 11 with lacerations greater than 3 cm deep or central or subcapsular hematoma more than 3 cm in diameter; and grade 4 in 11 with 3 or more lacerations more than 3 cm deep or foci of devascularized spleen. All children were managed nonoperatively.

Outcome.—All 15 grade 1 and 2 splenic injuries healed at follow-up, including 8 in patients who underwent follow-up within 4 months after injury. All but 1 grade 3 splenic injuries healed by 6 months. In all grade 4 splenic injuries, residual lesions were evident within 4 months, and complete healing occurred up to 11 months. Contrast-enhanced CT scans allowed clear visualization of 5 of 9 residual splenic injuries, including 4 that were depicted as healed injuries on non-enhanced CT scans. Splenic calcification was evident in a child with persistent abdominal pain (Fig 2).

Recommendations.—The optimal time for follow-up CT scanning of splenic injury should be based on the grade of splenic injury established at

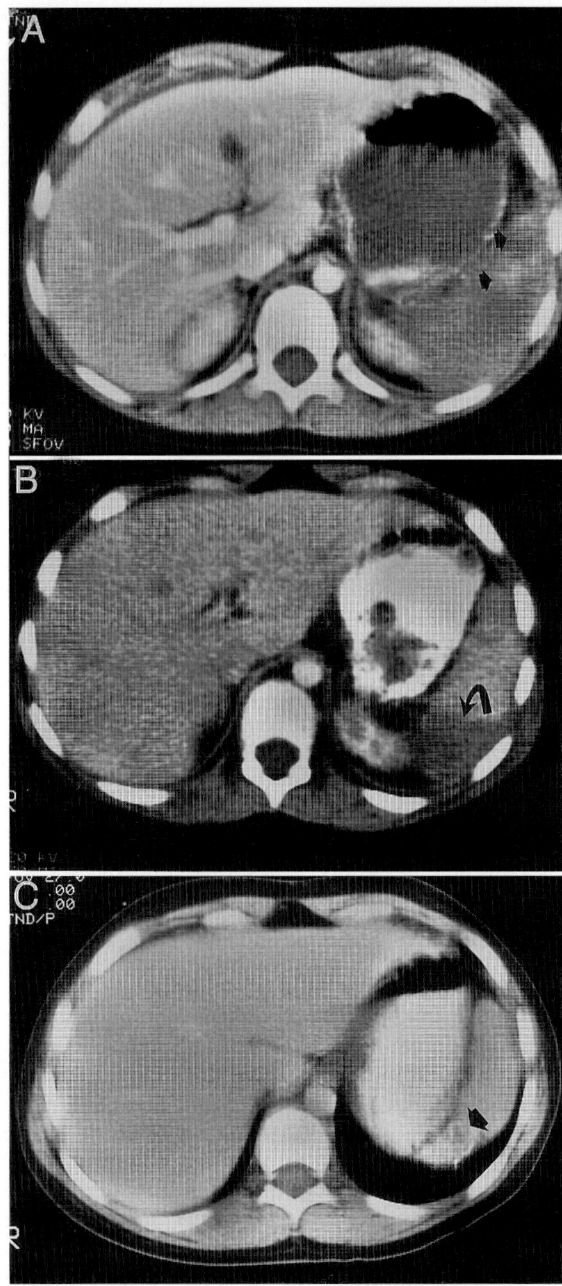

FIGURE 2.—Computed tomography scans of a 10-year-old boy with left-sided abdominal pain after a fall. **A,** initial CT scan shows a grade 4 splenic injury with devascularization of the majority of the spleen and 2 small foci (*arrows*) of enhancing splenic tissue. **B,** follow-up CT scan obtained 6 months after injury shows healing with persistent area of splenic injury posteriorly (*arrow*). **C,** second follow-up CT scan obtained 11 months after injury shows that the spleen has healed with calcification posteriorly (*arrow*). (Courtesy of Benya EC, Bulas DI, Eichelberger MR, et al; Splenic injury from blunt abdominal trauma in children: Follow-up evaluation with CT. *Radiology* 195:685–688, 1995; Radiological Society of North America.)

initial CT. Grade 1 and 2 splenic injuries may be scanned at 2 months, grade 3 at 3 months, and grade 4 at 6 months. If the injuries are unhealed, follow-up CT may be performed at 4 months (grade 1), 6 months (grade 2), and 9 months (grade 3).

▶ Computed tomography of the spleen is an appropriate and excellent example of use of CT as the primary imaging method to define the extent of intra-abdominal organ injury. The images in this article graphically document follow-up evaluation findings of the injured spleen by CT from which correlation of the rate of healing with 4 CT grades of splenic injury is made. Other recent articles that relate to the problem of splenic injury and its imaging are listed.[1–6]

L.W. Young, M.D.

References

1. Sclafani SJ, Shaftan GW, Scalea TM, et al: Nonoperative salvage of computed tomography-diagnosed splenic injuries: utilization of angiography for triage and embolization for hemostatis. *J Trauma* 39:818–825, 1995.
2. Ruess L, Sivit CJ, Eichelberger MR, et al: Blunt hepatic and splenic trauma in children: correlation of a CT injury severity scale with clinical outcome. *Pediatr Radiol* 25:321–325, 1995.
3. Roche BG, Bugmann P, Le Coultre C: Blunt injuries to liver, spleen, kidney and pancreas in pediatric patients. *Eur J Pediatr Surg* 2:154–156, 1992.
4. Pranikoff T, Hirschl RB, Schlesinger AE, et al: Resolution of splenic injury after nonoperative management. *J Pediatr Surg* 29:1366–1369, 1994.
5. Kohn JS, Clark DE, Isler RJ, et al: Is computed tomographic grading of splenic injury useful in the nonsurgical management of blunt trauma? *J Trauma* 36:385–389, 390 (discussion), 1994.
6. Choong RK, Grattan-Smith TM, Chohen RC, et al: Splenic injury in children: A 10 year experience. *J Paediatr Child Health* 29:192–195, 1993.

Doppler Ultrasound and Angiography of the Vasculature of the Liver in Children After Orthotopic Liver Transplantation: A Prospective Study

Kok T, Peeters PMJG, Hew JM, et al (Univ Hosp Groningen, The Netherlands)

Pediatr Radiol 25:517–524, 1995 4–48

Background.—Though Doppler ultrasound (US) is available, angiography remains a part of the protocol for assessing children after orthotopic liver transplantation (OLT) at some centers. The reliability of Doppler US for evaluating the patency of the hepatic artery, portal vein, and inferior vena cava and the anastomotic site of the portal vein in children after OLT was investigated.

Methods.—Thirty-eight children undergoing 40 transplants were included in the prospective study. In total, 59 paired Doppler US and angiographic assessments were available for comparison. Ten of these paired examinations were done on clinical demand, and the rest were performed according to protocol.

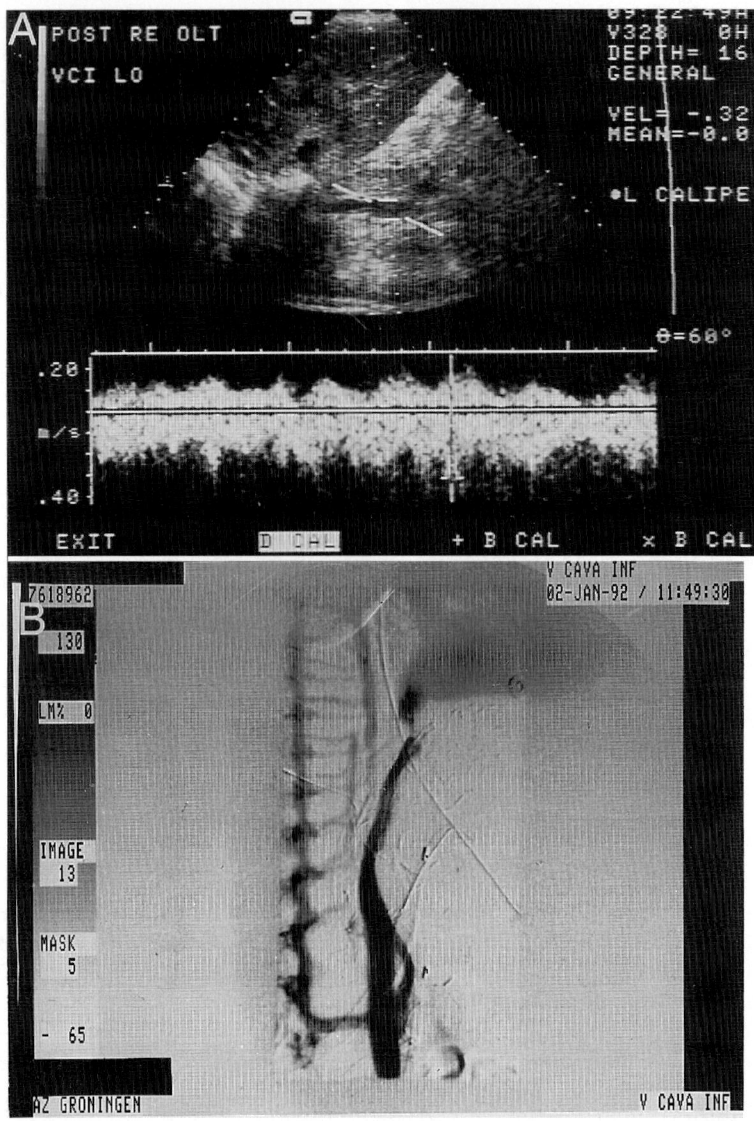

FIGURE 5.—A, Doppler ultrasound of reversed flow in the inferior vena cava in a child with the inferior vena cava syndrome. **B,** cavography of high-grade stenosis at the suprahepatic anastomosis. (*Pediatr Radiol*; Doppler ultrasound and angiography of the vasculature of the liver in children after orthotopic liver transplantation: A prospective study; Kok T, Peeters PMJG, Hew JM, et al; 25:517–524; Fig 5; 1995; Copyright notice of Springer-Verlag.)

Findings.—There was a good correlation between the examinations in demonstrating a patent hepatic artery, with a sensitivity of 96% and a specificity of 100%. Two hepatic artery flow false negative Doppler US findings were attributed to technical problems and rejection. Doppler US and angiography findings were in agreement in 58 of 59 assessments of portal vein patency. There was 1 portal vein occlusion false positive angiographic finding, which resulted from inadequate opacification. Doppler US depicted stenosis of the portal vein 3 times more often than angiography. Doppler US findings suggesting an abnormality in the inferior vena cava in 7 children were confirmed by cavography or surgery (Fig 5).

Conclusion.—Doppler US is reliable for assessing the patency of the hepatic artery, inferior vena cava, and portal vein and the anastomotic site of the portal vein. Doppler US appears to be the better method for demonstrating stenosis, though neither Doppler US nor angiography will serve as the gold standard for showing this abnormality. When stenosis is suspected on the basis of Doppler US or angiographic findings, the presence or absence of clinical signs of portal hypertension needs to be considered also.

► In follow-up of patients with OLT, angiography is the procedure of choice. This report shows Doppler US to be a correlative modality for examining these patients. Doppler ultrasonography is reliable for determining patency of the hepatic artery, the portal vein, the portal vein anastomosis, and the inferior vena cava. It is a necessary method to use before employing conventional angiography or cavography. It is no longer necessary to routinely perform the latter procedures. Other recent articles detail the use of color Doppler sonography to identify early signs of hepatic arterial or portal venous occlusion in the perioperative period of reduced-size hepatic allographs in children.[1, 2]

L.W. Young, M.D.

References

1. Donnelly LF, Babcock DS, Ryckman FC, et al: Reduced-size hepatic allograft vascular compression in children: Detection with color Doppler sonography. *AJR* 165:655–657, 1995.
2. Lomas DJ, Britton PD, Farman P, et al: Duplex Doppler ultrasound for the detection of vascular occlusion following liver transplantation in children. *Clin Radiol* 46:38–42, 1992.

The Value of Portal Vein Pulsatility on Duplex Sonograms as a Sign of Portal Hypertension in Children With Liver Disease

Westra SJ, Zaninovic AC, Vargas J (Univ of California, Los Angeles; Centro Radiologico "Fleming," Santiago de Chile; Ctr for the Health Sciences, Los Angeles)

AJR 165:167–172, 1995 4–49

Objective.—In patients with chronic liver disease, Doppler sonography provides useful information about hepatic vascular size, patency, and flow direction. Portal venous pressure cannot currently be detected noninvasively. Certain sonographic criteria are consistent with the presence of portal hypertension, including enlargement of the portal vein, lack of respiratory variation in portal venous flow, presence of paraumbilical veins and other collateral vessels, reversal of flow in the portal vein, and decreased antegrade flow volume in the portal vein. Experience suggests that children with chronic liver disease and portal hypertension may show markedly pulsatile waveforms in the portal vein during pretransplant sonographic evaluation. The significance of this finding was evaluated prospectively.

Methods.—The study included 38 children with end-stage hepatic decompensation. Chronic liver diseases were present in 36 patients, including failed Kasai's procedure for biliary atresia in 23; Alagille syndrome with biliary hypoplasia in 2; and Budd-Chiari syndrome, chronic active autoimmune hepatitis, neonatal hepatitis with cirrhosis, and hemochromatosis in 1 patient each. Each patient underwent color-assisted spectral Doppler waveform analysis of the hepatic artery and portal vein, with specified criteria for portal venous waveform pulsatility. The findings were compared with those of healthy controls and patients with acute viral hepatitis. Patients with 2 or more clinical or sonographic signs, including ascites, splenomegaly, collateral vessels, and flow reversal in the main portal vein, were considered to have portal hypertension.

Results.—Doppler imaging detected portal vein flow in 36 patients, all of whom showed portal vein pulsatility. Clinical or sonographic evidence of portal hypertension was noted in 34 patients. Two patients, both with large portosystemic shunts, had no portal vein flow detected in the liver hilum. The patients with end-stage liver disease showed significantly increased hepatic artery waveform pulsatility, with a mean resistive index of 0.89. Thirty-one percent of the patients had zero or reversed end-diastolic flow. Both control groups had no portal vein pulsatility and normal hepatic artery pulsatility. A pulsatile waveform in the portal vein was 94% sensitive and 90% specific in identifying children with end-stage liver disease and portal hypertension.

Conclusion.—The sonographic finding of portal vein waveform pulsatility can detect portal hypertension in children with end-stage liver disease. This finding may be useful in making clinical decisions about the timing of palliative therapy for portal hypertension and liver transplantation. It remains to be determined whether or not portal vein pulsatility is an early sign of portal hypertension. A prospective, longitudinal study of infants with biliary atresia will be needed to see if the degree of pulsatility is correlated with the severity of portal hypertension.

► The significantly high sensitivity and specificity value of portal vein waveform pulsatility for determining portal hypertension in end-stage liver disease justifies the use of this method in preference to angiography. Other recent articles also supportive of this viewpoint are listed.[1,2] Gallbladder varices[3,4] and cavernous transformation of the portal vein,[5] later findings in the portal hypertension spectrum, are also demonstrable by color Doppler.

L.W. Young, M.D.

References

1. Kozaiwa K, Tajiri H, Yoshimura N, et al: Utility of duplex Doppler ultrasound in evaluating portal hypertension in children. *J Pediatr Gastroenterol Nutr* 21:215–221, 1995.
2. de Vries PJ, Hoekstra JB, de Hooge P, et al: Portal venous flow and follow-up in patients with liver disease and healthy subjects. Assessment with duplex Doppler. *Scand J Gastroenterol* 29:172–177, 1994.
3. Helbich T, Breitenseher M, Heinz-Peer G, et al: Color Doppler ultrasound of gallbladder varicose veins in children. A rare sign of portal hypertension. *Ultraschall in der Medizin* 15:126–130, 1994.
4. Chawla Y, Dilawari JB, Katariya S: Gallbladder varices in portal vein thrombosis. *AJR* 162:643–645, 1994.
5. De Gaetano AM, Lafortune M, Patriquin H, et al: Cavernous transformation of the portal vein: patterns of intrahepatic and splanchnic collateral circulation detected with Doppler sonography. *AJR* 165:1151–1155, 1995.

Genitourinary System

Ultrasound Findings in Juvenile Nephronophthisis

Blowey DL, Querfeld U, Geary D, et al (Children's Mercy Hosp, Kansas City, Mo; Univ Children's Hosp, Cologne, Germany; Hosp for Sick Children, Toronto)

Pediatr Nephrol 10:22–24, 1996 4–50

Objective.—Children with the inherited renal disease juvenile nephronophthisis (JN) have polyuria, growth failure, anemia, and progressive renal failure. A correct diagnosis of JN is essential, not only for proper management of renal failure but also for purposes of genetic counseling. Renal medullary cysts with increased echogenicity has been suggested as a diagnostic ultrasound finding in JN, but the authors have seen several JN patients without such cysts. The ultrasound findings of 11 children with JN were reviewed.

Methods.—The children were 6 girls and 5 boys, mean age 9½ years at diagnosis. In most cases, the diagnosis of JN was made by the clinical history and renal histopathologic findings. The ultrasound findings for each patient were reviewed.

Results.—The initial ultrasound scan showed increased echogenicity with loss of corticomedullary differentiation in all patients but 1. The kidneys were of normal size or slightly smaller. No cysts were found in 9 of the patients, and the other 2 patients had only 1 cyst each. Follow-up scans performed 2 to 7 years later in 4 patients revealed visible renal cysts in 3 cases.

Conclusion.—Most patients with JN do not have renal medullary cysts on their initial ultrasound examination. Rather, the most frequent finding is increased echogenicity with loss of corticomedullary differentiation. The absence of visible cysts should not rule out the diagnosis of JN; cysts may develop later in the course, but these are not necessarily unique to JN.

▶ Although medullary cystic disease or JN morphologically contains small cysts, the usual initial modality, sonography, may not demonstrate such cysts in early childhood. Increased renal echogenicity is more often the finding as in this report. A recent article reports that thin-section CT detected some of these small cysts of medullary cystic disease.[1] Other recent articles on medullary cystic disease feature its genetic aspects.[2–8]

L.W. Young, M.D.

References

1. Elzouki AY, Al-Suhaibani H, Mirza K, et al: Thin-section computed tomography scans detect medullary cysts in patients believed to have juvenile nephronophthisis. *Am J Kidney Dis* 27:261–269, 1996.
2. Horie S: Hereditary tubulo-interstitial nephropathy. *Nippon Rinsho* 53:2064–2067, 1995.
3. Hildebrandt F, Singh-Sawhney I, Schnieders B, et al: Refined genetic mapping of a gene for familial juvenile nephronophthisis (NPH1) and physical mapping of linked markers. APN Study Group. *Genomics* 25:360–364, 1995.
4. Medhioub M, Cherif D, Benessy F, et al: Refined mapping of a gene (NPH1) causing familial juvenile nephronophthisis and evidence for genetic heterogeneity. *Genomics* 22:296–301, 1994.
5. Elzouki A, Mirza K: Clinical quiz. Familial juvenile nephronophthisis. *Pediatr Nephrol* 8:525–526, 1994.
6. Antignac C, Arduy CH, Beckmann JS, et al: A gene for familial juvenile nephronophthisis (recessive medullary cystic kidney disease) maps to chromosome 2p. *Nat Genet* 3:342–345, 1993.
7. Bernstein J: Glomerulocystic kidney disease—nosological considerations. *Pediatr Nephrol* 7:464–470, 1993.
8. Blowey DL, Alon U, Hellerstein S, et al: Radiological cases of the month. Juvenile nephronophthisis. *Am J Dis Child* 147:1117–1118, 1993.

Ureterocele Eversion With Vesicoureteral Reflux in Duplex Kidneys: Findings at Voiding Cystourethrography

Bellah RD, Long FR, Canning DA (Children's Hosp of Philadelphia)

AJR 165:409–413, 1995 4–51

Background.—Ureterocele eversion during voiding cystourethrography (VCUG) is the sudden appearance of a bladder diverticulum at the site of ureterocele compression. Its radiologic appearance is very similar to a congenital bladder diverticulum. Effective preoperative planning requires that ureterocele eversion with vesicoureteral reflux in duplex kidneys be distinguished from congenital bladder diverticula. The findings of ureterocele eversion and lower pole vesicoureteral reflux in duplex kidneys on VCUG were described to demonstrate how its appearance can be misleading.

Methods.—Twelve children with VCUGs demonstrating bladder diverticula with vesicoureteral reflux and ureteroceles associated with duplex systems at surgery were included in the study. Their medical records, sonograms, and cystograms were reviewed retrospectively.

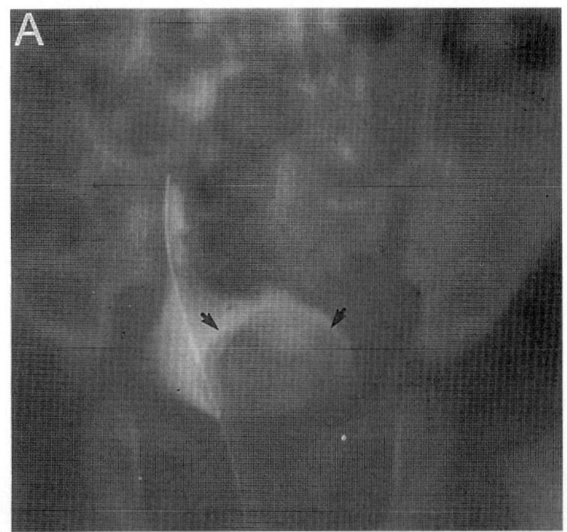

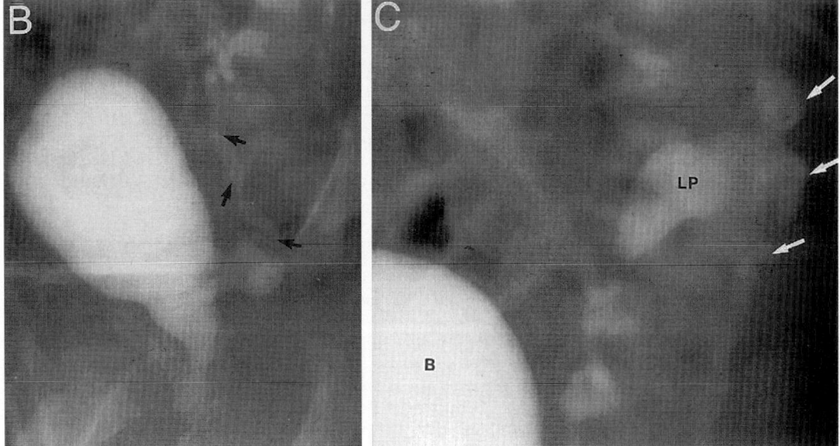

FIGURE 1.—Ureterocele eversion (2-month-old with typical appearance of ureterocele eversion and lower pole reflux). **A,** voiding cystourethrography (early filling) shows a left-sided ureterocele (*arrows*), **B,** during voiding, the ureterocele disappears and diverticulum appears. Note the lower pole ureter (*arrowheads*) entering the diverticulum. **C,** reflux occurs into the lower pole (*LP*) moiety of the left kidney. Bladder is *B*. Axis of the lower pole is tilted down, and only the lower pole component of calyces (*arrows*) is seen. The patient underwent cystoscopic ureterocele incision after recognition of ureterocele and eversion. (Courtesy of Bellah RD, Long FR, Canning DA: Ureterocele eversion with vesicoureteral reflux in duplex kidneys: Findings at voiding cystourethrography. *AJR* 165:409–413, 1995.)

Findings.—In 5 patients with unidentifiable ureteroceles or reflux occurring into what looked like single systems instead of lower poles of duplex systems, the diagnosis of ureterocele eversion with lower pole reflux was uncertain or misinterpreted as congenital bladder diverticula with reflux. Fluoroscopy identified ureterocele eversion with lower pole reflux in 2 patients in whom ureteroceles were not detected initially. Ureterocele was confirmed sonographically in 1 of these patients and by cystoscopy in the other (Figs 1 and 4).

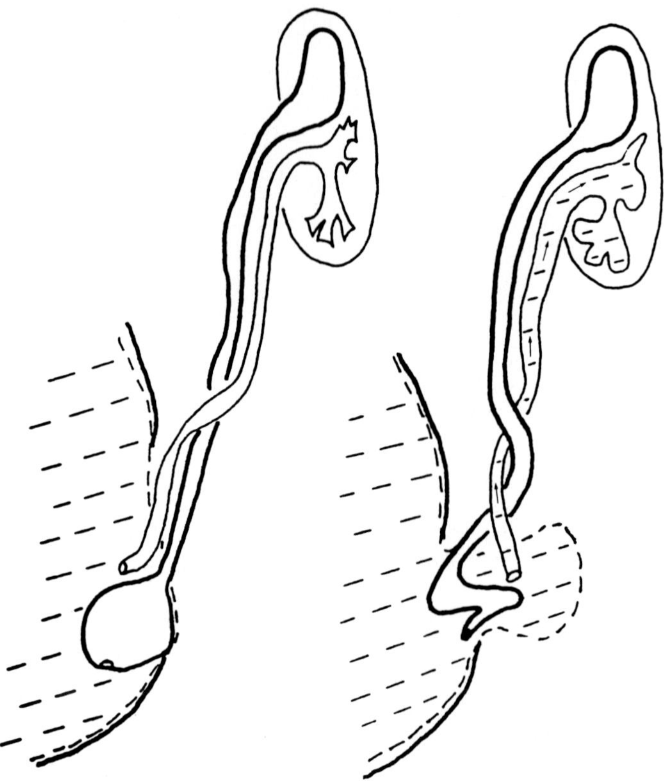

FIGURE 4.—Ureterocele eversion. During bladder filling (*left*), the ureterocele appears as a filling defect outlined by contrast (*dashes*). During voiding (*right*), the ureterocele is compressed, and the bladder mucosa at the ureteral hiatus protrudes. The entrance of the lower pole ureter is altered and repositioned such that lower pole reflux (*arrow*) occurs. (Courtesy of Bellah RD, Long FR, Canning DA: Ureterocele eversion with vesicoureteral reflux in duplex kidneys: Findings at voiding cystourethrography. *AJR* 165:409–413, 1995.)

Conclusion.—When a ureterocele is detected initially or the fluoroscopic appearance is typical, ureterocele eversion with lower pole vesicoureteral reflux is easily diagnosed on VCUG. However, it can be mistaken for a congenital paraureteral diverticulum with reflux into a single collecting system when the ureterocele is small or not initially identified or when the refluxed system is not interpreted as a lower pole moiety.

► Demonstration of unusual phenomenon of ureterocele eversion is important. The fluoroscopist must look for this phenomenon in real-time during VCUG. Otherwise, ureterocele eversion with lower pole reflux may be mistaken on fluoroscopic spot images for a paraureteral diverticulum at the ureterovesical junction. The reader is referred to the references listed for background on this unusual phenomenon.[1–4]

L.W. Young, M.D.

References

1. Cremin BJ, Funston MR, Aaronson IA: The intraureteric diverticulum: A manifestation of ureterocele intussusception. *Pediatr Radiol* 6:92–96, 1977.
2. Lebowitz RL, Avni FE: Misleading appearances in pediatric uroradiology. *Pediatr Radiol* 10:15–31, 1980.
3. Koyanagi T, Hisajima S, Goto T, et al: Everting ureteroceles: Radiographic and endoscopic observation, and surgical managment. *J Urol* 123:538–543, 1980.
4. Mandell J, Colodny AH, Lebowitz R, et al: Ureteroceles in infants and children. *J Urol* 123:921–926, 1980.

Pyourachus: CT Manifestations

Herman TE, Shackelford GD (Washington Univ, St Louis)
J Comput Assist Tomogr 19:440–443, 1995 4–52

Background.—Pyourachus, an infected urachal cyst, is often clinically mistaken for other abdominal inflammatory or neoplastic processes. The CT manifestations of this condition in 2 children with surgically proved pyourachus were described.

Case Reports.—Girl, 2½ years, was brought for medical assessment of intermittent severe abdominal pain. Diffuse abdominal guarding was noted on physical examination. Girl, 10 years, complained of abdominal discomfort and pain. Physical assessment of this patient revealed a large pelvic mass in the midline extending to the symphysis pubis. In these patients, the characteristics of CT examinations included midline masses located deep to the rectus abdominis muscle; conical shapes each extending from the tip at the umbilicus to a base over the bladder dome; peripheral inflammatory changes in subcutaneous tissues, rectus abdominis muscle, and mesenteric fat; and intraperitoneal fluid or abscess (Fig 1).

Conclusion.—The findings of pyourachus on abdominal CT are characteristic and should enable the differentiation of this entity from other abdominal-pelvic masses, including abdominal desmoplastic round cell tumor, undifferentiated non-Hodgkin's lymphoma, and intra-abdominal desmoid tumor. Urachal sinus and patent urachus are small-caliber tubular structures that are better investigated with fistulography or high-frequency sonography than CT.

▶ The major findings of pyourachus can be demonstrated with excretory urography, cystourethrography, and ultrasonography. Computed tomography demonstrates the most characteristic findings for a preoperative diagnosis of pyourachus. A clinical diagnosis of an infection or neoplastic process is

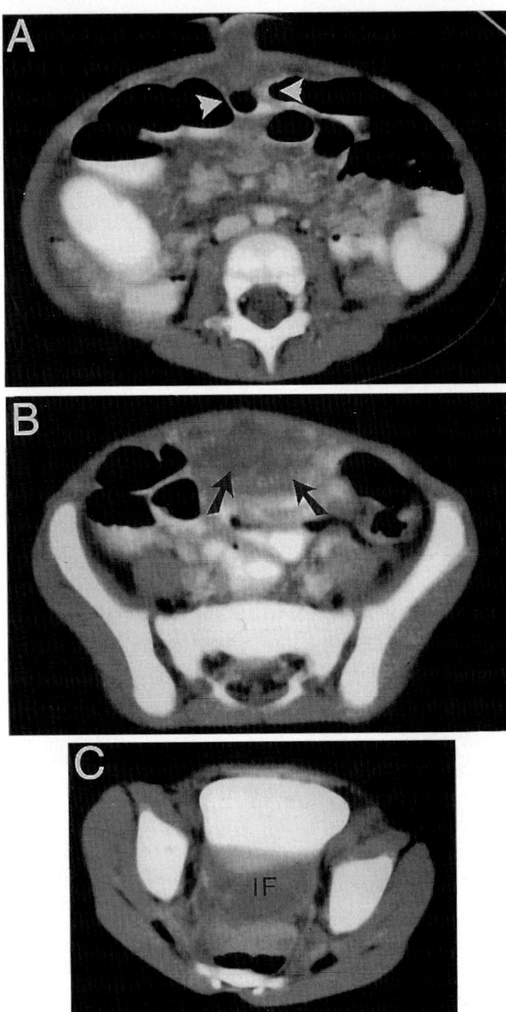

FIGURE 1.—Serial CT scans (**A**) at the level of the umbilicus, (**B**) just above the bladder dome, and (**C**) at the level of the urinary bladder. A hypodense mass (*arrows*, **B**) is present, extending in the midline just deep to the rectus abdominis muscles from the umbilicus (*arrowheads*, **A**) to the lower half of the pelvis. The mass is conical, with a larger diameter in cross section because it is scanned from the umbilicus to the lower half of the pelvis. Intraperitoneal fluid (*IF*) and mesenteric inflammatory changes are also present, which are more marked on the right side. Also noted is a fluid collection behind the urinary bladder in the peritoneal cul-de-sac. (Courtesy of Herman TE, Shackelford GD: Pyourachus: CT manifestations. *J Comput Assist Tomogr* 19:440–443, 1995.)

not unusual. Other recent reports feature the use of ultrasonography,[1, 2] and contrast medium fistulography.[1] Rarely the lesion may be diagnosed in an adult.[3]

L.W. Young, M.D.

References

1. Nagasaki A, Handa N, Hawanami T: Diagnosis of urachal anomalies in infancy and childhood by contrast fistulography, ultrasound and CT. *Pediatr Radiol* 21:321–323, 1991.
2. Yoshioka M, Ogino T, Shimada K, et al: A case of infected urachal cyst in an 8-year-old boy (review). *Hinyokika Kiyo-Acta Urologica Japonica* 37:183–185, 1991.
3. Ward TT, Saltzman E, Chiang S: Infected urachal remnants in the adult: Case report and review (review). *Clin Infect Dis* 16:26–29, 1993.

Uroradiologic Evaluation of Children With Urinary Tract Infection: Are Both Ultrasonography and Renal Cortical Scintigraphy Necessary?

Sreenarasimhaiah V, Alon US (Univ of Missouri, Kansas City)

J Pediatr 127:373–377, 1995 4–53

Objective.—The results of 3 investigative methods were compared in a prospective masked study of children with a clinical diagnosis of acute pyelonephritis. Fifty children aged 2 months to 15 years were entered into the study.

Methods.—All patients underwent renal scanning with technetium-99m–labeled glucoheptonate (GHS). All but 2 of them also underwent renal ultrasonography (RUS). Both imaging examinations were done within 2 to 4 days after admission to hospital. Two patients had IV pyelography, and 49 patients had voiding cystourethrography (VCUG).

Findings.—The findings of GHS were abnormal in 79% of the 48 patients who also had RUS, and the latter examination was abnormal in 42%. Findings of the 2 imaging methods were in agreement on the status of 57 of 96 renal units, 21 of which were abnormal. Voiding cystourethrography demonstated vesicoureteric reflux (VUR) in 4 renal units that had normal findings on both GHS and RUS. Fifteen children in all had VUR. In 7 kidneys only RUS was abnormal, usually demonstating mild to moderate pelvic dilation secondary to VUR. The combination of GHS and VCUG demonstrated abnormalities in all but 2 of 64 affected renal units.

Recommendation.—Renal ultrasonography has a number of advantages over renal scintigraphy, including its much lower cost, ready availability, and noninvasiveness. If GHS is to be part of the initial workup, it can be combined with VCUG and RUS left for use in a few selected patients.

▶ Comparison of findings of RUS, RUS and VCUG from examinations in children with urinary tract infection yields useful conclusions. The glucoheptonate scan routinely should be the initial screening method of choice for children with acute pyelonephritis. The radionuclide examination should be followed by VCUG in all cases, and RUS should be used only in special cases. Almost certainly some institutions prefer ultrasonography because the examination is easy to do and costs less. Glucoheptonate is used in preference to dimercaptosuccinic acid (DMSA), because glucoheptonate has additional imaging properties. The conclusions of this provocative article deserve careful consideration for wider implementation. Other recent related references concerning pyelonephritis and ultrasonography,[1, 2] additional support for use of DMSA,[2–5] the validity of a tailored excretory urogram to complement DMSA,[6] and the added value of ^{99m}Tc-DMSA single-photon emission CT are listed.

L.W. Young, M.D.

References

1. Pickworth FE, Carlin JB, Ditchfield MR, et al: Sonographic measurement of renal enlargement in children with acute pyelonephritis and time needed for resolution: Implications for renal growth assessment. *AJR* 165:405–408, 1995.
2. Majd M, Rushton HG: Renal cortical scintigraphy in the diagnosis of acute pyelonephritis (review). *Semin Nucl Med* 22:98–111, 1992.
3. Smellie JM: The intravenous urogram in the detection and evaluation of renal damage following urinary tract infection (review). *Pediatr Nephrol* 9:213–219, 1995. .
4. Tullus K, Fituri O, Linne T, et al: Urine interleukin-6 and interleukin-8 in children with acute pyelonephritis, in relation to DMSA scintigraphy in the acute phase and at 1-year follow-up. *Pediatr Radiol* 24:513–515, 1994.
5. Fukumoto Y, Hiraoka M, Takano T, et al: Acute tubulointerstitial nephritis in association with *Yersinia pseudotuberculosis* infection. *Pediatr Nephrol* 9:78–80, 1995.
6. Mastin ST, Drane WE, Iravani A: Tc-99m DMSA SPECT imaging in patients with acute symptoms or history of UTI. Comparison with ultrasonography. *Clin Nucl Med* 20:407–412, 1995

Congenital Mesoblastic Nephroma Metastatic to the Brain: A Report of Two Cases

Schlesinger AE, Rosenfield NS, Castle VP, et al (Texas Children's Hosp, Houston; Mem Sloan-Kettering Cancer Ctr, New York; Univ of Michigan, Ann Arbor)

Pediatr Radiol 25:73S–75S, 1995 4–54

Background.—Although congenital mesoblastic nephroma (CMN) was originally described as a benign neoplasm, a more aggressive, atypical form has since been recognized. The imaging findings of CMN that metastasized to the brain are reported.

Case Report.—Male infant, with a left renal mass seen on prenatal ultrasound examination, was found by CT to have a large, heterogeneous mass within the kidney. At 10 days of age, the patient underwent left nephrectomy, which revealed CMN of mixed classical and increased cellular pattern. Symptoms including decreased movement of the right extremities developed at 7 months of age; physical examination revealed an enlarged head circumference with a bulging anterior fontanel. A left cerebral mass with midline shift was seen on MRI. Craniotomy with gross total tumor resection was performed; the tumor had the same histologic characteristics as the primary tumor, which had not recurred. The tumor recurred despite chemotherapy.

Conclusion.—Brain metastases can occur in infants with CMN. Though recurrent disease and metastases are infrequent in patients with CMN, the radiologist should be aware of the possibility. Patients with CMN may be receiving more aggressive surveillance imaging studies in the future.

► There probably are no absolutes in medicine. Mesoblastic nephroma at one time was thought not to metastasize. Congenital mesoblastic nephroma metastatic to the brain perhaps gives company to malignant rhabdoid tumor.[1] Even rarely, Wilms' tumor spreads to the brain.[2] The association of Wilms' tumor with primary brain tumors in siblings has been reported recently.[2] Other recent pertinent articles on congenital mesoblastic nephroma are also listed.[3–7]

L.W. Young, M.D.

References

1. Cohn RD, Frank Y, Stanek AE, et al: Malignant rhabdoid tumor of the brain and kidney in a child: Clinical and pathologic features. *Pediatr Neurol* 13:65–68, 1995.
2. Rainov NG, Lubbe J, Renshaw J, et al: Association of Wilms' tumor with primary brain tumor in siblings. *J Neuropathol Exp Neurol* 54:214–223, 1995.
3. Becroft DM, Mauger DC, Skeen JE, et al: Good prognosis of cellular mesoblastic nephroma with hyperdiploidy and relaxation of imprinting of the maternal IGF2 gene. *Pediatr Pathol Lab Med* 15:679–688, 1995.
4. Lowery M, Issa B, Pysher T, et al: Cytogenetic findings in a case of congenital mesoblastic nephroma. *Cancer Genet Cytogenet* 84:113–115, 1995.
5. Martinez Ibanez V, Peiro Ibanez JL, Terradas M, et al: Does Bolande's malignant tumor exist? *Cir Pediatr* 7:25–29, 1994.
6. Newsham I, Dub D, Besnard-Guerin C, et al: Molecular sublocalization and characterization of the 11;22 translocation breakpoint in a malignant rhabdoid tumor. *Genomics* 19:433–440, 1994.
7. Litman DA, Bhuta S, Barsky SH: Synchronous occurrence of malignant rhabdoid tumor two decades after Wilms' tumor irradiation. *Am J Surg Pathol* 17:729–737, 1993.

Imaging of Solid Kidney Tumours in Children

Hugosson C, Nyman R, Jacobsson B, et al (King Faisal Specialist Hosp & Research Ctr, Riyadh, Saudi Arabia)
Acta Radiol 36:254–260, 1995 4–55

Background.—Solid renal tumors are the second most common retroperitoneal neoplasms in childhood. Ultrasound and CT have replaced the more traditional imaging modalities, including radiography, urography, inferior venocarnography, angiography, lymphangiography, radionuclide scintigraphy, in the assessment of renal masses. Few series of such tumors

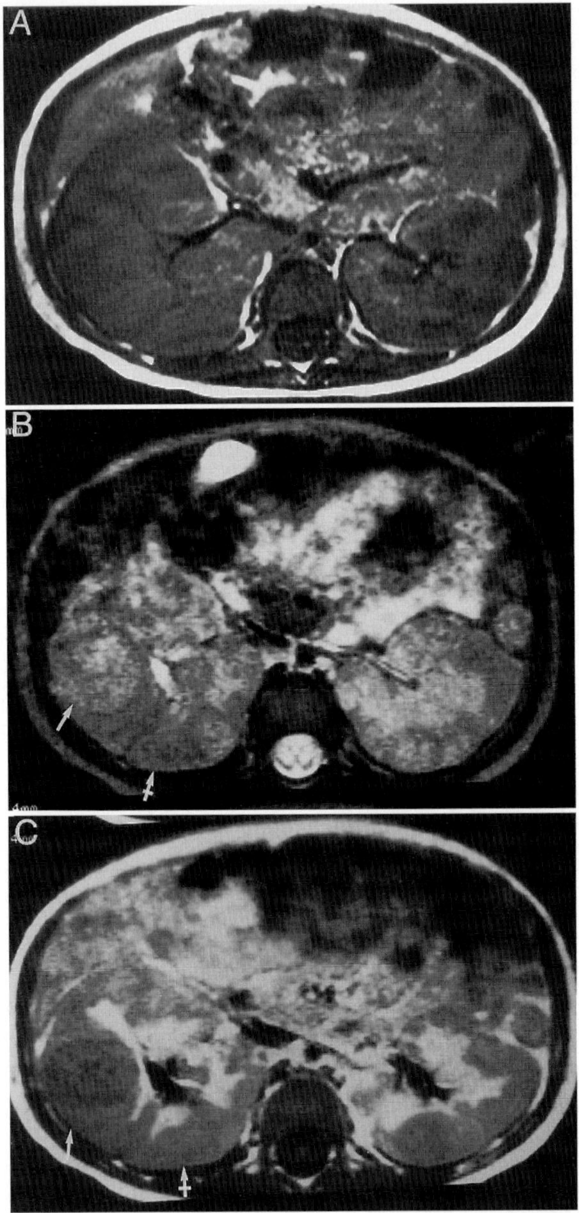

FIGURE 6.—Transverse MR images in a 1-year-old girl with bilateral nephroblastomatosis and Wilms' tumors. **A**, nonenhanced T1-weighted image demonstrating bilateral enlarged kidneys with heterogeneous signal intensity. **B**, T2-weighted image revealing cortical areas of increased signal intensity with biopsy-proven Wilms' tumor in both kidneys (*arrow*). The cortical areas with lower signal intensity most likely represent nephroblastomatosis (*crossed arrow*). **C**, enhanced T1-weighted image demonstrating lower enhancement in the areas of Wilms' tumor (*arrow*) compared with the nephroblastomatosis (*crossed arrow*). Centrally located areas of marked enhancement represent renal parenchyma. (Courtesy of Hugosson C, Nyman R, Jacobsson B, et al: Imaging of solid kidney tumours in children. *Acta Radiol* 36:254–260, 1995.)

evaluated by MRI have been reported. Ultrasound, CT, and MRI were compared in the assessment of solid renal masses in children.

Methods.—Eighteen children with 20 solid renal tumors were included in the study. The children ranged in age from 6 months to 12 years. Thirteen renal neoplasms were Wilms' tumors; 2, clear cell sarcomas of the kidney; 1, malignant rhabdoid tumor of the kidney; and 2, bilateral nephroblastomatosis with Wilms' tumor. Ultrasound, CT, and MRI were performed in all patients.

Findings.—Contrast-enhanced CT and contrast nonenhanced MR were equally accurate in determining tumor size and origin. However, these modalities did not reliably distinguish among NWTS stages I, II, and III disease. Ultrasound was only accurate in determining tumor size. Though MR features varied somewhat between Wilms' tumors and non-Wilms' tumors, contrast-enhanced MRI showed promise for distinguishing Wilms' tumors from nephroblastomatosis (Fig 6).

Conclusion.—Contrast-enhanced CT and non-enhanced MRI do not differ significantly in the assessment of primary renal tumors in children. Contrast-enhanced MRI may provide additional information in the evaluation of nephroblastomatosis complicated by Wilms' tumor. Ultrasound remains the primary modality for distinguishing cystic masses from solid renal tumors. For determining tumor size, origin, and stage, CT or MRI are the basic imaging modalities. However, these techniques appear to be incapable of accurately demonstrating a pseudocapsule.

► Imaging of solid kidney tumors in children with US, CT, and MRI has virtually replaced the traditional methods. Although all of the article is interesting, of special note is the information on nephroblastomatosis, which is demonstrated in Figure 6. Magnetic resonance imaging offers promise in being able to distinguish nephroblastomatosis from Wilms' tumor. However, for the other renal neoplasms, CT with contrast medium enhancement is probably just as good as MRI. Ultrasonography is a useful preliminary examination to distinguish cystic from solid aspects of a lesion. Additional lesions discussed are simple Wilms' tumor, renal cell sarcoma, and malignant rhabdoid tumor of the kidney. One aspect of this article, the staging of renal tumors, is confusingly presented. Criteria for staging as by the National Wilms' Tumor Study are not correctly referenced and are loosely defined. Other noteworthy recent references to a variety of pediatric renal tumors—rhabdoid tumor,[1] pediatric renal tumors and tumorlike lesions,[2] congenital mesoblastic nephroma,[3] multilocular cystic renal tumor,[4, 5] clear cell sarcoma,[5] and teratoid Wilms' tumor[6]—are listed.

L.W. Young, M.D.

References

1. Chung CJ, Lorenzo R, Rayder S, et al: Rhabdoid tumors of the kidney in children: CT findings. *AJR* 164:697–700, 1995.
2. Kissane JM, Dehner LP: Renal tumors and tumor-like lesions in pediatric patients (review). *Pediatr Nephrol* 6:365–382, 1992.

3. Tomlinson GE, Argyle JC, Velasco S, et al: Molecular characterization of congenital mesoblastic nephroma and its distinction from Wilms tumor. *Cancer* 70:2358–2361, 1992.
4. Agrons GA, Wagner BJ, Davidson AJ, et al: Multilocular cystic renal tumor in children: Radiologic-pathologic correlation. *Radiographics* 15:653–669, 1995.
5. Castillo OA, Boyle ET Jr, Kramer SA: Multilocular cysts of the kidney. A study of 29 patients and review of literature (review). *Urology* 37:156–162, 1991
6. Vujanic GM: Teratoid Wilms' tumor: Report of a unilateral case (review). *Pediatr Pathol* 11:303–309, 1991. .

Ovarian Torsion: Clinical and Imaging Presentation in Children

Meyer JS, Harmon CM, Harty MP, et al (Univ of Pennsylvania, Philadelphia)
J Pediatr Surg 30:1433–1436, 1995 4–56

Background.—Ovarian torsion, usually found in the first 3 decades of life, is an uncommon condition with a nonspecific clinical manifestation. In neonates, it is usually suggested by an abdominopelvic mass on prenatal ultrasound (US). In older girls, a variety of symptoms can occur, including nausea, vomiting, and pain. In such patients, imaging examinations are conducted for further assessment. The impact of imaging on the management of surgically confirmed ovarian torsion in 12 children was investigated.

Methods.—The 12 children had a total of 13 episodes of ovarian torsion. Three girls were neonates; 6 were premenarchal, and 3 were postmenarchal. The imaging modality of choice was US.

Findings.—Complex abdominopelvic cysts requiring surgery were demonstrated sonographically in all 3 neonates (Fig 1). Ultrasonography showed a solid mass strongly suggesting torsion in 5 of 10 episodes in older patients (Fig 2). Same-day surgery was performed in 3 patients. In 1, the involved ovary was salvaged. Another girl had a small piece of normal-appearing ovary left in situ. The low rate of ovarian salvage was attributed to the delay in clinical manifestation and the delay to treatment because of the nonspecific clinical and imaging findings.

Conclusion.—Ultrasonography is the imaging examination of choice for patients with possible ovarian torsion. Surgical delays can be reduced and the likelihood of ovarian salvage improved by a high level of clinical suspicion, prompt imaging, and familiarity with the various clinical and imaging manifestations of ovarian torsion.

► This is 1 of 2 excellent articles on this subject from the recent literature.[1] It must be emphasized that the sonographic findings are different in the prepubertal compared with the pubertal girl. The large cystic ovarian mass with layered debris is typical for torsion in neonates. The pattern is more of peripheral dilated cyst around a solid echogenic focus in adolescent girls. Although color Doppler depicts central vascular flow in some lesions, pe-

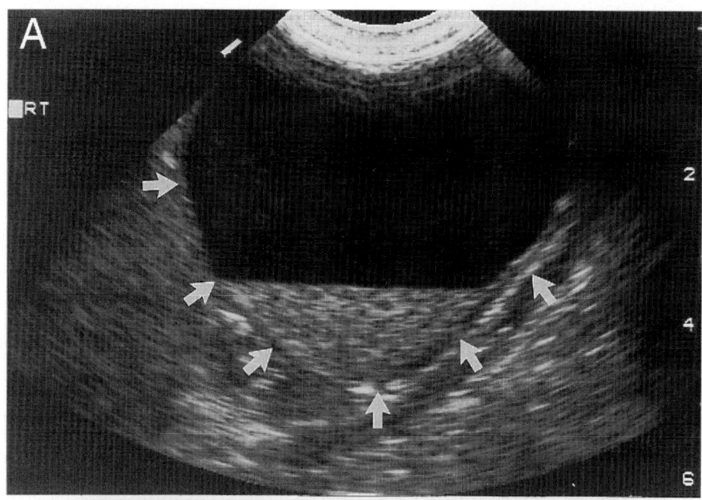

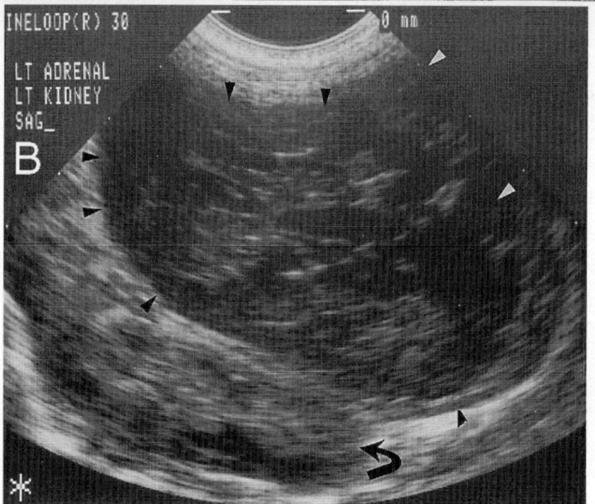

FIGURE 1.—Ultrasound images from neonates with ovarian torsion. **A,** debris-filled cystic mass (*arrows*). **B,** mixed mass (*arrowheads*) with cystic and solid components anterior to the left kidney (*curved arrows*). (Courtesy of Meyer JS, Harmon CM, Harty MP, et al: Ovarian torsion: Clinical and imaging presentation in children. *J Pediatr Surg* 30:1433–1436, 1995.)

ripheral vascular flow has been shown in others. Central vascular flow or peripheral vascular flow has not been specific to age. It is postulated that the presence of arterial waveforms in torsion may be because of the presence of symptoms before the occurrence of arterial occlusion or because of the existence of a dual ovarian blood supply.

L.W. Young, M.D.

References

1. Stark JE, Siegel MJ: Ovarian torsion in prepubertal and pubertal girls: Sonographic findings. *AJR* 163:1479–1482, 1994.

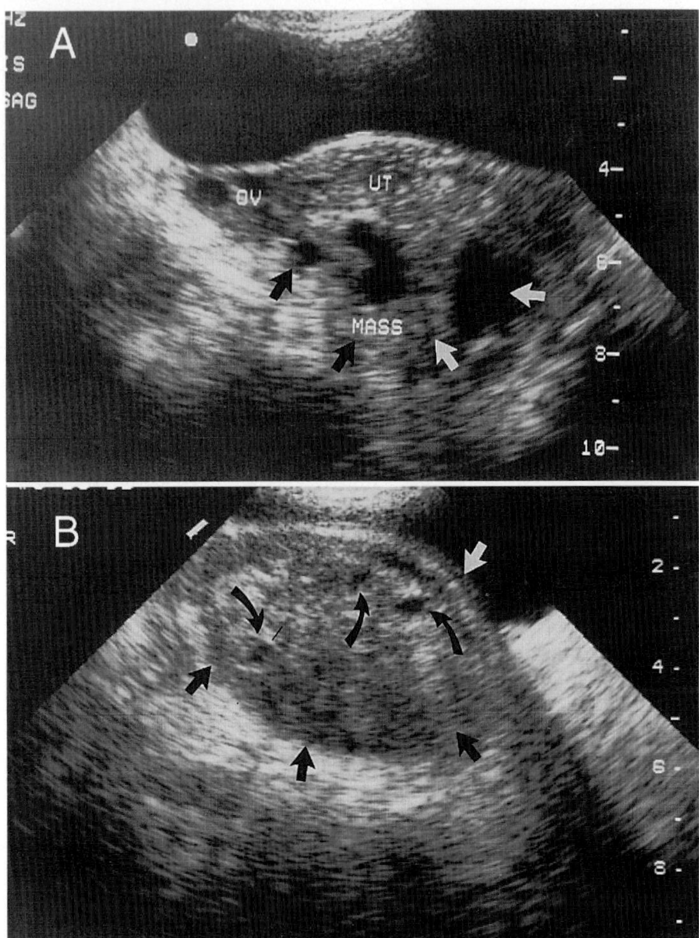

FIGURE 2.—Ultrasound images of masses from premenarchal patients. **A,** mass (*arrows*) with cystic and solid components posterior to the uterus (*UT*) and inferior to the ovary (*OV*). This patient had severe hematosalpinx, fallopian tube torsion, and early ovarian torsion. **B,** solid mass (*arrows*) with peripheral cysts (*curved arrows*). This is the most specific ultrasound appearance of ovarian torsion. (Courtesy of Meyer JS, Harmon CM, Harty MP, et al: Ovarian torsion: Clinical and imaging presentation in children. *J Pediatr Surg* 30:1433–1436, 1995.)

Suggested Reading

Fleischer AC, Stein SM, Cullinan JA, et al: Color Doppler sonography of adnexal torsion. *J Ultrasound Med* 14:523–528, 1995.

Quillin SP, Siegel MJ: Transabdominal color Doppler ultrasonography of the painful adolescent ovary. *J Ultrasound Med* 13:549–555, 1994.

Kimura I, Togashi K, Kawakami S, et al: Ovarian torsion: CT and MR imaging appearances. *Radiology* 190:337–341, 1994.

Rosado VM Jr, Trambert MA, Gosink BB, et al: Adnexal torsion: Diagnosis by using Doppler sonography. *AJR* 159:1251–1253, 1992.

Posttraumatic Arterial Priapism in Children: Management With Embolization

Miller SF, Chait PG, Burrows PE, et al (Hosp for Sick Children, Toronto; Children's Hosp, Boston; Univ of Medicine and Dentistry of New Jersey, Camden; et al)

Radiology 196:59–62, 1995 4–57

Purpose.—Most cases of priapism in children are painful, associated with venous obstruction and subsequent tissue ischemia. Posttraumatic priapism, in contrast, is caused by increased arterial inflow and is usually painless. The distinction between these 2 types is essential to make, because the treatments are different. The results of angiographic embolism for the management of posttraumatic priapism were reported, including the diagnostic use of color Doppler sonography.

Methods.—The patients were 5 boys, age 6 to 10 years, in whom priapism developed after blunt trauma to the perineum. None had any medical conditions associated with priapism. All patients underwent diagnostic angiography followed by selective embolization. In the last 3 patients in the series, color Doppler sonography was performed before angiography to see if it could aid in making the diagnosis and in guiding angiography and embolization.

Results.—Selective angiography made the diagnosis in all 5 patients: intracavernosal arteriovenous fistula in 2, pseudoaneurysm of the cavernosal artery in 2, and asymmetric cavernosal arterial flow in 1. Successful embolization was followed by prompt or delayed detumescence in all patients. Color Doppler sonography was diagnostic in all 3 patients who had it. The preangiographic study helped in detecting the causative lesion, localizing the abnormality, and assessing the effectiveness of embolization.

Conclusion.—For children with the rare problem of posttraumatic priapism, angiography with selective embolization is a safe and effective diagnostic/therapeutic procedure. Additional useful diagnostic information can be obtained by performing color Doppler sonography before angiography: The causative lesion can be identified and localized to a specific corpus, thus avoiding the need for diagnostic cavernosal aspiration.

► High-flow posttraumatic arterial priapism in children can be managed with angiography and selective embolization. Doppler sonography is an effective method to use to find the arterial lesion. Other recent articles on all types of priapism—low flow and high flow—are listed.[1–7]

L.W. Young, M.D.

References

1. Stock KW, Jacob AL, Kummer M, et al: High-flow priapism in a child: Treatment with superselective embolization. *AJR* 166:290–292, 1996.
2. Jameson JS, Terry TR, Bolia A, et al: An unusual case of priapism in a child: diagnosis and treatment. *Br J Urol* 77:462–463, 1996.
3. Miller ST, Rao SP, Dunn EK, et al: Priapism in children with sickle cell disease. *J Urol* 154:844–847, 1995.
4. Ramos CE, Park JS, Ritchey ML, et al: High flow priapism associated with sickle cell disease. *J Urol* 153:1619–1621, 1995.
5. Dewan PA, Lorenz C, Davies RP: Posttraumatic priapism in a 7-year-old boy. *Eur Urol* 25:85–87, 1994.
6. Bastuba MD, Saenz de Tejada I, Dinlenc CZ, et al: Arterial priapism: diagnosis, treatment and long-term followup. *J Urol* 151:1231–1237, 1994.
7. Ilkay AK, Levine LA: Conservative management of high-flow priapism. *Urology* 46:419–424, 1995.

Imaging Evaluation of Blunt Renal Trauma in Children: Diagnostic Accuracy of Intravenous Pyelography and Ultrasonography

Mayor B, Gudinchet F, Wicky S, et al (Univ Hosp, Lausanne, Switzerland)
Pediatr Radiol 25:214–218, 1995 4–58

Background.—Renal parenchymal injuries are present in 1.2% to 15% of all children with trauma. The main goal of renal injury management is to prevent complications such as bleeding, urinoma, infection, and hypertension and to preserve functioning renal parenchyma. Achieving this goal requires prompt diagnosis of renal damage, accurate staging, and optimal imaging.

Methods.—Forty-six consecutive children with blunt renal injury were included in a retrospective study of the diagnostic accuracy of different imaging methods. Ultrasonography (US), IV pyelography (IVP), and CT were performed. Doppler US had not been done in any emergent cases. The renal injuries included 25 contusions, 4 lacerations, 11 ruptures, and 6 pedicle injuries.

Findings.—In all types of renal injuries, the diagnostic accuracy of IVP was 80.8%, compared with 41% for US. Intravenous pyelography was diagnostic in 21 of 26 children and US in 16 of 39. Initial US findings included 16 false negatives for renal injury. Two children with false negative US findings had thrombosis of the main renal artery. Also, US resulted in an underdiagnosis of 5 patients with renal damage. Most injuries not detected by US were renal contusions. Five renal injuries were diagnosed by sonography only 24 to 48 hours after the trauma occurred. Initial IVP failed to show 5 renal contusions that were subsequently detected by US. Contrast-enhanced abdominal CT was performed on an emergent basis in 4 children, yielding correct diagnoses in all. None of the CT results were falsely positive. Six patients thought to have renal fracture or vascular injury underwent renal angiography without complication.

Conclusion.—Ultrasonography is less accurate than IVP in all types of renal injury. Thus, the 2 modalities should complement one another. In children with asymptomatic microscopic hematuria, IVP is of little value. Intravenous pyelography should be done as an emergent procedure in children with gross hematuria or clinically suspected isolated renal injury. Multiply injured children in stable condition suspected of having renal damage should undergo contrast-enhanced CT. If necessary, hemodynamically unstable children should have immediate exploratory laparotomy after appropriate imaging studies.

► Ultrasonography is diagnostically less accurate than IVP to examine for emergent renal injury from blunt trauma in children. However, CT is the imaging method used in most North American children's hospitals to examine for renal injury from blunt trauma. Just using figures from this article, one can appreciate the better demonstration of the injury by the CT image than by the IVP image in the same patient. Several relatively recent articles emphasize the use of CT for blunt injury to the kidney,[1–4] but CT may not demonstrate an occult vascular injury.

L.W. Young, M.D.

References

1. Stein JP, Kaji DM, Eastham J, et al: Blunt renal trauma in the pediatric population: Indications for radiographic evaluation. *Urology* 44:406–410, 1994.
2. Smith DP, Jerkins GR, Noe HN: Blunt renal trauma in children with the prune-belly syndrome. *J Urol* 153:1960–1961, 1995.
3. Abdalati H, Bulas DL, Sivit CL, et al: Blunt renal trauma in children: Healing of renal injuries and recommendations for imaging follow-up. *Pediatr Radiol* 24:573–576, 1994.
4. Baumann L, Greenfield SP, Aker J, et al: Nonoperative management of major blunt renal trauma in children: In-hospital morbidity and long-term follow-up. *J Urol* 148:691–693, 1992.

Renovascular Hypertension in Children: Curability Predicted With Negative Intrarenal Doppler US Results

Garel L, Dubois J, Robitaille P, et al (Hôpital Sainte-Justine, Montreal)
Radiology 195:401–405, 1995 4–59

Objective.—There is no general agreement on the ability of intrarenal Doppler ultrasound (US) to diagnose renal artery stenosis (RAS) in children. The results of intrarenal Doppler US and angiography results were compared with patient outcomes in a prospective study.

Methods.—Intrarenal Doppler US and then angiography were performed in 29 children (15 boys and 14 girls) aged 12 days to 15 years.

Results.—Doppler US and angiography results were positive for RAS in 15 children (group 1). Five patients in this group were cured by percutaneous transluminal angioplasty. In the other 10, severity of the vascular lesion precluded permanent cure. Doppler US results were negative for

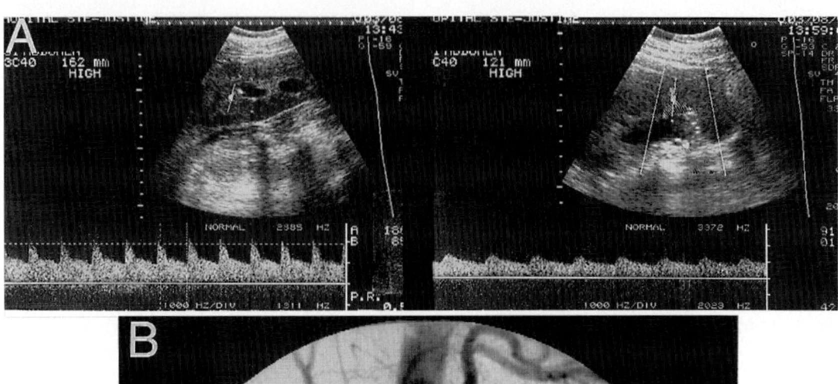

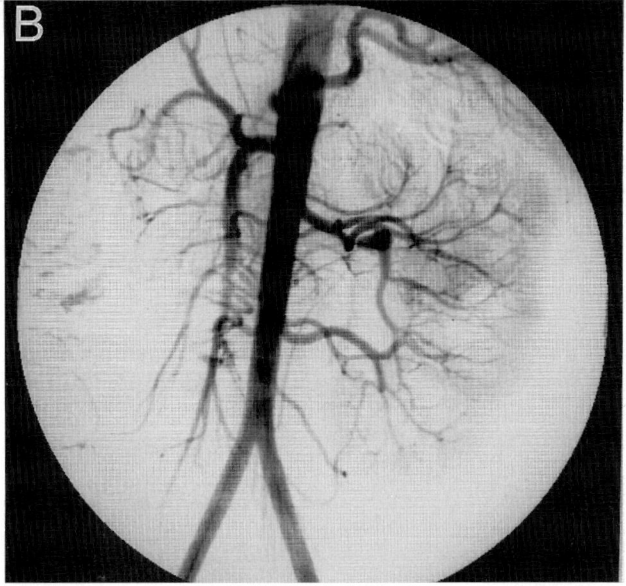

FIGURE 1.—Images of a 16-year-old girl who, at 9 years, underwent surgery on a solitary left kidney for pelviureteral junction obstruction. She was treated medically for years for high blood pressure (initial blood pressure reading 175/120 mm Hg), which was thought to be postsurgical in origin. **A**, intrarenal Doppler ultrasound scan shows the obvious difference between a normal and an abnormal waveform. *Left*, the normal waveform in the upper pole of the kidney shows a systolic upstroke with a sharp slope, an acute angle of the first peak, followed by a second midsystolic peak. *Right*, on the abnormal tracing in the midportion of the kidney, the systolic peak shows a smooth, round contour, with loss of the second peak. **B**, aortogram shows 4 left renal arteries with severe segmental renal artery stenosis (*arrow*). Percutaneous transluminal angioplasty was immediately effective. Blood pressure reading at 1-year follow-up was 110/70 mm Hg. (Courtesy of Garel L, Dubois J, Robitaille P, et al: Renovascular hypertension in children: Curability predicted with negative intrarenal Doppler US results. *Radiology* 195:401–405, 1995; Radiological Society of North America.)

RAS and angiographic evaluations positive for RAS in 14 children (group 2). In this group, only the 3 patients with neurofibromatosis were not cured by percutaneous transluminal angioplasty. Only 1 patient with accessory renal arteries had an RAS-positive Doppler US result before angiography (Fig 1, A and B). There was a significant association between cure and an RAS-negative Doppler US. Fourteen patients with hypertension and an RAS-negative Doppler US had multiple arteries and segmental lesions. The false RAS-negative Doppler US results for group 2 are similar to the 40% to 44% reported in the literature.

Conclusion.—In children with renovascular hypertension, cure by percutaneous transluminal angioplasty is more likely in those patients with an RAS-negative Doppler US.

▶ Intrarenal Doppler US is helpful in the evaluation of renovascular hypertension in children. In such patients, smoothing and rounding of the systolic peak is indicative of a poor prognosis, whereas a normal wave pattern is predictive of curability regardless of the angiographic findings. Doppler US findings are normal or inconclusive; selected segmental renal vein sampling and selective conventional renal arteriography are essential for diagnosis and managment.[1, 2] Doppler US contributes to a more directed arteriographic examination. Other authors[3, 4] advocate the use of captopril technetium-99m–diethylenetriamine pentaacetic acid renal scintigraphy, as well as digital subtraction or conventional renal angiography, in the evaluation of renovascular hypertension in children. In Tables 1 and 2 of the original article, causes of renovascular hypertension other than neurofibromatosis are listed.

L.W. Young, M.D.

References

1. Ellis D, Shapiro R, Scantleur VP, et al: Evaluation and management of bilateral renal artery stenosis in children: A case series and review. *Pediatr Nephrol* 9:259–267, 1995.
2. Deal JE, Snell MF, Barratt TM, et al: Renovascular disease in childhood. *J Pediatr* 121:378–384, 1992.
3. Guzzetta PC, Davis CF, Ruley EJ: Experience with bilateral renal artery stenosis as a cause of hypertension in childhood. *J Pediatr Surg* 26:532–534, 1991.
4. Hiner LB, Falkner B: Renovascular hypertension in children (review), *Pediatr Clin North Am* 40:123–140, 1993.

Systemic Oxalosis: Pathognomonic Renal and Specific Extrarenal Findings on US and CT

Akhan O, Özmen MN, Coskun M, et al (Hacetepe Univ, Turkey)
Pediatr Radiol 25:15–16, 1995 4–60

Introduction.—Renal abnormalities are generally the initial and most important manifestations of hyperoxaluria. Patients exhibit oxalosis, the deposition of calcium oxalate crystals in extrarenal tissues. The 2 patients reported here had primary hyperoxaluria, a rare autosomal recessive disorder, that was diagnosed with US and CT.

Case 1.—Boy, 5 years, was admitted with chronic renal failure. The second child of first-degree cousins, his older sister had died 2 years previously with similar pathosis. At admission he had proteinuria, a marked elevation of urine oxalate value (184 mg/L per

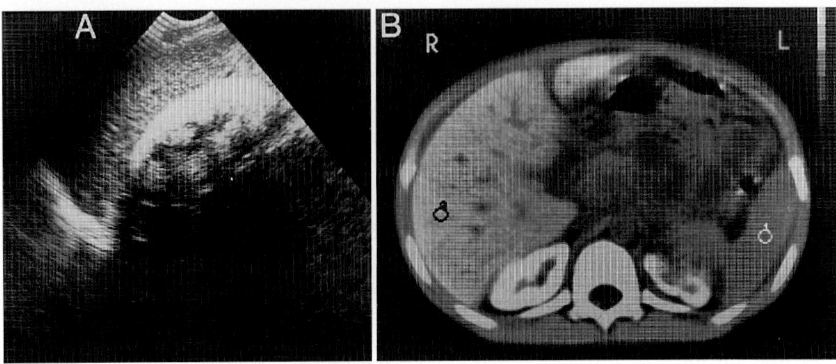

FIGURE 1.—Case 1. **A,** renal ultrasound shows a normal-sized kidney with markedly increased parenchymal echogenicity and loss of corticomedullary distinction. **B,** unenhanced CT scan demonstrates kidneys of almost bone density. Attenuation value of the liver is 112 HU and of the spleen is 53 HU. (*Pediatr Radiol;* Systemic oxalosis: Pathognomonic renal and specific extrarenal findings on US and CT; Akhan O, Özmen MN, Coskun M, et al; 25:15–16; Fig 1; 1995; Copyright notice of Springer-Verlag.)

24 hours), gross hematuria, and a metabolic acidosis. Dense kidneys and bilateral renal calculi were shown by abdominal radiography. Ultrasound revealed highly increased renal parenchymal echogenicity and almost total obliteration of corticomedullary differentiation. There was also an increase in liver echogenicity. CT unenhanced with intravenous contrast medium showed kidneys of almost bone density and markedly increased attenuation in the liver (Fig 1). The boy was treated with calcium carbonate and aluminum hydroxide gel, control of diet, and hemodialysis.

Case 2.—Girl, 9 years, was admitted for progressive renal failure. She was receiving peritoneal dialysis and had undergone several operations for recurrent renal calculi. Her parents were first-degree relatives; her 5-year-old sister died 4 years previously with similar symptoms. Abdominal radiography revealed bilateral dense kidneys with renal calculi. Ultrasound findings were similar to those of Case 1 and also included massive ascites and multiple gallstones. Echocardiography revealed a decrease in cardiac muscle contractility and pericardial effusion. Despite hemodialysis, she died of decompensated cardiac and renal failure.

Discussion.—Primary hyperoxaluria often manifests in childhood with progressive renal insufficiency resulting from recurrent calcium oxalate nephrolithiasis and nephrocalcinosis. Normal-sized kidneys with highly reflective echogenicity appear to be pathognomonic for the disease. Both of these patients had kidneys of normal size, with a uniformly dense cortex and medulla and markedly increased attenuation on CT. Liver features in both cases also suggested the presence of calcium oxalate crystal deposits. Cardiac muscle often shows increased echogenicity on US.

Progression of Bone Lesions in a Child With Primary Hyperoxaluria Type 1: Evaluation by Roentgenology and MRI

Vichi GF, Bongini U, Seracini D, et al ("A Meyer" Hosp, Florence, Italy; Univ of Florence, Italy)

Pediatr Radiol 25:102–104, 1995 4–61

Introduction.—Primary hyperoxaluria (PH) is a rare, inherited metabolic disorder characterized by declining renal function and subsequent deposit of calcium crystals in soft tissue and bone (oxalosis). The case presented here is followed by a discussion of the clinical and radiologic manifestations of PH type 1, which is caused by deficiency of peroxisomal alanine-glyoxylate aminotransferase (AGT) with hyperglycolic aciduria.

Case Report.—Boy, 5, was admitted because of recurrent urinary tract infections and passage of calcium oxalate stones. High urinary and blood oxalate levels led to a diagnosis of PH, confirmed as type 1 by the finding of a marked decrease in AGT activity on studies of a percutaneous liver biopsy specimen. The child experienced renal failure at age 6 and required hemodialysis by age 7. His kidneys were small and densely calcified, and severe, progressive skeletal disease was identified. Radiographs at age 8 revealed progression of bands and areas of rarefaction, together

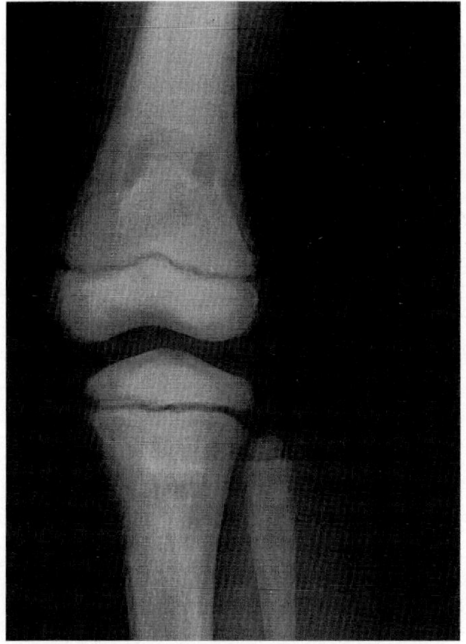

FIGURE 2.—C, progression of lesions on radiography. (Courtesy of Vichi GF, Bongini U, Seracini D, et al: Progression of bone lesions in a child with primary hyperoxaluria type 1: Evaluation by roentgenology and MRI. *Pediatr Radiol* 25:102–104, 1995.)

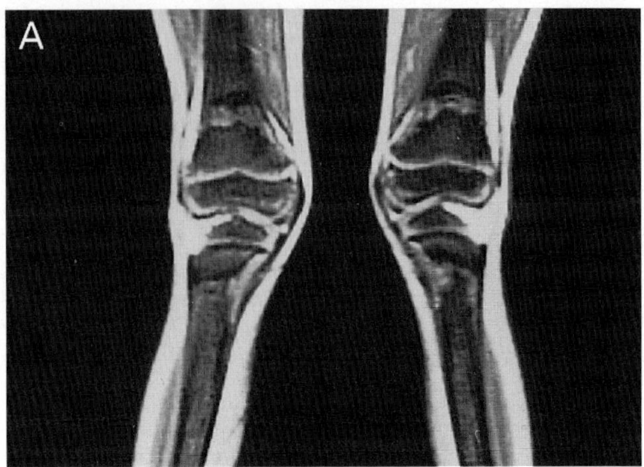

FIGURE 4.—A, coronal T1-weighted (TR 580/TE 26) MRI showing large transverse metaphyseal bands of high signal near the knee and similar longitudinal subperiosteal areas on the medial side of the proximal ends of the tibiae. Note the severe genu valgum. (Courtesy of Vichi GF, Bongini U, Seracini D, et al: Progression of bone lesions in a child with primary hyperoxaluria type 1: Evaluation by roentgenology and MRI. *Pediatr Radiol* 25:102–104, 1995.)

with subperiosteal cortical defects at the ends of long bones (Fig 2, C). At the same age MRI showed transverse bands of relatively high signal at the proximal end of the femora, tibiae, and fibulae (Fig 4, A). Other MRI findings included severe restriction of marrow channels, the result of thickening of cortical bone. A combined liver-kidney transplant is planned.

Discussion.—The most common of primary hyperoxalurias, PH type 1, results from a deficiency of the liver-specific enzyme AGT. Oxalate deposits in this child's bone, primarily at the corticomedullary level, led to severe deformity, knock knees, difficulty in walking, and bone pain. Cortical defects and transverse bands seen at skeletal imaging were the result of extensive bone marrow replacement by calcium oxalate crystals with pericrystalline giant cell granulomata. Because the in vitro response of residual AGT activity was negative in this patient, therapy with vitamin B_6 would not be effective. The child had not had fractures, perhaps because renal dialysis removed a large amount of oxalate.

▶ These recent articles on hyperoxaluria are noteworthy for different reasons. In the article by Akhan et al. (Abstract 4–60), renal, hepatic, and cardiac deposition of calcium oxalate crystals provide characteristic extraskeletal US and CT imaging findings of hyperoxaluria. In the article by Vichi et al., the radiographic progression of osseous lesions caused by the deposition of oxalate crystals in bone is emphasized radiographically, together with significant advanced MRI findings of the condition. The affected metaphyseal areas of altered primary spongiosa and excessive fibrosis as represented in the Figure are usually prone to fracture. A recent and good review article on hyperoxaluria is listed.[1]

L.W. Young, M.D.

Reference

1. Scheinman JI: Primary hyperoxaluria. *Miner Electrolyte Metab* 20:340–351, 1994.

5 Technical Developments, Economics, Education, and Quality

Introduction

Editing this section of the *YEAR BOOK* is both challenging and enlightening because it provides an overview of radiology that encompasses everything from job market assessment to the importance of visual patterns of radiologists in the detection of pathologic conditions. This grab bag of disconnected topics undoubtedly is representative of the dynamics of our field apart from organ-system radiology. Each year, the dramatic changes in the content of this chapter reflect the interests of the authors relevant to this particular time in the development of radiology. Of special note this year are the following topics:

- Continuing concern for the future of radiology, in general, and for the fate of academic radiology programs, in particular, in the environment of managed care
- Developing fear that we may be overproducing radiologists, with no scientific method to confirm this fear or solutions if it becomes a reality
- A sense that computer application will be a boon to radiology both in the clinical setting and in education
- A need to prove that radiology is a value-added specialty that is best practiced by trained radiologists
- Initial discussions of the importance of MR in the area of interventional radiology
- Concern about the impact of teleradiology on our field; will it be an asset or an adversary?

Three of the articles in this section would be of particular interest to those who are searching for answers concerning the future of our field. Staab (Abstract 5–1), Holman (Abstract 5–2), and Maynard (Abstract 5–3) discuss their views on the direction of radiology and the need for the academic radiology community to make changes if it is to survive the continued expansion of managed care as a means of controlling the cost of health care. Among major issues are the continued federal support of graduate medical education and the continued ability to use a portion of clinical income to fund research programs.

An important concern is the lack of information regarding the future demand for radiologists. Jonathan Sunshine of the American College of Radiology and colleagues (Abstract 5–7) are doing and excellent job of tracking job placement of radiologists who recently finished residencies and fellowships, as well as surveying practice groups about plans to add staff. However, no failsafe method exists to determine the need for radiologists 10 years from now. The uncertainty of the job market is compelling medical students to have second thoughts about radiology as a career, and for the first time in many years a large number of residency programs did not fill for 1997. We are accustomed to recruiting the best and brightest among medical students, and they have undoubtedly been major contributors to the advancement of radiology. If this lag in enthusiasm for radiology proves to be a trend, our field could be facing a serious problem in the next decade.

Communication in a timely manner from the radiologist to the referring clinician, and in many cases to the patient, is not a new subject but is one that must be addressed by radiologists. Good communication is essential for the satisfactory practice of radiology. In today's marketplace, where timeliness, appropriateness and "added value" are discussed daily, radiologists should take a second or even a third look at their communication pattern to see if it can be improved. As developing communication networks, such as high-speed information highways, becoming accessible to most radiologists, the necessary tools are in place for rapid communication of findings, written reports, and, in some cases, the actual images to the referring clinician. Radiologists must lead the way in optimizing the applications of these new communication pathways within their practice.

We hear the phrase "radiology by radiologists" frequently these days. The slogan is used to support the preeminence of trained radiologists for interpreting all imaging studies. In many circumstances, particularly the outpatient environment, clinicians have for years read their own films without overreading by a radiologist. With decreasing reimbursement brought on by managed care, attempts are being made to determine who is best able to interpret the images, who should be paid to do so, and what constitutes unnecessary duplication. Radiologists need to demonstrate unequivocally that they are available for the timely performance and interpretation of imaging studies and that they indeed add value in the process. Emergency room physicians, orthopedic surgeons, neurologists, and others will gladly step in to take our place unless we can substantiate our worth.

Picture archiving and communication systems (PACS) have been around for some time and have generated a lot of type but very little action. That situation is now changing. The technology is available to make filmless radiology, as predicted years ago by Paul Capp,[1] possible at last. After the discussion of digital imaging and PACS at the most recent Summer Meeting of the Intersociety Commission in Santa Fe, New Mexico, the attendees concluded that soft-copy quality is acceptable for interpreting studies and that the field of radiology should get on with the task of implementing a filmless environment. The military and the Veterans Administration hospitals are leading the way in providing that, with the enthusiastic participation of radiologists, adequate financing, and perseverance, a totally filmless system not only is possible but also is well worth the effort.

Computer literacy will be a must for radiologists. Not only is facility with computers necessary in the clinical practice of radiology, but conceivably much of our continuing education will be provided online over the Internet in the near future. Applications such as computer-assisted diagnosis are currently in their infancy, but in years to come they may be of considerable value to radiologists in their everyday practice.

On the horizon, specialized MR devices will be used as adjuncts to surgery. As the proper instruments become available at more medical centers, and as additional physicians (both radiologists and clinicians) become involved in the exploration of these techniques, major changes in interventional radiology may occur. These new developments warrant our diligent attention.

In spite of the managed care revolution, advances in our field continue undiminished. Even a cursory review of the radiology literature published last year, or attendance at 1 of the major radiology meetings, proves this point. The socioeconomic issues of our day can be both disconcerting and time consuming, but the science of radiology rolls on!

C. Douglas Maynard, M.D.

Reference

1. Capp MP: Radiology imaging—2000 A.D. *Radiology.* 138:541–550, 1981.

Academic Radiology, Manpower, and Continued Competence

Consensus Quest: Reshaping the Future of Radiology: RSNA Hartman Lecture/Eugene P. Pendergrass Horizons Lecture

Staab EV (Univ of Florida, Gainesville)

Radiology 198:643–650, 1996 5–1

Objective.—At a time of economic upheaval in medicine, radiologists must re-evaluate almost all of their beliefs, practices, habits, and ethics. The dramatic changes occurring are driven largely by economic factors that are lowering costs by limiting access to the health care system. A leading radiologist shares his thoughts about the future of radiology, emphasizing the need for a process of "continuing envisioning" of the future.

Future of Radiology.—Despite the uncertainty inherent in the changing medical environment, it is essential to rethink and respond to change in a positive way. Change brings new opportunities for radiologists to show their enthusiasm and creativity, to deepen their involvement, and to intensify their commitment. Key tasks include the identification and protection of what is valuable about radiology, and the development of a vision for the future. Radiologists will have to convince their colleagues about the inevitability of change and the importance of reshaping their profession.

Continuous Envisioning.—The major change in radiology's future will be the way in which practitioners consider their future and change it in a continuous process of envisioning. They will understand that they are able to influence the future by determining what they want it to be, and that creative thinking is needed to achieve discontinuous change. Future radiologists will apply "futures analysis" to all aspects of their profession, including education, work habits and places, communication, ethics, research, and technology. An example of this kind of initiative is provided by the FutuRAD group, which has made various efforts to inform radiologists about the prospects for change and the resulting impact on the radiologic profession, identity, and livelihood. Possible new roles and directions for radiologists include the exploration of their role as "information managers," improvement in residency curricula and training, greater radiologic involvement in therapeutics, and creative new techniques of research and reporting.

Conclusion.—The volatile medical environment promises major changes for the future of radiology. "Continuous envisioning" is presented as one way in which radiologists can actively envision and shape their own future. Although the challenges are great, so is the potential for reward.

► Ed Staab has been a leader in exploring the direction in which radiology is headed. His involvement with the FutuRad program of the Radiological Society of North America (RSNA) has inspired many people to start "envisioning." This article, which presents the Hartman Lecture that Ed gave at the 1995 annual meeting of the RSNA, challenges us all to pay more attention to the future of radiology and to devote less of our efforts to the present. You will not agree with everything Ed says, but you will be energized to think!

C.D. Maynard, M.D.

The Changing Face of Academic Radiology: Can It Survive Managed Care?

Holman BL (Harvard Med School, Boston)

Acad Radiol 2:1011–1015, 1995 5–2

Background.—The current golden age of academic radiology may be short lived as a result of sweeping changes in health care financing. The curtailment of training and research by academic programs to compete financially with community health facilities, cut hospital care costs, and meet the economic limitations created by revised standards of care, was discussed.

Discussion.—Shrinking clinical revenues and the long-term unreliability of industry financial support will require academic departments to focus their research efforts and to move away from organ-based and technology-based compartmentalization. Fewer faculty will be able to pursue research and more will become clinician-teachers. Research agendas must be modified to emphasize interdisciplinary projects. Vertical integration of services, use of a system-wide computerized radiology information service, and redistribution of imaging resources and personnel (including physicians) will be critical goals. Radiology training slots will decrease by up to 30%. Training will have to be customized to the different needs of clinicians, teachers, and researchers. Teaching, itself, must become a research priority. Radiologists must become active in lobbying for a steady source of money from third-party payers or government to fund postgraduate medical training.

Conclusion.—To maintain their academic mission, radiology teaching departments must take several steps. These include focusing research efforts and encouraging collaboration, finding innovative funding for research and teaching, reorganizing infrastructure and practices, and customizing training programs.

► This article provides a very thoughtful outline of both the problems to be faced and the opportunities available to radiology departments in academic medical centers under managed care. At first glance, these problems might seem to be limited solely to the more than 100 academic departments in the United States, but in reality, practicing radiologists in all nonteaching institutions or free-standing imaging centers should be equally concerned. The pool of trainees is the only source of future partners and any demise in the quality or numbers of trainees will greatly affect all radiologists, whether they are in academic medical centers or in nonacademic environments. Changes in graduate medical education pose a potentially serious threat to our specialty.

C.D. Maynard, M.D.

1995 AUR Hartman Centennial Lecture: Academic Radiology: Time for Action

Maynard CD (Wake Forest Univ, Winston-Salem, NC)
Acad Radiol 2:1097–1103, 1995 5–3

Background.—The action or inaction of academic radiology departments today will profoundly affect the future of radiology. Currently radiologists must cope with turf battles, reimbursement issues, questions about the appropriateness of studies, outcome measures, trainee numbers, job placement, job security, and many other difficult issues. Faculty and department chairpersons must be innovative and aggressive in facing the challenges of radiology today.

Time for Action.—To successfully face these challenges, academic radiology departments need to take action. Patient bases must be protected through institutional involvement and selected departmental outreach programs. Faculties need to be reorganized and their support earned to manage the changes that will result from health care reengineering. Residency and fellowship programs must be restructured to adapt positively to the needs of the new delivery system. Academic radiology departments must also take a stand on resident/fellow training, accreditation issues, and program length and composition. A national program should be developed to continue to attract the best medical students to radiology. More information is needed to best estimate work force requirements to eventually achieve the proper balance between supply and demand. Subspecialization in radiology, as well as research training, needs to be supported. Finally, academic radiologists need to support the Association of University Radiologists, Society of Chairmen of Academic Radiology Departments, and the Association of Program Directors in Radiology as the collective voice for academic radiology.

Conclusion.—Academic radiology is in the unique position of being the only supplier of human resources and research for the field of radiology. The faculty and chairpersons of academic radiology must take a stand on staff issues, changes in training programs, accreditation, certification, financing of graduate education, support for biomedical research, and all other matters important to academic programs.

► Academic radiology is under attack because of changes in the health care system. It is imperative that academic departments take a proactive role in securing the future for our field. To do so will require substantial changes in the function and organization, academic radiology departments, and philosophy of radiology chairmen and faculty. Resisting change wil greatly affect the future of our field. Now is not the time for us to be timid!

C.D. Maynard, M.D.

Social and Economic Issues in Radiology: Graduate Medical Education Financing: A Primer

Amis ES Jr, Lantos PRF (Albert Einstein College of Medicine, Bronx, NY; Montefiore Med Ctr, Bronx, NY)

Acad Radiol 3:507–511, 1996 5–4

Introduction.—Most training program directors and department chairpeople are unaware of the amount of graduate medical education funds that hospitals receive and must, therefore, often negotiate for fiscal resources under false assumptions. The source and extent of graduate medical education funding available to teaching hospitals was clarified.

History.—With the growth of available funds from Medicare and Medicaid and other third-party payments, graduate medical education expenses began to include salaries and fringe benefits of residents, partial salary support of faculty teaching residents, and overhead. The United States has more than 6,500 hospitals, yet about 30 are considered "major teaching hospitals," defined as having 25 or more trainees per 100 beds. A total of 1,250 hospitals get graduate medical education money.

Medicare.—Close to 40% of hospital care in the United States is supported through Medicare, with the remainder paid by private insurance, patients, and from other appropriations. Medicare reimburses hospitals according to direct costs, clearly identified as medical education in hospital accounting systems, and indirect costs, which are not so clearly identified, but are associated with such factors as increased severity of illness, need for latest technology, higher staffing ratios, larger standby capacity, and increased social work activities. Generally, the direct costs are apportioned as 55% to house staff, 26% to faculty, and 19% for other education expenses. The indirect costs are calculated using the ratio of a hospital's trainees to its beds, about an additional 7.65% for each 0.1 in the ratio of trainees to hospital beds, over and above the normal diagnosis-related group reimbursements made to a hospital. In 1992, the mean direct payment per resident was $18,600 and the mean indirect payment was $51,500, or a total of $70,100 per resident per year.

Future Funding.—Congress may oppose additional spending for graduate medical education because of pressure for reducing the deficit, particularly for trainees in specialties perceived to be in overabundance. This may result in hospital-mandated downsizing of specialty training programs.

► Payment for graduate medical education is certainly under discussion in Washington, D.C. This matter is not a simple one that can be easily resolved. Many hospitals rely on residents for delivering care and on the additional indirect funds associated with graduate medical education to help defray other expenses. Anyone with doubts about the complexity of the system should read this article!

C.D. Maynard, M.D.

The Initial Employment Status of Physicians Completing Training in 1994

Miller RS, Jonas HS, Whitcomb ME (American Med Assoc, Chicago; Assoc of American Med Colleges, Washington, DC)
JAMA 275:708–712, 1996 5–5

Introduction.—Most agree that the United States is on the verge of having an oversupply of physicians, and articles have indicated that some recent graduates have had problems finding employment. A survey was conducted to determine the career status of residents who completed graduate medical education training programs in selected specialties.

Methods.—Directors of 4,369 residency programs in 26 specialties and subspecialties were given a 1-page questionnaire. Directors identified how many resident physicians had completed the program, the known career status of those physicians, how many physicians had difficulty finding a practice position, the full-time clinical practice position characteristics, and how many physicians could not find full-time employment. Directors were also asked to give their perceptions of the likely trends of available practice opportunities for graduates and how resident positions would be changed.

Results.—The survey was completed by 3,090 program directors (70.7%) who reported on 15,999 resident physicians, 63.2% of whom were seeking a professional position. Most (92.9%) who were not seeking a position were pursuing additional training. Of the group seeking employment, the percentage who did not find a full-time position ranged from 0% in urology to 10.8% in pathology. Overall, about 70% of the entire group looking for employment found a position in their specialty. Physicians pursuing nongeneralist specialties had more problems than those pursuing generalist careers. Program directors of specialties perceived that their graduates will have more difficulty finding a full-time practice position during the next year.

Conclusion.—Physicians in some specialties are having difficulty finding a full-time position. Physicians entering practice in some specialties are being limited by market forces. The impact of physician oversupply is resulting in physician unemployment or underemployment for some specialties in some parts of the country.

▶ This article points out that concern about jobs exists not only in radiology but in other specialties as well. As the trend in this country moves toward managed care and a more prominent role for the primary care provider, opportunities may decline in other specialties.

C.D. Maynard, M.D.

Hiring by Radiology Groups in 1994

Deitch CH, Sunshine JH, Chan WC (American College of Radiology, Reston, Va; George Washington Univ, Washington, DC)

Radiology 198:359–364, 1996 5–6

Purpose.—For several years there has been concern that there may not be enough jobs for radiology trainees. The situation requires information on the number and types of positions available in radiology groups. Recent trends in hiring by radiology groups were studied.

Methods.—The findings were derived from a 1994 mail survey of U.S. radiology groups, conducted by the American College of Radiology (ACR). The response rate was 92%, with 341 groups responding. The findings were compared with a 1991 telephone survey, which included responses from 150 radiology groups.

Results.—The responses suggested that U.S. radiology groups sought to fill about 1,600 positions in 1994. This represented a 29% decline from the number of positions available in 1991; the percentage of groups seeking to hire radiologists declined as well. Fifty-two percent of the positions were in general diagnostic radiology, 31% were in the diagnostic subspecialties, and 15% were in radiation oncology. In both years, about three-fourths of the openings were filled. The likelihood of filling a position was no different between fields or subspecialties. Trainees rejected about 28% of offers made by the radiology groups.

Conclusion.—Surveys of radiology groups suggest that although the situation is not desparate, job opportunities for radiology trainees continue to decline. The difficulty of finding a position is about the same for trainees in all fields of radiology. Future studies will continue to monitor the employment market in radiology.

► Availability of jobs for diagnostic residents and fellows and for radiation oncology residents who have completed their training is a hot topic today and probably will continue to be so for some time. Are we training too many residents and fellows? Are jobs being put on hold because of uncertainty as to the effects of managed care? Surveys by the American College of Radiology are extremely important to help counsel medical students and to direct them in career choices. These decisions will affect our field for many years.

C.D. Maynard, M.D.

The Employment Market for 1995 Graduates of Diagnostic Radiology and Radiation Oncology Training

Sunshine JH, Burkhardt JH, Crewson PE, et al (American College of Radiology, Reston, Va; Univ of Cincinnati, Ohio; Med College of Wisconsin, Milwaukee; et al)

AJR 167:21–26, 1996 5–7

Objective.—There is great concern about the reported surplus of non–primary care physicians in the United States, and the unemployment rate among physicians has, in fact, been increasing. However, few studies have examined the problem of physician unemployment or underemployment or attempted to predict future trends. New graduates are particularly vulnerable to unemployment. The employment situation for diagnostic radiologists and radiation oncologists was studied with an emphasis on new graduates.

Methods.—In 1995 the American College of Radiology surveyed the directors of training programs in diagnostic radiology and radiation oncology. The directors were asked about how their 1995 graduates were doing in the employment market, as well as about future plans for their programs. A follow-up survey was conducted at the end of 1995. The findings were compared with those of a similar survey performed in 1994.

Results.—The response rate was 92%. At the end of 1995, the reported unemployment rate for fellows in diagnostic radiology was 0.6% ± 0.3%, less for trainees in other categories. About 90% of graduates were believed to have achieved a reasonably good match between their positions and their personal goals. The employment situation in 1995 was not significantly different from that in 1994 (Table 2). However, the program directors had become more pessimistic about the employment market. There were few significant differences in employment among the various subgroups of trainees, including those in different diagnostic subspecialties. The information on future plans suggested that the number of new graduates per year would not decrease substantially.

Conclusion.—Although unemployment among new radiology graduates is extremely low, training program directors continue to be pessimistic about the employment market. There are no significant differences in the employment situation across diagnostic subspecialties or between regions. Training programs are not planning major cuts in the number of available positions. The data suggest that the predicted surplus in the supply of radiologists may have been overstated.

► Exaggeration of the surplus of diagnostic radiologists and radiation oncologists will have a significant effect on the number of medical students choosing to enter these fields. Jonathan Sunshine, at the American College of Radiology, has the onerous task of trying to obtain meaningful data that all of us can use to plan for the future. Never before has the need for timely, accurate data on job opportunities and predictions for the future been more significant.

C.D. Maynard, M.D.

TABLE 2.—Employment Situation of Graduates in 1994 and 1995

Graduates	Residency Program Graduates						Fellowship Program Graduates			
	Diagnostic			Oncology			Diagnostic			Oncology†
	1994	1995	Significance*	1994	1995	Significance	1994	1995	Significance	1995
Number of graduates	135	919		24	149		77	482		26
Status as of April–May										
With commitments for positions (%)	97	95	NS	88	89	NS	86	83	NS	73
With jobs that fit training/goals (%)	88	87	NS	79	80	NS	73	72	NS	69
Job offers received (average no.)										
This year	2.2	2	NS	2.9	3.6	NS	2.1	1.8	NS	1.8
Last year	3.5	2.6		3.6	3.0		4.2	2.7		3.1
Status as of December follow-up										
With positions (%)	100	99.8	NS	100	100	NS	99	99.4	NS	100
With jobs that fit training/goals (%)	93	91	NS	96	90	NS	81	88	NS	85
Not included in December data										
Not in job market‡ [(no. (%)]		3 (0.3)			2 (1.3)			4 (0.8)		0 (0)
Status unknown§ [(no. (%)]		2 (0.2)			1 (0.7)			2 (0.4)		0 (0)

Note: $P > 0.05$; 2-tailed test.
* Statistical significance of difference between 1994 and 1995; 2-tailed probabilities.
† No 1994 graduates surveyed.
‡ Deliberately not working and not seeking work; consists mostly of women with infants or very young children.
§ Lost to follow-up.
Abbreviation: NS, not significant.
(Courtesy of Sunshine JH, Burkhardt JH, Crewson PE, et al: The employment market for 195 graduates of diagnostic radiology and radiation oncology training. *AJR* 167:21–26, 1996.)

Estimating Physician Workforce Requirements: The Devil Is in the Assumptions

Tarlov AR (Tufts Univ, Boston)

JAMA 274:1558–1560, 1995 5–8

Introduction.—An article by R.A. Cooper (Abstract 5–10) forecasting that the physician surplus will be trivial in the year 2000 and nonexistent by 2020 was discussed. This forecast contradicts several other studies predicting a physician surfeit because, Cooper says, these studies are based on insupportable assumptions. He believes that newer data on population projections, HMO staffing patterns, and physician work effort justify his projections.

Physician Supply and Demand for Services.—The author notes that projections of physician supply often agree, but estimates of requirements for their services rarely do. The latter are influenced by a complex of sometimes paradoxical and heterogeneous inputs spanning factors such as technological innovation, emergence of new diseases, demographic changes, management of medical services, and political ideology.

Consensual Realities.—Workforce policy formulation needs common ground that supersedes controversial assumptions. For example, the high U.S. per capita expenditures on health care are nevertheless accompanied by substandard health among Americans in many respects, so only modest expectations of the capacity of medical care to improve population health are warranted. A serious shortcoming of many models is that not all clinician groups have been integrated into projections of supply and requirements. Other factors that have an impact include financing medical and graduate medical education, medical school admissions, and geographic distribution, among others.

Key Assumption.—For most Americans, restraints on utilization of health services by managed care limit expansion of those services. Increases in requirements for physician services in the foreseeable future will be limited to levels that permit an annual expenditure increase of 1% to 2% above the consumer price index plus an allowance for increase in population size.

Conclusion.—Sweeping legislative and regulatory approaches to effect large corrections should be avoided, as should dependence solely on market forces or voluntary action. Modest private and public interventions to adjust the workforce supply should also be fashioned to attain other health goals as well.

► A warning is issued toward those who would like to orchestrate major changes in the numbers and types of physicians trained. The author does not believe accurate projections of need are possible. This subject is of considerable importance to radiology. Many in our field predict a major surplus, and this prediction is influencing the decisions of medical students as to whether to enter radiology. We cannot afford to have a shortage of radiologists in the future; the void would be quickly filled by eager clinicians trying to gain inroads into imaging. We should pay attention to the recommendation of people such as Tarlov and should not jump too quickly into decisions that might in the future harm our field.

C.D. Maynard, M.D.

Hospital Activities of Radiology Groups in the United States: Results of a 1992 ACR Survey

Bansal S, Sunshine JH (American College of Radiology, Reston, Va)
AJR 165:453–465, 1995 5–9

Introduction.—The American College of Radiology is the chief professional organization of radiologists in the United States and periodically surveys the profession. Data from the 1992 Group Practice Survey, the main survey of radiology groups, were presented and included the hospital activities of radiology groups.

Methods.—A random sample of radiology groups completed a detailed questionnaire for each hospital they practiced at. Results were weighted to make them representative of all hospitals where radiology groups practice.

Results.—An average of 47,800 diagnostic procedures was performed at hospitals by radiology groups in 1992. There was an average of 0.8 diagnostic procedure performed per inpatient day, but the number varied widely among hospitals. An average of 11,400 procedures were performed by a full-time equivalent diagnostic radiologist at a hospital, but, again, the number varied widely among hospitals. Radiology oncology services were performed principally at hospitals with more than 300 beds. There was an average of 380 new oncology patients annually at hospitals that offered radiation oncology services; these patients received an average of 8,435 fractions. At 42% of hospitals where radiologists provided diagnostic services, radiology groups accepted nonreferred patients for mammography. Radiologists provided 24-hour coverage for diagnostic radiology at 80% of hospitals.

Discussion.—The reported data may be useful for radiologists evaluating their own hospital activities. The averages do not reflect special situations that may exist at a given hospital and should not be taken as standards.

► With his timely research of practice patterns in the United States, Jonathan Sunshine of the American College of Radiology makes major contributions to our field every year. The information he provides in his surveys helps us to understand the changing practice of radiology and provides our training program directors with valuable data that assist them in determining changes that will be necessary to prepare radiology residents for the future. Changes are occurring so rapidly in health care delivery that we need all the help we can get to adjust to them. Thanks, Jonathan and staff!

C.D. Maynard, M.D.

Perspectives on the Physician Workforce to the Year 2020
Cooper RA (Med College of Wisconsin, Milwaukee)
JAMA 274:1534–1543, 1995 5–10

Objective.—There is increasing concern about a surplus of physicians in the United States, where fears of a shortage 2 decades ago prompted a doubling of the capacity to train new physicians. This survey was an attempt to assess the supply of and demand for physicians up to the year 2020. Future surpluses will depend in the main on how physicians are distributed geographically and also by the degree to which patients expect services from physicians that also will be offered by an increasing number of nonphysician clinicians (NPCs).

Perspectives.—Demand for physician services was examined by analyzing HMO experiences. Second, the distribution of physicians was studied in each state, allowing comparison of regional utilization patterns to national norms. Finally, the future supply of NPCs and their impact on physician services were addressed.

Supply and Demand.—The estimated need for physicians in 1993 was estimated at 205 per 100,000 population, and demand is expected to increase 18% by 2020. The supply of physicians is expected to increase more rapidly than demand at first, creating a 5% surplus of patient care physicians in 2000 and an 8% excess (62,100 physicians) in 2010. Later the gap will narrow. Presently the per capita distribution of physicians varies more than two-fold between states. There already are surpluses in some states, whereas shortages persist in others. The supply of NPCs is increasing and, by 2010, they are expected to number 60% of patient care physicians.

Demographics.—The average of patient visits per week has decreased about 15% in the past 15 years. Presently 22% of practicing physicians are older than 55, and this figure will rise to 38% in 2020. At the same time the proportion of female physicians will increase from 19% to 35%. Many physicians are assuming an employed status, and, on the average, those employed work fewer hours per week. It seems likely that both physician work efforts and the intensity of medical practice will continue to decline.

Summary.—There is no evidence of a substantial national surplus of physicians. Geographic distribution will be the chief determinant of whether or not there will be a surplus in a given region. In time, the major factor will be the extent to which patients continue to prefer to see physicians for services that also will be available from an increasing group of NPCs.

▶ No other professional group has devoted as much effort as physicians have in determining whether we are training the correct number for the future needs of our country. All past efforts have failed. It is important for the well-being of our specialty that we not be caught up in the fear of producing too many radiologists and, in response, cut our production either by decreasing the number of training slots or by scaring away medical students from entering our specialty. What would be worse than too many radiologists? Too few! A void would immediately be filled by untrained clinicians from other specialties.

C.D. Maynard, M.D.

The Continuing Competence Needs of Physicians: A Survey of the Medical Specialty Societies

McClennan BL, Herlihy CS (Washington Univ, St Louis; American College of Radiology, Reston, Va)

AJR 165:789–795, 1995 5–11

Background.—Increased emphasis on specialty recertification and physicians' demonstration of competency should be reflected in the programs and plans of the medical specialty societies. A questionnaire was sent to each specialty society to collect information on the societies' activities in these areas.

Methods.—Executive directors of each of the 25 members of the Council of Medical Specialty Societies were sent questionnaires. Areas of inquiry included existing recertification programs, interaction between societies and their specialty boards, collection and storage by the societies of members' continuing medical education (CME) credits, and the status of projects to evaluate clinical outcome data.

Results.—Of the 25 societies, 21 returned information suitable for study. Three sent no response. Ten societies reported existing recertification programs, 2 of which were voluntary. Several recertification pathways were offered, most commonly paper-pencil examinations but also others such as computerized examinations, practice audits, and continuing medical education programs. All but 1 of the 21 respondents mentioned the existence of society-sponsored competency programs, but only 2 societies' programs were even partially accepted by their boards for recertification. Forty percent of the societies had no data storage capability to record member CME and self-assessment results. Only half of the boards were developing programs for clinical outcome studies. When specialty society descriptions of their recertification services were compared with the descriptions published by their boards, it was obvious that the organizations did not communicate well. Boards tended to overestimate the degree to which societies were involved in recertification.

Conclusion.—The programs of medical specialty societies do not appear to adequately match the large changes taking place in assessing and documenting physicians' competence.

► As managed care becomes widespread, the need for radiologists to demonstrate continued competence will become a hot issue. The American College of Radiology has appointed a Task Force on Continued Competency to study the issue. Numerous methods of ensuring competency are available, each with obvious advantages and disadvantages. Some radiology organization must provide a method that is creditable, practical, economical, and fair—not an easy task. Many of the specialty boards now offer voluntary recertification, but recertification appears to work only when the initial certificate was time limited. At the moment, the American Board of Radiology is 1 of only 4 boards not issuing time-limited certificates. That will probably change in the near future.

C.D. Maynard, M.D.

Visual Scanning Patterns of Radiologists Searching Mammograms

Krupinski EA (Univ of Arizona, Tucson)

Acad Radiol 3:137–144, 1996 5–12

Introduction.—An analysis of undetected cancer in mammography showed that 43% was the result of lesions being overlooked, 52% was caused by misinterpretation, and 5% was caused by suboptimal technique. Whether the principles of search, detection, and decision making described for pulmonary nodule detection can be used for lesion detection in mammographies was investigated.

Methods.—Recordings were taken of the eye positions of 6 radiologists (3 radiology residents and 3 staff mammographers) as they searched 40 mammography images of 20 women for microcalcifications and masses in right and left breasts. They each read the set representing 20 mammographic cases in a 1-hour session. An eye-tracker was used to record their eye positions.

Results.—Prolonged gaze durations were associated with true positive and false positive decisions. Longer gaze durations were associated more with false negative decisions than with true negative decisions. Lesions were detected earlier by readers with more experience. Readers with less experience spent more time searching images and covering more image area. The experienced readers spent an average of 8.7 seconds on the lesion-containing side-by-side breast images, whereas the less experienced readers spent 16.7 seconds on these images.

Conclusion.—In mammography, gaze duration is a useful predictor of missed lesions. Gaze duration is a potential tool for perceptual feedback.

► Radiology needs to pay more attention to research in visual perception. We spend considerable effort on improving the resolution of our equipment. The truth is, however, that the capability of the radiologist who interprets a study is the most important element in the equation. How well the radiologist functions is critical. Hal Kundel, from the University of Pennsylvania, has led the way for many years in this area, but more articles like this one, which directs attention toward the science of visual perception, are needed.

C.D. Maynard, M.D.

Clinical Practice

Communication of the Urgent Finding
Berlin L (Rush Med College, Chicago)
AJR 166:513–515, 1996 5–13

Case Report.—Woman, age 23, with a history of Crohn's disease had multiple small-bowel resections, and her surgeon inserted a dual-lumen Groshong catheter into the superior vena cava via the right subclavian vein for hyperalimentation. A chest radiograph was obtained but was viewed by the surgeon without a consultation with the radiologist because of a series of communications mishaps. That evening, the patient received hyperalimentation fluid through the catheter, dyspnea and hypotension developed, and the patient went into shock and cardiopulmonary arrest and died. The catheter perforated the vena cava and the hyperalimentation fluid filled the right pleural cavity.

Malpractice.—The suit alleged that the radiologist was negligent for failing to communicate the possibility of vena cava perforation to the surgeon in a timely manner so that corrective action could have been taken. An expert for the plaintiff testified that the radiologist breached the standard of care by failing to immediately communicate his findings and that the radiologist showed a lack of concern for the patient by going home for the weekend and making no effort to contact anyone at the hospital during the weekend. The case was settled before trial.

Discussion.—The courts are expanding the radiologist's responsibilities in communicating information quickly to referring physicians, and even to patients if the patient's care requires it.

Summary.—The radiologist should phone a report to the referring physician immediately when there is reason to believe that a radiologic finding requires immediate treatment. If the referring physician cannot be found, an alternate physician should be located. If the alternate cannot be found, the patient should be informed and told to report to a hospital emergency department for care. Communication should be documented.

▶ Why this issue continues to be a point of discussion is hard to understand. One would assume that good common sense would be sufficient for deciding when to call the clinician. In our litigious society, however, it certainly behooves us to pay attention to the points raised by Dr. Berlin!

C.D. Maynard, M.D.

Disclosure of Imaging Findings to Patients Directly by Radiologists: Survey of Patients' Preferences

Schreiber MH, Leonard M Jr, Rieniets CY (Univ of Texas, Galveston)
AJR 165:467–469, 1995 5–14

Introduction.—Patients were questioned to determine whether they preferred to learn about results of imaging findings from the radiologist immediately after the studies or later from the referring physician.

Methods.—A questionnaire was distributed to 261 consecutive patients in the radiology department of a large university hospital. Several questions were designed to determine whether patients wanted the radiologist to tell them if the results were normal or abnormal; if they would prefer to hear results from their family physician, internist, or other primary care provider; and if they believed they were entitled to an explanation of their test results from the radiologist.

Results.—Overall approximately 98% of the patients wanted to hear normal findings from the radiologists and nearly 94% wanted the radiologist to tell them if results were abnormal. Between 2% and 6% did not want to hear results from the radiologists. Approximately 40% also wanted to hear results from their primary care providers. About 94% believed they were entitled to an explanation from the radiologist. Of those who wanted results only if they asked, about 65% also wanted results from their referring physician.

Conclusion.—The study indicates that the majority of patients want to hear results, normal or abnormal, from radiologists at the time of the examination. Recent legal opinions suggest, in fact, that the radiologist may be required to inform the patient. Certainly those who ask should be told results and results relayed promptly to the referring physician.

▶ Conclusions of this study may make our clinical colleagues somewhat uncomfortable, but we should listen to our patients. As we move closer toward the role of adjuncts to the primary care physicians, our interaction with patients will undoubtedly increase. The time we spend with the patients, however, will be beneficial to our field in the future. Patients may even get to know what radiologists do for them!

C.D. Maynard, M.D.

Radiology Reports: How Much Descriptive Detail Is Enough?

McLoughlin RF, So CB, Gray RR, et al (Foothills Hosp, Calgary, Alta, Canada)
AJR 165:803–806, 1995 5–15

Background.—Because information is the diagnostic radiologist's primary product, it is important to know if referring clinicians are receiving the information they believe they need. A series of scenarios, each with 3 increasingly complete report formats, was presented to clinicians to determine the information they preferred to receive.

Methods.—Four chest radiograph scenarios, with symptoms worsening from "none" to "dyspnea" and findings increasing from normal to complexly abnormal, were presented to each clinician. Two abdominal ultrasound imaging scenarios for right upper quadrant pain, with 1 result normal and 1 abnormal, were also presented. For each scenario, the 77 responding clinicians chose their preferred report among the 3 offered: a simple statement of diagnosis; a report of positive findings; and a complete description of technique, study quality, and all findings. Practice demographics of the respondents were collected.

Results.—In the absence of chest symptoms, the brief "normal" report was most commonly selected. However, with chest symptoms present, greater detail was requested by more than 90% of clinicians, primarily the brief report of positive findings. For the ultrasonography scenarios, the brief report of positive findings was again preferred by a majority. Of interest, for every scenario, one third of clinicians desired the most complete report. No physician characteristics, such as academic status and number of years in practice, were associated with specific preferences.

Conclusion.—Clinicians prefer different amounts of detail in radiology reports, depending on the clinical scenario. Nearly one third always prefer to receive a detailed report.

▶ These authors proved once again that you cannot please all of the people all of the time. Clinicians vary considerably in the amount of detail they want in a dictated report. It is important for radiologists to tailor their reports to suit the circumstances and the individual clinicians.

C.D. Maynard, M.D.

Explaining Variation in Radiologists' Reporting Times

Bryan S, Weatherburn G, Roddie M, et al (Brunel Univ Uxbridge, Middlesex, England; Hammersmith Hosp, London)

Br J Radiol 68:854–861, 1995 5–16

Background.—Significant resources are devoted to the reporting of radiologists' interpretations of images. Thus, managerial concerns about the planning and organization of the service are important. The reasons for time variations in senior radiologists' completion of radiologic reports were investigated.

Methods.—The reporting process at 1 hospital in the United Kingdom was observed for 25 days. Data were obtained on the time taken to write the report, the number and nature of all images interpreted, the experience of the radiologist, and the number of disturbances occurring.

Findings.—A total of 2,345 reports were completed during the observation period. Median report time was 117 sec. Reporting times tended to be significantly shorter during busy sessions. They were longer when radiologists were disturbed during the reporting process or when they were training junior radiologists during a reporting session. Surprisingly, reporting times for urgent and less urgent cases did not difffer significantly. Also, reporting times appeared to vary systematically depending on the day of the week and time of day.

Conclusion.—These findings confirm the importance of certain factors expected to cause variation in radiologists' reporting times. An unexpected finding was that the reporting times for cases designated urgent and nonurgent were comparable.

▶ As radiology is examined in light of the value added by specific procedures, studies similar to this 1 will no doubt conclude that on-line reporting for most cases, whether urgent or routine, will be necessary.

C.D. Maynard, M.D.

Capitated Contracting in Radiology: Negotiating Techniques, Financial Calculations, and Utilization Management

Levin DC, McArdle GH, Lockard CD (Jefferson Med College, Philadelphia; Thomas Jefferson Univ, Philadelphia)

Radiology 198:651–656, 1996 5–17

Introduction.—As fee-for-service payments to radiologists decline, capitated contracts in radiology are increasing, a pressure that has been driven primarily by managed care organizations. In this scenario, a radiology group is paid a fixed fee per member per month for each subscriber, regardless of the number of images performed on the subscriber. Radiologists perceive capitation as threatening because it transfers the risk of high use to the physicians. Some ideas were presented regarding capitated outpatient contracting, based on information from a single large practice in an academic institution.

Determining Fees.—Cost determinations can be subjective because the largest component of any radiology group's costs is the income earned by the radiologists, which can range from $75,000 to $475,000 per year. Fees should be determined using calculations based on revenues that are related to Medicare revenues. Fees for pediatric subscribers (0–19 years of age) would be lower and fees for those older than 65 years would be higher. Find out what percentage of patients fall into which age categories and determine a per subscriber fee based on a blend of the categories. In the Philadelphia area, the percentages are 62% adults, 33% pediatric-aged, and 5% Medicare-aged. The capitated fee incorporates technical and professional components, and the radiology group and the hospital should agree on the professional/technical split of the capitated fee. This should be based on the technical and professional relative value units assigned by the Medicare resource–based relative value scale. Generally, radiologists receive 30% to 40% of this fee.

Negotiating Contracts.—During negotiations, determine which procedures should be excluded from capitation. To lessen the risk of overutilization, exclude as many high-cost procedures as possible, such as MRI, all invasive procedures with surgical codes outside the 70000 series of the common procedural terminology, and cardiac nuclear medicine. Also exclude high-cost contrast agents used in imaging studies, or adjust the capitated fee accordingly. Define an "outpatient." Emergency department patients should be considered inpatients. Preadmission tests should also be negotiated.

Tracking Utilization.—Get utilization data. Larger managed care organizations in existence for years may have better data; however, these data may not be accurate because they may be based on the number of radiology claims. Radiologists have no incentives for submitting all claims because their reimbursement will not be increased. Utilization tracking should be conducted with a computer tracking program or a personal computer–based spreadsheet. Imaging guidelines and appropriateness criteria should be developed to control utilization of imaging by primary care physicians. Before imaging studies can be ordered, a consultation with a radiologist should be conducted to control utilization.

▶ We all need a primer on capitated contracts in radiology, and this is it!

C.D. Maynard, M.D.

Malpractice and Radiologists in Cook County, IL: Trends in 20 Years of Litigation

Berlin L, Berlin JW (Rush North Shore Med Ctr, Skokie, Ill; Northwestern Mem Hosp, Chicago)

AJR 165:781–788, 1995 5–18

Objective.—A review of malpractice litigation involving radiologic procedures or radiologists sought to identify trends among the types of lawsuits filed and to determine means of minimizing malpractice exposure and improving patient care. In contrast to previous reports, it dealt with malpractice lawsuits filed in a specific location during a limited time frame.

Methods.—Data on medical malpractice lawsuits filed in Cook County, Illinois, from January 1975 through December 1994 were obtained from the *Cook County Jury Verdict Reporter.* All lawsuits related to radiology were documented, analyzed, and categorized. Six case categories were identified: slip and fall, radiation oncology, failure to order a radiologic examination, complications, missed diagnoses, and miscellaneous.

Results.—During the 20-year period, 18,860 malpractice suits filed in Cook County had a medical or osteopathic physician as a defendant or codefendant. Annual increases were dramatic between 1975 and 1985 when tort reform in Illinois led to a reduction in the number of lawsuits. Yet from a low of 492 cases in 1986, the number of malpractice lawsuits rose again and reached 1,197 in 1994. The proportion of cases relating to radiology remained steady through the 20-year period, averaging 12% of the total. Decreases occurred in the categories of slip and fall, radiation oncology, and miscellaneous. Missed diagnoses, particularly of breast

TABLE 1.—Summary of Radiology-Related Malpractice Lawsuits, Cook County, Illinois, 1975–1994

Yr	All Malpractice Suits	Radiology-Related	Slip-and-Fall	Radiation Oncology	Failure to Order	Complications	Misses	Misc.
1975	847	129	10	39	18	13	37	12
1976	507	82	4	18	19	9	27	5
1977	443	66	6	5	14	11	24	6
1978	515	70	2	6	18	10	29	5
1979	755	118	10	13	26	20	42	7
5-year subtotal	3067	15% 465	7% 32	17% 81	20% 95	14% 63	34% 159	8% 35
1980	858	140	9	22	20	30	47	12
1981	906	114	7	12	15	22	48	10
1982	1103	127	9	10	23	27	52	6
1983	1312	138	2	4	12	28	81	11
1984	1393	168	8	8	43	32	69	8
5-year subtotal	5572	12% 687	5% 35	8% 56	16% 113	20% 139	43% 297	7% 47
1985	2364	222	8	12	28	51	93	30
1986	492	52	3	2	19	7	19	2
1987	717	64	3	1	10	8	36	6
1988	803	92	4	6	26	12	31	13
1989	809	83	7	2	24	13	27	10
5-year subtotal	5185	10% 513	5% 25	4% 23	21% 107	18% 91	40% 206	12% 61
1990	931	101	4	2	29	17	48	1
1991	932	111	3	3	21	12	66	6
1992	992	112	6	4	39	11	47	5
1993	984	97	4	5	28	11	45	4
1994	1197	133	3	4	50	17	55	4
5-year subtotal	5036	11% 554	4% 20	3% 18	30% 167	12% 68	47% 261	4% 20
Total	18860	12% 2219	5% 112	8% 178	22% 482	16% 361	42% 923	7% 163

(Courtesy of Berlin L, Berlin JW: Malpractice and radiologists in Cook County, IL: Trends in 20 years of litigation. *AJR* 165:781–788, 1995.)

cancer, increased from 34% to 47% of the total. The greatest percentage increase was in the category of failure to order a radiologic examination (Table 1), a category accounting for 16% of cases during 1980–1984 and for 30% of cases from 1990 through 1994. In keeping with radiologic advances, increases were seen in the number of lawsuits alleging failure to order angiography, MRI, and CT and in claims involving mammography.

Conclusion.—Tort reform measures in Illinois led to a temporary decrease in the number of malpractice lawsuits filed from 1986 through 1989. New measures passed by the state legislature in March 1995 may again lower the number of lawsuits, which rose to 1,197 in 1994. The proportion of suits related to radiology averaged 12% yearly and remained steady during the study period. A matter of concern in the climate of managed care and cost reduction is the growth in "failure to order" lawsuits. New imaging techniques, adherence to clinical practice standards and guidelines, and knowledge of relevant clinical history may improve the accuracy rate of radiologic procedures.

▶ This article should be read by all radiologists because it gives a good summary of the frequency of malpractice cases associated with radiologic examinations. Of particular interest is the increase in lawsuits related to the failure to order a study. This trend may have profound effect on radiology as we are asked to become gatekeepers in the new world of capitation.

C.D. Maynard, M.D.

Medical Malpractice Involving Radiologic Colon Examinations: A Review of 38 Recent Cases

Barloon TJ, Shumway J (Univ of Iowa Hosps and Clinics, Iowa City; Univ of Iowa College of Medicine, Iowa City)

AJR 165:343–346, 1995 5–19

Objective.—In an effort to reduce litigation resulting from radiologic contrast studies of the colon, medical malpractice claims reported in the past decade were reviewed and a number of risk prevention strategies were proposed.

Methods.—A search of legal journals and the computerized legal database WESTLAW for the period from 1985 to 1994 yielded 38 relevant cases. The published cases were from 18 different state civil courts and involved 52 allegations of malpractice. Colon or rectal perforation was the basis for litigation in 18 cases, and another 18 claims cited failure to diagnose colorectal cancer. One patient had an anaphylactic reaction during barium enema and another underwent surgery for colon cancer after barium enema films were mislabeled with her name (Table 1). Three patients died, and 15 experienced significant morbidity.

Results.—In 14 of 18 cases citing failure to diagnose colorectal cancer, the initial barium enema was interpreted as showing normal findings. Two patients were judged to have irritable or spastic bowel, and another was

TABLE 1.—Causes of Malpractice Claims Involving Contrast Examinations of the Colon

Malpractice Claim	No. of Allegations
Failure to diagnose colorectal cancer (18 patients)	
Perceptive error (barium enema interpretation: normal)	14
Technical error (failure to opacify and obtain views of cecum)	1
Interpretive error	
Barium enema interpretation: spastic bowel	2
Barium enema interpretation: diverticulosis	1
Colon or rectal perforation (18 patients)	
Failure to detect perforation in a timely manner	6
Delay in appropriate treatment	8
Rectal catheter inserted blindly by a nonphysician	3
Failure to use proper catheter	2
Overinflation of rectal or colostomy retention balloon	2
Improper insufflation of air into the colon	2
Failure to monitor procedure by fluoroscopy	2
Failure to recognize preexisting colon disease	2
Barium enema performed immediately after rectal biopsy	1
Barium enema performed immediately after perforation from colonoscopy	1
Barium enema continued after patient noted new abdominal pain	2
Improper elevation of barium reservoir	1
Miscellaneous (two patients)	
Anaphylactic reaction during barium enema	1
Barium enema films mislabeled with wrong name (patient underwent surgery for colon cancer)	1

(Courtesy of Barloon TJ, Shumway J: Medical malpractice involving radiologic colon examinations: A review of 38 recent cases. *AJR* 165:343–346, 1995.)

diagnosed with diverticulosis. Nonopacification of the cecum led to misinterpretation in the remaining case. Diagnosis was delayed in these cases by an average of 31 months. The most common site of missed colorectal cancers was the rectosigmoid area (9 cases). Colon perforation occurred at a number of sites, most commonly the extraperitoneal rectum (7 cases).

Discussion.—An awareness of the cause of litigation involving contrast studies of the colon may help radiologists to reduce malpractice claims. Risk prevention strategies include informing the patient of the nature of the examination and communicating results in a timely manner. A digital rectal examination to exclude tumors or rectal strictures should be performed before the barium examination, and fluoroscopic monitoring for tumors, strictures, and perforations is also advised. Patients who experience new abdominal pain during barium enema examination should be examined immediately for perforation; if perforation is detected, immediate surgical consultation is required. Complete filling and coating of all segments of the colon is mandatory is cases of suspected colorectal cancer. Latex retention balloons should be avoided because of the risk of allergic reactions and colostomy studies performed without a retention balloon. Finally, reviewing all barium enema examinations or having 2 people read the examination may reduce the number of missed colon cancers.

► This article should be read by everyone who performs barium enema examinations. It offers excellent advice on how to minimize the likelihood of a lawsuit resulting from the performance of these procedures. Although the authors focused on barium enemas, their recommendations for avoiding a medical malpractice suit have some application for all other radiologic examinations.

C.D. Maynard, M.D.

Radiology by Radiologists

Prospective Analysis of a Rapid Trauma Ultrasound Examination Performed by Emergency Physicians

Ma OJ, Mateer JR, Ogata M, et al (Med College of Wisconsin, Milwaukee; Kobe City Gen Hosp, Japan)

J Trauma: Injury Infect Crit Care 38:879–885, 1995 5–20

Introduction.—Trauma surgeons are gaining skill in the use of ultrasonography to evaluate patients with blunt trauma. However, few studies have evaluated the use of ultrasound to assess patients with blunt and penetrating trauma and to identify intracavitary hemorrhage outside of the intraperitoneal space. The use of ultrasound by emergency physicians to detect free peritoneal and thoracic fluid in patients with major blunt and penetrating torso trauma was evaluated.

Methods.—The prospective study included 245 patients with major blunt or penetrating trauma of the torso seen in a level I trauma center over a 1.5-year period. The emergency medicine residents and faculty were trained to perform a rapid trauma ultrasound examination of the torso to look for free intraperitoneal, retroperitoneal, pleural, and pericardial fluid. These examinations were performed immediately after the initial assessment by the trauma team using a 2.5- to 3.5-MHz probe. The sensitivity, specificity, and accuracy of the ultrasound examinations were calculated. The ultrasound findings were not used in making patient management decisions.

Results.—In a total of 975 intracavitary spaces examined, ultrasound demonstrated 64 positive findings for free fluid. Confirmation was obtained by CT scanning, peritoneal lavage, exploratory laparotomy, chest radiography, tube thoracostomy, or formal 2-dimensional echocardiography. The ultrasound examinations had a sensitivity of 90%, specificity of 99%, and accuracy of 99%. Review of videotapes by a surgical sonologist showed excellent agreement with the emergency physicians' interpretations. The ultrasound scans took an average of 4 minutes to perform.

Conclusion.—Ultrasound is an accurate adjunctive diagnostic technique for the identification of free peritoneal and thoracic fluid in patients with blunt and penetrating trauma. The scans can be quickly performed in the emergency department and accurately interpreted by emergency physicians. The role and techniques of ultrasound in the trauma center remain to be clarified further.

▶ The fact that emergency physicians are becoming more interested in learning to perform ultrasound procedures themselves is another reason for radiologists to provide around-the-clock coverage in emergency departments. Unfortunately, many radiology groups are too small to provide the coverage required. If radiologists are not available, the emergency physicians will try to fill the void.

C. D. Maynard, M.D.

A Prospective Study of Surgeon-Performed Ultrasound as the Primary Adjuvant Modality for Injured Patient Assessment

Rozycki GS, Ochsner MG, Schmidt JA, et al (Emory Univ, Atlanta, Ga; Mem Med Ctr, Savannah, Ga; Univ of Pennsylvania, Philadelphia)

J Trauma: Injury Infect Crit Care 39:492–500, 1995 5–21

Background.—Experienced surgeon sonographers may be able to successfully use focused ultrasound evaluations as a primary adjuvant modality to physical examination in patients with suspected thoracoabdominal injuries. The accuracy and efficacy of surgeon-performed ultrasound in the assessment of injured patients was prospectively evaluated.

Patients and Methods.—Ultrasound was performed by experienced surgeons and used as the main adjuvant modality to physical examination in 371 patients evaluated for chest and abdominal trauma over a 20-month period. Average patient age was 35 years, average Injury Severity Score was 10, and average Revised Trauma Score was 7.56. Positive or negative ultrasound findings for the detection of hemoperitoneum and pericardial effusion were recorded. Patients with positive findings underwent surgical exploration, whereas those with negative findings underwent repeat physical and ultrasound examinations 12 to 24 hours later, and were followed through discharge and as outpatients 1 week after discharge. Ultrasound findings were subsequently categorized as true-negative results (no fluid and continued negative physical examination), true-positive results (fluid identified, with subsequent confirmatory surgical findings), false-negative results (no fluid, but blood noted on therapeutic exploration and injuries identified that required repair), and false-positive results (fluid identified, but negative surgical findings).

Results.—Average ultrasound examination time was 2.5 minutes. There were 305 true-negative, 53 true-positive, 12 false-negative, and 1 false-positive result. Ultrasound therefore identified 53 of the 65 patients with significant injuries, yielding a sensitivity of 81.5% and a specificity of 99.7%.

Conclusions.—Ultrasound can be performed rapidly, provides accurate results, is noninvasive, and does not expose the patient to ionizing radiation. Costs associated with ultrasound examinations also are modest compared with other modalities, such as diagnostic peritoneal lavage and CT. For these reasons, ultrasound should be considered the preferred adjuvant modality to physical examination for the assessment of injured patients, particularly those with blunt thoracoabdominal and penetrating thoracic injuries.

► Our clinical colleagues find ultrasonography of considerable value in specific clinical emergency situations. Unless radiologists step up to provide this care in a timely fashion, clinicians will perform the studies themselves. Although radiologists should be the best qualified to perform these procedures, providing adequate radiology coverage in all emergency situations may be difficult. Still, we need to try.

C.D. Maynard, M.D.

Use of Sonography in Diagnosing Acute Appendicitis: Comparison of a Teaching Hospital and a Community Hospital

Sabra J, Roh M, Páez X, et al (Brown Univ, Providence, RI)

Acad Radiol 3:438–441, 1996 5–22

Introduction.—Patterns of use of sonography in diagnosing acute appendicitis were compared in a 715-bed university-affiliated teaching hospital with a 24-bed nonteaching hospital. It has been assumed that teaching hospitals order more tests per patient because of the inexperience of house officers. Whether the use of sonography was more frequent in a teaching hospital than in a community hospital, in light of rising health care costs, was investigated.

Methods.—A retrospective study was conducted of all cases of appendicitis seen in emergency departments of the teaching hospital (1993) and the community hospital (1992–1993). Patients ranged in age from 2 to 88 years. Pathology reports verified the diagnosis of appendicitis.

Results.—Sonography usage was 39.4% (61 of 155 patients) at the nonteaching hospital, whereas at the teaching hospital, sonography usage was 38.5% (65 of 169 patients). At both hospitals, sonograms were used more frequently for females than for males. Sonograms were given to 54.2% of the females and 23.3% of the males at the teaching hospital, whereas at the nonteaching hospital, sonograms were given to 43.6% of females and 35.1% of males.

Conclusion.—No significant difference was seen between nonteaching and teaching hospitals in the frequency of use of sonography in diagnosing appendicitis. Generally, sonography was used more for complicated or atypical cases.

► This article demonstrates the growing use of ultrasound in the emergency room. No significant difference was found between a teaching hospital and a nonteaching hospital with regard to the use of sonography in patients with appendicitis. Again, radiologists need to be available in both settings.

C.D. Maynard, M.D

Emergency Ultrasound Services as Perceived by Directors of Radiology and Emergency Departments

Heller M, Crocco T, Patterson J, et al (Univ of Pittsburgh, Pa)
Am J Emerg Med 13:430–431, 1995 5–23

Objective.—The availability of emergency US services and the attitudes of radiologists and emergency physicians (EPs) regarding the value of emergency ultrasound (US) were determined in a survey of emergency department (ED) directors of radiology at randomly selected hospitals. There has been concern that emergency US services are often not available, particularly after regular business hours.

Methods.—A 10-question survey was sent to 100 large teaching (T) hospitals and 100 small nonteaching (NT) hospitals throughout the United States. The survey was anonymous, but coding allowed responses to be identified as from T or NT hospitals and as from a director of a radiology department or a director of an ED. Surveys were returned from 106 institutions.

Results.—The rate of return was somewhat higher for T hospitals and ED directors than for NT hospitals and radiology departments. In-house, 24 hour-per-day US services were uncommon in both types of institutions. Directors of EDs were significantly more likely than directors of radiology to report that US was "immediately" available fewer than 40 hours per week (Table 1). Directors of radiology and ED directors also differed significantly in their perceptions of the value of increased US availability and in the desirability of having EPs perform US examinations (Table 2).

Discussion.—This sample of approximately 4% of the 5,000 EDs in the United States suggests that emergency US services are rarely available in both T and NT hospitals. Radiologists and EPs differ considerably in their

TABLE 1.—Ultrasound Availability

	Teaching		Nonteaching	
	ED%	RAD%	ED%	RAD%
In-house ultrasound 24/h/d	15	22	0	10
On-call or in-house ultrasound 24 h/d	86	86	70	72
Ultrasound "immediately" available <40 h/wk	22*	9*	59†	21†

* $P < 0.05$.
† $P < 0.001$.
Abbreviations: ED, emergency department; *RAD*, radiology department.
(Courtesy of Heller M, Crocco T, Patterson J, et al: Emergency ultrasound services as perceived by directors of radiology and emergency departments. *Am J Emerg Med* 13:430–431, 1995.)

TABLE 2.—Attitudes Toward Emergency Department Ultrasound

	Teaching		Nonteaching	
	ED%	RAD%	ED%	RAD%
"Significant" value of increased ultrasound availability	80*	64*	77*	52*
Knowledge of impact in specific case	48*	13*	50†	15†
Ultrasound performed now by EPs	6	2	0	0
Ultrasound by EPs				
"Bad idea"	20†	88†	38†	80†
"Makes sense"	52†	0†	33†	0†

* $P < 0.05$.
† $P < 0.001$.
Abbreviations: ED, emergency department; *RAD*, radiology department; *EPs*, emergency physicians.
(Courtesy of Heller M, Crocco T, Patterson J, et al: Emergency ultrasound services as perceived by directors of radiology and emergency departments. *Am J Emerg Med* 13:430–431, 1995.)

views of the need for such services. Whereas ED directors perceive emergency US to have clinical value, directors of radiology departments do not advocate the use of US by EPs.

► If this survey accurately depicts the perception on the part of radiology and ED heads about the value of US procedures in emergency situations, the move by EPs to obtain experience with US in specific clinical situations is easily understood. If this assessment is correct, and the attitude of radiologists persists, these procedures will ultimately be lost to the EPs. I know that would not be in the best interests of the field of radiology, and I doubt that it would be in the best interests of the patient.

C.D. Maynard, M.D.

Comparative Analysis of Radiographic Interpretation of Orthopedic Films: Is There Redundancy?

Turen CH, Mark JB, Bozman R (Univ of Maryland, Baltimore; Naval Med Ctr, Portsmouth, Va)

J Trauma 39:720–721, 1995 5–24

Background.—Stringent economic conditions have prompted the reassessment of the need for many health care procedures. Radiologists' and orthopedists' interpretations of plain orthopedic films were compared prospectively to illuminate possible areas of unnecessary patient cost resulting from redundant services.

Methods.—Orthopedic surgical and radiology attending physicians independently interpreted 507 consecutive radiographic studies of acute orthopedic injuries in 438 patients. The physicians did not perform physical examinations of the patients.

Findings.—Both groups' readings were very sensitive and specific. There were no significant differences between them. The mean cost of the radiologists' interpretations in the local area was about $16,100. There was no cost associated with orthopedists' readings.

Conclusion.—Radiologist interpretation of the radiographic studies of patients with acute orthopedic injuries is redundant, constituting an unnecessary expense to patients. Eliminating this redundant service on a national level could result in a health care cost savings of millions of dollars.

▶ We will hear similar reports in the future as capitation becomes a major method of reimbursing physicians. Several factors should be considered, however, before we jump to the conclusion that radiologists have no legitimate role in the interpretation of orthopedic films. In addition to providing an expert diagnostic opinion on individual cases, the radiologist often provides quality control for the procedure, makes the official report on the case, and serves as a consultant to orthopedic surgeons in unusual cases. Furthermore, radiologists interpret orthopedic films for family practitioners, general internists, pediatricians, and other physicians. A physician will always be needed to serve in this capacity, and a radiologist, by training, is most qualified to do so.

C.D. Maynard, M.D.

Radiologic Interpretation by Family Physicians in an Office Practice Setting

Bergus GR, Franken EA Jr, Koch TJ, et al (Univ of Iowa, Iowa City)

J Fam Pract 41:352–356, 1995 5–25

Introduction.—Many family physicians interpret radiographs in their offices; however, studies on the performance of their interpretation of radiographs are scant. The performance of family physicians in interpreting radiographs ordered in a free-standing family practice office was investigated.

Methods.—Radiographic studies performed in a family practice office were evaluated during a 3-year period. The analysis included 1,674 radiographic studies, and each was interpreted by the family physician ordering the study and by a radiologist. The studies were accepted as having been correctly interpreted if the interpretations between the physicians agreed. When interpretations did not agree, the study was re-examined. The study also evaluated whether there were any differences in quality of analysis based on the body part imaged and whether the disease was identified.

Results.—There were correct interpretations of 92.4% of the radiographic studies by family physicians. The family physicians' accuracy with chest films (89.3%) was lower than their accuracy with extremity films (96%) (Table 1). Normal films were more likely to be correctly interpreted by family physicians than abnormal films (95.2% vs. 85.9%). Correct interpretations were given by family physicians in 35% of the cases that resulted in initial disagreements of interpretations.

TABLE 1.—Accuracy of Family Physicians at Interpreting Normal and Abnormal Radiographic Studies in an Office Setting

	Accurate Interpretation by Family Physicians, %		
Type of Radiograph	Normal Radiographs	Abnormal Radiographs	Total Radiographs*
Chest (n = 898)†	93.6	80.0	89.3
Extremity (n = 776)‡	96.8	93.8	96.0
Total (N = 1674)†	95.2	85.9	92.4

* $P < 0.001$ comparing accurate interpretation of chest vs. extremity films.
† $P < 0.001$ comparing accurate interpretation of normal vs. abnormal radiographs.
‡ $P = 0.06$ comparing accurate interpretation of normal vs. abnormal radiographs.
(Bergus GR, Franken EA Jr, Koch TJ, et al: Radiologic interpretation by family physicians in an office practice setting. *J Fam Pract* 41:352–356, 1995. Reprinted by permission of Appleton & Lange, Inc.)

Conclusion.—In an office setting, family physicians had a high degree of accuracy in interpreting radiologic films, and they were correct in more than one third of the discrepant cases. Extremity films were inherently easier to interpret than chest films, which may be the result of the greater variety of subtle findings and abnormalities found on chest radiographs. The performance of family physicians may vary in different practice settings, depending on the body part being imaged and the prevalence of disease.

► Considerable plain film radiology is done in offices of family practitioners, where many of the films are not read by a radiologist. How accurately these clinicians interpret these films has always been of concern to radiologists. This article seems to indicate that family practitioners interpret films fairly well. As teleradiology of plain films becomes more affordable, we need to further establish the value of having these studies over-read by radiologists, as this task could be accomplished in a timely fashion.

C.D. Maynard, M.D.

Added Value of Radiologist Consultation to Family Practitioners in the Outpatient Setting

Franken EA Jr, Bergus GR, Koch TJ, et al (Univ of Iowa, Iowa City)
Radiology 197:759–762, 1995 5–26

Background.—Many family physicians interpret radiographs obtained in their own office-based units. Frequently radiologists are consulted to reread these films. The benefit of this radiologist consultation was investigated.

Methods.—A total of 1,674 radiographs of the chest and extremity, read by both family physicians and radiologists, were reviewed. The readings of the 2 physician groups were discrepant in 196 cases.

Findings.—The overall sensitivities of the readings were 92% for radiologists and 86% for family physicians, respectively. Specificities between

TABLE 1.—Summary of Findings in All Cases

Radiographic Finding	True-Positive Finding		False-Negative Finding		True-Negative Finding		False-Positive Finding	
	FP	Radiologist	FP	Radiologist	FP	Radiologist	FP	Radiologist
Chest								
Normal (n = 613)	0	0	0	0	575	586	38	27
Abnormal (n = 285)								
Pneumonia (n = 127)	105	111	22	16	0	0	0	0
"Complicated" pneumonia (n = 9)	5	6	4	3	0	0	0	0
Congestive heart failure (n = 34)	26	31	8	3	0	0	0	0
Mass (n = 15)	5	15	10	0	0	0	0	0
Other (n = 100)	87	92	13	8	0	0	0	0
Extremities								
Normal (n = 566)	0	0	0	0	548	552	18	14
Abnormal (n = 210)								
Fracture (n = 183)	178	173	5	10	0	0	0	0
Other (n = 27)	19	26	12	6	0	0	0	0

Abbreviation: FP, family practitioner.
(Courtesy of Franken EA Jr, Bergus GR, Koch TJ, et al: Added value of radiologist consultation to family practitioners in the outpatient setting. *Radiology* 197:759–762, 1995.)

the 2 groups did not differ significantly. The accuracy of the radiologist and family physician readings of extremity radiographs did not differ significantly. For chest films, radiologists' sensitivity (89%) was substantially greater than that of family physicians' (80%). Radiologic consultation was especially beneficial for detecting pneumonia and masses (Table 1).

Conclusion.—The difference between radiologists' and family physicians' readings of extremity radiographs was negligible, suggesting that the radiologist's role for such studies can be limited to individual consultations. However, radiologists' review of all chest radiographs continues to be important.

► Radiologists must interpret cases in "real time" to be most valuable in specific clinical situations. The radiologist should be consulting with the primary care physician while the patient is being evaluated and before treatment is undertaken. Technological advances in telecommunications ultimately will make this scenario economically feasible. Although the role of the radiologist often is to verify what the primary care physician suspects, the radiologist frequently adds useful information in a timely fashion.

C.D. Maynard, M.D.

Responses to a Payment Policy Denying Professional Charges for Diagnostic Imaging by Nonradiologist Physicians

Hillman BJ, Olson GT, Colbert RW, et al (Univ of Virginia, Charlottesville; FIRST HEALTH Strategies Inc, Pittsburgh, Pa; United Mine Workers of American Health and Retirement Funds, Washington, DC)

JAMA 274:885–887, 1995 5–27

Background.—In an attempt to control diagnostic imaging costs, the United Mine Workers of America Health and Retirement Funds (the funds) stopped reimbursing billings for the professional component of imaging studies to any physicians but radiologists. The effect of the new policy on annual imaging rates and cost to the Funds was studied.

Methods.—Claims from 20 counties, containing 45% of all beneficiaries, were reviewed. The number of professional, technical, and global (professional and technical combined) reimbursements and their cost were calculated for the year before and the year after the policy change. Results were adjusted to account for a 6% decrease in the number of beneficiaries between the 2 years.

Results.—In 1993, after the policy change, the funds paid 12% more for diagnostic imaging than in 1992. The increase per beneficiary was 23%. There was a 41% increase in allowed claims per beneficiary, with the largest percentage change for technical services and the largest change in number of claims for professional services.

Conclusion.—A major objective of the new policy, to decrease the cost of diagnostic imaging, was not realized. The reason for the increased cost and number of claims is not clear but is probably multifactorial.

► An attempt to decrease the cost of imaging services by paying only for the radiologist's interpretation backfired on the United Mine Workers of America Health and Retirement Funds. If this is the expected outcome of such actions, third-party payers are not likely to adopt this approach as a general policy.

C.D. Maynard, M.D.

Picture Archiving and Communications Systems and Teleradiology

Making Filmless Radiology Work

Siegel EL, Diaconis JN, Pomerantz S, et al (Univ of Maryland, Baltimore)
J Digit Imaging 8:151–155, 1995 5–28

Introduction.—Abandoning film for digital imaging faces many obstacles including economic constraints, concerns about image quality and time required for interpreting images, and overcoming inertia associated with new paradigm shifts. The Baltimore Veterans Affairs Medical Center has had digital imaging for 2 years, including computed radiography, digital angiography, digital fluoroscopy, ultrasound, CT, and MRI. They use a picture archiving and communication system.

Transition.—Radiologists took about 5 months to convert to soft-copy interpretation. During the transition period, films were printed that were generated by the computed radiography laser imagers and given to the radiologists with old film jacket to have for comparison when doing their soft-copy interpretations. Maximum speed was generally achieved in about 2–3 weeks with the picture archiving and communication system.

Speed and quality.—Radiologists spend slightly more time reading the soft-copy images compared with convention film; however, their overall productivity has increased up to 30%. The paradoxical increase in productivity is the result of easier and more rapid access to old images and reports and the elimination of interruptions by clinicians and file-room staff looking for films. Radiologists need to take more breaks with the new system (every 40 to 50 minutes) than with the conventional system (every 1 to 2 hours). The radiologists' perception of the image quality of the new system is positive and of quality comparable to that achieved by the top 10% to 20% of films.

Conclusion.—Sufficient funding, including money set aside for maintenance and upgrades, must be available to make the switch to computed radiography. Adequate back-up systems are necessary to allow continued operation with the new system, as are an adequate number of work stations to allow for convenient access to any health care workers. Films of the last 5 years must be stored on line. The chief of the radiology department must endorse this system. Short-term pain resulting from making the switch from reading conventional films to interpreting soft copies will result in long-term gain.

► Paul Capp[1] predicted that radiology would be filmless by the year 2000. It seems that all of the technical requirements to reach that goal are in place or evolving. The missing element is the fact that radiologists must embrace the technique. Before this will happen, it must be demonstrated that filmless radiology saves time, is as accurate as current film/screen systems, is affordable, and is cost effective.

C.D. Maynard, M.D.

Reference

1. Capp MP: Radiology—2000 A.D. *Radiology* 138:541–550, 1981.

PACS: A Phased Implementation Strategy

Stewart BK (Univ of Washington, Seattle)

Adm Radiol Nov:10–16, 1995 5–29

Purpose.—The past 15 years have seen major back-and-forth shifts in enthusiasm for the concept of Picture Archiving and Communication Systems (PACS). PACS systems have been on the leading edge of the information technology curve and, until recently, have tended to be unreliable and non–cost-effective. It is still difficult to measure the benefits of PACS and the difficulties involved in full-scale implementation. In the managed care era, PACS may offer benefits beyond those historically expected from "filmless radiology." A staged approach to the implementation of PACS was described.

PACS Implementation.—The question facing health care centers is not whether they should implement PACS, but when they will have to do so to remain competitive and efficient. Centers should not wait for a fully developed system to arrive. Rather, they should implement PACS in phases—using modular components that can be expanded by increments—with the ultimate goal of integrating those components into a hospital-wide image and information management system. The 3-phase approach starts with acquiring the basic connectivity infrastructure by developing mini-PACS applications. This is followed by "going filmless" for nuclear medicine, CT, MRI, and ultrasound, and connecting to an RIS. The final phase seeks to achieve a long-term archive, an on-line medical record through connection with an HIS/CIS and filmless archiving for plain film radiography and other x-ray studies. At the author's hospital, the plan is to invest in Ethernet technology and convert to Asynchronous Transfer Mode technology in the future. Medium-term storage of images will be an important consideration in filmless operation. Most likely, this will involve storage of about 1 year's worth of images on a number of magneto-optic disks in a "jukebox"-style data base. The final phase of implementation will include such tasks as long-term archiving and high-resolution softcopy imaging.

Discussion.—A staged approach to the implementation of PACS technology is recommended. Institutions can take steps now to be ready for the PACS of tomorrow. The author's institution is still in the first phase of implementation, but some of the elements required for the second phase are already in place. Considerable work remains to be done for the final stages of implementation, however, especially in the development of intelligent software tools.

▶ Picture Archiving and Communication Systems it seems, have been around for an eternity. Without question, the hype has far surpassed the results. I remain convinced, however, that the advantages of this technology will be important to radiology as we launch efforts to provide care in extensive networks of practices and hospitals. We must focus on the demonstrated value-added aspects of PACS. Areas such as teleradiology, which provides coverage in remote sites, communication systems that send chest images to critical care units, and mini-PACS for the digital modalities are good places to start. Full-fledged PACS will come with time.

C.D. Maynard, M.D.

Prospective Study of a PACS: Information Flow and Clinical Action in a Medical Intensive Care Unit

Kundel HL, Seshadri SB, Langlotz CP, et al (Univ of Pennsylvania, Philadelphia)

Radiology 199:143–149, 1996 5–30

Background.—Picture archiving and communication systems (PACS) are supposed to avoid some of the difficult challenges posed in the management of large-volume imaging operations. The authors have reported that the use of a PACS in the medical ICU setting can decrease the time needed to take certain clinical actions and reduce consultation with radiology staff. However, this research had several limitations. A larger, prospective comparison of a digital PACS with a standard film-only system was therefore conducted.

Methods.—The study used a sequential design to compare the two systems in a random sample of nonroutine, bedside chest radiographs. The film-only system used either conventional analog film or computed radiography (CR) hard copies. The PACS system used CR images, which could be viewed on a multiviewer in the radiology department and on a workstation in the medical ICU. Three main events were timed from the completion of each examination: the time to image display, the time to encounters with image information, and the time to actions prompted by the image.

Results.—Seventy-five percent of images could be viewed on the workstation within 20 minutes of completion of the study. The time to display

75% of the images on the multiviewer was 1.8 hours. Use of the workstation did not reduce the time until staff accessed the image information. However, it did reduce the time until they took clinical action. Radiologists were consulted about 90% of images with the film-only system, compared to 28% with the workstation.

Conclusions.—Implementation of a PACS in the medical ICU setting can improve the delivery of chest radiographs. The PACS also shortens the time until actions based on imaging studies are taken and reduces consultation with radiologists. Future reports will address the incremental costs associated with PACS, as well as the accuracy of electronic display.

▶ This report demonstrates that a PACS can be useful in selected settings such as intensive care units, and in additional situations such as emergency department coverage and teleradiology from off-site facilities.

C.D. Maynard, M.D.

Off-Hours Interpretation of Radiologic Images of Patients Admitted to the Emergency Department: Efficacy of Teleradiology

DeCorato DR, Kagetsu NJ, Ablow RC (St Luke's-Roosevelt Hosp Ctr, New York)

AJR 165:1293–1296, 1995 5–31

Objective.—The effectiveness of a teleradiology system in off-site interpretation of radiological studies from a hospital emergency department was evaluated.

Background.—In many emergency departments, nonradiologists make an initial interpretation of radiologic studies during off-hours. It is unclear if delayed interpretations provided by radiologists increase the quality of care. Teleradiology systems offer an alternative to this problem.

Methods.—A total of 812 radiologic studies performed at a hospital during off-hours were digitized and transmitted to the radiology department at a second hospital, where they were interpreted by radiology residents. These interpretations were compared with the official interpretations made by a certified radiologist at the original hospital.

Results.—Clinically significant discrepancies occurred in 5% of images. Of these, 2% resulted from interobserver error, 2% from digital image reader error, 0.4% from inadequate digital image, and 0.2% resulted from film reader error. Inadequate digital images sometimes resulted from underpenetrated radiographs or drifting of the laser digitizer.

Conclusion.—The accuracy of interpretation was 99.6%. The teleradiology equipment used is reliable and effective for interpretation of emergency department radiologic studies made during off-hours.

▶ Whether radiologists view teleradiology as an asset or an enemy depends on how it is used. In the future, radiographs obtained in the emergency setting must be read on line for the radiologist to be reimbursed; otherwise, the clinician who originally interprets the radiograph (e.g., the emergency room physician) and not the radiologist who reads the study after the fact will be compensated by the third-party carrier. The Health Care Financing Administration is certainly moving in that direction. Done properly by radiologists, teleradiology can provide on-line emergency room consults, offering the emergency room physician and the patient the benefit of our expertise. Small radiology groups can join together to provide the service, or they can contract with teleradiology services that are being developed throughout the country. The technology is here; it is up to us to apply it appropriately.

C.D. Maynard, M.D.

Medical-Legal Issues in Teleradiology

Berger SB, Cepelewicz BB (Yale Univ, New Haven, Conn)

AJR 166:505–510, 1996 5–32

Objective.—Teleradiology refers to the transmission of images from a local site to a remote site for interpretation. The availability of high-speed, high-definition digital imaging will have a major impact on the field of teleradiology. Some of the important medicolegal issues pertaining to teleradiology—including privacy, licensing, credentialing, liability, and fraud—were reviewed.

Privacy.—Though it is often claimed that electronic systems provide improved security, no system is perfect, and the health care professional is still responsible for the maintainance and enforcement of the network security system. Currently, privacy laws vary by state, but a federal privacy protection code, or Uniform State Medical Information Code, has been proposed.

Licensure.—Under the current system, physicians consulting by teleradiology would have to be licensed in more than one state. One possible solution is to create a national licensure system in which the patient is considered as being "electronically transferred" to the consulting physician in another state. License to practice in other states could be obtained by reciprocity or by endorsement. Some states have consultation exemptions, which range in scope from very narrow to very broad. Of these states, some are considering closing their consultation exceptions to protect local radiologists from the perceived threat of teleradiology.

Credentialing.—Similar problems are raised by the issue of credentialing; some staff physicians fear that their privileges will be ignored in favor of noncredentialed telemedicine specialists. In one scenario proposed by the Joint Commission on Accreditation of Healthcare Organizations, the consulting physician would act as an adjunct for the local physician, though the consultant would still face potential liability involvement. At least one company's managed care plans is already requiring enrolled workers to use a teleradiology system for routine imaging instead of local radiologists.

Malpractice Liability.—So far, there is no experience with malpractice issues related to teleradiology. A number of significant issues could apply, however, including whether any information is lost in the image received by the teleradiology consultant and whether the standards of the local or remote community prevail. New standards for the minimally acceptable level of image transmission may be required, and the question of whether the digitized image becomes part of the patient record will have to be addressed. Another possibility is that a local physician could be held responsible for failing to consult with an available teleradiology specialist.

Discussion.—Teleradiology offers the potential for higher-quality health care with significant cost savings. However, it also brings up a spectrum of untested medicolegal issues. There are still some ways in which teleradiology consultants may limit their risk, especially by complying with the American College of Radiology Standard on Teleradiology. The teleradiologist always retains responsibility for making sure that the image transmitted is adequate for diagnostic purposes.

▶ This is a must-read article for anyone who is currently involved in teleradiology, or who is contemplating involvement in this area. The authors raise all the relevant issues. At present, obstacles to the applications of this technology are numerous, but as telemedicine evolves, many of these problems will disappear.

C.D. Maynard, M.D.

Computers

Invited Review: Computer Aids for Decision-Making in Diagnostic Radiology: A Literature Review

Taylor P (Advanced Computation Lab, London)

Br J Radiol 68:945–957, 1995 5–33

Introduction.—It is now possible for computer systems to capture, store, transmit, and display radiologic images, thereby aiding in decision making in diagnostic radiology. The issues involved in designing these systems and criteria for evaluating them, and 5 different types of decision support systems were discussed.

Issues and Criteria.—The first issue common to all decision support systems is the need for a decision aid. An aid is needed when interpretation requires the expertise of a specialist, when many images are generated, or when interpretation is very difficult. The next issue is the constraints placed on the computer system by the medical domain and the clinical setting in which the system is used. Another issue is the mechanism of retrieving information. These issues result in four general criteria for evaluating computerized decision aids: need, practicality, veracity, and relevance. Veracity suggests that the decision support is based on information that is accurate, complete, and within limits that are understood. Relevance suggests that the system provides information that is known to improve decision making.

Decision Support Systems.—The earliest computer decision aids were based on numerical methods and used statistical data. These aids used various mathematical equations describing how probabilities should be combined to improve decision making. Image databases store large numbers of images to assist the radiologist and should be able to retrieve the images rapidly based on their visual content. Expert systems use information that represents clinical knowledge that is combined with information supplied by the user to create inferences. Image processing systems mathematically transform digital images for quantitative measurements, image enhancement, object recognition, segmentation, three-dimensional reconstruction, and tomography. Image understanding systems use image processing to create a symbolic representation of the image.

Conclusion.—Despite research in medical imaging, the human visual system is still better at detecting structure than any computer. Our capacity to design tools to enhance this interpretive skill is limited by our understanding of the human perceptual system. The medical domains that might benefit most from computer technology are not necessarily the domains for which computerized decision aids are easily designed. Systems that require lengthy interaction and are not integrated into the normal routine of the clinician will not be readily accepted or used.

▶ This article nicely summarizes the uses of computers as aids in the diagnostic process. Electronic computers cannot replace the human computer (the radiologist) any time soon, but they can be tremendous assets in the decision-making process.

C.D. Maynard, M.D.

Value of On-Line Informational Databases in a Radiology Department

Frank MS, Berge RE (Univ of Washington, Seattle)

AJR 164:1537–1539, 1995 5–34

Introduction.—Staff in radiology departments routinely use much paper-based information, such as telephone numbers and emergency procedures. All such information was transferred to computer databases accessible from any hospital computer terminal. The value of this on-line system was discussed.

Materials.—On-line information includes emergency procedures, premedication protocols, operational guidelines, protocol manuals, and telephone and pager directories. Two computer programs create, update, and access the databases. Data are stored and accessed in a hierarchy. Access to most information does not require a password.

Discussion.—On-line information can be updated quicker than paper-based information, cannot be misplaced, and is simultaneously available to all users. Often many computer terminals are available in hospitals that use information systems. Personnel are more easily held accountable for consistency when there is 1 clear source of procedures and protocols. Radiologists and technologists can access the same information when conferring by telephone, and data can be accessed from remote sites by modem. Response from staff has been favorable. Paperbased versions of crucial information are maintained in case of computer failure. Down time is 12 hours per 6 months. Specific hardware and software information is also included.

► Computer systems are commonplace in radiology departments, and we have the experience and expertise to use them to advantage in patient care. As information management in medicine increases in importance, radiologists should be leading the way.

C.D. Maynard, M.D.

Teaching Skeletal Radiology With Use of Computer-Assisted Instruction With Interactive Videodisc

Chew FS, Smirniotopoulos JG (Armed Forces Inst of Pathology, Washington, DC)

J Bone Joint Surg (Am) 77A:1080–1086, 1995 5–35

Objective.—The effectiveness and logistical practicality of using computer-assisted instruction with an interactive videodisc to teach the radiology of musculoskeletal injuries to orthopedic surgery residents were evaluated.

Methods.—Eleven residents in orthopedic surgery completed the study. Each resident completed a pretest, used the computer-videodisc program to learn the principles of radiology of skeletal injuries, and then completed a posttest. The program was designed in such a way that the resident could control the images on the videodisc monitor, which were coordinated with the instruction on the computer screen. In addition, a single, still image could be displayed. The program responded to actions of the user by sounds and screen displays indicating the accuracy of the user's response. Each work station, consisting of a computer, monitor, and videodisc player, cost less than $2,000.

Results.—The difference between pretest and posttest scores was significant. Before using the training program, the residents answered 56% of the test questions correctly compared with 86% after the training. The effect size of 3.57 is interpreted as important in educational research. The residents reported that the computer-videodisc program increased their interest in the subject being studied and was better than other educational tools traditionally used. The cost of this program is lower than commercially available conventional radiograph teaching files. Also, with this program, information is easily updated and maintained, and the images cannot be lost or misfiled.

Conclusion.—The interactive computer-videodisc training program in skeletal radiology is effective, affordable, and well received by the users.

▶ Chew and Smirniotopoulos are leading the way in computer instruction for radiology. There is little doubt that computer instruction will speed up the acquisition of knowledge. Perhaps we should be trying to develop a system that will help our radiology residents learn radiology faster so that we can shorten the total time required to become certified. A more revolutionary approach might be to let them learn at their own speed and finish their programs at different times, depending on what they have learned!

C.D. Maynard, M.D.

An Internet-Based Nuclear Medicine Teaching File

Wallis JW, Miller MM, Miller TR, et al (Washington Univ, St Louis)
J Nucl Med 36:1520–1527, 1995 5–36

Background.—A network-accessible electronic teaching file has several advantages over a traditional film-based file. Cases are more easily indexed and accessed, are readily available over any distance, cannot be lost from files, and can display dynamic studies. An Internet-based nuclear medicine teaching file using a Mosaic application for image display and searching was studied for its suitability.

Description.—A World Wide Web server, configured to run on a UNIX work station, is connected to the hospital network and, using a microwave relay, to an Internet gateway on a nearby campus. Access to the teaching file is possible from Apple Macintosh and IBM-PC compatible computers and from UNIX work stations. Data can be displayed with diagnoses or as unknown cases. Hypertext Markup Language links text to appropriate images and other text pages. Case entry uses a specific form, displayed on the screen, and requires the use of a password. Cases are reviewed by faculty before release onto the network. Direct image transfer to the teaching file from clinical interpretation work stations is possible.

Results.—Access time is generally less than 10 sec using Ethernet or Internet. Access using a 14.4K modem requires about 50 sec. Initial entry of a simple nuclear medicine case requires around 10 minutes. Pre-entry research and text writing can, of course, take much longer. Utilizing image compression, a 300 by 400 pixel whole-body bone scintigraph can be stored in 56K bytes. A relatively complex case with multiple images fills around 1.25 megabytes.

Conclusion.—This Teaching File-Web application allows ease of access, ease of new case entry, and widespread availability of a collection of nuclear medicine teaching cases.

▶ The use of the Internet to provide teaching files for radiology trainees is becoming commonplace. With time there will be a considerable amount of material in all areas of radiology for teaching programs to be accessed over the Net. Perhaps 1 of the major radiology scientific societies, such as the Radiological Society of North America, the American Roentgen Ray Society, or the American College of Radiology, should coordinate the plethora of teaching files that are springing up. It would seem to me that some type of quality control is needed to ensure that the case files are accurate representations of the entity. Obviously participation in electronic teaching files should be voluntary.

C.D. Maynard, M.D.

Interventional Radiology

Interactive MR-Guided Biopsy in an Open-Configuration MR Imaging System

Silverman SG, Collick BD, Figueira MR, et al (Brigham and Women's Hosp, Boston; Gen Electric Med Systems, Waukesha, Wis)
Radiology 197:175–181, 1995 5–37

Purpose.—Magnetic resonance imaging has several potential advantages for use in guided percutaneous biopsy and interventions. Anticipating this application of MRI, the investigators have developed an open-configuration MRI system with an integrated optical tracking system for

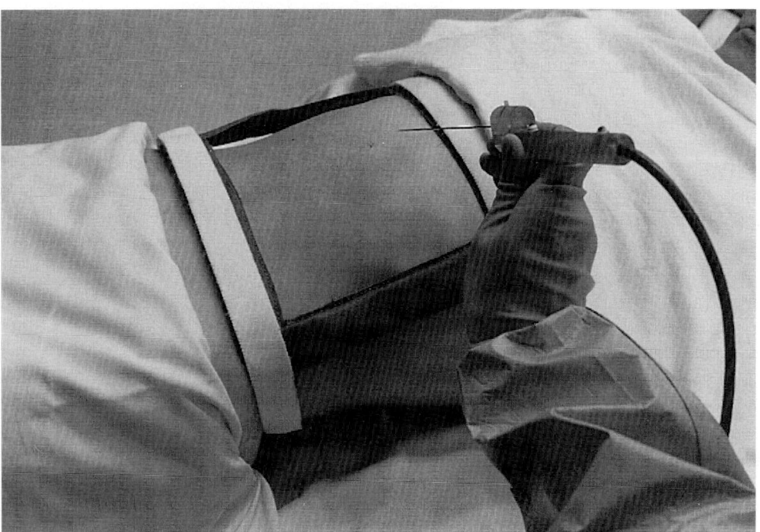

FIGURE 1.—Transmit/receive flexible surface coil used in the MR system positioned on a volunteer in the preparation area outside the interventional MR suite to demonstrate the typical position used for imaging and biopsy of liver lesions. The rectangular region is the surface area in which the cutaneous entry route is chosen. (Courtesy of Silverman SG, Collick BD, Figueira MR, et al: Interactive MR-guided biopsy in an open-configuration MR imaging system. *Radiology* 197:175–181, 1995; Radiological Society of North America.)

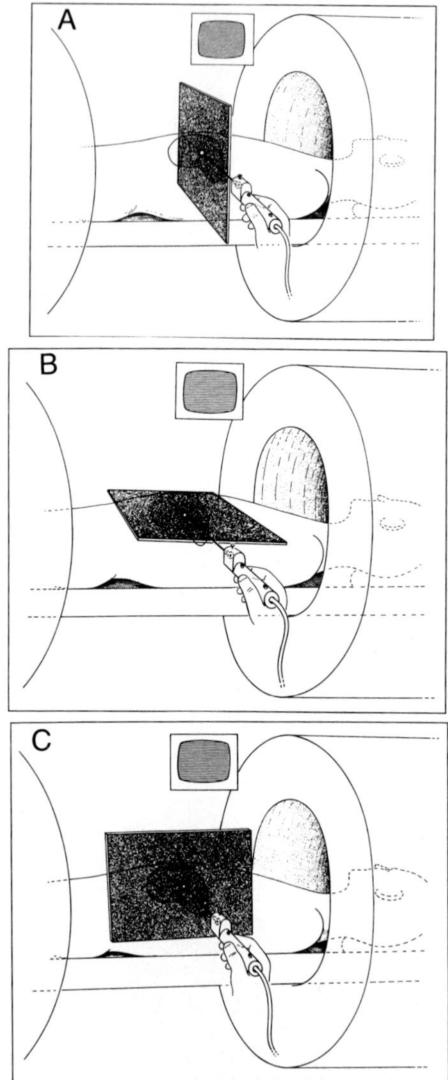

FIGURE 2.—Diagrammatic representation of an interactive MR-guided liver biopsy in the MR system to depict the 3 orthogonal planes used in interactive imaging. The 3 orthogonal planes shown on the video display include (**A**) in-plane 90 degrees, which results in an image that is in the plane of the long axis of the needle and is perpendicular to the floor; (**B**) in-plane 0 degree, which results in an image that is both in the plane of the long axis of the needle and in a plane that is 90 degrees to the in-plane 90-degree view; and (**C**) perpendicular plane, which results in an image that is perpendicular to the long axis of the needle at the level of the needle tip. (Courtesy of Silverman SG, Collick BD, Figueira MR, et al: Interactive MR-guided biopsy in an open-configuration MR imaging system. *Radiology* 197:175–181, 1995; Radiological Society of North America.)

frameless stereotaxic guidance. The application of this system for percutaneous biopsy was reported, including an evaluation of its spatial accuracy.

Methods.—The open-configuration MRI system was used to perform percutaneous biopsies in 28 patients. In this system, a hand-held probe attached to the biopsy needle was used for interactive control of the image planes (Fig 1). The needle was advanced in 3 orthogonal planes using an icon integrated into the image for guidance (Fig 2). The spatial accuracy of the system was evaluated in in vitro studies.

Results.—The system's accuracy was greatest near the isocenter. Within a 2.5-cm sphere around the isocenter, the maximum measured error was 3.1 mm. The biopsies resulted in the retrieval of diagnostic tissue from 25 patients, including liver, lymph node, and renal biopsies.

Conclusion.—The findings demonstrate the safety and accuracy of MR-guided biopsy using a frameless stereotaxic technique. The interactive system provides nearly real-time image feedback for use in performing MR-guided biopsies and placing probes for MR-guided therapies. The ability to provide an interactive, 1-step method of localization and targeting is 1 of the system's major advantages.

► This technology could play a major role in interventional radiology in future years. Innovations will undoubtedly occur as more such MR devices are installed. Before the technique can reach its full potential, physicians from disciplines other than radiology will have to become excited about its prospects.

C.D. Maynard, M.D.

Superconducting Open-Configuration MR Imaging System for Image-Guided Therapy

Schenck JF, Jolesz FA, Roemer PB, et al (Gen Electric Co, Schenectady, NY; GE Med Systems, Waukesha, Wis; Brigham and Women's Hosp, Boston)

Radiology 195:805–814, 1995 5–38

Rationale.—A lack of accessibility to patients undergoing MRI has limited the intraoperative use of conventional superconducting imagers. An openly configured superconducting MRI system that provides direct vertical access to the patient was developed. The interventional radiologist is able to acquire high-quality images in nearly real time while standing or seated within the magnet.

Device.—The magnet is designed with coils in separate but communicating cryostats to provide a spherical imaging volume 30 cm in diameter with a 56-cm gap at the center for access to the patient (Fig 1). Niobium tin was used as the superconducting material in place of niobium titanium to widen the region of access. The magnet was designed to operate safely at fields up to 1 tesla. A 3-dimensional digitizer system is incorporated to

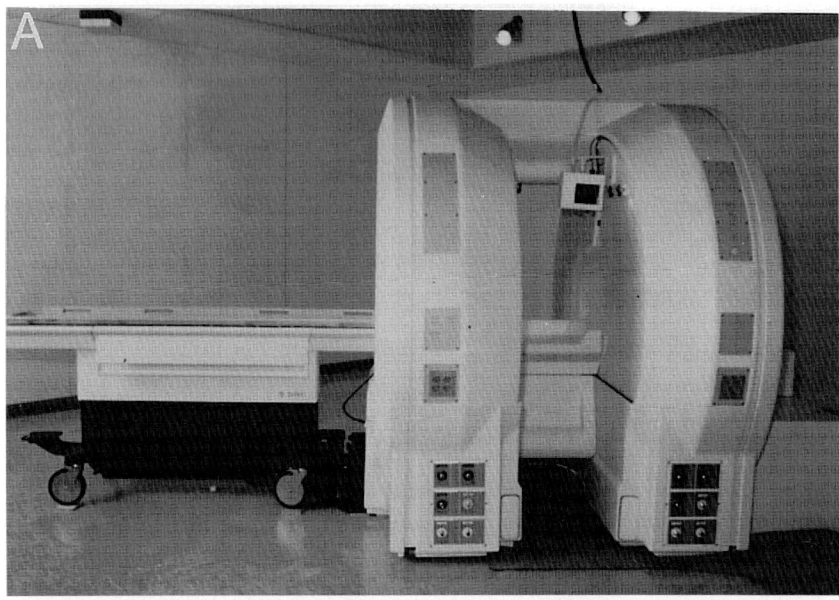

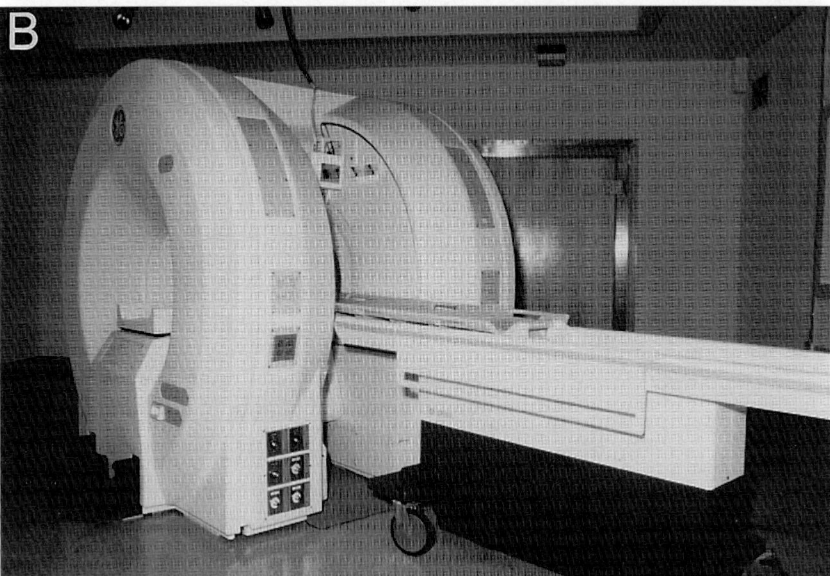

FIGURE 1.—Open-magnet system. The magnet is constructed by using 2 interconnected cryostats with an opening between them to permit clinical access to the patient during imaging. Depending on the procedure to be performed, the patient table may be positioned (**A**) along the axis of the imager or (**B**) perpendicular to this axis. (Courtesy of Schenck JF, Jolesz FA, Roemer PB, et al: Superconducting open-configuration MR imaging system for image-guided therapy. *Radiology* 195:805–814, 1995; Radiological Society of North America.)

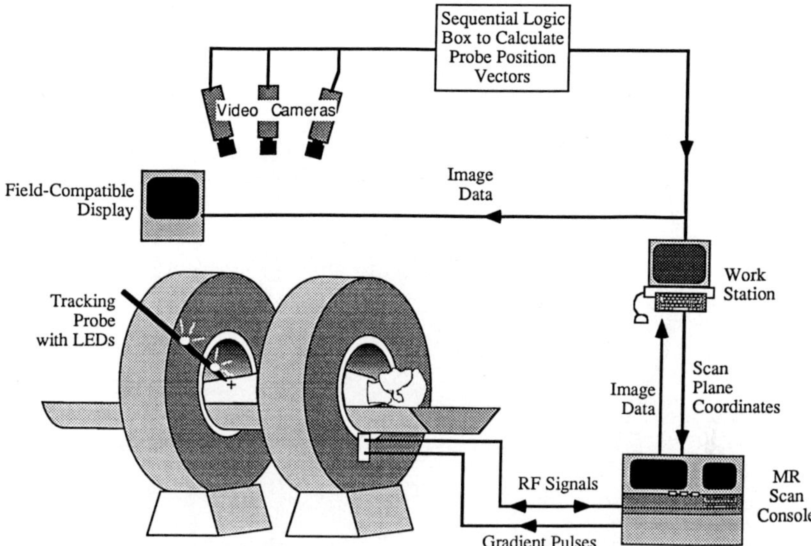

FIGURE 3.—Schema of interactive image control shows an open-magnet design that permits direct clinical access to the patient and simultaneous control of the MRI process. Light-emitting diodes on the probes are visualized by the television cameras and allow calculation of the 3-dimensional location of the probe tip. From within the magnet, the clinician can control the image plane and can view the resulting images on the field-compatible liquid crystal monitor. *Abbreviations: RF,* radio–frequency; *LEDs,* light-emitting diodes. (Courtesy of Schenck JF, Jolesz FA, Roemer PB, et al: Superconducting open-configuration MR imaging system for image-guided therapy. *Radiology* 195:805–814, 1995; Radiological Society of North America.)

allow interactive selection of the image plane (Fig 3). An operator of median height has ready access to the patient (Fig 5), and the patient may be imaged while sitting (Fig 6).

Application.—The magnet homogeneity was 12.3 ppm. The gradient field was linear to within 1% over an imaging area 30 cm in diameter. The signal/noise ratio was 10% greater than with a comparable 0.5-tesla superconducting device. Images were acquired of a number of anatomical regions using routine pulse sequences. In addition, fast gradient–recalled echo images were obtained at a rate of 1 every 1.5 sec. Within the 30–cm diameter region, images were comparable to or slightly better than those obtained using a conventional 0.5-tesla imager. A tracking technique using pulsed-gradient fields was used for real-time monitoring of the position of needles, catheters, drains, and the like. It was possible to display the coil position graphically by interleaving the coil-localizing pulse sequence with a conventional imaging sequence.

Conclusion.—This MR imager allows interactive image control and nearly real-time imaging rates while maintaining continuous direct contact with the patient.

▶ This is a revolutionary step for MRI and 1 that will propel the use of MR more deeply into interventional radiology. Success will depend on innovative

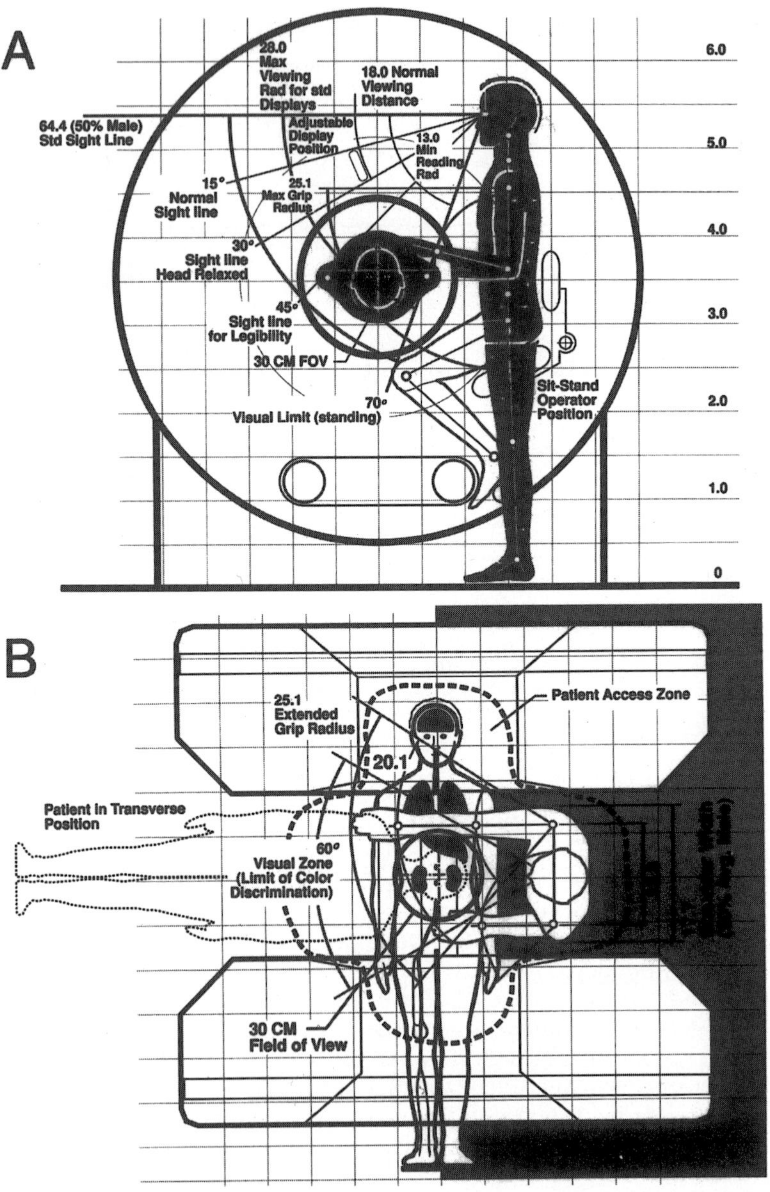

FIGURE 5.—Clinical access and working zones. Effective MRI is possible over a spherical volume, at the center of the magnet, approximately 30 cm in diameter. The clinician may stand or sit at the patient's side or head. Regions of the patient accessible to the vision and reach for a male operator of median height (48 inches) are shown for the (**A**) vertical and (**B**) horizontal planes. Values on the *y* axis are in feet. *Abbreviations: std,* standard; *FOV,* field of view. (Courtesy of Schenck JF, Jolesz FA, Roemer PB, et al: Superconducting open-configuration MR imaging system for image-guided therapy. *Radiology* 195:805–814, 1995; Radiological Society of North America.)

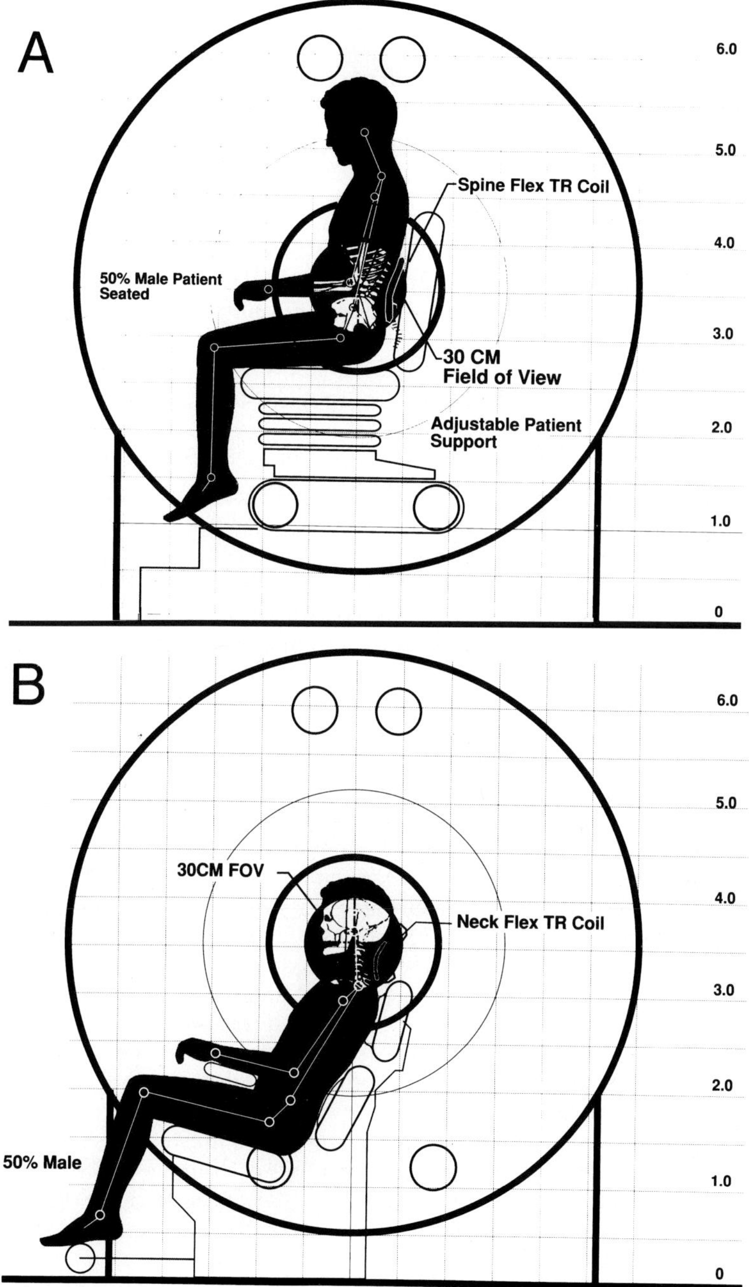

FIGURE 6.—Patient positioning options. Unlike conventional superconducting systems, spine images may be obtained in patients who are upright. Values on the *y* axis are in feet. **A,** lumbar spine may be imaged with the patient seated. It is also possible to image this region with the patient standing. **B,** if the sitting position is lowered, the cervical spine may also be imaged with the patient upright. *Abbreviations: TR,* recovery time; *FOV,* field of view. (Courtesy of Schenck JF, Jolesz FA, Roemer PB, et al: Superconducting open-configuration MR imaging system for image-guided therapy. *Radiology* 195:805–814, 1995; Radiological Society of North America.)

applications not only by radiologists but by surgeons as well. For this technology to gain widespread use, however, applications must be demonstrated in areas where conventional CT and ultrasonography cannot do an equally good job.

C.D. Maynard, M.D.

Participation by Radiologists and Other Specialists in Percutaneous Vascular and Nonvascular Interventions: Findings From a Seven-State Database

Levin DC, Flanders SJ, Spettell CM, et al (Jefferson Med College, Philadelphia; Athena Advanced Healthcare Solutions, Indianapolis, Ind)

Radiology 196:51–54, 1995 5–39

Introduction.—The performance of percutaneous interventions by nonradiologic specialists has been a matter of controversy for more than 10 years. Few data are available, however, on the extent to which nonradiologic specialists actually perform these procedures. A 1992 Medicare claims database from 7 states was used to determine the percentages of various types of percutaneous interventional procedures performed by both radiologists and other specialists.

Methods.—All Medicare Part B claims from 7 midwestern and southern states were analyzed for the study. Of approximately 70 million claims and $2.8 billion in Medicare physician reimbursements, 4% were related to radiology. Codes that do not pertain to the physical act of performing the procedure were excluded by analyzing only the surgical procedure codes. The assessed codes were in 4 broad categories: noncardiac percutaneous transluminal angioplasty (PTA), nonvascular percutaneous abdominal interventions, percutaneous genitourinary tract interventions, and non-vascular percutaneous thoracic interventions.

Results.—Radiologists performed the majority of all noncardiac PTAs (Table 1) and were well represented in all categories of surgical codes. They participated in 92.7% of renal cyst aspirations, 90.5% of biliary decompression procedures, 87.7% of abdominal or retroperitoneal biopsies, 84.2% of lung or mediastinal biopsies, and from 74% to 78% of noncardiac angioplasties, pancreatic biopsies, and upper urinary tract decompressions. Fewer radiologists were involved in liver biopsy (43.7%), renal biopsy (38.4%), certain types of abscess drainages (38.2%), and thoracentesis with tube insertion (29.4%). The role of radiologists was minimal in thoracenteses without tube insertion (4.7%) and in tube thoracostomy (1.7%).

Conclusion.—Radiologists clearly dominate in noncardiac PTA and in the percutaneous treatment of biliary and upper urinary tract obstruction. Participation in percutaneous biopsies was higher for pancreatic and abdominal or retroperitoneal biopsies than for liver and renal biopsies. Because instruction in percutaneous interventions is provided almost

TABLE 1.—Percentage of Noncardiac Percutaneous Transluminal Angioplasties Performed by Radiologists and Other Specialists

Procedure Type and CPT-4 Code	No. of Procedures	Specialty Group Radiologists	Cardiologists	Surgeons	Others
Lower extremity angioplasty	3,123	2,302 (73.7)	417 (13.4)	315 (10.1)	89 (2.8)
Tibioperoneal trunk PTA 35470					
Aortic PTA 35472					
Iliac PTA 35473					
Femoropopliteal PTA 35474					
Renal PTA 35471	453	350 (77.3)	64 (14.1)	35 (7.7)	4 (0.9)
Venous PTA 35476	568	510 (89.8)	3 (0.5)	53 (9.3)	2 (0.4)
Brachiocephalic PTA 35475	184	163 (88.6)	14 (7.6)	6 (3.3)	1 (0.5)
All Noncardiac PTA	4,328	3,325 (76.8)	498 (11.5)	409 (9.5)	96 (2.2)

Note: Numbers in parentheses are percentages.
Abbreviation: CPT-4, Common Procedural Terminology version 4.
(Courtesy of Levin DC, Flanders SJ, Spettell CM, et al: Participation by radiologists and other specialists in percutaneous vascular and nonvascular interventions: Findings from a seven-state database. *Radiology* 196:51–54, 1995; Radiological Society of North America.)

solely by radiology departments, there is concern that physicians in other disciplines may not be properly trained.

▶ This study confirms the primary role of radiologists in the area of noncardiac vascular and nonvascular interventional procedures. Impetus for this role has been gained by the introduction of such procedures into diagnostic radiology training programs and the existence for many years of fellowship programs in radiology departments to train individuals in the performance of these procedures. Further evidence that these procedures are truly in the domain of radiology was provided by 2 recent actions. The Accreditation Council on Graduate Medical Education agreed to accredit training programs in this area of radiology, and the American Board of Medical Specialties voted to allow the American Board of Radiology to issue Certificates of Added Qualification in vascular and interventional procedures.

C.D. Maynard, M.D.

6 Neuroradiology

Introduction

It was a very productive year for the neurosciences in general. As we move through the midportion of the "Decade of the Brain," we seem to be undergoing a "midlife crisis" of sorts. Much of our effort in imaging has been spent in refinements of MRI, which is a very mature technology. Many exciting new pulse sequence strategies have been developed, and MR angiography (MRA) and spectroscopy (MRS) continue to advance. Yet, despite this, we need to re-evaluate the role of CT, and we revisit many classic conditions—albeit with the "twist" of better image quality or vastly larger patient populations.

Some of our advances are heavily predicated on other specialties. For example, the neuropathologists of the World Health Organization gave us a better understanding of CNS neoplasms with their 1993 revision of the classification system. This allowed us to report on newly established tumor entities, such as dysembryoplastic neuroectodermal tumors and hemangiopericytomas. Lastly, much effort has gone into the evaluation of neurodegenerative disorders (both inherited and inflammatory), and interest has been renewed in cerebrovascular diseases (CVD) and screening methods for CVD.

James G. Smirniotopoulos, M.D.

Primary and Secondary Brain and Spinal Cord Neoplasms

Intracranial Subependymomas: CT and MR Imaging Features in 24 Cases

Chiechi MV, Smirniotopoulos JG, Jones RV (Armed Forces Inst of Pathology, Washington DC; Georgetown Univ, Washington, DC)

AJR 165:1245–1250, 1995 6–1

Introduction.—The term "subependymoma" denotes a tumor of the fourth ventricle that grows slowly and often is discovered incidentally at autopsy in elderly men. It is important to identify these lesions preoperatively, inasmuch as they reportedly do not recur after being totally resected. Subependymomas appear to be radiosensitive tumors.

Objective.—The CT and MR findings were reviewed in 24 patients, 17 men and 7 women with an average age of 48 years, who had a pathologically confirmed intracranial subependymoma and related symptoms.

Findings.—Eighteen of the 24 tumors were 3 cm or more in their largest dimension. Fourteen masses were in the lateral ventricle, and 13 of them at least partially obstructed 1 or both foramina of Monro. These tumors appeared to be attached to the septum pellucidim. Four of the 6 smaller lesions were in the fourth ventricle. All but 3 of the 24 patients had hydrocephalus, which in 16 cases was moderate or severe. The CT densities varied but most lesions in the lateral ventricle were hypodense. Only 1 of 10 tumors at this site enhanced appreciably. All lateral ventricular tumors were hypointense relative to cortical gray matter on T1-weighted MR images. Four of 6 fourth ventricular tumors also were hypointense. All lateral ventricular masses were hyperintense on T2-weighted images. Tumors in the posterior fossa were heterogeneously enhanced by contrast injection, whereas most lateral ventricular masses showed minimal if any enhancement.

Conclusions.—A lack of calcification and appreciable contrast enhancement permits subependymomas of the lateral ventricle to be distinguished from other tumors at this site. Fourth ventricular subependymomas, however, are not as readily identified.

▶ This the first report in the radiology literature of a series of patients with the subependymoma (SEP) variant of ependymoma. Although this variant is well known as a typically asymptomatic mass of the fourth ventricle, its occurrence within the lateral ventricle is uncommonly noted. The authors present the findings of 24 cases, all symptomatic. An unusual, and unexplained, observation is the difference between the characteristics of this lesion when it appears above, vs. below, the tentorium cerebelli. Lateral ventricular subependymomas were found to be noncalcified lesions without significant contrast enhancement, yet those of the fourth ventricle commonly enhanced and showed both radiologic and pathologic calcification.

J.G. Smirniotopoulos, M.D.

Computerized Tomography: Guided Stereotactic Surgery for Brainstem Masses: A Risk-Benefit Analysis in 71 Patients

Rajshekhar V, Chandy MJ (Christian Med College and Hosp, Vellore, India)

J Neurosurg 82:976–981, 1995 6–2

Objective.—The ability of MR imaging to precisely delineate brainstem lesions without the artifacts that make CT problematic has led some to question whether all brainstem masses have to be verified histologically. The benefits and risks of a policy of CT-guided stereotactic surgery for all intrinsic brainstem masses were examined.

Series.—Seventy-one patients seen in the years 1987–1993 with isolated masses intrinsic to the brainstem underwent 72 CT-guided stereotactic procedures. The patients ranged in age from 2.5 to 67 years, but nearly three fourths were younger than 18 years of age.

Methods.—All patients had contrast CT studies preoperatively, and 16 patients had MR imaging as well. Local anesthesia was used for 12 of the 72 procedures. Most often a precoronal burr hole was used for entry. A 1.2-mm-diameter sheath was passed to the target, and 1 mm^3 of tissue was obtained with a cup forceps when biopsy was indicated. Cystic masses were gently aspirated.

Results.—A large majority of the masses were diffuse, and 62% of them were contrast enhanced. All but 1 of the 69 biopsies were positive. Benign masses including tuberculomas and epidermoid cysts were discovered in 9 patients. In 8 cases it was possible to aspirate fluid from a cystic mass, and this was clinically beneficial to 4 patients with benign lesions and 2 with neoplasms. In all, 13 patients (18%) were thought to have benefited from the procedure. Benign lesions were most frequent in patients having focal or ring-enhancing masses. One patient deteriorated neurologically after surgery, but there were no treatment-related deaths.

Conclusions.—Image-guided stereotactic biopsy is indicated as the initial approach to most patients having intrinsic brainstem masses. The risk is minimal. All focal and enhancing masses should be evaluated histologically. Diffuse, hypodense, non-enhancing masses should be examined by gadolinium-enhanced MR imaging.

▶ The use of brainstem biopsy for treatment decision-making in brainstem lesions is controversial. Because of the potential for significant morbidity, therapeutic decisions may be based on clinical and imaging findings alone, without histologic confirmation. Therapy for suspected high-grade gliomas usually includes radiation treatments. The trend toward fewer biopsies has been advanced by refinements in imaging technique and diagnostic analysis. This paper, an analysis of 71 patients who had biopsies with CT stereotactic guidance, suggests a compelling re-evaluation of the need for brainstem biopsy. In addition, stereotactic aspiration of the cystic component of some lesions had a therapeutic effect in diminishing the volume of these lesions. The authors conclude: "The main value...lies in the identification of benign masses in a significant proportion of patients..."

J.G. Smirniotopoulos, M.D.

Intracranial Metastatic Melanoma: Correlation Between MR Imaging Characteristics and Melanin Content

Isiklar I, Leeds NE, Fuller GN, et al (Univ of Texas, Houston)
AJR 165:1503–1512, 1995 6–3

Objective.—It has been suggested that patients with melanoma who have melanotic vs. amelanotic brain metastases can be distinguished by analysis of specific MRI patterns. This hypothesis was tested in a large series of patients with melanoma, including correlation with the findings of surgically resected metastases.

Methods.—The retrospective study included 30 patients with histologically confirmed intracerebral melanoma. The MRI findings were classified into 4 patterns: a melanotic pattern, with hyperintense lesions in relation to cortex on T1-weighted images; an amelanotic pattern, with lesions that were hypointense or isointense in relation to cortex; an indeterminate or mixed pattern; and a hematoma pattern.

Results.—Of 52 lesions identified, 10 were classified as melanotic, 16 as amelanotic, 11 as indeterminate, and 5 as hematoma. Seventy percent of the lesions with a melanotic pattern included more than 10% melanin-containing cells. Fifty-six percent of those with an amelanotic pattern contained histologically identifiable melanin, but never in more than 10% of cells. The lesions in the indeterminate group were either amelanotic or contained less than 10% melanotic cells.

Conclusions.—In patients with melanoma, few intracranial metastases demonstrated the MRI pattern linked to melanotic melanoma. The MRI pattern previously linked to amelanotic melanoma is nonspecific, because melanin can be found in most lesions showing this imaging pattern.

► Thirty patients with intracerebral melanoma were reviewed, looking for the melanotic pattern (bright on T1, dark on T2 compared to cortex). In this series, 7 of 10 patients with the melanotic pattern had more than 10% melanin-containing cells; 7 of 8 patients with more than 10% melanin-containing cells had the expected melanotic pattern of signal intensity. However, 9 of 16 patients without this pattern also had some melanin (but in less than 10% of cells) and only 6 of 13 without melanin had the amelanotic pattern. Thus, although here is some correlation, interpretation of the presence or absence of the melanotic pattern should be made circumspectly.

J.G. Smirniotopoulos, M.D.

Pineoblastoma in Adults

Chang SM, Lillis-Hearne PK, Larson DA, et al (Univ of California, San Francisco; Brook Army Med Ctr, Fort Sam Houston, Tex)
Neurosurgery 37:383–391, 1995 6–4

Introduction.—Tumors of the pineal region are 10 times more frequent in children than adults. In adults, pineocytomas and pineoblastomas—the latter being more malignant and less differentiated—account for less than 15% of pineal region tumors. Pineoblastomas are classified and treated as supratentorial primitive neuroectodermal tumors (PNETS). A series of adult patients with pineoblastomas are reported in whom the entire neuraxis was staged at diagnosis.

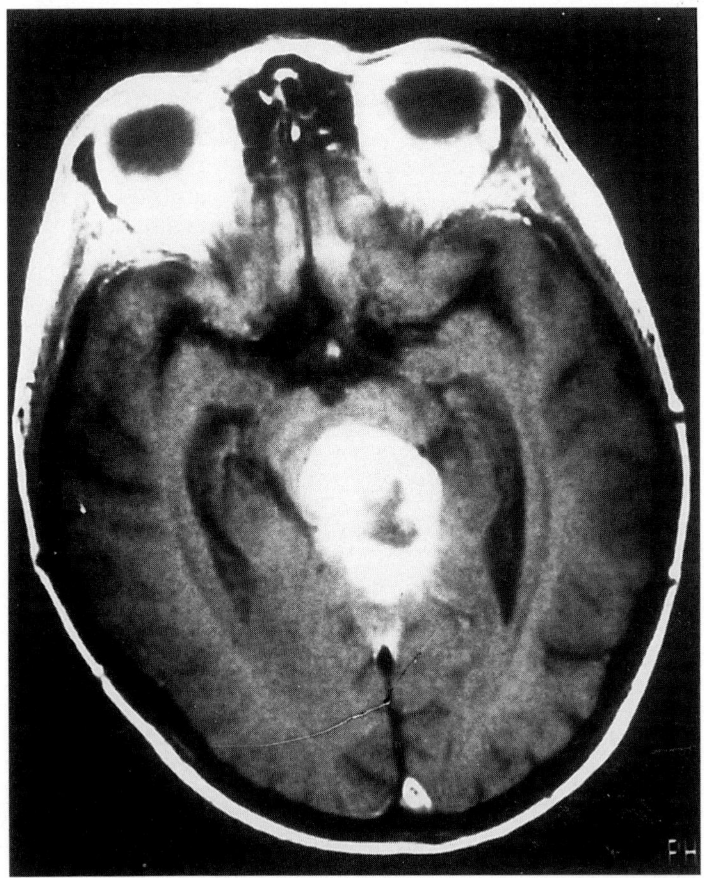

FIGURE 1.—Gadolinium-enhanced axial MR image of the brain, showing a large enhancing mass in the pineal region at the time of diagnosis in patient 4. (Courtesy of Chang SM, Lillis-Hearne PK, Larson DA, et al: Pineoblastoma in adults. *Neurosurgery* 37:383–391, 1995.)

Patients.—Eleven patients older than 16 years of age with histologically proven pineoblastoma were seen during a 17-year period at 1 center. They were identified from a series of 54 patients with tumors of the pineal region. Nine patients had pineoblastomas and 2 had mixed pineocytoma and pineoblastoma. All had obstructive hydrocephalus at presentation. The initial staging included spinal MRI in 9 patients, myelography in 1, and CSF examination in 10. Focal tumors were present in 5 patients and disseminated disease in 4. Two patients had spinal metastases apparent on MRI but no tumor cells in the CSF, and 2 had tumor cells in the CSF but a normal MRI scan or myelogram. Because of the supratentorial location of their tumors, all patients were considered poor risks. The 5 patients with disseminated disease at diagnosis all had recurrent disease develop

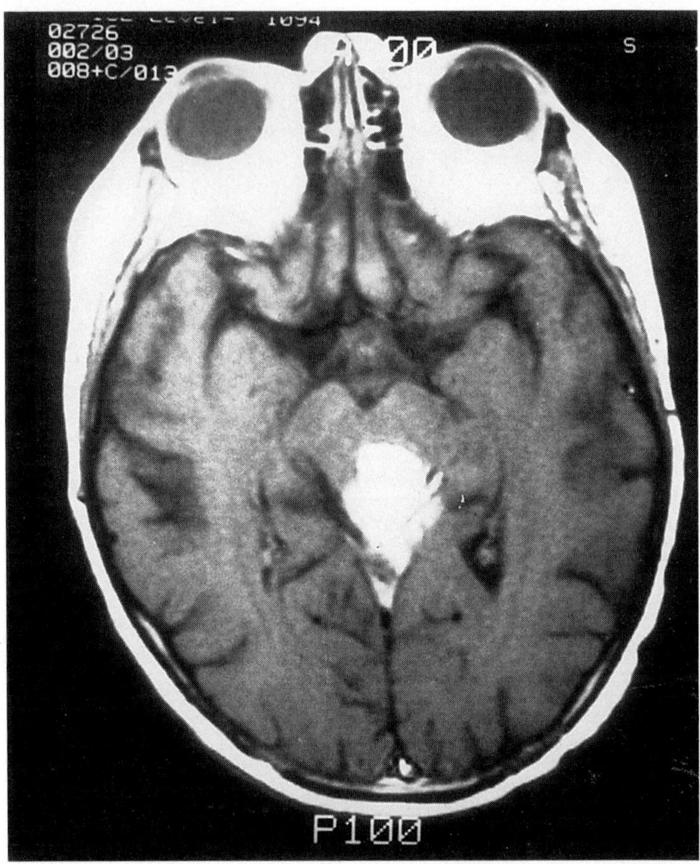

FIGURE 2.—Magnetic resonance image of the brain after craniospinal irradiation, showing a decrease in the enhancing mass in patient 4. (Courtesy of Chang SM, Lillis-Hearne PK, Larson DA, et al: Pineoblastoma in adults. *Neurosurgery* 37:383–391, 1995.)

within 8 to 49 months. In contrast, the 5 patients with negatively staged pineoblastoma were all alive and progression free at a median follow-up of 26 months.

Conclusions.—The first study of adult pineoblastoma to include complete neuraxial staging at the time of diagnosis suggests that the extent of disease at that time is a major prognostic factor. Staging should include a CSF examination as well as spinal MRI. Because pineal parenchyma tumors are so rare, their histologic, biological, and clinical features are not fully defined. They are prone to wide metastasis throughout the CSF pathways, like other PNETs. The benefits of craniospinal irradiation followed by systemic chemotherapy remain unclear (Figs 1 and 2).

► We normally consider that PNETs are seen only in children. However, up to one third of cerebellar PNETs (medulloblastomas) will be diagnosed in patients between 15 and 30 years of age. Now, we must add another type of PNET to the list of those that develop in adults—pineoblastomea. The authors did not attempt to discern diagnostic criteria for these lesions; indeed, by reporting the adult presentation of pineoblastoma, they have deleted 1 of the criteria formerly used to exclude this lesion, i.e., the patients age. As would be expected, metastatic disease at the time of presentation was an ominous sign, and, the authors have recommended that all patients have adequate evaluation of the spine and CSF.

J.G. Smirniotopoulos, M.D.

Proton Magnetic Resonance Spectroscopy in Patients With Glial Tumors: A Multicenter Study

Negendank WG, Sauter R, Brown TR, et al (Fox Chase Cancer Ctr, Philadelphia; Wayne State Univ, Detroit; Mallinkrodt Inst, St Louis, Mo; et al)
J Neurosurg 84:449–458, 1996 6–5

Background.—Histopathologic and molecular biological study of brain tumors may provide prognostically relevant information. Proton ^{1}H-nuclear MR (NMR) spectroscopy has been used to study the metabolic function of brain tumors. So far, attempts at using ^{1}H-MR spectroscopy to distinguish grades of glial tumors have had problems with variation and overlap. A cooperative group using identical acquisition techniques was formed to assess the use of in vivo metabolic imaging with ^{1}H-MR spectroscopy to characterize glial brain tumors.

Methods.—Fifteen eligible institutions using similar equipment provided blinded, centralized MR spectroscopy data on patients with glial tumors. The analysis included independent central review of MR spectroscopy voxel placement, composition and contamination by brain, histopathologic typing according to current World Health Organization criteria, and clinical data. All proton ^{1}H-MR spectroscopic studies were performed using a spin-echo technique to obtain spectra from 8-cc voxels in the tumor. When possible, spectra were obtained from the contralateral brain as well. Data from the contralateral brain were available in 41 of the 86 assessable patients.

Results.—Compared with normal brain tissue, the glial tumors showed significantly elevated intensities of choline signals, decreased intensities of creatine signals, and decreased intensities of *N-acetylaspartate*. Astrocytomas and anaplastic astrocytomas had the highest choline signal intensities, whereas glioblastomas had the lowest creatine signal intensities. Great variation was noted within each glial tumor subtype, whether expressed relative to brain or as within-tumor ratios. Because of these overlaps, the technique could not accurately differentiate between low-and high-grade tumors. Voxel contamination by brain tissue significantly affected the metabolite concentrations and ratios, but the overlaps were still present on analysis of cases with minimal contamination. Whereas lactate was an infrequent finding that occurred in all tumor grades, mobile lipids were found in 41% of high-grade tumors. The mean amounts of lactate were higher in glioblastomas.

Conclusions.—The findings of a standard ^{1}H-MR spectroscopic technique in patients with glial tumors are evaluated. The various types and grades of glial tumors appear to be metabolically heterogeneous, and the technique cannot distinguish between high- and low-grade tumors. However, this and other recent studies suggest that the ^{1}H-MR spectroscopic in vivo finding of mobile lipids may be an independent prognostic factor in individual patients.

▶ This article was a multicenter review of the utility of proton H-MR spectroscopy in grading glial tumors. As with many other studies of MR spectroscopy, the limitations included a relatively large voxel size (8 cc), which allowed frequent contamination of tumor signal by brain. As in several previous small reports, there was a correlation between elevated choline signal and an associated decrease in creatine and *N*-acetylaspartate compared to normal brain. Although these trends were greatest in glioblastomas, there was considerable variation, which limited the ability to predict tumor grade. However, mobile lipids occurred in almost half (41%) of high-grade tumors. These mobile lipids appear to reflect microscopic tumor necrosis, which is a histologic hallmark of glioblastoma multiforme. The authors have suggested that the presence of mobile lipids on MR spectroscopy may have predictive value in patients' survival.

J.G. Smirniotopoulos, M.D.

MR Imaging of Myxopapillary Ependymoma: Findings and Value to Determine Extent of Tumor and Its Relation to Intraspinal Structures

Wippold FJ II, Smirniotopoulos JG, Moran CJ, et al (Washington Univ, St Louis, Mo; Uniformed Services Univ, Bethesda, Md; Armed Forces Inst of Pathology, Washington, DC; et al)

AJR 165:1263–1267, 1995 6–6

Purpose.—Myxopapillary ependymomas are highly vascular tumors that cause such symptoms and signs as back pain and lower extremity radiculopathy. These are similar to the findings in patients with disk disease, and because of this, the correct diagnosis may be delayed. An MRI study of myxopapillary ependymoma is reported.

Methods.—The retrospective study included 20 patients with 24 confirmed myxopapillary ependymomas. Magnetic resonance imaging studies from these patients were analyzed to determine the typical MRI features of these tumors and the value of MRI in identifying the tumor, evaluating its extent, and assessing its relationship to intraspinal structures.

Results.—All patients had masses detected on MRI—solitary masses in 17 patients and multiple lesions in 3. Twenty-one of the 24 lesions appeared as predominantly intradural extramedullary masses, 2 as intramedullary masses, and 1 as an extradural postsacral mass. The most common site was the level of the L2 vertebral body, and the tumors spanned an average of 4 vertebral segments; none extended above the T9 level. Expansion of the spinal canal was noted in most tumors extending over 5 or more vertebral segments, and 2 tumors extended into the neural foramina. The T1-weighted sequences showed an isointense tumor signal in 12 patients, a hypointense signal in 3 patients, and a hyperintense signal in 1 patient. All tumors were hyperintense on T2-weighted sequences, and all enhanced after contrast administration.

Conclusions.—Magnetic resonance imaging can detect myxopapillary ependymomas, evaluate the extent of these tumors, and define their relationship to intraspinal structures. The findings are not specific, but the presence of a large, intensely enhancing, intradural extramedullary thoracolumbar mass extending across several vertebral levels suggests the diagnosis of myxopapillary ependymoma. In this situation, the complete MRI examination should include the entire thoracolumbar region and IV contrast administration.

► Myxopapillary ependymoma is the most common mass of the conus medullaris/cauda equina region of the spinal cord. However, the imaging characteristics are nonspecific. The myxopapillary type of ependymoma, because of its hypervascularity, commonly has imaging characteristics that include evidence of blood breakdown products. Thus, T1 and T2 shortening are common. The lesions are often extensive on initial presentation and may span several vertebral segments.

J.G. Smirniotopoulos, M.D.

MR of Malignant Optic Glioma of Adulthood

Millar WS, Tartaglino LM, Sergott RC, et al (Thomas Jeffeson Univ, Philadelphia; Wills Eye Hosp, Philadelphia)

AJNR 16:1673–1676, 1995 6–7

Objective.—The initial clinical presentation of malignant optic glioma in adults can mimic that of optic neuritis. A case of malignant optic glioma of adulthood is reported, focusing on the MRI findings.

Man, 60, was evaluated for a 3-week history of blurred vision in his right eye. Magnetic resonance images revealed nonspecific enlargement and enhancement of the optic nerve, suggesting the diagnosis of optic neuritis. Medial decompression orbitotomy was performed after the patient failed to respond to IV steroids. Six weeks later, vision in the right eye decreased dramatically, with central retinal artery occlusion. Another course of IV steroids was given; MRI showed no change in the right optic nerve abnormality. Six months later, when mildly decreased visual acuity of the left eye developed, MRI scans revealed a large mass involving both optic nerves and the optic chiasm, with invasion of the hypothalamus and seeding of the ependyma. Anaplastic astrocytoma was diagnosed on excisional biopsy of the right optic nerve. The patient died of progressive tumor 5 months later.

Discussion.—In malignant optic glioma of adulthood, the signs suggestive of an intraorbital mass are either absent or appear late in the clinical course. Magnetic resonance imaging thus takes on a major role in early diagnosis. If the diagnosis of malignant optic glioma of adulthood is considered, it may alter the course of this rapidly progressive, fatal malignancy.

► Optic nerve disease in adults is usually not a glioma, but acute optic neuritis (which may be "proven" by a response to corticosteroids).

Optic pathway gliomas in children are usually low grade, and associated with neurofibromatosis type 1. Adult optic gliomas are rare (30 cases reported since 1900), without association with neurofibromatosis, and a mean age of 52 years.

J.G. Smirniotopoulos, M.D.

Development of Intracranial Meningiomas at the Site of Cranial Fractures: Remarks on 15 Cases

Artico M, Cervoni L, Carloia S, et al (Univ of Rome)

Acta Neurochir (Wien) 136:132–134, 1995 6–8

Background.—Trauma as a cause of tumor, especially meningioma and glioma, is controversial. Fifteen patients with posttraumatic intracranial meningioma were reviewed to address the possible correlation between trauma and tumor onset.

Patients and Findings.—The patients were selected for review using previously published criteria. The patients were 9 men and 6 women aged 13 to 69 years. All patients had had head trauma characterized by a loss of consciousness and bone fracture on plain films and CT scans. The causes of trauma included motor vehicle accidents, domestic accidents, and blows to the head from a hammer, pickaxe, stick, and falling roof tile. The interval between trauma and the onset of tumor ranged from 4 to 45 years, with a mean of 4 years. Meningioma occurred most frequently in the cerebral convexity. Complete tumor removal was possible in all patients. Eleven tumors were World Health Organization histologic grade I; 3, grade II; and 1, grade III. Mean follow-up was 15 years, with a range of 5 to 40 years. Four patients died of unrelated causes. The 11 survivors are currently in good neurologic condition.

Conclusions.—Head trauma may contribute to the development of meningioma in some patients. Both neuroradiologic and macroscopic findings indicated that the meningioma occurred at the same site as the trauma in the patients reviewed. Moreover, the trauma produced a bone fracture near the suture in all of these patients.

▶ Trauma has frequently been cited as a putative cause for intracranial meningiomas, although this theory is often challenged. This paper reviews 37 cases (3%) of patients with a history of trauma, culled from 1,109 patients with meningioma, treated between 1951 and 1988. Trauma was believed to be an etiologic factor in 15 (1%) patients with meningioma. The authors of this series were careful to include only those patients in whom the trauma was significant, localized (and documented) near the site of the meningioma, and where the interval between trauma and tumor was "significant."

J.G. Smirniotopoulos, M.D.

Dysembryoplastic Neuroepithelial Tumors: MR and CT Evaluation

Ostertun B, Wolf HK, Campos MG, et al (Univ of Bonn, Germany)

AJNR 17:419–430, 1996 6–9

Background.—Dysembryoplastic neuroepithelial tumor (DNT) is a benign multinodular lesion with glial and neuronal elements, which has several features in common with gangliogliomas and glioneuronal malformations. The MRI and CT findings in 16 patients were reviewed to identify criteria distinguishing DNT from gangliogliomas and glioneuronal malformations.

Methods.—The records of 16 patients with DNT who underwent surgery during a 7-year period were reviewed, including the CT scans for 10 patients and the MRI studies of all 16 patients. Six of the patients underwent 2 or more CT or MR studies between 1.5 and 13 years before undergoing surgery.

Results.—The DNT locations were in the temporal lobe in 14 of the patients and in the frontal lobe in 2 patients. All of the patients had cortical involvement, and 10 also had subcortical white matter involvement. There were signal abnormalities in the MRI studies of all 16 patients. In 9 patients, the DNTs were seen as space-occupying lesions, whereas there was no mass effect in the remaining 7 patients. The lesion margins were sharp in 8 patients and poorly defined in 8 patients. All of the DNTs had inhomogeneous signal intensities, consistent with a cystic or semiliquid structure. Solid components were detected in 11 tumors. The CT scans in 10 patients revealed sharp margins on 9 lesions and poorly defined margins on 1 lesion. Tumor density was homogeneous in 4 patients and inhomogeneous in 6 patients. There was a mass effect in 7 patients. Six patients had hypodense areas resembling CSF, suggesting cyst-like lesions. Of the 6 patients with serial preoperative CT or MR studies, there was evidence of significant change in the DNT in 2 patients, which revealed growth of a calcified tumor area in 1 patient and growth and extension of the cystic tumor parts in the other patient.

Conclusions.—Dysembryoplastic neuroepithelial tumors may be differentiated from gangliogliomas and glioneuronal malformations by their multicystic appearance on MRI studies. This appearance corresponds to the multinodular architecture and the myxoid matrix of these lesions.

▶ This paper evaluates DNTs and is another study that shows they are all intracortical lesions, with 14 of 16 occurring in the temporal lobes. Seizures are the most likely presentation (or do we only find the ones causing seizures). The lesions were of predominantly low attenuation on CT and high signal on T2-weighted MR—presumbably from the myxoid matrix of these tumors. Contrast enhancement was reported in 6 cases and 2 of these showed lesion progression over time. However, in this series, none of the lesions was associated with calvarial changes, and 1 lesion had prominent calcifications.

J.G. Smirniotopoulos, M.D.

Radiologic Appearance of the Dysembryoplastic Neuroepithelial Tumor

Kuroiwa T, Bergey GK, Rothman MI, et al (Univ of Maryland, Baltimore)

Radiology 197:233–238, 1995 6–10

Objective.—Patients with dysembryoplastic neuroepithelial tumor (DNT) usually have intractable partial complex seizures. Because this benign tumor can be confused with astrocytoma and mixed oligoastrocytoma, recognition of its characteristics is important to avoid unnecessary radiation or chemotherapeutic treatment. The MR and CT radiologic features of DNT were reviewed and compared.

Methods.—The records of 10 DNT patients (5 men), aged 2 to 43 years, with intractable seizures, were retrospectively reviewed. Computed tomography of 5- and 10-mm-thick sections was performed before surgery on 6 patients, including contrast-enhanced studies in 4, and MR imaging was performed on all 10 patients, including gadolinium enhanced studies in 7.

Results.—Clinical summaries and radiologic findings were tabulated. Tumors were found in the frontal lobe in 4 patients, the parietal lobe in 2, and the temporal lobe in 4 with hippocampal involvement in 2. Computed tomography visualized a low attenuation mass in all cases except 1. The T1 weighted MR images of DNT had decreased signal intensity, whereas T2 weighted images demonstrated increased signal intensity. "Thick gyriform" or "nodular" findings were observed on both T1- and T2-weighted images of all 10 patients. No peritumoral edema was found. In 8 of 10 patients, lobular tumor margins were well demarcated on T2-weighted images. The CT scans of 4 of 6 patients (67%) and MR images of 6 of 10 patients (60%) showed thinning of the adjacent calvaria.

Conclusion.—An accurate diagnosis of DNT may be difficult using imaging modalities alone, but the radiologic features described may serve to distinguish DNT from other gliomas.

► The DNT is a newly accepted intracortical neoplasm of childhood. These lesions are often associated with seizures and present the opportunity for surgical cure. This review of 10 patients confirms the findings in previous reports that the lesions are typically superficial and often intracortical (100%); they increase water content (low attenuation on CT, high signal intensity on T2-weighted MR) present a high incidence of scalloped remodeling of the inner table of the skull (60%); and, occasionally the lesions may enhance (2 of 7).

J.G. Smirniotopoulos, M.D.

Phakomatoses

Neurofibromatosis Type 1: Pathologic Substrate of High-Signal-Intensity Foci in the Brain

DiPaolo DP, Zimmerman RA, Rorke LB, et al (Children's Hosp of Philadelphia)
Radiology 195:721–724, 1995 6–11

Objective.—Patients with neurofibromatosis type 1 (NF-1), also known as von Recklinghausen disease, have several different types of intracranial lesions. The most common type is high-signal intensity foci observed on long repetition time (TR) MRI scans. These lesions are assumed to be nonneoplastic, but no definitive radiologic-pathologic correlation has been established. The radiologic and necropsy findings of 3 patients with NF-1 with these characteristic lesions were compared.

Methods.—The study included 3 girls—two 10-year-olds and 1 newborn—with NF-1 and abnormal hyperintense lesions on long TR images of the brain. The 2 older girls had the classic hyperintensities of the internal capsules and globus pallidus, whereas the newborn had diffuse white matter hyperintensities of the supratentorial and infratentorial regions. All patients underwent necropsy after death, and the radiologic and pathologic findings of the high signal intensity foci were correlated.

Results.—The high signal intensity areas proved to represent areas of spongiform myelinopathy or vacuolar myelin change. The absence of stainable material suggested that this tissue was filled with water during life. Areas appearing as large lesions on long TR images appeared to represent a coalescence of smaller vacuoles.

Conclusions.—A radiologic-pathologic correlation of the characteristic hyperintense foci seen on T2-weighted MRI scans in patients with NF-1 is presented. These lesions correspond to areas of consistent intramyelinic spongiotic or vacuolar change. The vacuoles are probably filled with fluid during life, which explains why the lesions appear as high signal intensity areas on T2-weighted scans.

► For several years, we have seen the unidentified bright objects (UBOs) of neurofibromatosis type 1 (von Recklinghausen disease). However, until now, the nature of these lesions has eluded rigorous analysis. This article suggests that the majority of these T2 hyperintensities represents "intramyelinic edema" and that the T1 hyperintensities are due to the well-known (but seemingly paradoxical) effect of microcalcifications.

J.G. Smirniotopoulos, M.D.

Spinal Tumors in Patients With Neurofibromatosis Type 2: MR Imaging Study of Frequency, Multiplicity, and Variety

Mautner V-F, Tatagiba M, Lindenau M, et al (Allgemeines Krankenhaus Hamburg Ochsenzoll, Germany; Nordstadtkrankenhaus Hannover, Germany; Hamburg-Othmarschen MRI Inst, Germany; et al)

AJR 165:951–955, 1995 6–12

Background.—Neurofibromatosis type 2 (NF2), a rare autosomal dominant disorder, results in various CNS tumors. Vestibular schwannomas are the hallmark of the disease. Patients with a single symptomatic spinal tumor sometimes have multiple asymptomatic spinal lesions. The frequency, multiplicity, and variety of spinal tumors in patients with NF2 were reported.

Methods.—Seventy-three patients with NF2 underwent MR imaging of the whole spinal canal. The patients' ages ranged from 4 to 69 years. Nineteen patients had a total of 22 histologically proven spinal tumors.

Findings.—Eighty-nine percent of the patients showed evidence of spinal tumors on MR images. Intramedullary tumors were seen on MR in 23

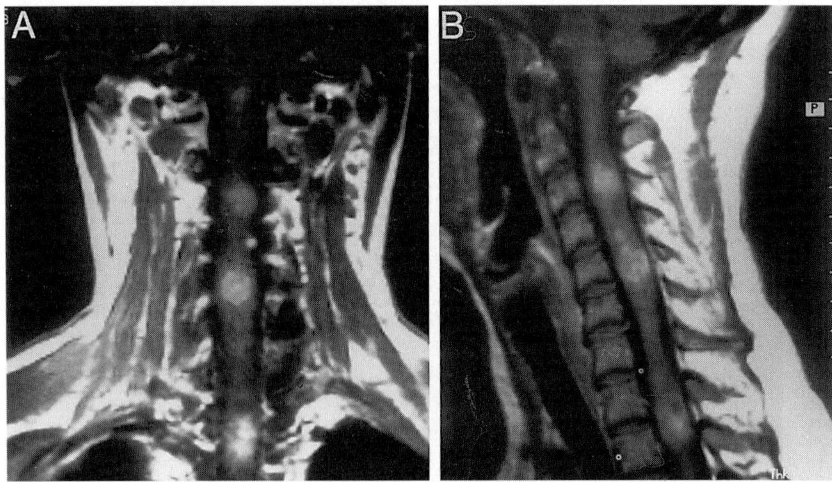

FIGURE 3.—Presumed astrocytomas. A 31-year-old woman with atactic gait disturbance. **A,** T1-weighted coronal MR image (SE500/15 [TR/TE]) shows 3 intramedullary masses with intense contract enhancement centrally and diffuse contrast enhancement peripherally. **B,** T1-weighted sagittal MR image (SE 500/15) confirms intramedullary localization of contrast-enhancing tumors up to upper thoracic spine. Multiple intramedullary tumors are a feature of neurofibromatosis type 2. (Courtesy of Mautner V-F, Tatagiba M, Lindenau M, et al: Spinal tumors in patients with neurofibromatosis type 2: MR imaging study of frequency, multiplicity, and variety. *AJR* 165:951–955, 1995.)

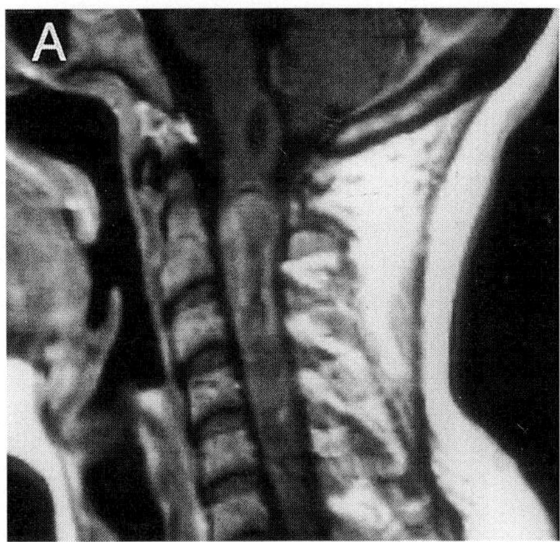

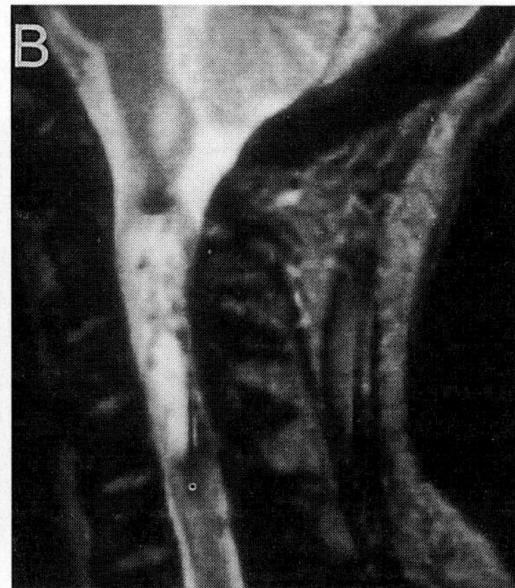

FIGURE 4.—Histopathologically proven ependymoma. A 42-year-old woman with intractable neck pain. **A,** T1-weighted sagittal MR image (SE 500/15 [TR/TE]) after administration of contrast material shows intramedullary tumor reaching from C1 to C4 with peripheral contrast enhancement and cystic tumor area reaching medulla oblongata. Spinal ependymomas belong to spectrum of neurofibromatosis type 2. **B,** flash 2-dimensional MR image (gradient-recalled echo 340/18, 18° flip angle) shows clear demarcation of nodular intramedullary tumor. Cranially and caudally, caplike black hemosiderin borders are visible. (Courtesy of Mautner V-F, Tatagiba M, Lindenau M, et al: Spinal tumors in patients with neurofibromatosis type 2: MR imaging study of frequency, multiplicity, and variety. *AJR* 165:951–955, 1995.)

patients (Fig 3), including 3 pathologically proven ependymomas. Extradural and intradural extramedullary tumors were seen on the cervical spine images of 36 patients, on thoracic spine images of 40, and on lumbar spine images of 49. These tumors were meningiomas, schwannomas, or neurofibromas, types that could not be differentiated by neuroradiologic findings. Ten schwannomas, 7 meningiomas, and 2 neurofibromas were proved pathologically. Imaging demonstrated extradural extramedullary tumors in the cervical spine of 12 patients, the thoracic spine of 5, and the lumbar spine of 18. Two patients had a syrinx associated with a tumor. Tumor type was confirmed by histologic assessment in 19 patients.

Conclusions.—Spinal tumors are common in patients with NF2. These tumors are often multiple and of a variety of histologic types. The presence of multiple spinal tumors of different pathologic types strongly suggests NF2. Detecting spinal tumors in patients who do not meet the diagnostic criteria for NF2 may enable the diagnosis in at-risk family members, thus permitting appropriate genetic counseling.

▶ This important paper demonstrates the need for adequate evaluation of the spine in patients with NF2. Neurofibromatosis type 2 is one tenth as common as von Recklinghausen disease (NF1) and was formerly called "central neurofibromatosis" because of the absence of cutaneous and spinal lesions. However, this classification is no longer valid. Skin lesions have been reported in NF2, and this paper now establishes the very high incidence (89%) of intraspinal masses. Unlike NF1, which is characterized by intra-axial tumors of the optic nerve and brain (astrocytomas), the intracranial lesions of NF2 are usually extra-axial, including the index lesions, bilateral vestibular schwannomas. Similarly, although both types of neurofibromatosis have nerve sheath tumors, the lesions of NF1 are neurofibromas, whereas those in NF2 are schwannomas. This article suggests that a patient with newly diagnosed NF2 would benefit from an initial screening examination of the spine (by MR), even if asymptomatic. Four types of intraspinal tumors were found: intramedullary gliomas (in this series all the pathologically proven lesions were ependymomas); and extramedullary schwannomas, meningiomas, and occasional neurofibromas. In contrast, in NF1, the overwhelming spinal burden is from extramedullary masses that are neurofibromas such that von Recklinghausen disease is a "true" neurofibromatosis. However, we are prompted to say that NF2 is not a "neurofibromatosis," but is rather the MISME syndrome (Multiple inherited schwannomas, meningiomas, and ependymomas).

J.G. Smirniotopoulos, M.D.

Brainstem Tumors in Patients With Neurofibromatosis Type 1: A Distinct Clinical Entity

Molloy PT, Bilaniuk LT, Vaughan SN, et al (Children's Hosp of Philadelphia)
Neurology 45:1897–1902, 1995 6–13

Background.—In patients with neurofibromatosis type 1 (NF1), brainstem tumors and other intracranial abnormalities can be detected by MRI. However, brainstem tumors may be confused with increased T2 signal abnormalities known as "unidentified bright objects" (UBOs), which are commonly observed in the brainstem of patients with NF1. Clinically, these tumors may be confused with non-NF1 brainstem tumors. Brainstem tumors in patients with NF1 are discussed as a distinct subtype of tumors.

Patients.—Seventeen NF1 patients with neuroimaging evidence of brainstem tumors—the largest such series studied to date—were analyzed. The mean follow-up period was 59 months. Eighty-eight percent of patients had neurologic manifestations of brainstem dysfunction, including dysarthria, cranial neuropathies, and gross motor incoordination. Eighty-two percent had tumors located mainly in the medulla, whereas patients without NF1 were more likely to have tumors in the pontine location. At diagnosis, 7 of the NF1 patients required shunt placement for hydrocephalus. Although radiographic signs of tumor progression were seen in 6 patients, clinical progression occurred in just 3.

Outcomes.—Partial surgical resection was performed in 2 patients with progressive symptoms. These tumors proved to be fibrillary or anaplastic astrocytomas. Of 3 patients treated with radiation therapy and/or chemotherapy, 2 died. Of the 15 survivors, 14 required no adjuvant therapy.

Conclusions.—Brainstem tumors occurring in patients with NF1 appear to be a distinct clinical entity. These tumors are much less aggressive than the pontine tumors observed in patients without NF1, but are more likely to cause symptoms than the brainstem UBOs that accompany NF1. Brainstem tumors in patients with NF1 should be managed conservatively, with close clinical and radiologic follow-up for progression.

► Neurofibromatosis type 1 (von Recklinghausen disease) causes multiple lesions that are histologically neoplastic. In NF1, many tumors behave in an indolent fashion, even though they may be multiple. True brainstem neoplasms should be distinguished from nonneoplastic lesions. However, this article emphasizes that pontine astrocytomas, although more symptomatic than brainstem UBOs, are "much less aggressive than non-NF1 pontine tumors."

J.G. Smirniotopoulos, M.D.

Epilepsy

Frequency and Characteristics of Dual Pathology in Patients With Lesional Epilepsy

Cendes F, Cook MJ, Watson C, et al (McGill Univ, Montreal; Natl Hosp for Neurology and Neurosurgery, London; Univ of California, Sacramento)
Neurology 45:2058–2064, 1995 6–14

Background.—Some patients with epilepsy have "dual pathology" i.e., coexistent mesial temporal sclerosis (MTS), which is neuronal loss and gliosis involving the hippocampus, along with extrahippocampal lesions. The contribution of the repetitive partial seizures and the extrahippocampal lesion to the development of hippocampus sclerosis remains unclear. A series of patients with partial epilepsy was studied to clarify the frequency and clinical characteristics of dual pathology.

Methods.—The study included 167 (87 females and 80 males, mean age 33 years) patients from 3 centers with temporal or extratemporal partial epilepsy and identifiable lesions. Forty-eight patients had neuronal migration disorders (NMDs), 52 had low-grade tumors, 34 had vascular malformations, 16 had porencephalic cysts, and 17 had gliotic lesions resulting from early cerebral insults. Each patient underwent MRI volumetric studies by using 1.5-or 3.0-mm coronal images to seek an atrophic hippocampal formation (HF), indicating dual pathology. The same imaging study was performed in 44 age-matched controls.

Results.—The MRI studies showed atrophic HF in 15% of patients. Seventeen percent of lesions involving temporal areas and 14% of lesions involving extratemporal areas had abnormal HF volumes. Hippocampal atrophy was frequently associated with febrile seizures of early childhood; it was unrelated to age at onset or duration of epilepsy. Only 9% of patients with vascular lesions and 2% of those with low-grade tumors had hippocampal atrophy, compared to 25% of patients with NMDs, 31% of those with porencephalic cysts, and 24% of those with reactive gliosis. The relationship between NMD and hippocampal atrophy was independent of the distances between the lesion and the HF. In contrast, for patients with vascular malformations and other lesions, dual pathology occurred when the lesion was close to the HF.

Conclusions.—Among patients with partial epilepsy, dual pathology is more frequent in those with certain types of lesions, namely NMD, porencephalic cysts, or reactive gliosis. These associations could arise from a common pathogenic mechanism during prenatal or perinatal development, such as associated developmental abnormalities or a predisposition to prolonged febrile convulsions. More study of patients with dual pathology is needed to clarify the pathogenesis of MTS and to improve planning for the surgical treatment of lesional epilepsies.

▶ This article serves as strong reminder that we must constantly search for "tandem lesions" in all patients. There has long been a debate about whether MTS can be a cause or an effect of a seizure disorder, or both. In this series of 167 patients with "identifiable lesions" as cause of seizures, 25 (15%) had MTS as a dual pathology or second lesion. The authors speculate that the MTS association can be the result of a potentiating effect of the primary lesion in producing febrile seizures. The MTS being a consequence of those febrile seizures. This concept is supported by the more common association of hippocampal atrophy in patients with congenital lesions such as migration disorders (25%), porencephaly (31%), "reactive gliosis" 23.5%), and a less common association with low-grade neoplasms (2%) and vascular causes of seizures.

J.G. Smirniotopoulos, M.D.

Cerebrovascular Diseases

Moyamoya Disease: Diagnostic Accuracy of MRI

Yamada I, Suzuki S, Matsushima Y (Tokyo Med and Dental Univ)
Neuroradiology 37:356–361, 1995 6–15

Objective.—The rare cerebrovascular occlusive condition, moyamoya disease, is most frequently encountered in Japan but does occur elsewhere. Patients with moyamoya disease may undergo MRI to obtain vascular information without the need for contrast medium, but no studies of its diagnostic accuracy have been reported. The MRI findings of 30 patients with moyamoya disease are described and compared with the angiographic findings.

Methods.—The patients were 19 women and 11 men, average age, 14 years. Three patients had undergone external to internal carotid artery bypass surgery. All patients underwent both MRI and transfemoral cerebral angiography. The MRI findings in occlusive lesions, collateral vessels, and parenchymal lesions were assessed for their diagnostic value.

Findings.—Bilateral occlusion or stenosis of the supraclinoid internal carotid artery and the proximal anterior and middle cerebral arteries were clearly demonstrated by MRI in every patient (Figs 1 and 2). In 73% of the

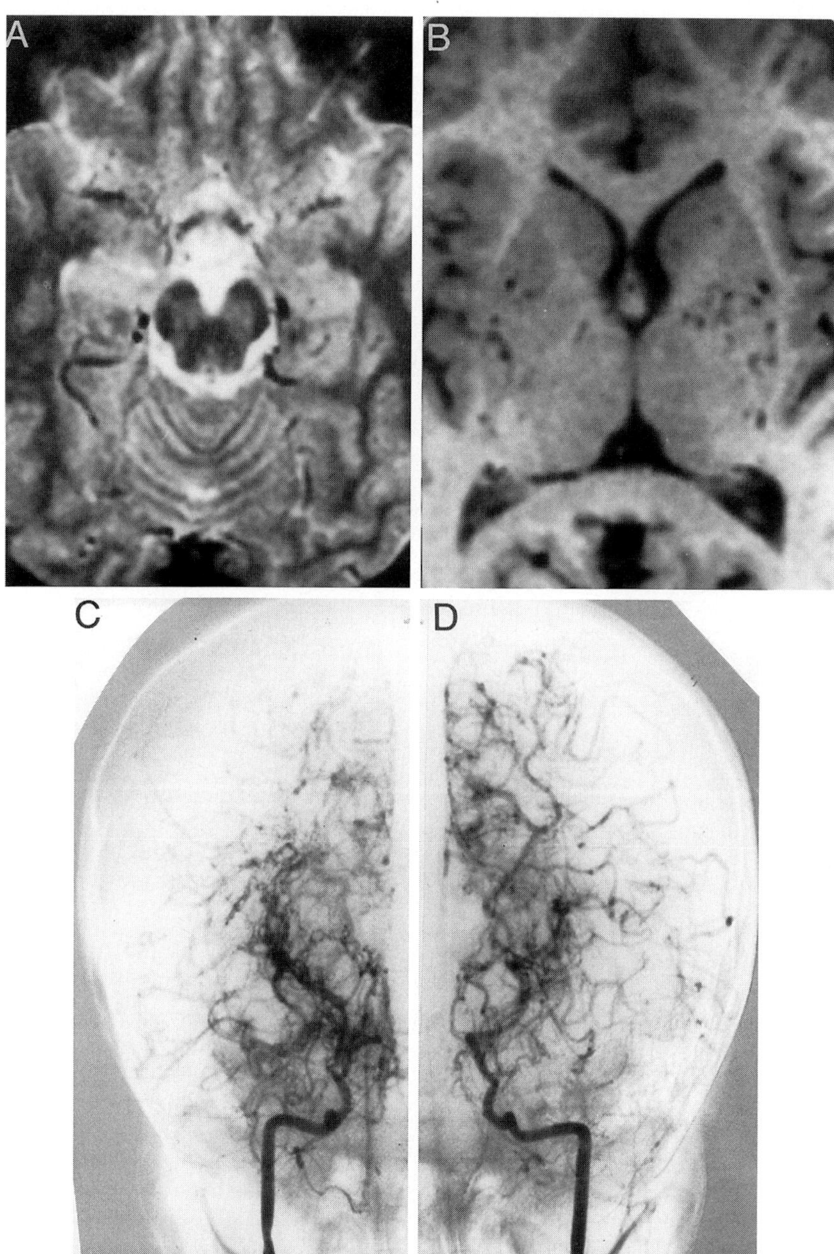

FIGURE 1.—A 7-year-old boy. **A**, axial T2-weighted image shows that the supraclinoid internal carotid artery and proximal anterior cerebral artery and middle cerebral artery are occluded bilaterally. **B**, axial T1-weighted image shows marked bilateral moyamoya vessels. **C** and **D**, right and left internal carotid arteriography, frontal projections, shows that both internal carotid arteries are occluded in the distal supraclinoid portion and the anterior and middle cerebral arteries in their proximal portions. Marked moyamoya vessels are seen. (*Neuroradiology*, Moyamoya disease: Diagnostic accuracy of MRI. Yamada I, Suzuki S, Matsushima Y, Vol 37:356–361, 1995, copyright notice of Springer-Verlag.)

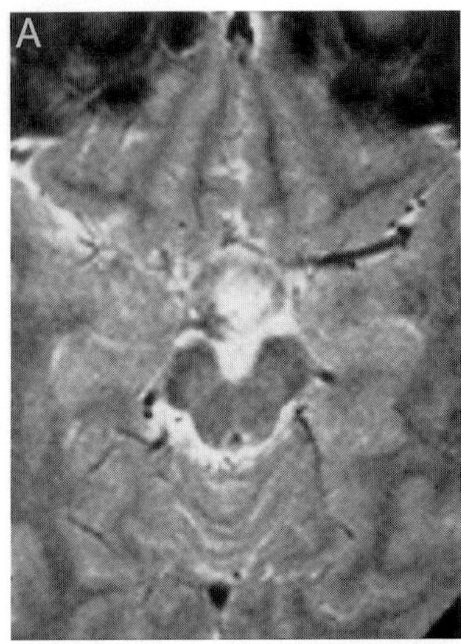

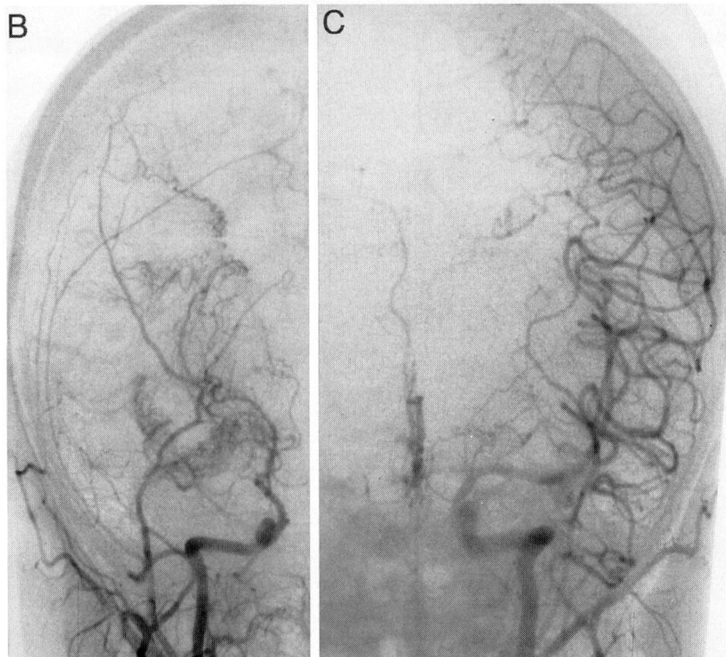

FIGURE 2.—A 9-year-old boy. **A**, axial T2-weighted image shows that the right internal carotid artery, anterior cerebral artery, and middle cerebral artery are completely occluded; the proximal left anterior cerebral artery is stenotic, although the proximal middle cerebral artery is normal in caliber. **B**, right internal carotid arteriogram, frontal projection, shows that the internal carotid artery is occluded in its distal supraclinoid portion and the anterior cerebral artery and middle cerebral artery in the proximal portions. Moderate moyamoya vessels are seen. **C**, left internal carotid arteriogram shows that the proximal anterior cerebral artery is so stenotic that its branches are poorly seen, although the proximal middle cerebral artery and the supraclinoid internal carotid artery are normal in caliber. (*Neuroradiology*, Moyamoya disease: Diagnostic accuracy of MRI. Yamada I, Suzuki S, Matsushima Y, Vol 37:356–361, 1995, copyright notice of Springer-Verlag.)

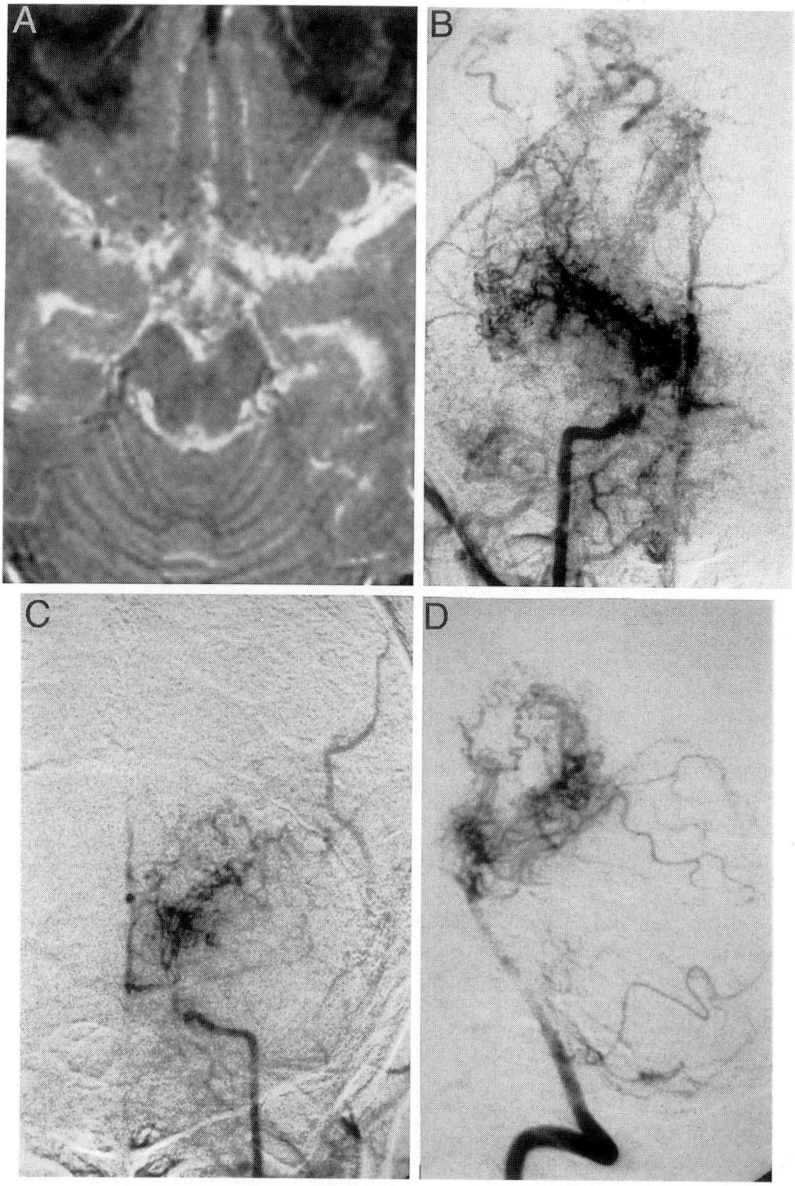

FIGURE 3.—A 13-year-old girl. **A**, axial T2-weighted image shows that the supraclinoid internal carotid artery and the proximal anterior cerebral artery, middle cerebral artery and posterior cerebral arteries are occluded bilaterally. **B**, right internal carotid arteriogram, frontal projection, shows that the internal carotid artery is occluded in its distal supraclinoid portion and the anterior cerebral artery and middle cerebral artery in their proximal portions. Marked moyamoya vessels are seen. **C**, left internal carotid arteriogram, frontal projection, shows that the supraclinoid internal carotid artery and the proximal anterior cerebral artery and middle cerebral artery are markedly stenotic. Moderate moyamoya vessels are seen. **D**, left vertebral arteriogram, lateral projection, shows that both posterior cerebral arteries are occluded proximally. Marked moyamoya vessels are seen. (*Neuroradiology*, Moyamoya disease: Diagnostic accuracy of MRI. Yamada I, Suzuki S, Matsushima Y, Vol 37:356–361, Figure 3, 1995, copyright notice of Springer-Verlag.)

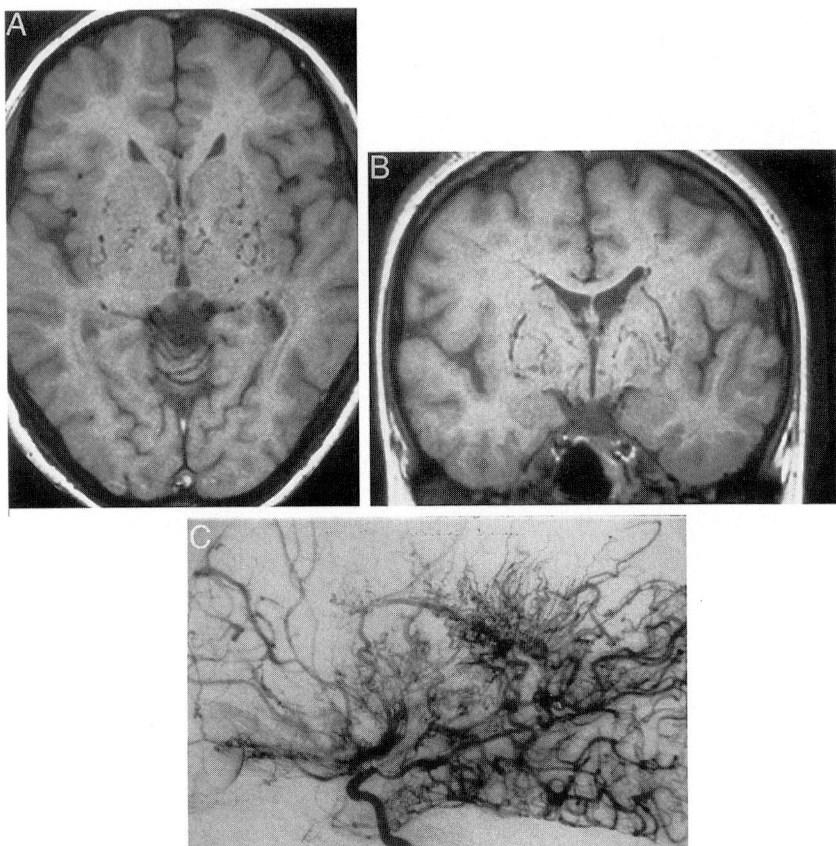

FIGURE 4.—A 12-year-old girl. **A** and **B**, axial and coronal T1-weighted images show marked moyamoya vessels bilaterally. The coronal image shows the full extent of moyamoya vessels from the chiasmatic cistern to the basal ganglia and deep white matter. **C**, right internal carotid arteriogram, lateral projection, shows that the internal carotid artery is occluded in its distal supraclinoid portion. Marked moyamoya vessels extend from the chiasmatic cistern, and the medullary arteries of the deep white matter are seen. The left internal arteriogram was similar. (*Neuroradiology*, Moyamoya disease: Diagnostic accuracy of MRI. Yamada I, Suzuki S, Matsushima Y, Vol 37:356–361, Figure 4, 1995, copyright notice of Springer-Verlag.)

arteries studied, MRI and angiography agreed as to the extent of the occlusion. Magnetic resonance imaging overestimated the extent of occlusive disease in 8 of 60 supraclinoid internal carotid arteries (Fig 3). Basal cerebral moyamoya vessels were clearly depicted by MRI, especially coronal images (Fig 4). Also, MRI was able to identify 45 of 71 large leptomeningeal and transdural collateral vessels. Eighty percent of hemispheres had parenchymal lesions demonstrated by MRI. There was good correlation between the extent of occlusion in the anterior circulation and white matter infarcts and between occlusion in the posterior circulation and cortical and/or subcortical infarcts.

Conclusions.—The MRI findings in patients with moyamoya disease are evaluated. Magnetic resonance imaging is moderately successful in depicting occlusive disease, staging, and assessing the collateral vessels. Because it can also demonstrate parenchymal lesions, it has a role in the follow-up as well as the diagnosis of patients with moyamoya disease.

► The authors report 30 cases of moyamoya disease studied by MRI. Moyamoya disease is an idiopathic, slowly progressing vasculopathy producing progressive occlusion of intracranial cerebral vessels and accompanying hypertrophy of multiple small collateral vessels. Magnetic resonance imaging clearly demonstrated the diagnostic features of bilateral supraclinoid carotid occlusions/stenosis in all patients. In 54 of 60 cerebral hemispheres, moyamoya vessels (dilated tubular signal voids in the basal ganglia, deep white matter, and cisterns) were demonstrated.

J.G. Smirniotopoulos, M.D.

Patients With Polycystic Kidney Disease Would Benefit From Routine Magnetic Resonance Angiographic Screening for Intracerebral Aneurysms: A Decision Analysis

Butler WE, Barker FG II, Crowell RM (Harvard Med School, Boston; Massachusetts Gen Hosp, Boston; Berkshire Associates, Pittsfield, Mass)

Neurosurgery 38:506–516, 1996 6–16

Purpose.—Patients with autosomal dominant polycystic kidney disease (ADPKD) have elevated rates of cerebral aneurysm and subarachnoid hemorrhage. A 1983 decision analysis suggested no benefit of routine arteriography to screen for cerebral aneurysms in patients with ADPKD. However, since then, MR angiography has emerged as a potentially useful MRI screening technique. A new decision analysis study was performed to see if MRI would be useful in screening ADPKD patients for intracerebral aneurysms.

Methods.—The study used a Markov model to compare MRI screening, followed by neurosurgical management for patients found to have intracerebral aneurysms, with no screening. Patients without screening received cerebrovascular interventions only after subarachnoid hemorrhage occurred. The prevalence of asymptomatic intracerebral aneurysms in patients with ADPKD was estimated at 15% based on previous clinical reports. The estimated annual incidence of aneurysmal rupture was 1.6%, with an associated morbidity of 70% and mortality of 56%. The risk of transfemoral arteriography was set at 0.2%, and the morbidity and mortality of surgery for an unruptured aneurysm were estimated at 4.1% and 1.0%, respectively.

Results.—The results suggested that MRI screening for intracerebral aneurysms would save 1 additional life-year without neurologic disability for a 20-year-old patient with ADPKD. The decision model proved sensitive to changes in the prevalence of aneurysms, the annual incidence of

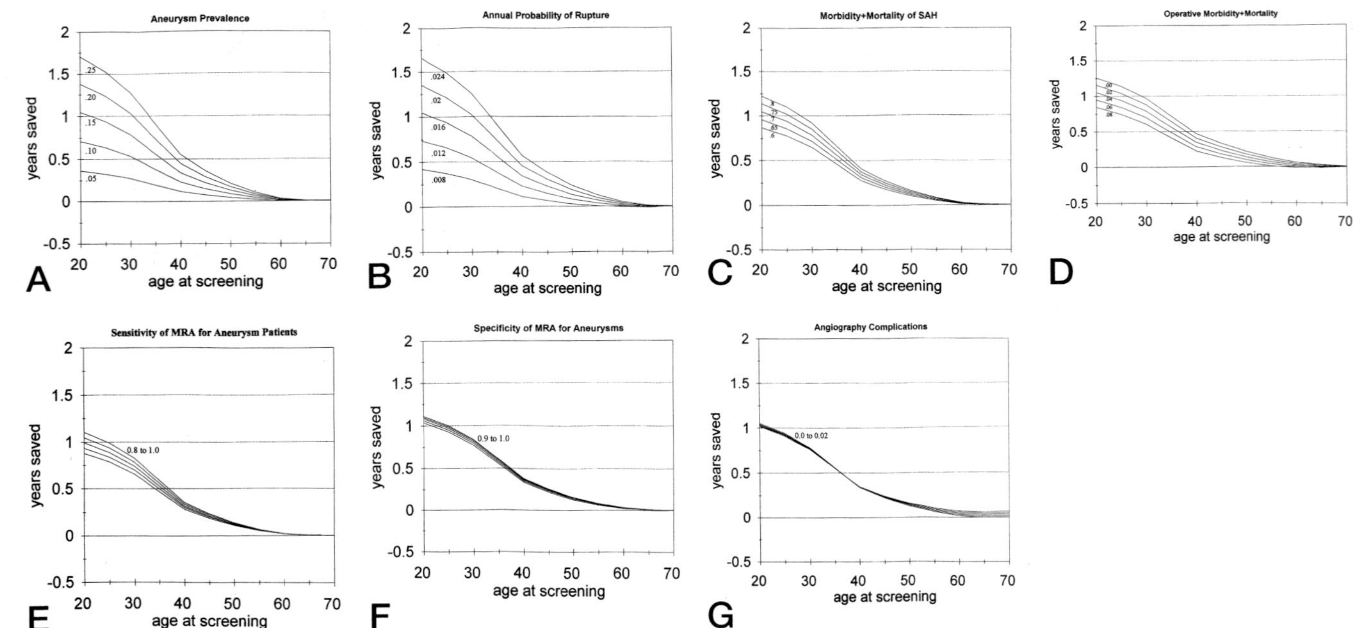

FIGURE 3.—Sensitivity analyses for prevalence of aneurysms (**A**), annual probability of rupture (**B**), probability that a rupture is fatal or disabling (**C**), operative complications (**D**), sensitivity of MRI to aneurysms (**E**), specificity of MRI for aneurysms (**F**), and probability of angiography complications (**G**). Each graph (**A–G**) consists of a family of curves that is generated by systematically varying the value of the corresponding parameter and recalculating the years of life saved without neurologic deficit. When space between the curves permits, the parameter value is placed under the corresponding curve. (Courtesy of Butler WE, Barker FG II, Crowell RM: Patients with polycystic kidney disease would benefit from routine magnetic resonance angiographic screening for intracerebral aneurysms: A decision analysis. *Neurosurgery* 38:506–516, 1996.)

rupture, and the morbidity and mortality after rupture (Fig 3) Cost analysis suggested that screening carried a net financial benefit across the range of plausible assumptions.

Conclusions.—Routine MRI screening for intracerebral aneurysms appears likely to improve life expectancy for patients with ADPKD. It would be especially valuable for patients with a personal or family history of such aneurysms. For a patient with an asymptomatic aneurysm detected by this screening approach, surgical treatment would be expected to add about 10 years of life expectancy.

► Another of the controversies concerning aneurysms is the efficacy of screening an asymptomatic population at risk. One such readily identifiable population is patients with ADPKD. Several classic articles, including 1 by Levy et al. (cited by the authors as their reference no. 34) have repeatedly suggested that the cumulative risk of aneurysmal rupture in asymptomatic patients was roughly the same as the risk of angiographic screening. This led many, but not all, to conclude that screening the asymptomatic patient was an unnecessary risk, even with an appropriate family history (e.g., ADPKD). However, the considerations of risk were turned upside down with the advent of noninvasive screening using MR, MR angiography (MRA), and now CT angiography (CTA). Although this paper is a "meta-analysis" of the published literature, the conclusion is no less valid. It should also be emphasized that the target population considered in the statistical predictions of this study were theoretical 20-year-old subjects. Despite this, there is a distinct attraction toward using a noninvasive imaging modality that itself carries no measurable risk (i.e., MRA without contrast). In the face of the declining charges for MR and MRA, it is difficult to present a cogent argument against the use of noninvasive screening for these patients.

J.G. Smirniotopoulos, M.D.

The Negative Angiogram in Subarachnoid Haemorrhage

Duong H, Melançon D, Tampieri D, et al (Montreal Gen Hosp; Montreal Neurological Inst)

Neuroradiology 38:15–19, 1996 6–17

Background.—In some patients with acute, nontraumatic subarachnoid hemorrhage (SAH), no cause can be identified even with thorough neuroradiologic studies. Survival is somewhat lower than expected in these patients, who are usually treated empirically. A 10-year experience with patients for whom no cause of SAH can be found is presented.

Findings.—The authors' hospital performed cerebral angiography in 295 patients with acute SAH from 1983 to 1992. On review, cerebral panangiography was negative in 31% of patients. A second or third angiogram found an aneurysm in 5 patients, for a false negative rate of 5%. Fifty-five percent of the patients with negative angiograms had only a small amount of SAH on CT scan. There were few complications of conservative treatment in this group of patients, and 93% had recovered completely by the time of hospital discharge.

Conclusions.—The outcomes of patients with subarachnoid hemorrhage and negative angiograms are reviewed. The results appear to be especially good for patients with perimesencephalic SAH. The causes of SAH in these patients are still unknown.

▶ One of the most enduring controversies in neuroimaging is the extent of the workup required for patients who have SAH. The classic teaching is that the initial angiogram, even when well performed and including selective injections of both carotid and vertebral arteries, may fail to demonstrate intracranial aneurysms. This failure can be related to small size of the aneurysm, spasm of the vessels and/or the aneurysm neck, and thrombosis of the aneurysms. This paper reviewed a consecutive series of 295 patients, acquired entirely in the modern angiographic era (1983–1992). Almost one third (31%) had a negative initial arteriogram. The number of subsequently disclosed aneurysms (on follow-up second and/or third arteriograms) gave a total false negative rate of 5% for the initial negative evaluation. This article also confirms earlier observations that suggest a more benign course for patients with subarachnoid hemorrhage limited to the perimesencephalic cisterns.

J.G. Smirniotopoulos, M.D.

Factors That Predict the Bleeding Risk of Cerebral Arteriovenous Malformations

Pollock BE, Flickinger JC, Lunsford LD, et al (Univ of Pittsburgh, Pa)

Stroke 27:1–6, 1996 6–18

Introduction.—Left untreated, arteriovenous malformations (AVMs) have an overall 2% to 4% annual hemorrhage rate. Although several risk factors predisposing to bleeding of AVMs have been suggested, their relative importance is unknown. Risk factors for bleeding of AVMs were examined in a retrospective study.

Methods.—Clinical and angiographic data from 315 patients undergoing stereotactic radiosurgery were analyzed. The study addressed the natural history of untreated AVMs, so the bleeding rate after radiosurgery was not included. Half the patient data, the analysis cohort, was used to evaluate bleeding risk factors and to create bleeding risk groups. The other half, the test cohort, was then used to test the risk groups identified.

Results.—The AVMs had a mean volume of 4 mL and a maximum diameter of about 2 cm. In 10,348 patient-years there were 196 initial hemorrhages; the annual initial bleed rate was thus 1.89%. During 591 patient-years in these 196 patients, 44 patients had a repeat bleed; the annual rebleed rate was thus 7.45%, and the overall crude annual bleed rate was 2.4%. Several risk factors were identified on univariate analysis (Table 2), but only 3 were significantly associated with hemorrhage on

TABLE 2.—Univariate Analysis of Arteriovenous Malformation Factors Predictive of Hemorrhage

Factor	Higher Risk Group	*P*
Sex	Male	.377
Age	Increases with age	.620
Presentation	Hemorrhage	<.001
Volume	<4.0 mL	.062
Morphology	Diffuse	.010
No. of draining veins	One	.002
Piat/ependymal	Yes	.169
Related aneurysm	Yes	.626
Varix	Yes	.123

(Courtesy of Pollock BE, Flickinger JC, Lunsford LD, et al: Factors that predict the bleeding risk of cerebral arteriovenous malformations. *Stroke* 27:1–6, 1996.)

multivariate analysis: a previous bleed, relative risk (RR) 9.09; a single draining vein, RR 1.66; and a diffuse AVM morphology, RR 1.64. Four risk groups were identified on the basis of these factors. These groups, and their annual bleeding rates, were low-risk, 0.99%; intermediate-low-risk, 2.22%; intermediate-high-risk, 3.72%; and high-risk, 8.94%.

Conclusions.—Bleeding risk varies considerably among patients with AVMs. Based on their clinical and angiographic characteristics, these patients can be categorized as to their risk of AVM bleeding. Management decisions should be based on the factors corresponding to low vs. high risk of hemorrhage, as well as the treatment-related morbidity.

► The risk of bleeding from aneurysms that occur with rupture is roughly 4% per year. This article suggests that a similar risk of bleeding and/or rebleeding exists for AVMs. The patients included in the study underwent stereotactic radiosurgery of known AVMs. Three factors appear to be associated with a high risk of hemorrhage: previous bleeding, a more diffuse blood supply (multiple arterial feeders), and a single draining vein. The authors commented about the relationship between the arterial pressure to the AVM and the venous pressure draining the AVM, to the chance of rupture. In addition, there was little if any correlation between overall AVM size, and the presence of associated aneurysms in the feeding vessels. One complicating factor, regarding the lack of association between size and risk of bleeding, is related to the initial complaint that allows the discovery of the AVM in the first place. In other words, a small AVM may be identified because of hemorrhage, whereas a larger AVM may produce signs and symptoms related to mass effect in the absence of hemorrhage. Thus, a small AVM (without hemorrhage) may not be recognized at all and may really have only a minimal risk of hemorrhage. However, the small lesions that occur with hemorrhage have already revealed a more ominous character.

J.G. Smirniotopoulos, M.D.

Case Reports: Recurrent Hypertensive Intracerebral Hemorrhage

Misra UK, Kalita J (Sanjay Gandhi Postgraduate Inst, Lucknow, India)

Am J Med Sci 310:156–157, 1995 6–19

Background.—Hypertension is the most important risk factor in the development of spontaneous intracerebral hemorrhage (ICH). It has been assumed that hypertensive ICH is a 1-time event. However, 5 patients with recurrent hypertensive ICH are described.

Case Reports.—Between 1991 and 1993, 105 patients were seen with hypertensive ICH. Five of these patients had a recurrence. Two patients had moderate hypertension and 3 had severe hypertension. Blood pressure was poorly controlled in all 5 patients. The 5 patients had a total of 11 episodes of hypertensive ICH. All but 1 patient had recurrent hemorrhage in a site different from the first. The sites were ganglionic in 9 episodes, pontine in 1, and lobar in 1. The patients all had normal blood urea, serum creatinine concentrations, and bleeding and coagulation parameters. They also all had grade II hypertensive retinopathy, left ventricular hypertrophy, and elevated proteinuria. There was good recovery even after the second hemorrhage in 4 of the 5 patients.

Discussion.—The assumption that hypertensive ICH was not recurrent was based on large, clinically detected hematomas and autopsy confirmation. However, CT can detect smaller hemorrhages with atypical clinical signs. These patients have a good chance for recovery. Their longer survival increases the possibility of recurrence. The patients all had moderate-to-severe, uncontrolled hypertension and clinical signs consistent with long-term hypertension, suggesting that continued hypertension may be a risk factor for recurrent hypertensive ICH.

Sensitivity of New-Generation Computed Tomography in Subarachnoid Hemorrhage

Sames TA, Storrow AB, Finkelstein JA, et al (Joint Military Med Ctrs, San Antonio, Tex)

Acad Emerg Med 3:16–20, 1996 6–20

Objective.—The sensitivity of newer-generation CT scanners for detecting acute, nontraumatic subarachnoid hemorrhage and the need for lumbar puncture in patients with normal CT scans from these scanners were evaluated.

Background.—Acute, nontraumatic subarachnoid hemorrhage is often encountered in the emergency department and has an overall mortality of 50%. Currently, lumbar puncture is recommended when subarachnoid hemorrhage is suspected in patients with normal CT scans because the sensitivity of older-generation CT scanners is 90% for detecting this disease. The newer designs and improved computer technology of newer-generation scanners result in better performance and resolution.

Methods.—The medical records of patients with subarachnoid hemorrhage were reviewed. Patients with head trauma within 24 hours of symptom onset were excluded. Group 1 consisted of patients with symptoms for less than 24 hours before scanning, and group 2 consisted of those with symptoms for more than 24 hours before scanning. The sensitivity of newer-generation CT scanners was determined.

Results.—The records of 181 patients were reviewed. For patients in group 1, the sensitivity of the newer-generation CT scanners for detecting subarachnoid hemorrhage was 93.1%. For patients in group 2, the sensitivity was 83.8%. Overall sensitivity was 91.2%. In all patients with subarachnoid hemorrhage not detected by newer-generation CT scanners, lumbar puncture was used to diagnose the disease. There was no association between the resolution of the scanners and sensitivity for subarachnoid hemorrhage.

Conclusions.—In detecting subarachnoid hemorrhage, initial interpretation of these scans from newer-generation CT scanners did not approach 100% sensitivity. The sensitivity decreased as more time passed between symptom onset and initial scan. Lumbar puncture is recommended for patients with suspected subarachnoid hemorrhage with normal findings on CT scans.

▶ This is a review of the sensitivity of modern scanners for non-traumatic subarachnoid hemorrhage. Computed tomography had a sensitivity of 93% in the first 24 hours which dropped to 84% after 24 hours. Although the combined sensitivity is 91%, this study suggests a continued role for lumbar puncture in patients with a negative CT scan.

J.G. Smirniotopoulos, M.D.

A Founder Mutation as a Cause of Cerebral Cavernous Malformation in Hispanic Americans

Günel M, Awad IA, Finberg K, et al (Yale Univ, New Haven, Conn; Univ of New Mexico, Albuquerque; Stanford Univ, Palo Alto; et al)

N Engl J Med 334:946–951, 1996 6–21

Background.—Cerebral cavernous malformation is characterized by abnormal vascular spaces with a lining of a single layer of endothelium and no intervening neural parenchyma or mature vessel-wall elements. It can cause headaches, seizures, and cerebral hemorrhage. Both familial and sporadic cases have been found, particularly among Hispanic Americans of Mexican descent. Previous studies have discovered a causative gene on the long arm of chromosome 7. A linkage study was performed with segregation of genetic markers in patients with both familial and sporadic disease.

Methods.—Genomic DNA was extracted from the venous blood of 57 patients with cerebral cavernous malformation, diagnosed either by surgery or MRI, and of 47 unrelated, healthy controls. Of these 57 patients, 47 were members of 14 kindreds with familial cavernous malformation and 10 were sporadic cases. The genotypes on chromosome 7q were determined with polymerase chain reaction, and haplotypes were constructed.

Results.—All of the affected members, but none of the unaffected members, of 1 family inherited allele 6 of locus D7S657. Markers D6S492 and D7S479 were not completely cosegregated, indicating disease gene location in a 7-cM segment between D7S492 and D7S479, were found in all 47 chromosomes from the kindreds, but in only 4 of the 98 chromosomes from the Hispanic control subjects. Identical haplotypes were found in affected patients from 10 kindreds, with the affected patients from the other 4 kindreds having haplotypes with a portion of the interval that contained the cavernous-malformation gene. In addition, the entire conserved haplotype was found in 33 asymptomatic subjects from the kindreds. Eight of the 10 sporadic patients also had the entire conserved haplotype, and the other 2 had part of the conserved haplotype containing the cavernous-malformation gene.

Conclusions.—Virtually all cases of either familial or sporadic cavernous malformation in Hispanic Americans of Mexican descent were caused by inheritance of the same mutation from a common ancestor. Further study is needed to identify the mutation, which can form the basis of a genetic screening test.

▶ This is not really an imaging paper, but I wanted to include it because it is a strong reminder of how neuroradiologists must now learn genetics and molecular biology to remain competent. Numerous articles have shown a high incidence of autosomal dominant inheritance for cavernous hemangiomas among Hispanic Americans of Mexican ancestry. This classic article from the *New England Journal of Medicine* now documents that the reported association is not only valid and true, but may be the result of a "founder mutation." The molecular biology of multiple cavernous hemangiomas suggests that the abnormal chromosome is number 7, and that the nearby genetic markers suggest that the 47 individuals studied, from 14 different "unrelated" kindreds, most probably have a single common ancestor—the "founder" of cavernous hemangiomas.

J.G. Smirniotopoulos, M.D.

Leukoencephalopathy and Other Inflammatory Disorders

MR Findings in Adult-Onset Adrenoleukodystrophy

Kumar AJ, Köhler W, Kruse B, et al (Johns Hopkins Med Insts, Baltimore, Md; Moabit Hosp, Berlin; Kennedy Krieger Inst, Baltimore, Md)
AJNR 16:1227–1237, 1995 6–22

Background.—Adrenoleukodystrophy (ALD) is an X-linked disorder associated with increased, very long chain saturated fatty acids in the brain and adrenal gland, red blood cells, and plasma attributed to defective peroxisomal fatty acid oxidation. The phenotypic expression of ALD varies widely, ranging from the most severe childhood cerebral form to the milder adult forms. The adult neurologic variant affects approximately 30% of men and 15% to 20% of women heterozygotes. The most common form is adrenomyeloneuropathy (AMN), which involves mainly the spinal cord and peripheral nerves with mild-to-absent inflammatory response in cerebral white matter. The MR findings of the brain and spinal cord in adult-onset ALD were examined.

Methods.—Magnetic resonance imaging of the brain was performed in 164 adult patients, aged 19 to 74 years, with clinically and biochemically proven ALD. In 30 patients, MR of the spine was also performed.

Findings.—The brain MR findings were abnormal in 46% of male and in 20% of female heterozygotes. The brain abnormalities consisted of varying degrees of demyelination of the cerebral white matter in 46 patients, corpus callosum in 25, corticospinal tracts in 46, visual tracts in 31, and auditory tracts in 18. Diffuse spinal cord atrophy, mainly in the thoracic regions, were evident on MRI in 18 of 20 men and 8 of 10 women. There were no focal T2-weighted abnormalities in the spinal cord.

Correlation of the MR findings with clinical features allowed tentative subdivision of adult-onset ALD into 4 subtypes that appeared to differ with respect to prognosis and possible pathogenesis. Sixty-five men had "pure" AMN with normal brain MR findings and disease confined to the spinal cord and peripheral nerves. Another 16 male patients with AMN had adrenoleukomyeloneuropathy type 1 (ALMN 1) with brain MR abnormality confined to the long fiber tract systems, mainly bilateral involvement of the corticospinal tract. In this group, the more than 25-year interval between onset of neurologic symptoms and tract degeneration represented a "dying-back" mechanism of these long tracts, possibly due to a defective axonal protein transport secondary to metabolic alterations of the perikarya. Thirty-two male patients with AMN had ALMN 2 with diffuse lobar cerebral involvement. The most common pattern was a bilateral parieto-occipital involvement extending across the splenium of the corpus callosum in combination with bilateral pyramidal tract involvement in the brainstem and internal capsule. Six patients had adult cerebral ALD with severe lobar white matter demyelination and/or severe brain atrophy and a severe and rapidly progressive course.

Summary.—The clinical course in adult phenotypes of ALD differs significantly. The evaluation of the brain with MR allows differentiation of adult ALD phenotypes for prognostic considerations; it also enables patient selection for experimental dietary therapy and bone marrow therapy, which can be effective if given in the early stages of the disease.

▶ Adrenoleukodystrophy is X-linked, and affects the white matter, adrenal cortex, and testis, accumulation of very long chain saturated fatty acids in the brain and adrenal gland, red blood cells and plasma due to peroxisomal disorder. Gene mapping is to Xq28 (long arm of the X chromosome). Adrenoleukodystrophy varies from a severe childhood form (often fatal in the first decade) to a milder adult type (survival to eighth decade). The childhood type has a presentation by 7.1 years, progressing to a vegetative state and death associated with large areas of demyelination. Adult forms include AMN as the most common, characterized by spinal cord and peripheral nerve problems, without a significant white matter lesion. Adrenomyeloneuropathy has a mean onset of 27.6 years with lower extremity spasticity and weakness, sphincter and sexual dysfunction, and it slowly progresses for decades.

J.G. Smirniotopoulos, M.D.

A Reversible Posterior Leukoencephalopathy Syndrome

Hinchey J, Chaves C, Appignani B, et al (New England Med Ctr, Boston; Tufts Univ, Boston; Hôpital Sainte Anne, Paris)

N Engl J Med 334:494–500, 1996 6–23

Introduction.—Some hospitalized patients will have a reversible syndrome consisting of headache, altered mental function, seizures, and visual loss. Imaging studies suggest that this complication is related to a predominantly posterior leukoencephalopathy. Toward fuller characterization of this reversible posterior leukoencephalopathy, 15 cases are reviewed.

Findings.—The 15 patients were identified by review of patients undergoing CT and MRI at 2 hospitals during a 7-year period. Seven patients were receiving immunosuppressive therapy at the time the reversible posterior leukoencephalopathy syndrome developed, and 4 had acute hypertensive encephalopathy associated with kidney disease. In total, 12 of the patients were found to have abrupt rises in blood pressure and 8 to have some form of renal impairment. The extensive, bilateral white matter abnormalities noted on CT and MRI were consistent with edema. Treatment consisted of antihypertensive medications and withdrawal of immunosuppressive therapy for patients who are receiving it. All patients' neurologic symptoms disappeared within 2 weeks.

Conclusions.—The clinical and neuroimaging findings of reversible posterior leukoencephalopathy syndrome are reviewed. This complication appears mainly in patients with immunosuppression, renal insufficiency, or hypertension. The imaging findings in this condition suggest subcortical edema without infarction.

► Just when you thought it was safe to look at the white matter, a new disease crops up. This article presents the findings in 15 patients of a reversible syndrome of primarily white matter edema involving the posterior portions of the cerebral hemispheres. This is associated with appropriate clinical findings of loss of vision, as well as altered mental status, seizures, and headache. In the 15 patients reported, these findings were reversible; the patients had an acute illness requiring hospitalization, and almost half (7 of 15) were immune suppressed. These findings were reversible with control of the patients' hypertension and/or withdrawal of immunosuppressive medication. Because half the patients were hypertensive, it is appropriate to make a comparison with both hypertensive encephalopathy and eclampsia. Both of those conditions are associated with transient and reversible cerebral edema and occasionally with petechial hemorrhages. Just as in this series of patients, the posterior portions of the cerebral hemispheres (parietal, occipital lobes) bear the brunt of the insult; the pathophysiology in eclampsia and hypertensive encephalopathy appear to be related to endothelial dysfunction, including both spasm and blood-brain barrier breakdown. The authors propose that the mechanism in the immunosuppressed patients is endothelial and/or neurotoxicity. It is important to recognize this new cause of primarily posterior white matter disease, because it may be reversible with control of hypertension or by temporary withdrawal of immunosuppressive therapy.

J.G. Smirniotopoulos, M.D.

Changes in the Amount of Diseased White Matter Over Time in Patients With Relapsing-Remitting Multiple Sclerosis

Stone LA, Albert PS, Smith ME, et al (NIH, Bethesda, Md; Cornell Univ, New York)

Neurology 45:1808–1814, 1995 6–24

Objective.—In patients with multiple sclerosis (MS), MRI is a sensitive technique for assessing diseased tissue. The T2-weighted images can detect diseased white matter (WM), whereas contrast-enhanced T1-weighted images can depict active disease as reflected by abnormalities of the blood-brain barrier (BBB). Contrast-enhanced MRI can show active disease in patients with mild relapsing-remitting MS, even early in the course of disease and during periods of clinical stability. Changes in the amount of WM abnormalities over time were assessed in patients with mild relapsing-remitting multiple sclerosis (RRMS).

Methods.—The study included 7 patients with clinically definite but mild RRMS—baseline Expanded Disability Status Scale scores were no more than 3.0. All patients had frequent contrast-enhancing lesions on

MRI. The patients underwent monthly MRI imaging for 26 to 36 months using a 1.5 T scanner. Both T2- and T1-weighted images were included in calculating the area of increased WM signal in each MRI study. The changes in WM abnormalities were tracked over time, and their relationship to other MRI and clinical findings were evaluated.

Results.—There was considerable fluctuation in the amount of WM abnormalities over time, reflecting BBB breakdown, measurement error, and other factors. However, the overall amount of abnormal WM increased in all 7 patients. This increase was best appreciated by comparing the mean of the first 6 months of measurement with that of the final 6 months, or by linear regression modeling. There was no consistent relationship between the magnitude of change in WM abnormalities and the degree of clinical worsening.

Conclusions.—Amounts of abnormal WM, as assessed by MRI, increase over time in patients with mild RRMS. The findings suggest that accumulation of abnormal WM could be a useful technique for assessing disease activity in patients with MS. The value of this approach could be enhanced by the development of simpler and faster methods of counting or measuring disease activity in the brains of patients with MS.

▶ Seven patients imaged monthly for a total of 26–36 months, were reviewed and analyzed with image processing software. All patients showed fluctuations in lesions, with an overall progressive increase in the amount of abnormal WM over time. This paper suggests that automated techniques may improve sensitivity over a more simple visual assessment.

J.G. Smirniotopoulos, M.D.

AIDS-Associated Cytomegalovirus Infection Mimicking Central Nervous System Tumors: A Diagnostic Challenge

Moulignier A, Mikol J, Gonzalez-Canali G, et al (Hôpital de l'Institut Pasteur, Paris; Hôpital Lariboisière, Paris; Hôpital Saint-Louis, Paris; et al)
Clin Infect Dis 22:626–631, 1996 6–25

Introduction.—Cytomegalovirus (CMV) infection is very common in patients with HIV infection—it is found in 40% of patients with end-stage AIDS and in 90% of autopsy cases. It can be very difficult to diagnose CMV infection of the CNS, because imaging studies are usually normal and CMV is rarely cultured from cerebrospinal fluid. Three unusual cases of CMV infection of the CNS masquerading as tumors are reported.

Patients.—Of 543 HIV-1-infected patients with CMV infections, 37 had clinical evidence of neurologic involvement. Three of these patients had MRI studies showing unusual gadolinium ring-enhanced, space-occupying lesions that mimicked CNS tumors. All of the patients were profoundly immunosuppressed, with a mean CD4 cell count of 13/mm^3. One patient had spinal cord enlargement of the spinal cord, whereas the other 2 had ring-enhanced mass lesions of the cerebral hemispheres. All patients had marked edema and a mass effect. The presence of active CMV infection was confirmed by image-guided stereotactic biopsy in all 3 patients, and all patients responded to specific anti-CMV therapy. Focal intraparenchymal lesions consistent with marked focal necrosis were present, probably reflecting severe and long-standing immunosuppression.

Discussion.—Ring-enhanced, space-occupying mass lesions are an unusual presentation of HIV-related CMV infection. Magnetic resonance imaging should clarify the diagnosis in these cases, leading to improved outcomes. A slowly progressive CNS lesion that does not respond to antitoxoplasmic therapy could be a CMV abscess or "cytomegaloviroma." Biopsy is indicated in these cases.

▶ This article is yet another reminder of how difficult it is to predict the nature of mass lesions in patients with AIDS. From the Pasteur Institute in France, the authors noted that half the 37 patients with neurologic symptoms had CNS involvement and half had peripheral disease. The appearance of these infectious lesions in 3 patients could not be distinguished from a neoplasm. Thus, re-emphasizing the need for biopsy in certain patients with AIDS.

J.G.Smirniotopoulos, M.D.

Callosal Bleeding in a Case of Marchiafava-Bignami Disease

Kamaki M, Kawamura M, Moriya H, et al (Tokyo Metropolitan Hiroo Gen Hosp; Showa Univ, Japan; Chiba Univ, Japan)

J Neurol Sci 136:86–89, 1996 6–26

Background.—There have been only rare reports of callosal bleeding in patients with Marchiafava-Bignami disease (MBD). These cases have all been confirmed with autopsy findings. A case is reported in which there was CT and MRI evidence of hemorrhagic necrosis of the corpus callosum.

Case Report.—Woman, 43, was brought to the hospital unconscious. She had a history of heavy drinking for 20 years, coldness and pain in her toes for 3 years, and forgetfulness for 2 months. Neurologic findings included delirium, mildly hypertonic muscles, and urinary incontinence. One month later, she had normal consciousness and muscle tone, but residual dysarthria, orientation deficits, and memory loss. She later had multiple syndromes develop indicating interhemispheric disconnection during a 7-year period. During the hyperacute stage (within the first 24 hours), CT revealed a low-density area in the anterior half of the corpus callosum; the hypodensity increased during the subacute and chronic stages in this area. The density of the posterior half of the corpus callosum was low in the hyperacute stage, became high during the subacute stage, and was extremely low during the chronic stage. The MRI showed very low signal intensity on T1-

weighted images and high signal intensity on T2-weighted images in the anterior half of the corpus callosum. The posterior half of the corpus callosum revealed low signal intensity on both T1-and T2-weighted images. The very low signal intensity in the corpus callosum on the T2-weighted images remained 6 years after the onset.

Discussion.—It is likely that the low density on CT and high signal intensity on T2-weighted MRI in the hyperacute stage of MBD reveals the edema of the entire corpus callosum, whereas the extremely hypodense and hypointense CT and MRI findings during the subacute stage are suggestive of the cystic lesion typical of MBD. The areas of high density and high intensity during this stage also demonstrate hemorrhagic lesions in the trunk and splenium of the corpus callosum. The very low signal intensities on T2-weighted images during the chronic stage indicate the deposition of hemosiderin, consistent with hemorrhagic necrosis in the corpus callosum.

▶ This case report documents acute hemorrhage into the corpus callosum in a case of MBD. Rather than being the "classic" Italian red wine drinker, the patient in this study consumed Japanese rice wine. Serial images including both CT and MR, showed the subacute (29 days) development of hemorrhage into the splenium at the same time that edema was still noted in the middle layers from the genu through the middle third of the corpus callosum.

J.G. Smirniotopoulos, M.D.

An Autopsy Case of Marchiafava-Bignami Disease With Peculiar Chronological CT Changes in the Corpus Callosum: Neuroradiopathological Correlations

Shiota J-I, Nakano I, Kawamura M, et al (Ushioda Gen Hosp, Yokohama, Japan; Tokyo Metropolitan Inst; Showa Univ, Japan; et al)

J Neurol Sci 136:90–93, 1996 6–27

Background.—Patients with Marchiafava-Bignami disease (MBD) are known to have necrosis of the central portion of the corpus callosum, anterior commissure, and optic chiasm. The serial CTs obtained in a patient with MBD were compared with the neuropathologic findings during autopsy.

Case Report.—Man, 40, died of respiratory failure. Five years earlier, he had become suddenly comatose. After recovering consciousness, he had disorientation, personality change, dysarthria, pyramidal tract signs, and frontal lobe symptoms. All but the dysarthria resolved within 3 months. X-ray, CT, and MRI studies were obtained, revealing a hypodense lesion in the corpus callosum on day 2, which became isodense on day 14, and returned to hypodense. The serial studies had findings consistent with necrosis in the corpus callosum, leading to a diagnosis of MBD. The autopsy revealed a cystic lesion in the corpus callosum corresponding to the MRI findings. A histologic examination revealed a corpus callosum missing nerve fibers but with a cyst cavity lined with astrocytes swollen with hemosiderin pigments.

Discussion.—The hemosiderin pigments engulfed in astrocytes in the cyst wall of the corpus callosum provided evidence of hemorrhage in the corpus callosum between days 2 and 14 of the disease. The neuroimaging studies demonstrated evidence of bleeding at corresponding sites and of extravasation of small amounts of blood. Callosal bleeding may therefore be more common in patients with MBD and may be involved in the disease's pathomechanism.

▶ This article presents excellent radiologic/pathologic correlation of MBD which typically affects the central corpus callosum, anterior commissure, and optic chiasm.

The patient reported here consumed sake, rather than wine. The lesions identified at autopsy, as in the case reported in the article by Kamaki et al., included histologic findings suggestive of old hemorrhage. Taken together, these 2 articles prove that MBD can clearly be associated with callosal hemorrhages that are probably petechial in nature. Petechial hemorrhages into an area of previous low attenuation could produce an appearance on CT suggesting resolution of edema.

J.G. Smirniotopoulos, M.D.

Clinical Case Seminar: Lymphocytic Hypophysitis: Clinicopathological Findings

Thodou E, Asa SL, Kontogeorgos G, et al (Mount Sinai Hosp, Ont, Canada; St Michael's Hosp, Ont, Canada; Wellesley Hosp, Ont, Canada)

J Clin Endocrinol Metab 80:2302–2311, 1995 6–28

Objective.—The rare pituitary inflammatory lesion, lymphocytic hypophysitis, may have a clinically acute outcome and sometimes leads to severe complications or death. Histologic examination is the only way to make the definitive diagnosis. Sixteen cases of lymphocytic adenohypophysitis—the largest series reported to date—are described.

Patients.—The patients were 14 women and 2 men, mean age 31 and 42 years, respectively. Seventy-one percent of the women were seen during pregnancy. An expanding pituitary sellar mass was noted in 56% of cases, anterior pituitary hypofunction in 63%, and diabetes insipidus in 19%. In 19% of patients, progressive undiagnosed hypopituitarism led to death. Thirty-eight percent of the patients had hyperprolactinemia, and 1 had elevated growth hormone levels leading to IGF-1 excess.

A pituitary mass mimicking adenoma was seen on MRI in 83% of patients, and an associated autoimmune thyroiditis was seen in 25%. Morphologic and immunohistochemical studies revealed a polyclonal lymphoplasmacytic infiltrate with occasional neutrophils, eosinophils, and macrophages. Focal or diffuse adenohypophysial destruction of varying severity with associated fibrosis occurred as a result of the inflammatory process. In at least 1 patient with diabetes insipidus, the inflammatory infiltrate involved the neurohypophysis.

Conclusions.—The clinicopathologic features of lymphocytic hypophysitis are described. This diagnosis should be considered in women who have pituitary enlargement during the peripartum period and in patients with pituitary hormone deficiency and/or excess and a coexisting autoimmune disorder. Lymphocytic hypophysitis should probably also be considered in patients with rapidly growing pituitary masses and compressive symptoms, with or without pituitary hormone dysfunction. For many patients, it may be possible to avoid aggressive pituitary surgery by giving conservative treatment on the basis of clinical suspicion.

▶ Lymphocytic hypophysitis has been reported in more than 100 cases in the literature. The process is thought to be autoimmune and may be associated with other immune phenomena, such as thyroiditis. The majority of patients, although not all, are pregnant or postpartum; however, men are rarely affected. Although uncommon, it is a well-known cause of both endocrine and imaging abnormalities of the pituitary gland. The mass effect can be striking, mimicking the appearance of a pituitary adenoma, sarcoid, or Langerhans' histiocytosis. More than half the patients have symptoms of a sellar mass and/or decreased pituitary function. However, due either to a presumed "stalk-effect" or to concomitant pregnancy, some patients may have elevated prolactin levels. This entity should always be considered in the setting of gestational pituitary mass lesions and may be treated by bromocriptine, corticosteroids, or surgical decompression.

J.G. Smirniotopoulos, M.D.

Miscellaneous Topics

Surgery for Seizures

Engel J Jr (Univ of California, Los Angeles)
N Engl J Med 334:647–652, 1996 6–29

Background.—Patients who continue to have seizures despite taking antiepileptic drugs account for three fourths of the costs of epilepsy in the United States. Although many patients with such refractory epilepsy can benefit from surgical treatment, few are referred to epilepsy surgery centers. A review of surgical treatment for epilepsy is presented, focusing on the preoperative evaluation, early intervention, and surgical results.

Preoperative Evaluation.—The presurgical workup for patients with epilepsy seeks to identify the brain area responsible for the seizures and to show that it can be removed without any neurologic or cognitive deficits. The evaluation usually includes interictal EEG to localize areas of interictal epileptic excitability; long-term video EEG monitoring to determine ictal electrical activity and clinical symptoms; MRI or other studies to detect structural abnormalities; positron emission tomography, single-photon emission CT, neuropsychological tests to evaluate for nonepileptic dysfunction; and cortical mapping and other studies of normal cortical function. The specific diagnostic approaches used depend on the surgical intervention being considered. With modern diagnostic techniques, such as MRI and positron emission tomography, surgery has become possible for patients previously considered to have "cryptogenic" epilepsy. With continued advances, such as outpatient ictal EEG recording, magnetoencephalography, MR spectroscopy, and functional MRI, presurgical evaluation of patients with epilepsy will become less expensive.

Early Intervention.—Although the patients referred for epilepsy surgery will most likely have very frequent seizures that do not respond to drug therapy, many patients with less frequent but disabling seizures may also benefit. Certain syndromes, such as mesial temporal-lobe epilepsy, discrete structural lesions, and diffuse hemispheric disturbances, are known to respond poorly to medical therapy but well to surgery. Other surgically remediable seizure syndromes will likely be identified with continued advances in diagnosis and surgical treatment. In addition, even patients without known surgically remediable syndromes may benefit from referral to an epilepsy surgery center.

Outcomes.—The available data show steady improvement in the results of epilepsy surgery. Disability is less likely if the patients receive surgical treatment early in the course of their epileptic disorder. Complications are relatively rare; functional brain mapping before surgery may help to avoid unacceptable language, memory, or neurologic disturbances. With microsurgery and other advances, even complex procedures such as hemispherectomy and corpus callostomy have become feasible options.

Discussion.—The current status of surgery for medically refractory epilepsy is reviewed. Surgical treatment is now a safe and effective option for many patients with disabling seizure disorders. More effort is needed to make this form of treatment more widely accepted and available.

► There are more than 100 epilepsy surgery centers throughout the world. Radiology plays an important role in the preoperative evaluation and localization of lesions for proposed seizure control surgery. In addition to anatomical information derived from MRI, positron-emission tomography can demonstrate areas of abnormal glucose uptake, and single photon emission CT imaging may show areas of altered cerebral blood flow. More extensive and specific resections can be performed when functional information through cortical localization is added to these tests. In the past, noninvasive electrical monitoring was often complemented by invasive stereotactic depth or perceptual electrodes. However, the current state of functional and anatomical localization of seizure activity may eliminate the need for depth electrodes in almost all patients. As we have learned more about the plasticity of the human brain and the destructive effects of seizure activity, more clinicians and patients have turned to seizure control surgery. The goal of this surgery, as with medical treatment for seizures, includes not only the reduction in incidence or the elimination of seizure activity, but also the prevention or elimination of the psychological problems associated with seizures. It has also been recognized that seizure activity in and of itself may cause secondary changes in the brain. The identification of a surgically amenable lesion is based primarily on recognition of focal EEG abnormalities, a structural lesion seen on MRI, or an interictal region of hypometabolism. However, it is possible for a patient to have multiple lesions, and for the epilepsy to be the result of a lesion that is occult on imaging studies; therefore, structural lesions without electrical lateralization should be considered carefully.

Overall, the outcome for seizure control surgery has shown significant improvement. More than one half of patients are seizure free, and fewer than 20% have no significant improvement after surgery.

J.G. Smirniotopoulos, M.D.

MR of Oculomotor Nerve Palsy

Blake PY, Mark AS, Kattah J, et al (Georgetown Univ, Washington, DC; Washington Hosp Ctr, DC)

AJNR 16:1665–1672, 1995 6–30

Introduction.—After the sixth cranial nerve, the oculomotor nerve is involved most often in patients who have diplopia or ptosis. The history often reveals diabetic vascular disease, hypertension, systemic inflammatory disease, or malignancy. The site of the lesion often is obscure, however, especially in a patient with diabetes or hypertension with pupil-sparing third nerve palsy. This condition traditionally is ascribed to microvascular ischemia in the peripheral part of the nerve, but recently brainstem infarction has been implicated.

Objective.—The MR findings were reviewed in 50 patients from a number of centers who had oculomotor nerve palsy. The pupil was spared in 43 of them. Magnetic resonance imaging (Fig 1) was performed with and without gadopentate dimeglumine.

Findings.—Thirty-two patients had abnormalities on MR imaging. The third nerve was enhanced in 9 of 11 patients who had involvement in the subarachnoid space. Involvement of the cavernous sinus represented either extension of a mass, such as a pituitary adenoma, or increased tissue within the sinus. The nerve was enhanced in 6 of these 15 patients. Only 1 patient with positive imaging findings had a history of hypertension. None of the patients had diabetes. Examples of MR abnormalities are shown in Figures 2 and 9.

Discussion.—Magnetic resonance imaging is able to depict a wide range of disorders affecting the third cranial nerve. If patients with intrinsic oculomotor nerve involvement undergo MR imaging at an early stage,

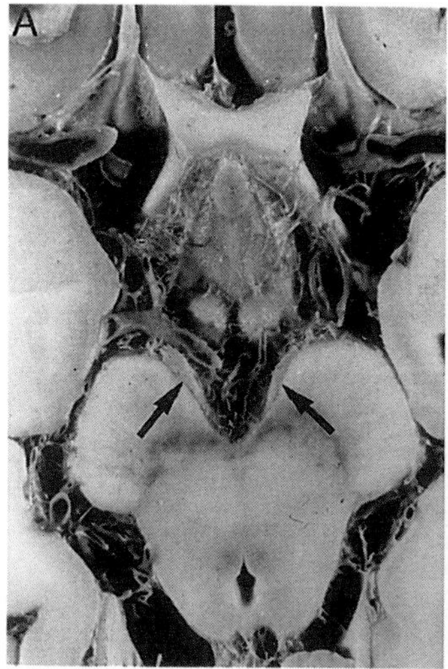

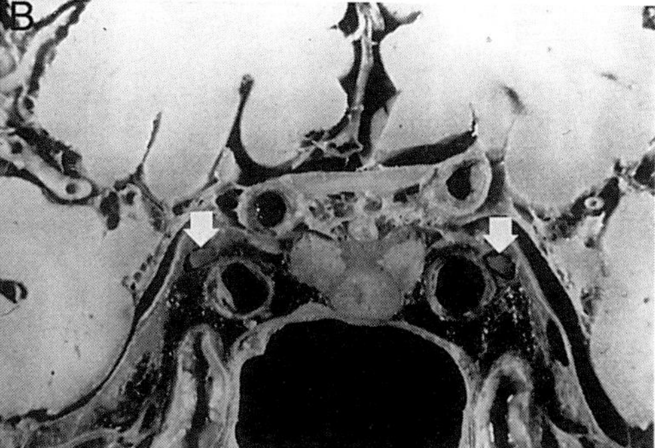

FIGURE 1.—**A**, normal anatomy is demonstrated in this axial anatomical section through the interpeduncular cistern. Note the cisternal segment of the oculomotor nerve (*arrow*). **B**, coronal anatomical section through the posterior aspect of the cavernous sinus. The oculomotor nerve (*arrow*) is located immediately above and lateral to the cavernous carotid artery. (Figure 1 courtesy of Jack DeGroot, M.D.) (Courtesy of PY Blake, AS Mark, JJ Kattah, M Kolsky: MR of oculomotor nerve palsy. *AJNR* 16:1665–1672, 1995. Copyright by American Society of Neuroradiology.)

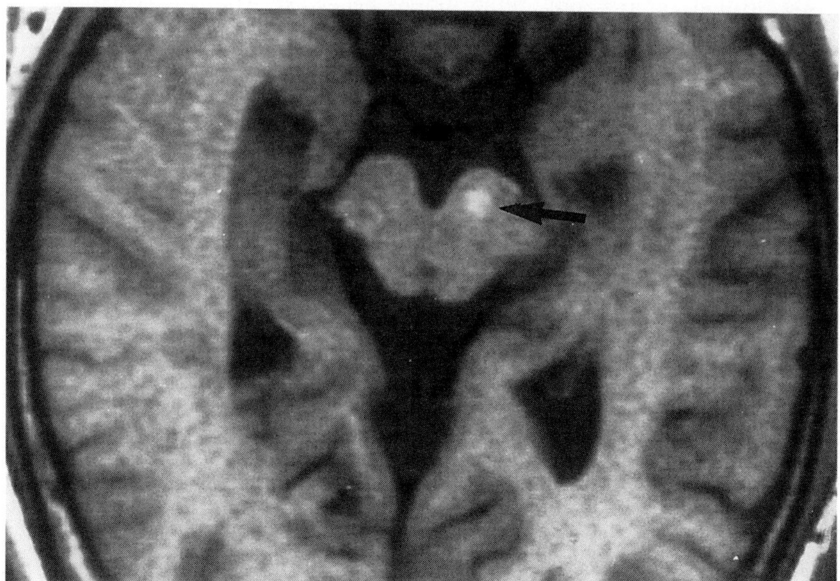

FIGURE 2.—Fascicular lesion in a 40-year-old HIV-positive man. Axial T1-weighted image demonstrates a small hyperintense lesion (*arrow*) that was present on both the T1-weighted images and the T2-weighted images. This appearance is consistent with a hemorrhagic lesion of unclear cause in this patient. (Courtesy of PY Blake, AS Mark, JJ Kattah, M Kolsky: MR of oculomotor nerve palsy. *AJNR* 16:1665-1672, 1995. Copyright by American Society of Neuroradiology.)

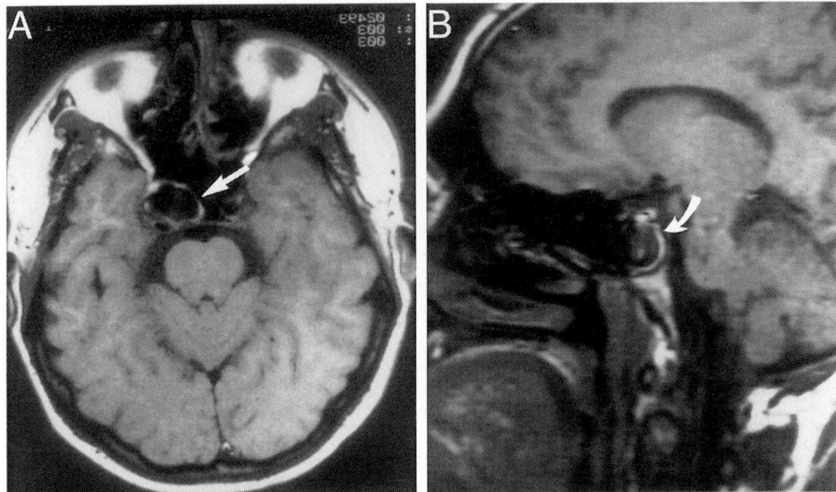

FIGURE 9.—A 40-year-old woman with right cranial nerve III and cranial nerve IV palsies. **A**, axial T1-weighted image demonstrates a 1.5-cm right cavernous carotid aneurysm (*arrow*). **B**, sagittal T1-weighted image demonstrates right cavernous carotid aneurysm (*curved arrow*). (Courtesy of PY Blake, AS Mark, JJ Kattah, M Kolsky: MR of oculomotor nerve palsy. *AJNR* 16:1665–1672, 1995. Copyright by American Society of Neuroradiology.)

conventional angiography might not be necessary. The MR enhancement caused by demyelinating processes resembles that seen in demyelinating optic neuropathy. Diabetic or ischemic third nerve palsy probably reflects the results of demyelination and subsequent remyelination.

► This excellent article presents the imaging findings in a series of 50 patients with oculomotor (CNN 3) palsy. A wide variety of lesions are illustrated. In addition to providing a summary of the conditions associated with CNN 3 palsy, the article reviews the pertinent neuroanatomy and some important physiology (e.g., the preservation of pupillary constriction in patients with microvascular diseases like diabetes and hypertension). The authors also present a plan for the evaluation of new onset of oculomotor palsy that includes initial MR imaging in those patients without a history of subarachnoid hemorrhage or microvascular disease.

J.G. Smirniotopoulos, M.D.

One Hundred and Twenty-Seven Cases of Acute Subdural Haematoma Operated On: Correlation Between CT Scan Findings and Outcome

Massaro F, Lanotte M, Faccani G, et al (CTO Hosp, Torino, Italy)

Acta Neurochir (Wien) 138:185–191, 1996 6–31

Introduction—Even with rapid transport and aggressive diagnosis and treatment, acute subdural hematoma (ASH) has a mortality of 50% to 90%. One factor affecting the morbidity and mortality of ASH could be differences in the type of associated cerebral lesions. The association between CT scan findings and outcome was evaluated in 127 consecutive cases of ASH.

Methods.—The patients were identified from a review of 1,688 patients with head injuries treated over a 10-year period. Of these, 127 had ASH requiring surgery for a midline shift of greater than 5 mm, as seen on the admission CT scan. Fifty-seven percent of the patients with ASH died, and 23% had functional recovery. The findings of the admission CT scan were analyzed for their impact on morbidity and mortality. Other factors were analyzed as well, including mechanism of injury, age, neurologic presentation, and delay from injury to intervention.

Results.—The neurologic presentation, as indicated by the Glasgow Coma Scale (GCS), was significantly related to patient outcome. The mortality rate was 0% patients with an admission GCS of 13 or greater, 42% for those with a GCS of 9–12, and 68% for those with a GCS of less than 8. The admission CT findings were also a significant prognostic factor—the functional recovery rate was 32% in patients with pure ASH, 20% in those with satellite ASH, and 12% in those with associated ASH. Mortality was 62%, 52%, and 63%, respectively. The time to operative clot removal was not a significant factor, and neither were mechanism of injury, age, or sex.

Conclusions.—In patients with ASH, the extent of primary brain injury—as indicated by the admission CT scan and GCS—is the most important prognostic factor. The time to clot removal was not significant in this study; however, the analysis did not consider such factors as the rapidity of hematoma development and brain decompensation or the presence of additional direct brain lesions. Rapid evacuation may improve the outcome for patients with pure ASH and a lucid interval who do not have additional direct brain lesions.

▶ The diagnosis of epidural hematoma conjures up images of coma, herniation, and death. However, it is the ASH that actually has the worst prognosis. This paper and several others continue to emphasize that the mortality of ASH is very high (almost 60%) and that the poor outcome is due to mostly to underlying primary brain injuries, rather than to the ASH itself.

J.G. Smirniotopoulos, M.D.

Annotated Bibliography

JOHN H. REES, M.D.

Deweer B, Lehèricy S, Pillon B, et al: Memory disorders in probable Alzheimer's disease: The role of hippocampal atrophy as shown with MRI. *J Neurol Neurosurg Psychiatry* 58:590–597, 1995.

► Memory loss is 1 of the primary clinical components of most dementias. This study shows a direct relationship between hippocampal volume as measured by MRI, and degrees of memory impairment measured on various clinical tests.

Ellaszlw M, Rankin RN, Fox AJ, et al: Accuracy and prognostic consequences of ultrasonography in identifying severe carotid artery stenosis. *Stroke* 26:1747–1752, 1995.

► The lack of correlation between the risk of stroke and ultrasonographic findings shown in 1,011 patients from the North American Symptomatic Carotid Endarterectomy Trial is strong evidence in favor of the continuing use of catheter angiography in the preoperative assessment of patients being considered for endarterectomy. We should remember, however, that these patients were examined in 1989 and 1991.

González RG, Fischman AJ, Guimaraes AR, et al: Functional MR in the evaluation of dementia: Correlation of abnormal dynamic cerebral blood volume measurements with changes in cerebral metabolism on positron emission tomography with fludeoxyglucose F 18. *AJNR* 16:1763–1770, 1995.

► Two imaging modalities that show some promise in evaluation of patients with dementia are positron-emission tomography (PET) and functional MRI (fMRI). The PET scans display the uptake of F-18-labeled glucose, and fMRI can show, among other things, variable rates of cerebral blood flow. This study shows strong correlation between fMRI measurements of cerebral blood volume and PET images of the glucose metabolic rates in patients with Alzheimer's disease (AD), which is the most common cause of dementia. This correlation is of interest, primarily because fMRI techniques are more widely available than PET scans, which require reasonable proximity to a cyclotron.

Patel MR, Kuntz KM, Klufas RA, et al: Preoperative assessment of the carotid bifurcation: Can magnetic resonance angiography and duplex ultrasonography replace contrast arteriography? *Stroke* 26:1753–1758, 1995.

► Three-dimensional time-of-flight MR angiography (3D TOF MRA) is compared to duplex sonography and catheter angiography individually, and the combination of 3D TOF MRA and ultrasound is compared with angiography in the evaluation of carotid stenosis. The 3D TOF MRA is found to be the most sensitive and specific noninvasive test, and if both MRA and ultrasound are done and are concordant, no additional information is gained from angiography. If MRA and ultrasound are discordant, angiography may be needed for clarification. Using this algorithm, catheter angiography is needed in only 16% of cases. The cost-effectiveness of performing both MRA and ultrasound and then angiography in 16% of patients is not analyzed in this article.

Read SL, Miller BL, Mena I, et al: SPECT in demenita: Clinical and pathological correlation. *Geriatr Soc* 43:1243–1247, 1995.

► Single photon emission CT (SPECT) is a widely available nuclear medicine study most commonly used for spine and body imaging. Its use in the brain has been called "the poor man's PET scan" because the most commonly used agent, HMPAO or Ceretec, acts as a perfusion agent and produces images similar to PET images, which reflect metabolic activity. This study correlates SPECT findings with neuropathologic findings in 27 patients with various types of dementia. In general, Alzheimer's disease is seen as a clearly recognizable pattern of SPECT, although certain lookalikes are described. One of the great values of this study is that it correlates imaging findings with neuropathologic findings. This minimizes the variability found in the clinical assessment of dementias.

Srinivasan J, Mayberg MR, Weiss DG, et al: Duplex accuracy compared with angiography in the Veterans Affairs Cooperative Studies Trial for symptomatic carotid stenosis. *Neurosurg* 36 (4):648–655, 1995.
► There is a strong correlation between duplex ultrasound examinations and angiography for stenoses greater than 50% in this study performed by the Veterans Administration between 1989 and 1991. However, much higher rates of discordance are noted in lower grades of stenosis, where ultrasound frequently underestimates the degree of narrowing. Angiography is nevertheless felt to be the final standard for patients who are surgical candidates.

Shonk TK, Moats RA, Gifford P, et al: Probable Alzheimer's disease: Diagnosis with proton MR spectroscopy. *Radiology* 195:65–72, 1995.
► Magnetic resonance spectroscopy (MRS), also known as proton spectroscopy, is a technique that has been used for decades in laboratory analysis and has been applied only recently to clinical imaging. By measuring the concentrations of various metabolites within brain tissue, a variety of pathologic conditions can be detected with some accuracy. In this study, MRS differentiated patients with mild-to-moderate Alzheimer's disease (AD) from normal patients with 83% sensitivity and 98% specificity. This study does not claim that MRS is superior or even equal to clinical findings in the initial diagnosis of AD, but does show a high degree of correlation.

Vanninen R, Manninen H, Soimakallio S: Imaging of carotid artery stenosis: Clinical efficacy and cost-effectiveness. *AJNR* 16:1875–1883, 1995.
► This cost-effectiveness analysis shows the value of using ultrasound as a screening test for patients who have suffered transient ischemic attacks or nondisabling strokes, and that should be followed by catheter angiography as the definitive preoperative procedure. Until, and unless, MR angiography is proven to be a definitive preoperative examination on its own, these authors recommend we continue to use ultrasound followed by angiography.

Subject Index*

A

* *All entries refer to the year and page number(s) for data appearing in this and previous editions of the* Year Book.

B

C

D

E

G

H

I

J

K

L

N

O

Q

R

S

T

U

V

W

X

Z

Author Index

A

B

C

D

L

M

N